L105 MES

Cefn Coed Library

Z003997

WITHDRAWN 19/06/24

The Mesolimbic Dopamine System: From Motivation to Action

The Mesolimbic Dopamine System: From Motivation to Action

Edited by

PAUL WILLNER
Psychology Department, City of London Polytechnic, London, UK

and

JØRGEN SCHEEL-KRÜGER
Psychopharmacological Research Laboratory, St Hans Hospital, Roskilde, Denmark

JOHN WILEY & SONS
Chichester · New York · Brisbane · Toronto · Singapore

Copyright © 1991 by John Wiley & Sons Ltd.
Baffins Lane, Chichester,
West Sussex PO19 1UD, England

All rights reserved.

No part of this book may be reproduced by any means,
or transmitted, or translated into a machine language
without the written permission of the publisher.

Other Wiley Editorial Offices

John Wiley & Sons, Inc., 605 Third Avenue,
New York, NY 10158–0012, USA

Jacaranda Wiley Ltd, G.P.O. Box 859, Brisbane,
Queensland 4001, Australia

John Wiley & Sons (Canada) Ltd, 22 Worcester Road,
Rexdale, Ontario M9W 1L1, Canada

John Wiley & Sons (SEA) Pte Ltd, 37 Jalan Pemimpin 05–04,
Block B, Union Industrial Building, Singapore 2057

Library of Congress Cataloging-in-Publication Data

The mesolimbic dopamine system: from motivation to action / editors, Paul Willner, Jørgen
Scheel-Krüger.
p.   cm.
Based on a workshop held in September 1989 under the auspices of the European
Behavioral Pharmacology Society.
Includes bibliographical references.
Includes index.
ISBN 0 471 92886 0
1. Limbic system—Congresses.   2. Dopaminergic mechanisms—Congresses.
3. Psychopharmacology—Congresses.   4. Dopamine—Physiological effect—Congresses.
I. Willner, Paul. II. Scheel–Krüger, Jørgen.   III. European Behavioral Pharmacology
Society.
[DNLM: 1. Dopamine—congresses.   2. Limbic System—congresses.
WL 314 M582 1989]
QP383.2.M47 1991
615'.78—dc20
DNLM/DLC
for Library of Congress   90-12986
                                                                              CIP

British Library Cataloguing in Publication Data

The mesolimbic dopamine system: from motivation to action.
1. Medicine. Psychopharmacology. Neuropsychiatry
I. Willner, Paul   II. Scheel-Krüger, Jørgen
615.7
616.8

ISBN 0 471 92886 0

Phototypeset by Photo·graphics, Honiton, Devon
Printed and bound by Biddles Ltd, Guildford

For Heather and Birgit

Contents

Contributors

E. Acquas Institute of Experimental Pharmacology and Toxicology, University of Cagliari, 09100 Cagliari, Sardinia, Italy

S. Ahlenius Department of Neuropharmacology, Astra Research Centre, S-151 85 Sodertalje, Sweden

P.H. Andersen Departments of Behavioral Pharmacology and Biochemical Pharmacology, CNS Division, Novo Nordisk A/S, DK-2880 Bagsvaerd, Denmark

H. Anisman Psychology Department, Carleton University, Ottawa, Ontario, Canada K1S 5B6

R.J. Beninger Department of Psychology, Queen's University, Kingston, Canada K7L 3N6

H.W. Berendse Department of Anatomy and Embryology, Vrije Universiteit, Van der Boechorststraat 7, 1081 BT Amsterdam, The Netherlands

C.D. Blaha Department of Psychology and Division of Neurological Sciences, Department of Psychiatry, University of British Columbia, Vancouver BC, Canada V6T 1Y7

G. Blanc Chaire de Neuropharmacologie, INSERM U.114, College de France, 11 Place Marcelin-Berthelot, 75005 Paris Cedex 05, France

M.A. Bozarth Department of Psychology, State University of New York at Buffalo, Buffalo, NY 14260, USA

M.S. Buchsbaum Department of Psychiatry, Brain Imaging Center, UC Irvine, Irvine CA 92717, USA

W.E. BUNNEY, JR   *Department of Psychiatry, Brain Imaging Center, UC Irvine, Irvine CA 92717, USA*

L. BURGWALD   *Department of Psychiatry, Brain Imaging Center, UC Irvine, Irvine CA 92717, USA*

M. CADOR   *INSERM U.259, Université de Bordeaux II, Domaine de Carreire, rue Camille Saint-Saëns, 33077 Bordeaux Cedex, France*

E. CARBONI   *Institute of Experimental Pharmacology and Toxicology, University of Cagliari, 09100 Cagliari, Sardinia, Italy*

A.R. COOLS   *Department of Pharmacology, University of Nijmegen, PO Box 9101, 6500 HB Nijmegen, The Netherlands*

S.J. COOPER   *School of Psychology, University of Birmingham, Birmingham B15 2TT, UK*

J.-M. DEMINIÈRE   *Psychobiologie des Comportements Adaptatifs, INSERM U.259, Université de Bordeaux II, Domaine de Carreire, rue Camille Saint-Saëns, 33077 Bordeaux Cedex, France*

G. DI CHIARA   *Institute of Experimental Pharmacology and Toxicology, University of Cagliari, 09100 Cagliari, Sardinia, Italy*

B.A. ELLENBROEK   *Department of Pharmacology, University of Nijmegen, PO Box 9101, 6500 HB Nijmegen, The Netherlands*

B.J. EVERITT   *Department of Anatomy, University of Cambridge, Downing Street, Cambridge CB2 3EB, UK*

H.C. FIBIGER   *Division of Neurological Sciences, Department of Psychiatry, The University of British Columbia, 2255 Wesbrook Mall, Vancouver BC, Canada V6T 1W5*

J. GLOWINSKI   *Chaire de Neuropharmacologie, INSERM U.114, College de France, 11 Place Marcelin-Berthelot, 75005 Paris Cedex 05, France*

H.J. GROENEWEGEN   *Department of Anatomy and Embryology, Vrije Universiteit, Van der Boechorststraat 7, 1081 BT Amsterdam, The Netherlands*

S.N. HABER   *Department of Anatomy and Neurobiology, University of Rochester, Wilson Boulevard, Rochester NY 14627, USA*

D. Hervé   *Chaire de Neuropharmacologie, INSERM U.114, College de France, 11 Place Marcelin-Berthelot, 75005 Paris Cedex 05, France*

C.B. Hubner   *NIMH/BPB, Building 10, Room 3N212, Rockville Pike, Bethesda, MD 20892, USA*

G.F. Koob   *Department of Neuropharmacology, Research Institute of Scripps Clinic, 10666 No. Torrey Pines Road, La Jolla CA 92037, USA*

M. Le Moal   *Psychobiologie des Comportements Adaptatifs, INSERM U.259, Université de Bordeaux II, Domaine de Carreire, rue Camille Saint-Saëns, 33077 Bordeaux Cedex, France*

A.H.M. Lohman   *Department of Anatomy and Embryology, Vrije Universiteit, Van der Boechorststraat 7, 1081 BT Amsterdam, The Netherlands*

S. Maccari   *Psychobiologie des Comportements Adaptatifs, INSERM U.259, Université de Bordeaux II, Domaine de Carreire, rue Camille Saint-Saëns, 33077 Bordeaux Cedex, France*

G.E. Meredith   *Department of Anatomy and Embryology, Vrije Universiteit, Van der Boechorststraat 7, 1081 BT Amsterdam, The Netherlands*

G.J. Mogenson   *Department of Physiology, The University of Western Ontario, London, Ontario, Canada N6A 5C1*

P. Mormède   *Psychobiologie des Comportements Adaptatifs, INSERM U.259, Université de Bordeaux II, Domaine de Carreire, rue Camille Saint-Saëns, 33077 Bordeaux Cedex, France*

R. Muscat   *Department of Psychology, City of London Polytechnic, Old Castle Street, London E1 7NT, UK*

E.B. Nielsen   *Departments of Behavioral Pharmacology and Biochemical Pharmacology, CNS Division, Novo Nordisk A/S, DK-2880 Bagsvaerd, Denmark*

M. Papp   *Department of Psychology, City of London Polytechnic, Old Castle Street, London E1 7NT, UK*

A. Pert   *Biological Psychiatry Branch, National Institute of Mental Health, 9000 Rockville Pike, Bethesda MD 20892, USA*

J.G. Pfaus   *Department of Psychology, University of British Colum-*
                      bia, Vancouver BC, Canada V6T 1Y7

A.G. Phillips   *Department of Psychology, University of British Colum-*
                      bia, Vancouver BC, Canada V6T 1Y7

G. Phillips   *Department of Psychology, City of London Polytechnic,*
                      Old Castle Street, London E1 7NT, UK

P.V. Piazza   *Psychobiologie des Comportements Adaptatifs,*
                      INSERM U.259, Université de Bordeaux II, Domaine
                      de Carreire, rue Camille Saint-Saëns, 33077 Bordeaux
                      Cedex, France

G. Ploeger   *Department of Pharmacology, University of Nijmegen,*
                      PO Box 9101, 6500 HB Nijmegen, The Netherlands

R.M. Post   *Biological Psychiatry Branch, National Institute of*
                      Mental Health, Building 10, Room 3N212, 9000 Rock-
                      ville Pike, Bethesda MD 20892, USA

S. Potkin   *Department of Psychiatry, Brain Imaging Center, UC*
                      Irvine, Irvine CA 92717, USA

L. Pulvirenti   *Behavioral Pharmacology Unit, Department of Neurol-*
                      ogy, University of Pavia, Via Palestro 3, Pavia 27100,
                      Italy

C. Reynolds   *Department of Psychiatry, Brain Imaging Center, UC*
                      Irvine, Irvine CA 92717, USA

T.W. Robbins   *Department of Experimental Psychology, University of*
                      Cambridge, Downing Street, Cambridge CB2 3EB, UK

J.D. Salamone   *Department of Psychology, University of Connecticut,*
                      Storrs CT 06269-1020, USA

D. Sampson   *Department of Psychology, City of London Polytechnic,*
                      Old Castle Street, London E1 7NT, UK

J. Scheel-Krüger   *Psychopharmacological Research Laboratory, St Hans*
                      Hospital, DK-4000 Roskilde, Denmark

H. Simon   *Psychobiologie des Comportements Adaptatifs,*
                      INSERM U.259, Université de Bordeaux II, Domaine
                      de Carreire, rue Camille Saint-Saëns, 33077 Bordeaux
                      Cedex, France

L. Stinus   *INSERM U.259, Université de Bordeaux II, Domaine de Carreire, rue Camille Saint-Saëns, 33077 Bordeaux Cedex, France*

N.R. Swerdlow   *Department of Psychiatry, University of California, San Diego, La Jolla, CA 92093, USA*

R.J. Tafalla   *Department of Psychiatry, Brain Imaging Center, UC Irvine, Irvine CA 92717, USA*

J.-P. Tassin   *Chaire de Neuropharmacologie, INSERM U.114, College de France, 11 Place Marcelin-Berthelot, 75005 Paris Cedex 05, France*

M. Trenary   *Department of Psychiatry, Brain Imaging Center, UC Irvine, Irvine CA 92717, USA*

F. Trovero   *Chaire de Neuropharmacologie, INSERM U.114, College de France, 11 Place Marcelin-Berthelot, 75005 Paris Cedex 05, France*

R. van den Bos   *Department of Pharmacology, University of Nijmegen, PO Box 9101, 6500 HB Nijmegen, The Netherlands*

P. Vezina   *Chaire de Neuropharmacologie, INSERM U.114, College de France, 11 Place Marcelin-Berthelot, 75005 Paris Cedex 05, France*

P. Voorn   *Department of Anatomy and Embryology, Vrije Universiteit, Van der Boechorststraat 7, 1081 BT Amsterdam, The Netherlands*

S.R.B. Weiss   *Biological Psychiatry Branch, National Institute of Mental Health, 9000 Rockville Pike, Bethesda MD 20892, USA*

F.J. White   *Wayne State University School of Medicine, Department of Psychiatry, Cellular and Clinical Neurobiology Program, Neuropsychopharmacology Laboratory, Lafayette Clinic, 951 E. Lafayette, Detroit MI 48207, USA*

P. Willner   *Department of Psychology, City of London Polytechnic, Old Castle Street, London E1 7NT, UK*

J.G. Wolters   *Department of Anatomy and Embryology, Vrije Universiteit, Van der Boechorststraat 7, 1081 BT Amsterdam, The Netherlands*

C.C. YIM — *Department of Physiology, The University of Western Ontario, London, Ontario, Canada N6A 5C1*

R.M. ZACHARKO — *Psychology Department, Carleton University, Ottawa, Ontario, Canada K1S 5B6*

Preface

This book originated in Krakow, Poland, on a sunny day in May 1988, in the aftermath of the first Polish/Swedish Symposium on Structure and Function in Neuropharmacology. (We trust that there will be many more, although the palace near Warsaw where the meeting was held has since burned to the ground.) The Editors, neither of whom is either Swedish or Polish, were accompanied in Krakow as guests of the Institute of Pharmacology of the Polish Academy of Sciences by a Swede, Sven Ahlenius. Meeting as a group for the first time, and coming to the mesolimbic system from rather different places, we all agreed immediately that sufficient progress had been made in understanding its functioning to attempt a vertical integration from neuroanatomy to psychopathology. We decided on the spot to translate this motivation into action by means of two parallel projects, a workshop and a book.

Upon our return home, we searched for a suitable venue for the meeting, which we had decided should be a Mediterranean island, to tempt participants and to prevent them straying too far away. We rapidly agreed on Malta, and recruited Richard Muscat, whose knowledge of local conditions and customs was to prove invaluable, to the organizing committee. Arrangements for the meeting proceeded at an alarming pace: Lex Cools and Chris Fibiger joined the committee, and, barely 16 months from conception, the workshop took place in September 1989 under the auspices of the European Behavioural Pharmacology Society, and attended by more than 130 enthusiastic participants.

This book is based primarily on the papers presented at that conference. However, it is far from being simply an account of the proceedings. Most of the chapters were prepared in draft form in advance of the meeting, and were extensively reworked in the light of information received, exchanged and debated. We hope that the end-product is a coherent synthesis of the operation of the mesolimbic dopamine system in health and in mental disorder.

The enterprise would not have been possible were it not for the generous support of a number of pharmaceutical companies who provided financial assistance for the workshop. We have great pleasure in taking this opportunity to thank: Astra, Sweden; Boehringer Ingelheim, FRG; Bristol-Myers, USA; Duphar, The Netherlands; Glaxo, UK; Lilly, UK; Lundbeck, Denmark; Merck, Sharp and Dohme, UK; Novo-Nordisk, Denmark; Organon, The Netherlands; Roussel, France; Schering, FRG; Servier, France; and Smith, Kline and French, UK. We are also most grateful to the Ministries of Health and Tourism of the Republic of Malta, and to the various friends, colleagues and total strangers who (among other things) rescued us from the brink of some barely credible disasters. Heather Reid, Birgit Scheel-Kruger and Sue Muscat provided a constant haven of calm and reassuring support (ably assisted at the meeting by Matthew and Jessica Willner-Reid and Henrik Scheel-Kruger). Turning now to this book, our admiration goes out to our chapter authors, both for their acceptance and supremely competent execution of their brief, and for their toleration of our exasperating editorial interventions. Above all, we thank our fellow members of the workshop organizing committee, Lex Cools, Chris Fibiger, and especially our comrades through thick and thin, Sven Ahlenius and Richard Muscat who shared all of the stress and so deserve to share fully in the credit.

Paul Willner and Jørgen Scheel-Krüger
London and Roskilde
May 1990

INTRODUCTION

1

The Mesolimbic Dopamine System

PAUL WILLNER[1], SVEN AHLENIUS[2], RICHARD MUSCAT[1] AND JØRGEN SCHEEL-KRÜGER[3]

[1]Department of Psychology, City of London Polytechnic, Old Castle Street, London E1 7NT, UK; [2]Department of Neuropharmacology, Astra Research Centre, S-151 85 Sodertalje, Sweden; [3]Psychopharmacological Research Laboratory, St Hans Hospital, DK-4000 Roskilde, Denmark

In the late 1950s, converging evidence from different sources, biochemical, histochemical and pharmacological, identified dopamine (DA) as a neurotransmitter in the central nervous system. Although diffuse plexuses of DA terminals could be seen in vast territories of the brain and spinal cord, the initial mapping of a nigrostriatal, a mesolimbic (though not so named at the time), and a tuberoinfundibular DA pathway proved very powerful. Thus, these subdivisions had different and separate clinical implications: the nigrostriatal pathway was involved in extrapyramidal motor function; the tuberoinfundibular pathway (intrinsic to the hypothalamus) was involved in neuroendocrine regulation; and the mesolimbic pathway was suggested to be important for cognitive functions and motivation (Anden et al., 1966, 1969; Fuxe and Hökfelt, 1969).

Further details of ascending and descending projections were later provided (Lindvall and Bjorklund, 1983). Some of the ascending projections were found to terminate in the prefrontal and cingulate cortices, parts of the hippocampus, and the amygdala. These projections, like the previously described projections to the basal forebrain (nucleus accumbens, bed nucleus of the stria terminalis and diagonal band of Broca), had their origin in the ventral tegmental area (VTA), in a cell group labelled A10 by Dahlstrom and Fuxe (1965). Since these forebrain structures were interlinked in the so-called limbic system, a somewhat diffuse assembly of phylogenetically old structures ('the reptile brain') known to be intimately involved in

The Mesolimbic Dopamine System: From Motivation to Action.
Edited by P. Willner and J. Scheel-Krüger

© 1991 John Wiley & Sons Ltd

motivation and affect (MacLean, 1949; Nauta, 1986), the ascending DA projection from the A10 area was called the mesolimbic DA pathway (Ungerstedt, 1970).

A separation of nigrostriatally-mediated extrapyramidal effects from other, presumably more cognitive and mesolimbic, functions, is supported by the observation that neuroleptic-induced Parkinsonism, in people, can usually be antagonized by anti-cholinergics without serious loss of clinical anti-schizophrenic efficacy (McEvoy, 1983). The significance of this observation is reinforced by the observation in laboratory studies that the effects of DA receptor blocking anti-psychotics on neostriatal, but not on limbic, DA turnover is antagonized by anti-cholinergics (Anden, 1972). Continued experimental research has provided further details of the functional separation between the two mesencephalic DA projections (Robbins and Everitt, 1982). Taken together, the experimental evidence generally supports the original notion that the nigrostriatal pathway is involved in extrapyramidal and cognitive functions (Cools, 1980; Divac, 1984), whereas the mesolimbic trajectory supports a variety of behavioural functions related to motivation and reward. This volume presents the current status of mesolimbic dopaminergic functions, their morphological and biochemical substrates, and their possible clinical implications.

STRUCTURE AND FUNCTION OF THE MESOLIMBIC SYSTEM

The initial animal experiments on functional correlates of brain dopaminergic neurotransmission (Anden et al., 1969) provided the basis for a rapidly growing field of research; it is worth noting that the development of modern psychopharmacology is, to a large extent, linked to these efforts. The development of specific and selective chemical tools for manipulating DA synapses greatly aided in this process. As a consequence, it also became possible to describe changes in animal behaviour resulting from selective interference with normal brain functions. The use of such models has been of considerable value in the development of new drugs in the fields of Parkinsonism and schizophrenia (Randrup and Munkvad, 1967, 1968; Carlsson, 1978; Iversen and Iversen, 1981; Ahlenius and Archer, 1985).

Progress was most rapid in relation to the well-defined nigrostriatal DA pathway and its association with extrapyramidal motor functions in laboratory studies, and with the clinical syndrome of Parkinson's disease (Carlsson, 1959; Ehringer and Hornykiewicz, 1960). In animal experiments, increases or decreases in nigrostriatal DA transmission were found to result in clear behavioural signs of stereotypy and catalepsy, respectively (Scheel-Krüger and Randrup, 1967; Randrup and Munkvad, 1967; Fog et al., 1968). The functions of the mesolimbic projection proved more elusive, at least initially.

Two obvious factors may account for this: in contrast to the nigrostriatal pathway, the mesolimbic pathway ramifies more widely to a number of different forebrain structures, each with different functional connotations; also, the proposed motivational functions are more difficult to define. Needless to say, these difficulties do not simplify the task of relating results obtained in animal experiments to human mental functions and dysfunctions.

Following the clear delineation of the neuroanatomical projections of the A10 DA cell body area, it then became possible to consider the mode of operation of the mesolimbic DA system in relation to the other brain structures with which this system interacts. Two major concepts emerged and these have served to integrate much of the subsequent anatomical, physiological and behavioural data. They concern the parallel organization of information transmission through the basal ganglia, and the role of the major target structure of the mesolimbic DA system, the nucleus accumbens, as a functional interface between the limbic system and the motor system.

It is now clear that the major components of the forebrain, the cerebral cortex, basal ganglia and thalamus, are organized in parallel circuits, which operate by similar principles, but differ functionally to the extent that their input systems differ. Thus, the dorsal striatum is innervated by sensory and motor areas of the cortex, and projects back to those cortical areas via the dorsal pallidum, while the ventral striatum is innervated by prefrontal and limbic cortical areas, and projects back to those areas via the ventral pallidum; within each of these major divisions, a number of distinct subcircuits have been identified (Nauta, 1986; Alexander et al., 1986; see Groenewegen et al., Chapter 2, this volume).

In addition to its input from the frontal cortex, the other major afferent projections to the nucleus accumbens are from the amygdala and the hippocampus. These three projections, which represent the major output pathways of the limbic system, are themselves all innervated by the mesolimbic DA system, and their terminal regions within the nucleus accumbens overlap with one another, and with the mesolimbic DA afferents (see Cador et al., Chapter 9, this volume, Figure 2). This pattern of organization suggests two things: that the nucleus accumbens is the major interface through which limbic structures influence motor output systems, and that these limbic influences over behaviour are controlled and modulated by the mesolimbic DA system (Nauta and Domesick, 1979; Mogenson et al., 1982). Electrophysiological studies have amply confirmed this concept of the role of mesolimbic DA (Mogenson and Yim, 1981; Mogenson and Yang, 1987; Mogenson and Yim, Chapter 4, this volume).

While the broad outlines of the functional anatomy of the limbic forebrain are gradually becoming clearer, a number of other problems have emerged that are as yet unresolved. One such is the compartmental organization of the striatum, which, in the ventral region, is characterized by a matrix rich in DA and other classical neurotransmitters, enclosing patches which contain little DA but which are enriched in neuropeptides (Graybiel, 1989). A related issue is the co-localization within mesolimbic DA neurons, and the co-release with DA, of the peptides neurotensin and cholecystokinin (CCK) (Hökfelt et al., 1980). CCK has been shown to be a functional DA antagonist (see Mogenson and Yim, Chapter 4, this volume); there is a suspicion that changes in the balance of DA and peptide release may contribute to long-term adaptations involving the mesolimbic system, but little evidence with which to assess this possibility.

The past decade has also seen major advances in our understanding of presynaptic and postsynaptic DA receptor systems. Nevertheless, the functional significance of the distinction between the D1 and D2 receptor subtypes, and of the interactions between them, has not yet been established (Clark and White, 1987; White, Chapter 3, this volume). It is also unclear what significance to place on the absence, or lesser density, of inhibitory presynaptic autoreceptors on the DA cells projecting to the frontal cortex, which leads to these cells having firing rates and DA turnover substantially higher than is found in the subcortical DA projections (Chiodo et al., 1984; White, Chapter 3, this volume): the answer to this question may emerge from studies of the interaction between the frontal cortex and ventral striatum (Tassin et al., Chapter 7, this volume), which is at present poorly understood. Finally, we are only beginning to explore the interactions, at the levels of both the VTA and the nucleus accumbens, between the mesolimbic DA system and other systems of neurochemically defined neurons: interactions with noradrenaline (NA), serotonin (5HT), GABA, and opioid peptides are the focus of intense current investigation (White, Chapter 3; Cools et al., Chapter 6; Cooper, Chapter 13, this volume).

The current status of these and other problems are explored in detail in the first section of this book. In the opening chapters, Groenewegen et al. (Chapter 2) review the functional anatomy of the ventral striatum, and White (Chapter 3) reviews factors influencing the electrophysiological activity of mesolimbic DA neurons, and their target cells in the nucleus accumbens. The next two chapters consider the role of the nucleus accumbens as a limbic–motor interface: Mogenson and Yim (Chapter 4) discuss the modulatory action of DA on afferents from the amygdala and hippocampus, and Pulvirenti et al. (Chapter 5) trace out the efferent systems leading to locomotor behaviour. The final two chapters in this section explore the interactions between mesolimbic DA and other systems: Cools et al. (Chapter 6) focus on DA–NA interactions in the ventral striatum, and Tassin et al. (Chapter 7) consider the interaction between the mesolimbic and mesocortical DA projections.

BEHAVIOURAL PHARMACOLOGY OF MESOLIMBIC DOPAMINE

The behavioural pharmacology of the mesolimbic DA system revolves around psychomotor stimulants and neuroleptic drugs, and as such, has a long history: two of the earliest observations in behavioural pharmacology were the selective blockade of conditioned avoidance responding by neuroleptics (the unconditioned escape response being far more resistant to disruption) (Cook et al., 1955), and the locomotor activating effects of amphetamine. However, the recognition that these actions were mediated by DA systems was relatively slow: as recently as 1970 it was the case that 'the exact mechanisms by which d-amphetamine stimulates the CNS remain largely unexplained' (Maickel et al., 1970). This state of uncertainty was rapidly and decisively resolved by the introduction of the selective neurotoxin 6-hydroxy-dopamine (6-OHDA) (Ungerstedt, 1968); by 1975, it was clear that amphetamine caused stereotyped behaviour by releasing DA in the dorsal striatum, and locomotor activity by releasing DA in the nucleus accumbens (Kelly et al., 1975). Around the same time, the introduction of new families of neuroleptics with a narrower spectrum of activity than the earlier phenothiazines confirmed that DA receptor antagonism is responsible for the major behavioural actions of these drugs (Creese and Snyder, 1978).

Despite the wealth of early literature describing the effects of neuroleptics in aversive paradigms (and the widespread use of the conditioned avoidance paradigm within the pharmaceutical industry, in neuroleptic screening programmes), and despite the demonstration that appetitively and aversively motivated behaviours are equally sensitive to suppression by neuroleptics (Waller and Waller, 1962), recent research has focused largely on the role of DA in rewarded behaviour.

These efforts were stimulated primarily by the formulation by Wise and colleagues of the 'dopamine hypothesis of reward' (Wise et al., 1978; Wise, 1982; Wise and Rompre, 1989; Bozarth, Chapter 12, this volume). The hypothesis that the mesolimbic DA system functions as a 'reward pathway' was originally advanced on the basis of an apparent similarity between the effects on rewarded behaviour of neuroleptic treatment and those of non-reward (Wise et al., 1978). It subsequently emerged that this parallel is rather limited, and its interpretation remains controversial (Tombaugh et al., 1980; Willner et al., Chapter 10, this volume). However, the hypothesis has a number of other, independent roots, some of which, such as the potentiation of conditioned reinforcement by DA-releasing drugs (Hill, 1970; Robbins, 1975; Cador et al., Chapter 9, this volume), are more robust.

The major evidence implicating the mesolimbic DA system in reward comes from studies of intracranial self-stimulation (ICSS) and drug self-administration (Liebman and Cooper, 1989; Bozarth, Chapter 12, this volume). As with most functions of brain DA, ICSS was originally attributed, wrongly, to forebrain NA projections. It subsequently became apparent that mesolimbic DA neurons form an essential substrate for ICSS at many, though not all, electrode sites (Phillips and Fibiger, 1989). In the case of the classical ICSS sites in lateral hypothalamus, the ICSS electrode stimulates a descending system of fibres which terminate in the VTA and activate DA cells trans-synaptically (Shizgal and Murray, 1989). Similarly, the release of DA in the nucleus accumbens is essential for the rewarding properties of stimulant drugs. The situation with regard to other drugs with rewarding properties, particularly opiates, is more complex, but is broadly consistent with a central role for the mesolimbic DA system (Bozarth, Chapter 12; Cooper, Chapter 13; Di Chiara et al., Chapter 14, this volume).

As noted earlier, the construction of this impressive body of evidence on the involvement of the mesolimbic DA system in reward has proceeded in relative isolation, with little or no consideration of how these data might be integrated with the evidence that in many respects, neuroleptics have exactly comparable effects on aversively motivated behaviours. This paradox is addressed by several of the contributors to this book, but has not as yet been convincingly resolved (but see below).

The recent development of techniques such as brain dialysis (Di Chiara et al., Chapter 14, this volume) and *in vivo* electrochemistry (Phillips et al., Chapter 8, this volume) has made it possible to ask the fundamental, but overlooked, question of whether rewards do actually activate the mesolimbic DA system. In the first chapter of Part 2 (Chapter 8), Phillips et al. argue that the system is not in fact activated by rewards, but rather by stimuli that precede and predict the delivery of rewards. Although somewhat tangential to much earlier thinking, there is an excellent functional logic to this conclusion: activation of the mesolimbic system elicits forward loco-motion, which, in the preparatory phase of appetitive behaviour, causes approach to reward-related cues, and, ultimately, to the reward itself. An important aspect of this emerging picture is that DA plays an essential role in the process by which neutral stimuli that are associated with rewards acquire incentive properties, such that they are later able to activate the mesolimbic system. In the second chapter of part 2 (Chapter 9), Cador et al. describe the interaction between the amygdala and ventral striatum that is crucial in this process.

Other chapters are concerned with the neuropharmacology of rewarded behaviour. In the first of two chapters dealing with the behavioural effects of DA antagonists, Willner et al. (Chapter 10) discuss the problem of demonstrating that neuroleptics impair the reward process, as distinct from a more prosaic impairment of motor behaviour; in the second, Beninger (Chapter 11) reviews the relative contributions of D1 and D2 receptor systems, and proposes a theoretical model in which the acquisition of incentive motivation is mediated by changes in the sensitivity of postsynaptic D1 receptors. The final three chapters in this section deal with the rewarding and aversive effects of psychoactive drugs: Bozarth (Chapter 12) reviews the evidence that the mesolimbic DA system is the crucial substrate for the rewarding properties of medial forebrain bundle ICSS, psychomotor stimulants and other drugs of abuse; Cooper (Chapter 13) presents a detailed analysis of the interaction of endogenous and exogenous opioids with the mesolimbic DA system; and Di Chiara et al. (Chapter 14) assess the role of the mesolimbic system in drug-induced place preferences and aversions.

MESOLIMBIC DYSFUNCTION

Much of the excitement of research in this area stems from the obvious relevance of mesolimbic DA to psychopathological disorders. It is apparent from the foregoing discussion that the mesolimbic DA system is likely to prove one of the major brain substrates of drug abuse. In addition, however, there is also powerful evidence implicating this system in both schizophrenia and affective disorders.

The DA hypothesis of schizophrenia was originally proposed on the basis of two lines of pharmacological evidence, the DA receptor antagonist properties of anti-schizophrenic drugs (Creese and Snyder, 1978), and the ability of amphetamine and other DA agonists to elicit a syndrome indistinguishable from paranoid schizophrenia (Randrup and Munkvad, 1967, 1968; Snyder, 1973). Subsequently, Crow and colleagues delineated two schizophrenic subsyndromes, and suggested that Type I schizophrenia (positive symptoms) was associated with an increase in DA receptors, while Type II schizophrenia (negative symptoms) was associated with brain damage (Crow, 1980; Crow and Johnstone, 1986). The claim that neuroleptics are selectively active against positive symptoms of schizophrenia (Crow, 1980) has been questioned (Kane and Meyerhoff, 1989). Nevertheless, a number of studies have supported the notion that DA receptor numbers are elevated in schizophrenia, though this finding remains controversial, and there are problems in its interpretation (Fibiger, Chapter 24, this volume).

Although these data suggest that schizophrenia may involve hyperactivity of DA function, they do not differentiate between the nigrostriatal and mesolimbic projections. However, other evidence points clearly to a mesolimbic substrate: for example, the reversal by anti-cholinergics of neuroleptic effects in the dorsal striatum (Anden, 1972), without loss of clinical efficacy (Manos et al., 1981; McEvoy, 1983; Bamrak et al., 1986; but see Singh et al., 1987). The most persuasive evidence comes from the so-called atypical neuroleptic drugs, which are anti-schizophrenic without causing Parkinsonian side effects, and act selectively at mesolimbic sites (White and Wang, 1983).

Ideas of dopaminergic involvement in affective disorders developed in parallel to the research on schizophrenia, and in relative isolation from it. The roots of a DA hypothesis of depression go back to a spate of reports in the 1950s that depression was caused as a side effect of treatment with the catecholamine-depleting anti-hypertensive, reserpine (see Willner, 1983). However, the implications of this observation were for many years overshadowed by the apparent failure of tricyclic anti-depressants to interact with DA synapses. This situation was radically altered by the discovery that, after long-term administration, tricyclics (and other anti-depressants) increase the functional responsiveness of mesolimbic DA receptors (Willner, 1983; Willner et al., Chapter 15, this volume). When combined with the emerging evidence of the crucial role of mesolimbic DA in responsiveness to rewards, the implication that the mesolimbic system might be dysfunctional in depression was inescapable.

As noted by Willner et al. in the first chapter of Part 3 (Chapter 15), the direct clinical support for this hypothesis is weak (though perhaps no more so than for other biochemical hypotheses of depression); however, it receives strong support from animal models of depression. In the following chapter (Chapter 16), Zacharko and Anisman review the evidence that the mesolimbic DA system is powerfully activated not only by stimuli associated with rewards, but also by stress. Both chapters demonstrate that stressors can cause an anti-depressant-reversible decrease in responsiveness to rewards, which is mediated through the mesolimbic DA system.

It is perhaps surprising that DA hypotheses of depression have been so unfashionable when DA agonists are well known to elicit manic-like states. In Chapter 17, Post et al. assess the psychomotor stimulant model of mania, and consider the evidence that vulnerability to mania may involve a process of sensitization similar to that observed with repreated administration of amphetamine or cocaine. Along related lines, but with an orientation to the drug abuse implications of these data, Piazza et al. (Chapter 18) present evidence that differences between animals in mesolimbic DA activity determine their degree of vulnerability to acquire amphetamine self-administration.

Three further chapters review the current status of the DA hypothesis of schizophrenia. First, Robbins (Chapter 19) considerably extends the scope of the hypothesis by discussing the cognitive dysfunctions in schizophrenia and Parkinsonism (which, according to a simple DA hypothesis, should be diametrical opposites, but in fact are not), in the context of the functional interconnections between the striatum and frontal cortex. In the second chapter, Buchsbaum et al. (Chapter 20) present evidence from recent PET scanning studies of DA function in the brains of schizophrenic patients. Finally, Nielsen and Andersen (Chapter 21) review current approaches to the development of neuroleptic drugs with novel mechanisms of action.

FROM MOTIVATION TO ACTION

Research on the mesolimbic DA system is notable in several respects. This pathway is unique in its involvement in so wide a range of major psychological disorders. It also illustrates par excellence the multidisciplinary character of behavioural neuroscience, and the constant and productive interplay between its many components. Not least is the inherent philosophical challenge of the brain mechanisms responsible for translating motivation into action. The final section of this book consists of three chapters that draw on the earlier material to summarize and synthesize the state of our current understanding of the role of the mesolimbic DA system in normal and abnormal brain function.

In the first of these chapters (Chapter 22), Scheel-Kruger and Willner review the structure and function of the mesolimbic system in an overview of the afferent systems innervating the VTA, the integrative functions of the ventral striatum, and its efferent projections, feeding forward to the motor system and back to frontal cortex and limbic structures. The central concern of this chapter is to analyse the behavioural functions of the frontal cortex, amygdala and hippocampus, and the role of the mesolimbic DA system in integrating and coordinating the transmission of information from those structures through the limbic–motor interface.

In the following chapter (Chapter 23), Salamone presents a behavioural counterpart of the anatomical model, an analysis of the complex hierarchical organization of sensorimotor behaviour, leading to a hierarchical and multiprocess model of motivation. Although simplistic models of behaviour are much preferred by most neuroscientists, it is argued that, in this area at least, simple models have outlived their usefulness, and future progress will depend on the adoption of models that more accurately recognize and reflect the complexity of motivated behaviour. This approach moves us on from identifying the mesolimbic DA system as a reward pathway to fractionating the construct of 'reward' and asking with which aspect(s) the system is concerned. One immediate benefit is a potential resolution of the paradoxical and troublesome involvement of this same system in stress. The solution may be to accept that subjective euphoria is a higher order construct, which is not derived directly from activity in the mesolimbic DA system. It is then apparent that activation of the system, whether by reward-related incentive stimuli or by stress, leads to active behaviour that has reinforcing consequences in both cases: the delivery of a reward following the successful execution of a sequence of appetitive behaviour, or stress reduction following the successful execution of an avoidance or escape response.

In the final chapter, Fibiger addresses the crucial clinical paradox which looms in the background but is rarely acknowledged: how to reconcile the apparent involvement of the mesolimbic DA system in both affective disorders and schizophrenia. This problem is parallel, in many respects, to that of reconciling the roles of the mesolimbic system in both reward and stress, but as is often the case with clinical issues, is more complex. Nevertheless, the route to a solution may involve a similar strategy of identifying the specific aspects of the clinical disorders that are DA-dependent. The success of this strategy illustrates a more general principle, that progress in biological psychiatry may be better served by the analysis of specific symptoms than by the traditional syndromal approach.

The mesolimbic DA system is increasingly emerging as a predominant focus in the attempt to understand the brain mechanisms underlying motivated behaviour. This book, and in particular, its final three chapters, provides an overview of the area that we hope will serve to define the broad outlines of future research.

REFERENCES

Ahlenius, S. and Archer, T. (1985) Normal and abnormal animal behaviour: importance of catecholamine release by nerve impulses for the maintenance of normal behaviour. In: Gilles, R. and Balthazar, J. (eds) *Neurobiology*. Berlin and Heidelberg: Springer, pp. 329–343.

Alexander, G.E., DeLong, M.R. and Strick, P.L. (1986) Parallel organization of functionally segregated circuits linking basal ganglia and cortex. *Annual Review of Neuroscience* **9**, 357–381.

Anden, N.E. (1972) Dopamine turnover in the corpus striatum and the limbic system after treatment with neuroleptic and antiacetylcholine drugs. *Journal of Pharmacy and Pharmacology* **24**, 905–906.

Anden, N.E., Dahlstrom, A., Fuxe, K., Larsson, K., Olson, L. and Ungerstedt, U. (1966) Ascending monoamine neurons to the telencephalon and diencephalon. *Acta Physiologica Scandinavica* **67**, 313–326.

Anden, N.E., Carlsson, A. and Haggendal, J. (1969) Adrenergic mechanisms. *Annual Review of Pharmacology* **9**, 119–134.

Bamrak, J., Kumar, V., Krska, J. and Soni, S. (1986) Interactions between procyclidine and neuroleptic drugs. *British Journal of Psychiatry* **149**, 726–733.

Carlsson, A. (1959) The occurrence, distribution and physiological role of catecholamines in the nervous system. *Pharmacological Reviews* **11**, 490–493.

Carlsson, A. (1978) Mechanism of action of neuroleptic drugs. In: Lipton, M.A., DiMascio, A. and Killam, K.F. (eds) *Psychopharmacology: A Generation of Progress*. New York: Raven, pp. 1057–1070.

Chiodo, L.A., Bannon, M.J., Grace, A.A., Roth, R.H. and Bunney, B.S. (1984) Evidence for the absence of impulse regulating somatodendritic and synthesis-modulating nerve terminal autoreceptors on subpopulations of mesocortical dopamine neurons. *Neuroscience* **12**, 1–16.

Clark, D. and White, F.J. (1987). D1 dopamine receptor—the search for a function: a critical evaluation of the D1/D2 dopamine receptor classification and its functional implications. *Synapse* **1**, 347–388.

Cook, L., Weidley, E., Morris, R. and Mattis, P. (1955) Neuropharmacological and behavioral effects of chlorpromazine. *Journal of Pharmacology and Experimental Therapeutics* **113**, 1–11.

Cools, A.R. (1980) Role of the neostriatal dopaminergic activity in sequencing and selecting behavioural strategies: facilitation of process involved in selecting the best strategy in a stressful situation. *Behavioural Brain Research* **7**, 361–378.

Creese, I. and Snyder, S.H. (1978) Behavioral and biochemical properties of the dopamine receptor. In: Lipton, M.A., DiMascio, A. and Killam, K.F. (eds) *Psychopharmacology: A Generation of Progress*. New York: Raven, pp. 377–388.

Crow, T.J. (1980) Positive and negative schizophrenic symptoms and the role of dopamine. *British Journal of Psychiatry* **137**, 383–386.

Crow, T.J. and Johnstone, E.C. (1986) Schizophrenia: nature of the disease process and its biological correlates. In: Mountcastle, V.B. and Plum, F. (eds) *Handbook of Physiology: The Nervous System*, Vol. V. Baltimore: American Physiological Society, pp. 843–869.

Dahlstrom, A. and Fuxe, K. (1965) Evidence for the existence of monoamine neurons in the central nervous system. I. Demonstration of monoamines in the cell bodies of brain stem neurons. *Acta Physiologica Scandinavica* **232**, 1–55 (suppl).

Divac, A. (1984) The neostriatum viewed orthogonally. In: Evered, D. and O'Connor, M. (eds) *Functions of the Basal Ganglia*. London: Pitman, CIBA Foundation Symposium, pp. 201–215.

Ehringer, H. and Hornykiewicz, O. (1960) Verteilung von Noradrenalin und Dopamin (3-Hydroxytytamin) im Gehirn des Menschen und ihr Verhalten bei Erkrankung des Extrapyramidalen Systems. *Klinische Wochenschrift* **38**, 1236–1239.

Fog, R.L., Randrup, A. and Munkvad, I. (1968) Neuroleptic action of quaternary chlorpromazine and related drugs injected into various brain areas in rats. *Psychopharmacology* **12**, 428–432.

Fuxe, K. and Hökfelt, T. (1969) Catecholamines in the hypothalamus and the pituitary gland. In: Ganong, W.F. and Martini, L. (eds) *Frontiers in Neuroendocrinology*. New York: Oxford University Press, pp. 47–96.

Graybiel, A. (1989) Dopaminergic and cholinergic systems in the striatum. In: Crossman, A.S. and Sambrook, M.A. (eds) *Neuronal Mechanisms in Disorders of Movement*. London: Libbey, pp. 3–15.

Hill, R.T. (1970) Facilitation of conditioned reinforcement as a mechanism of psychomotor stimulation In: Costa, E. and Garattini, S. (eds) *Amphetamines and Related Compounds*. New York: Raven, pp. 781–795.

Hökfelt, T., Skirboll, L., Rehfeld, J.F., Goldstein, M., Markey, K. and Dann, O. (1980) A subpopulation of mesencephalic dopamine neurons projecting to limbic areas contains a cholecystokinin-like peptide: evidence from immunohistochemistry combined with retrograde tracing. *Neuroscience* **5**, 2093–2124.

Iversen, S.D. and Iversen, L.L. (1981) *Behavioural Pharmacology*. Oxford: Oxford University Press.

Kane, J.M. and Meyerhoff, D. (1989) Do negative symptoms respond to pharmacological treatment? *British Journal of Psychiatry* **155**, 115–118 (suppl. 7).

Kelly, P.H., Seviour, P.W. and Iversen, S.D. (1975) Amphetamine and apomorphine responses following 6-OHDA lesions of the nucleus accumbens septi and corpus striatum. *Brain Research* **94**, 507–522.

Liebman, J.M. and Cooper, S.J. *The Neuropharmacological Basis of Reward*. Oxford: Oxford University Press.

Lindvall, O. and Bjorklund, A. (1983) Dopamine- and norepinephrine-containing neuron systems: their anatomy in the rat brain. In: Emson, P.C. (ed) *Chemical Neuroanatomy*. New York: Raven, pp. 229–255.

MacLean, P.D. (1949) Psychosomatic disease and the 'visceral brain': recent developments bearing on the Papez theory of emotion. *Psychosomatic Medicine* **11**, 338–353.

Maickel, R.P., Cox, R.H., Ksir, C.J., Snodgrass, W.R. and Miller, F.P. (1970) Some aspects of the behavioral pharmacology of the amphetamines. In: Costa, E. and Garattini, S. (eds) *Amphetamines and Related Compounds*. New York: Raven, pp. 747–759.

Manos, N., Gkiouzepas, J. and Logothetis, J. (1981) The need for continuous use of antiparkinsonian medication with chronic schizophrenic patients receiving long-term neurleptic therapy. *American Journal of Psychiatry* **138**, 184–188.

McEvoy, J.P. (1983) The clinical use of anticholinergic drugs as treatment for extrapyramidal side effects of neuroleptic drugs. *Journal of Clinical Psychopharmacology* **3**, 288–302.

Mogenson, G.J. and Yang, C.R. (1987) Dopamine modulation of limbic and cortical inputs to striatal neurons. In: Chiodo, L.A. and Freeman, A.S. (eds) *Neurophysiology of Dopaminergic Systems: Current Status and Clinical Perspectives*. Detroit: Lakeshore Publishing Co., pp. 237–251.

Mogenson, G.J. and Yim, C.Y. (1981) Electrophysiological and neuropharmacological behavioral studies of the nucleus accumbens and implications for its role as a limbic-motor interface. In: Chronister, R.B. and DeFrance, J.F. (eds) *The Neurobiology of the Amygdala*. Brunswick, ME: Haer Institute, pp. 210–229.

Mogenson, G.J., Jones, D.L. and Yim, C.Y. (1982) From motivation to action: functional interface between the limbic system and the motor system. *Progress in Neurobiology* **14**, 69–97.

Nauta, W.J.H. (1986) Circuitous connections linking cerebral cortex, limbic system and corpus striatum. In: Doane, B.K. and Livingston, K.E. (eds) *The Limbic System: Functional Organization and Clinical Disorders*. New York: Raven, pp. 43–54.

Nauta, W.J.H. and Domesick, V.B. (1979) The anatomy of the extrapyramidal system. In: Fuxe, K. and Calne, D.B. (eds) *Dopaminergic Ergot Derivatives and Motor Function*. Oxford: Pergamon, pp. 3–22.

Phillips, A.G. and Fibiger, H.C. (1989) Neuroanatomical bases of intracranial self-stimulation: untangling the Gordian knot. In: Liebman, J.M. and Cooper, S.J. (eds) *The Neuropharmacological Basis of Reward*. Oxford: Oxford University Press, pp. 66–105.

Randrup, A. and Munkvad, I. (1967) Stereotyped activities produced by amphetamine in several animal species and man. *Psychopharmacology* **11**, 200–310.

Randrup, A. and Munkvad, I. (1968) Behavioural stereotypies induced by pharmacological agents. *Pharmakopsychiatrie/Neuro-Psychopharmakologie* **1**, 18–26.

Robbins, T.W. (1975) The potentiation of conditioned reinforcement by psychomotor stimulant drugs: a test of Hill's hypothesis. *Psychopharmacology* **45**, 103–114.

Robbins, T.W. and Everitt, B.J. (1982) Functional studies of the central catecholamines. *International Review of Neurobiology* **23**, 303–365.

Scheel-Krüger, J. and Randrup, A. (1967) Stereotyped hyperactive behaviour produced by dopamine in the absence of noradrenaline. *Life Science* **6**, 1389–1398.

Shizgal, P. and Murray, B. (1989) Neuronal basis of intracranial self-stimulation. In: Liebman, J.M. and Cooper, S.J. (eds) *The Neuropharmacological Basis of Reward*. Oxford: Oxford University Press, pp. 106–163.

Singh, M.M., Kay, S.R. and Opler, A.A. (1987) Anticholinergic–neuroleptic antagonism in terms of positive and negative symptoms of schizophrenia: implications for psychobiological subtyping. *Psychological Medicine* **17**, 39–48.

Snyder, S.H. (1973) Amphetamine psychosis: a 'model' schizophrenia mediated by catecholamines. *American Journal of Psychiatry* **130**, 61–67.

Tombaugh, T.N., Anisman, H. and Tombaugh, J. (1980) Extinction and dopamine receptor blockade after intermittent reinforcement training: failure to find functional equivalence. *Psychopharmacology* **70**, 19–28.

Ungerstedt, U. (1968) 6-Hydroxy-dopamine induced degeneration of central mono-amine neurons. *European Journal of Pharmacology* **5**, 107–112.

Ungerstedt, U. (1970) Stereotaxic mapping of the monoamine pathway in the rat brain. *Acta Physiologica Scandinavica* **367**, 1–48 (suppl).

Waller, M.B. and Waller, P.F. (1962) Effects of chlorpromazine on appetitive and aversive components of a multiple schedule. *Journal of the Experimental Analysis of Behavior* **5**, 259–264.

White, F.J. and Wang, R.Y. (1983) Differential effects of classical and atypical antipsychotic drugs on A9 and A10 dopamine neurons. *Science* **221**, 1054–1056.

Willner, P. (1983) Dopamine and depression: a review of recent evidence. *Brain Research Reviews* **6**, 211–224.

Wise, R.A. (1982) Neuroleptics and operant behavior: the anhedonia hypothesis. *Behavioral and Brain Sciences* **5**, 39–88.

Wise, R.A. and Rompre, P.-P. (1989) Brain dopamine and reward. *Annual Review of Psychology* **40**, 191–225.

Wise, R.A., Spindler, J., De Wit, H. and Gerber, G.J. (1978) Neuroleptic-induced 'anhedonia' in rats: pimozide blocks the reward quality of food. *Science* **201**, 262–264.

Part 1

STRUCTURE AND FUNCTION OF THE MESOLIMBIC SYSTEM

2

Functional Anatomy of the Ventral, Limbic System-Innervated Striatum

H.J. GROENEWEGEN[1], H.W. BERENDSE[1],
G.E. MEREDITH[1], S.N. HABER[2], P. VOORN[1],
J.G. WOLTERS[1] AND A.H.M. LOHMAN[1]

[1]Department of Anatomy and Embryology, Vrije Universiteit, Van der Boechorststraat 7, 1081 BT Amsterdam, The Netherlands; [2]Department of Anatomy and Neurobiology, University of Rochester, 601 Elmwood Ave. Rochester NY 14642, USA.

INTRODUCTION

The participation of the basal ganglia in the functions of the brain has been associated primarily with motor aspects. However, the exact role of these nuclei, which encompass the striatum, the pallidal complex, the subthalamic nucleus and the substantia nigra, is still an enigma, and it has been argued that for a proper understanding of their actions, sensory aspects have received too little attention (Schneider, 1987). Moreover, it has become widely accepted that the basal ganglia are also involved in cognitive, mnemonic and limbic functions. In line with this notion, the hypothesis has been advanced that disturbances of specific parts of the basal ganglia lead to psychiatric states, such as schizophrenia, mania, depression and obsessive/compulsive disorders (Willner, 1983; Swerdlow and Koob, 1987). Furthermore, the fact that the gross motor disturbances, as seen for instance in Parkinson's disease, may be accompanied by sensory, cognitive and affective deficits has received greater attention in the last few years (Robbins, Chapter 19, this volume).

The main contribution of morphological studies to the acceptance of a non-motor role for the basal ganglia has been the demonstration that

The Mesolimbic Dopamine System: From Motivation to Action.
Edited by P. Willner and J. Scheel-Krüger

© 1991 John Wiley & Sons Ltd

information from functionally diverse parts of several forebrain structures, i.e. the cortical mantle, including the motor-, sensory- and association-cortical areas, the midline and intralaminar nuclei of the thalamus, and limbic structures such as the amygdala and the hippocampus, is channelled through different parts of the basal ganglia according to a similar organizational principle (Heimer and Wilson, 1975; Nauta, 1979; Nauta, 1986b). This has led to the idea that the connections of the major components of the forebrain, being the cortex, the basal ganglia and the thalamus, are organized in a number of parallel circuits (Alexander et al., 1986). These circuits are probably concerned with particular functions or sets of functions, ranging from simple movements for those parts of the basal ganglia related to the sensorimotor cortex through more complicated sequences of movements to complex behavioral patterns for those parts of the basal ganglia related to the association and limbic cortical areas (Nauta, 1986a).

The striatum may be considered as the main 'input structure' of the basal ganglia, since it receives projections not only from the cortex, the thalamus and limbic structures, but also from serotonergic and dopaminergic nuclei in the midbrain. As discussed in other chapters in this volume, dopamine (DA) plays a crucial role in the regulation of the transfer of information from these inputs to the output structures of the striatum, i.e. the pallidal complex and the substantia nigra. The wide distribution of the DA input throughout the functionally heterogeneous striatum possibly explains the involvement of this transmitter system, not only in a great variety of motor and complex behavioral functions but also in the neurological and psychiatric dysfunctions mentioned above.

If the assumption that the basal ganglia are involved in a wide range of functions is correct, the important question arises as to whether and how the different input systems interact with each other. Are there indeed parallel, segregated pathways through the nuclei of the basal ganglia that subserve different functions, ranging from motor through cognitive to limbic, or does a great deal of limbic/motor integration take place at the level of the basal ganglia, in particular in the striatum? Although data from anatomical studies can never provide the ultimate answer to this question, knowledge of the 'morphological basis' may help to design functional experimental approaches.

The present account is a review of a number of important organizational aspects of the striatum, i.e. its input/output relations, both at the light and the electron microscopical level, and its compartmental structure. The main focus will be on the ventral, limbic system-innervated part of the striatum, since in this region information from the amygdala, the hippocampal region and the prefrontal cortex converges and interacts with the DA input from the ventral tegmental area. The data concerning the ventral striatum will be related to our knowledge of the structural organization of the dorsal striatum, i.e. the caudate-putamen complex.

THE PARALLEL ORGANIZATION OF THE DORSAL AND THE VENTRAL STRIATOPALLIDAL SYSTEMS

The idea that the nucleus accumbens and parts of the olfactory tubercle are to be considered an integral part of the striatum, i.e. the ventral striatum, and that certain regions in the substantia innominata are of pallidal nature, i.e. the ventral pallidum, was put forward by Heimer and Wilson (1975) some 15 years ago. However, only recently have the connections of these structures with other parts of the brain been studied systematically. It was clear from earlier studies that the projections from the ventral striatum to the ventral pallidum parallel those from the dorsal striatum (caudate-putamen complex) to the globus pallidus (Heimer and Wilson, 1975; Nauta et al., 1978). More recently, the connectivity between the striatal and the pallidal elements of the olfactory tubercle was described in more detail (Heimer et al., 1987; Zahm and Heimer, 1987). In addition, it has been demonstrated that the projections from the dorsally located globus pallidus (external pallidal segment in the rat) to the subthalamic nucleus, the substantia nigra and the striatum, are paralleled by projections from the ventral pallidum to the same structures, although to different parts (Haber et al., 1985; Walker et al., 1989; Groenewegen and Berendse, 1990; Zahm, 1989; Figure 1). The ventral pallidum has immunohistochemical characteristics of both the external and the internal (entopeduncular nucleus in the rat) segments of the dorsal pallidal complex, since it contains a mixed plexus of enkephalin- and substance P-woolly fibers (Haber and Nauta, 1983). If, on the basis of this, the ventral pallidum can be considered to represent the two segments of the dorsal pallidum, the parallels between the dorsal and ventral pallidofugal pathways are even more striking. Thus, the entopeduncular nucleus and the ventral pallidum project to the thalamus, respectively to the ventral anterior and the mediodorsal nuclei, and also to the lateral habenula (Figure 1; Herkenham and Nauta, 1977; Young et al., 1984; Haber et al., 1985; Zahm and Heimer, 1987; Zahm et al., 1987; Groenewegen, 1988). Efferent projections from the ventral pallidum to the basolateral nucleus of the amygdala appear to be unique for this part of the pallidal complex. However, these projections largely stem from the cholinergic cell population in the ventral pallidum (Grove et al., 1983; Carlsen et al., 1985; Grove, 1988) which most likely forms an extension of the cholinergic magnocellular nuclear complex into the ventral pallidal area.

The consequence of the parallel arrangement of the dorsal and ventral striatopallidofugal systems is that information carried through the two sectors

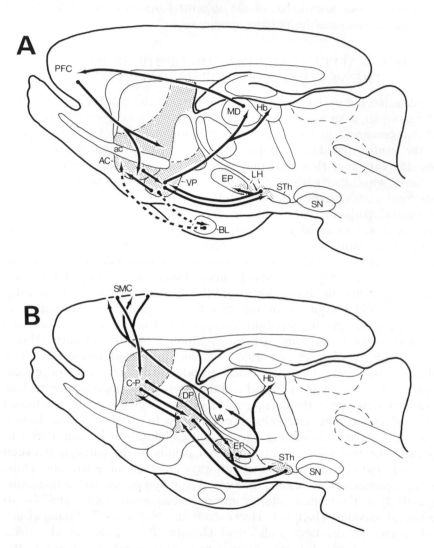

Figure 1. Schematic representation showing the parallel organization of the ventral (**A**) and dorsal (**B**) corticostriatopallidothalamic pathways in the rat. The reciprocal connections between the pallidal complex and the subthalamic nucleus are also indicated for both systems. AC, nucleus accumbens; ac, anterior commissure; BL, basolateral amygdaloid nucleus; C-P, caudate-putamen; DP, dorsal pallidum; EP, entopeduncular nucleus; Hb, habenula; LH, lateral hypothalamus; MD, mediodorsal thalamic nucleus; PFC, prefrontal cortex; SMC, sensorimotor cortex; SN, substantia nigra; STh, subthalamic nucleus; VA, ventral anterior thalamic nucleus; VP, ventral pallidum

of the striatum is conveyed to different frontal cortical areas (Nauta, 1986b). The (pre)motor cortex is reached by way of the ventral anterior thalamic nucleus and the prefrontal cortex through the mediodorsal nucleus. This concept of a parallel organization of the basal ganglia–thalamocortical circuits contrasts with the classical view of a convergence of information from all parts of the cortical mantle through the basal ganglia to the (pre)motor cortex (DeLong and Georgopoulos, 1981; Goldman-Rakic and Selemon, 1986; Alexander et al., 1986). Thus, each circuit has a specific, functionally distinct region of the frontal cortex as a nodal point and further involves anatomically distinct sectors of the striatum, the pallidum and the thalamus. It might be emphasized here that there are no corticostriatopallidothalamic loops directed towards cortical areas caudal to the frontal lobe.

The clearest example of a 'functional loop' is the 'motor circuit', which in the primate focuses on the supplementary motor area and includes the putamen, the ventrolateral part of the internal segment of the globus pallidus, and the medial and oral parts of the ventrolateral thalamic nucleus (DeLong and Georgopoulos, 1981). Apart from this 'motor circuit', Alexander et al. (1986) have proposed the existence of an 'oculomotor circuit' and of several 'complex or associational circuits' that involve distinct regions of the prefrontal cortex. Recent evidence suggests that in the monkey an additional 'limbic loop' can be defined which involves the medial magnocellular portion of the mediodorsal thalamic nucleus and the medial orbitofrontal cortex (Goldman-Rakic and Porrino, 1985; Russchen et al., 1987; Haber et al., 1990). This loop further involves the most ventral and medial part of the striatum and the medial part of the ventral pallidum (Russchen et al., 1987; Haber et al., 1990). The ventromedial part of the striatum in the monkey receives projections from the hippocampus and the amygdala (Poletti and Creswell, 1977; Russchen et al., 1985).

In the rat, projections from the prefrontal, premotor and sensorimotor cortical areas to the striatum are arranged such that the mediolateral and dorsoventral axes are to a large degree maintained (Beckstead, 1979; Sesack et al., 1989; McGeorge and Faull, 1989). As in the monkey (Selemon and Goldman-Rakic, 1985), most cortical areas in the rat project throughout the entire rostrocaudal length of the caudate-putamen complex. In turn, the projections from the medial part of the caudate-putamen and from different parts of the ventral striatum to the pallidal complex show a high degree of topographical organization (Gerfen, 1985; Heimer et al., 1987; Berendse and Groenewegen, unpublished observations). The projections from the ventral pallidum and the medial part of the globus pallidus to the mediodorsal thalamic nucleus, and the reciprocal relationship of the mediodorsal nucleus with the prefrontal cortex are also fairly strictly topographically organized (Beckstead, 1979; Groenewegen, 1988). In the rat, therefore, the corticostriatofugal pathways are also organized in a number of parallel circuits, four of which are exemplified in Figure 2. This is a schematic

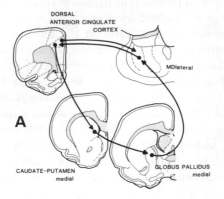

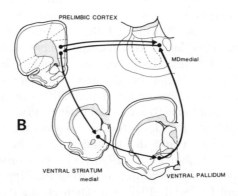

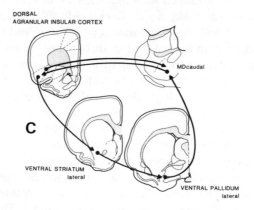

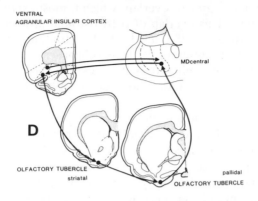

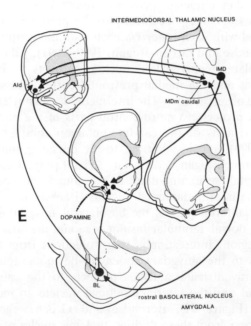

Figure 2. A–D. Schematic diagrams of four parallel corticostriatopallidothalamic circuits in the rat. Note that each circuit involves different subregions of the medial or lateral prefrontal cortex, the ventral striatum or the medial caudate-putamen, the ventral pallidum (VP) or the medial globus pallidus, and the mediodorsal thalamic nucleus (MD). **E.** Convergence of the projections from the intermediodorsal thalamic nucleus (IMD) and the rostral part of the basolateral amygdaloid nucleus (BL) on the lateral prefrontal cortex and the lateral part of the ventral striatum which, in turn, are connected with each other. Note that the intermediodorsal thalamic nucleus projects, in addition, to the rostral basolateral amygdaloid nucleus. Ald, dorsal agranular insular cortex

representation, since the prefrontal cortical projection areas in the striatum show a considerable degree of overlap, which is most extensive in the caudal half of the striatum. This overlap of corticostriatal projections may provide a way of integrating, at the level of the striatum, information which is conducted through different cortical–subcortical loops. Integration of information carried through different loops can also take place through corticocortical connections (Alexander et al., 1986; Groenewegen et al., 1990a).

It may thus be concluded that parallel processing is an important organizational principle in cortical–subcortical relations, as it is for cortico-cortical connections (Goldman-Rakic, 1988; Selemon and Goldman-Rakic, 1988). For the rat, this can be further illustrated by the organization of the projections from the amygdala and the midline/intralaminar thalamic complex to both the striatum and the prefrontal cortex. For example, the anterior paraventricular thalamic nucleus projects strongly to the medial part of the nucleus accumbens and very specifically to the prelimbic cortex, two areas that are connected with each other *via* corticostriatal projections (Berendse et al., 1988; Berendse and Groenewegen, 1990, 1991). Likewise, the caudal part of the basolateral amygdaloid nucleus projects to both the medial nucleus accumbens and the medial prefrontal cortex (Russchen and Price, 1984; unpublished observations). The intermediodorsal nucleus of the midline thalamic complex projects to more central parts of the nucleus accumbens and to adjacent regions of the caudate-putamen complex (Berendse and Groenewegen, 1990) and, in addition, to the dorsal agranular insular area (Berendse and Groenewegen, 1991). The striatal projections of this part of the lateral prefrontal cortex distribute to the same region of the striatum as the fibers from the intermediodorsal nucleus (Beckstead, 1979; Figure 2E). Furthermore, the anterior part of the basolateral amygdaloid nucleus sends fibers to both the dorsal agranular insular area and the striatal target region of this cortical region. Interestingly, the projections from the intralaminar thalamic complex to the amygdala appear to be topographically organized such that the paraventricular nucleus projects to the caudal part of the basolateral nucleus and the intermediodorsal nucleus to more rostral parts of this nucleus (Figure 2E; Berendse and Groenewegen, unpublished observations). Fibers from these midline thalamic nuclei reach, in addition, other amygdaloid nuclei. Nevertheless, in the thalamic projections to the basolateral nucleus, the parallelism in the cortical–subcortical relationships is maintained (Groenewegen et al., 1990a).

The specific functions of the various loops are at present unknown, but most probably they depend upon the information that enters these circuits both at the level of the cortex and of the striatum. In this respect it is important to note that in the rat the corticostriatal projections from the frontal lobe, including the prefrontal, premotor/supplementary motor and motor cortices cover almost the entire striatum in a topographical manner (Beckstead, 1979; McGeorge and Faull, 1989; our own unpublished observations). In addition, virtually all striatal regions receive inputs from more caudally located cortical areas in the hemisphere, i.e. the parietal, the temporal and/or the occipital cortices. The patterns, in which frontal cortical projections and inputs from other cortical areas converge in the striatum of the rat, are incompletely known. It has been found that certain cortical areas in the monkey, which are interconnected *via* corticocortical projections, have overlapping projection areas in the striatum (Yeterian and VanHoesen, 1978). Employing double anterograde tracing techniques in the monkey, Selemon and Goldman-Rakic (1985) concluded that the interrelationship of striatal projections from cortical areas that are interconnected, range from almost segregated projection fields (in case of projections from dorsolateral prefrontal and orbital cortices) to extensive overlap of terminal areas (in case of projections from frontal and temporal cortices). Within the areas of convergence, the discontinuous prefrontal and temporal terminal fields are arranged in an interdigitating rather than in an overlapping manner (Selemon and Goldman-Rakic, 1985). This also holds for the ventral striatum of the rat. For example, the hippocampus and entorhinal cortex are connected with the medial part of the prefrontal cortex, i.e. the prelimbic and infralimbic areas. These four cortical areas project in an overlapping manner to a medial and ventral sector of the nucleus accumbens and the caudate-putamen. The lateral prefrontal cortex, i.e. the dorsal and ventral agranular insular areas, and the perirhinal cortex are also strongly interconnected. Their termination area in the striatum includes a more central and lateral sector in the nucleus accumbens and the caudate-putamen (Beckstead, 1979; Reep and Winans, 1982; Witter et al., 1989; unpublished observations). How the terminal fields of converging corticostriatal fibers exactly relate to each other remains to be established. Preliminary results in our laboratory suggest that in the rat the terminal fields of, for example, the ventral subiculum and the prelimbic area are complementary in the medial part of the nucleus accumbens. This arrangement appears to be comparable with the interdigitating patterns of terminals from the dorsolateral prefrontal and the temporal cortical areas in the caudate nucleus of the monkey (Selemon and Goldman-Rakic, 1985). The compartmental structure of the striatum, discussed below, may play a role in integrating information from the different, interdigitating cortical areas.

It is important to realize that at the level of the striatum, DA input might influence the transmission of information through all functionally different cortical–subcortical circuits. As will be discussed below (see section on Synaptic Organization), DA terminals on striatal output neurons are in a position to modulate selectively the transmission of cortical information through the striatum.

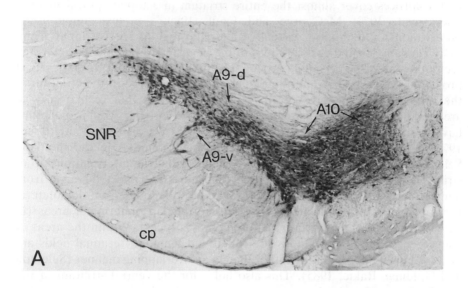

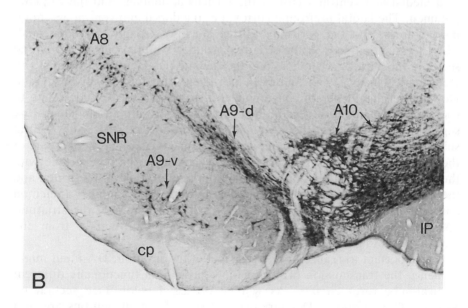

A remarkable exception to the basic principle of the parallel organization of circuits involving the different nuclei of the basal ganglia is the arrangement that exists between the striatum and the pallidal complex on the one hand, and the DA cell groups of the substantia nigra on the other. As noted previously (Nauta et al., 1978; Domesick, 1981; Nauta and Domesick, 1979, 1984), the ventral striatum is predominantly innervated by the DA neurons of the ventral tegmental area, but the return projections from the ventral striatum to the ventral mesencephalon terminate primarily in the medial part of the substantia nigra and only to a minor degree in the ventral tegmental area. The ventral striatum seems therefore to be in a position to influence the DA input of the dorsal striatum (Nauta and Domesick, 1979, 1984; Somogyi et al., 1981b). Recent studies in our laboratory have confirmed and extended these conclusions. We combined the tracing of the efferent connections of the ventral striatum and the ventral pallidum, based on the anterograde transport of the lectin *Phaseolus vulgaris*-leucoagglutinin (PHA-L), with the

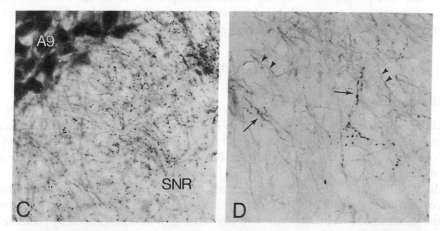

Figure 3. A and **B**. Low power photomicrographs of coronal sections through the ventral mesencephalon stained with a DA anti-serum to show the location of the different DA cell groups. Note the difference between the dorsal (A9-d) and the ventral (A9-v) cell groups of the pars compacta. **C** and **D**. High-power photomicrographs (120 ×) of double-immunostained sections of the substantia nigra following injections of the anterograde tracer *Phaseolus vulgaris*-leucoagglutinin (PHA-L) in the ventral striatum (**C**) and in the ventral pallidum (**D**). PHA-L-labeled fibers and terminals are stained black, and the dopaminergic cell bodies (A9 in **C**) and dendrites are stained brown to allow for a clear distinction between the two types of immunostained elements. Note the rather random distribution of the striatonigral fibers and terminals in (**C**) and the close appositions (arrows) between pallidonigral fibers and dopaminergic dendrites in (**D**). Arrowheads point at dopaminergic dendrites. cp, cerebral peduncle; IP, interpeduncular nucleus; SNR, substantia nigra, pars reticulata

immunohistochemical detection of DA in the ventral mesencephalon. It could be confirmed that the ventral striatum projects to the DA cell groups A10, A9 and A8 as well as to the medial part of the pars reticulata of the substantia nigra (Nauta et al., 1978; see also section on Compartmental Organization). The pars reticulata of the substantia nigra in the rat is traversed by vertically orientated DA dendrites (Figure 3A and B). In the DA cell groups, the ventral striatal fibers and their terminals establish close appositions with cell bodies and dendrites of the DA neurons, but in the pars reticulata such appositions between fibers from the ventral striatum and DA dendrites are relatively infrequent (Figure 3C). By contrast, large boutons on axons arising from the ventral pallidum frequently establish close appositions with DA cells, both in the pars compacta and in the pars reticulata of the substantia nigra (Figure 3D). These results imply that the ventral striatum can exert a direct influence on the DA cells in the mesencephalon, although an indirect influence *via* the pallidum must also be taken into account (Figure 4). By these connections and, subsequently, by the DA projection from the substantia nigra to the dorsal striatum, the ventral striatum appears to be able to modulate, at the level of the striatum, the information transfer in other circuits that involve the basal ganglia.

COMPARTMENTAL ORGANIZATION OF THE STRIATUM

Dorsal Striatum

Beginning with the observation in 1972 by Olson et al. that the DA fibers in the striatum of young postnatal rats are inhomogeneously distributed, forming an island/matrix pattern, it has gradually become clear that most of the neurochemical substances in the striatum have a compartmental distribution. The demonstration in the monkey that fibers from frontal cortical areas terminate in a patchy manner in the striatum suggests that the connections of the striatum are also arranged inhomogeneously (Künzle, 1975; Goldman and Nauta, 1977). Since the striatum in most species is rather homogeneous cytoarchitectonically (*cf.*, however, Goldman-Rakic, 1982), evidence for a compartmentation has been primarily derived from (immuno)histochemical studies.

Immunohistochemical Compartmentation

The enzyme acetylcholinesterase (AChE) shows a clear differential regional activity (Butcher and Hodge, 1976). On the basis of the discontinuous staining pattern of this enzyme, Graybiel and Ragsdale (1978, 1983) defined the so-called 'striosomes' as the principal units of the striatum: lightly staining striosomes against a darker stained background, the 'matrix', could

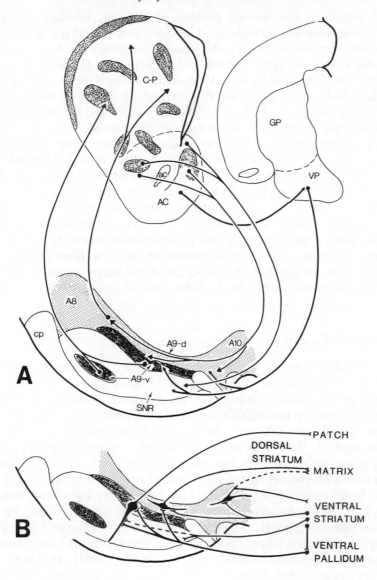

Figure 4. The distribution of ventral striatal and ventral pallidal fibers in the DA cell groups of the substantia nigra. In addition, the projections from the different DA cell groups to the patch and matrix compartments in the dorsal striatum are indicated. The scheme in (**A**) emphasizes the general distribution of these projection systems, whereas (**B**) focuses on the possible synaptic relationships. A9-d, dorsal cell groups; A9-v, ventral cell groups; AC, nucleus accumbens; ac, anterior commissure; C-P, caudate-putamen complex; cp, cerebral peduncle; GP, globus pallidus; SNR, substantia nigra, pars reticulata; VP, ventral pallidum

be identified in the caudate nucleus of the cat, monkey and human. Subsequent (immuno)histochemical studies showed that the distribution of many neuroactive substances in the striatum correlates in one way or another with the striosome/matrix pattern (e.g. enkephalin: Graybiel et al., 1981; neurotensin: Zahm and Heimer, 1988; somatostatin: Gerfen, 1985; Chesselet and Graybiel, 1986; substance P: Graybiel et al., 1981; calcium-binding protein: Gerfen et al., 1985; DA: Voorn et al., 1986; see also Figure 5D). For example, AChE-poor striosomes in the caudate nucleus of the cat correspond to patches of high enkephalin-like immunoreactivity (Graybiel et al., 1981). Several types of receptors, such as opioid (Herkenham and Pert, 1981), cholinergic (muscarinic; Nastuk and Graybiel, 1988), DA (Besson et al., 1988; Beckstead et al., 1988; Loopuyt, 1989) and benzodiazepine (Faull and Villiger, 1986), are also inhomogeneously distributed in patterns that, to a certain degree, correspond to the striosome/matrix arrangement. Furthermore, regions of high enkephalin-immunoreactivity or low AChE activity (striosomes), as seen in transverse tissue sections of the caudate nucleus of the cat, appear, in three-dimensional reconstructions, to form an intricate labyrinth (Groves et al., 1988; Desban et al., 1989).

Connectivity Patterns

A relationship between the termination patterns of frontal corticostriatal fibers and island/matrix patterns in the cytoarchitecture of the caudate nucleus of the monkey was described by Goldman-Rakic in 1982. The precise relationship between cortical afferents and the compartments depends on the specific cortical area, the region of the striatum and the animal species studied. Prefrontal corticostriatal fibers terminate preferentially in AChE-poor striosomes in the cat (Ragsdale and Graybiel, 1981) or enkephalin-rich patches in the rat (Gerfen, 1984), whereas in the monkey, fibers from comparable cortical areas appear to avoid the striosomes (Graybiel, 1984a). Since prefrontal cortical areas, which are associated with limbic structures, appear to terminate preferentially in opioid receptor-rich patches, these patches have been viewed as limbic-related islands embedded in a more sensorimotor-related matrix (Gerfen, 1984). However, recent evidence suggests that, in the rat, the specific compartment in the striatum in which fibers from a certain cortical area terminate depends primarily on the layers of origin in the cortex and, to a lesser degree, on the cortical area of origin (Gerfen, 1989). Thus, fibers from neurons in superficial layer V and layers II and III of the prelimbic cortex terminate in the striatal matrix, whereas axons from neurons in deep layer V and layer VI end in the patches. A similar arrangement holds for the projections from the cingular and motor cortices. However, the inputs from the prelimbic cortex to the patches are denser than those from the cingular and motor cortical areas in their respective striatal terminal fields. The opposite is true for the inputs from these cortical areas to the matrix (Gerfen, 1989).

Recent tracing studies in several species have shown that the connections between the striatum and the substantia nigra, including the ascending DA pathways, are organized compartmentally (rat: Gerfen et al., 1987a; cat: Jimenez-Castellanos and Graybiel, 1987, 1989; monkey: Feigenbaum-Langer and Graybiel, 1989). Figure 3 shows the subdivision of the groups of midbrain DA neurons in the rat. First, there is the classical parcellation into the ventral tegmental area (A10), the pars compacta of the substantia nigra (A9), and the retrorubral area (A8). Within the A9 cell group, differences in morphology, location and neurochemistry of the neurons lead to a further subdivision. As shown by Gerfen et al. (1987a, b), there is a dorsal tier of A9 DA neurons (A9-d) which extend their dendrites predominantly in a horizontal direction (see also Figure 3) and exhibit immunoreactivity for calcium-binding protein (CaBP, calbindin-D_{28kDa}). A smaller population of DA neurons located in the ventral part of the pars compacta of the substantia nigra (A9-v) have dendrites that are orientated vertically and extend ventrally into the pars reticulata (see also Figure 3). These ventral A9 DA neurons of the pars compacta, together with a substantial population of the scattered DA neurons in the ventral part of the pars reticulata, are devoid of CaBP (Gerfen et al., 1987a, b). Using anterograde tracing methods, Gerfen et al. (1987a) demonstrated that the dorsal tier of DA cells in the pars compacta, like the adjacent neuronal cell groups A10 and A8, project to the striatal matrix. The more ventrally located DA neurons in both the pars compacta and the pars reticulata of the substantia nigra send their axons to the striatal patches (Gerfen et al., 1987a). These results thus suggest the existence of two neurochemically different DA systems, differentially projecting to the patch and matrix compartments of the striatum. In turn, neurons in the matrix compartment of the striatum project to the pars reticulata of the substantia nigra, avoiding the areas with populations of DA perikarya in A9 and the ventrally located DA cells in the pars reticulata (Gerfen, 1985). By contrast, striatal patch neurons appear to project primarily to the ventrally located A9 DA neurons and the DA neurons in the pars reticulata of the substantia nigra (Gerfen, 1985; Gerfen et al., 1987a). These data indicate that the connections of the patches and the ventral DA neurons are arranged in a reciprocal fashion, whereas striatal projections arising in the matrix affect the output zone of the substantia nigra, the pars reticulata. As discussed above, one of the inputs to the dorsal DA neurons that send projections to the matrix of the dorsal striatum is the ventral striatopallidal system (Figure 4).

Ventral Striatum

The ventral striatum is, like the dorsal striatum, neurochemically a heterogeneous structure. On the basis of the distribution patterns of several neuroactive substances, the nucleus accumbens, which is the most prominent representative of the ventral striatum, can be subdivided into a 'shell' and a 'core' region (Zaborszky et al., 1985; Voorn et al., 1989). In contrast to the dorsal striatum, the nucleus accumbens appears to be cytoarchitectonically heterogeneous, since it contains clusters of small neurons in its medial and ventral parts (Herkenham et al., 1984). These inhomogeneities in the cytoarchitecture accentuate the subdivision of the nucleus in the two regions mentioned above. The shell contains cell-poor regions with a loose arrangement of neurons. Cell clusters line the dorsal and lateral borders of the shell and are dispersed ventrally and medially within the shell (Domesick, 1981; Herkenham et al., 1984). In the central core of the nucleus accumbens, neurons are in general more closely packed and more homogeneously distributed than in the shell.

Cell clusters in the nucleus accumbens appear to coincide with dense opioid receptor patches and regions of low AChE activity, and are avoided by fibers from the midline and intralaminar thalamic nuclei and the ventral tegmental area (Herkenham et al., 1984). The latter observation was confirmed by Voorn et al. (1986) who showed that DA fibers are concentrated in cell-poor regions in the nucleus accumbens. However, this is not a general rule, since in the same study it was found that, in the extreme dorsomedial corner of the caudal nucleus accumbens, a cell-dense area is strongly innervated by DA fibers. Moreover, in the border region between the nucleus accumbens and the caudate-putamen complex, small patches of sparse DA innervation have no clear cytoarchitectonic counterparts (Figure 5).

Immunohistochemical Compartmentation

The compartmental structure of the ventral striatum has recently been further elucidated using immunohistochemical methods for localizing various neurochemical substances (Voorn et al., 1986, 1989; Meredith et al., 1989). Immunohistochemistry of different substances, such as DA, enkephalin, substance P, choline acetyltransferase (ChAT) and CaBP, was carried out on adjacent sections of the same brain (Voorn et al., 1989) or, by means of double-label procedures, on the same tissue section (Meredith et al., 1989). Furthermore, the use of double-label immunohistochemistry has enabled us to determine the relationship between a number of inputs and outputs of the ventral striatum and its compartmental structure (Groenewegen et al., 1987, 1989; Berendse et al., 1988; Berendse and Groenewegen, 1990).

Immunoreactivity for the opioid peptide enkephalin in the nucleus

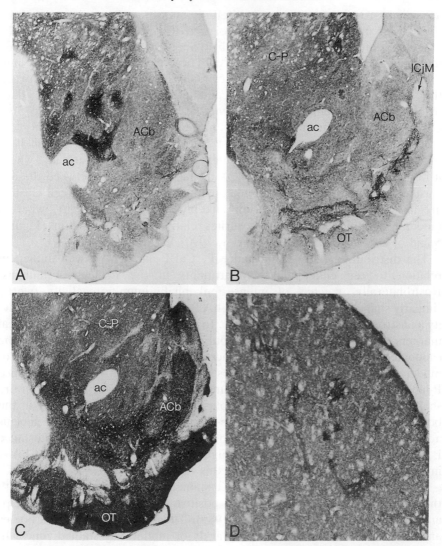

Figure 5. A and **B**. Low-power photomicrographs to show the distribution of enkephalin-immunoreactivity in the ventral striatum of the rat. Note the relatively large, dark patches in the rostrolateral part of the nucleus accumbens (ACb) and the moderate staining in the shell region of the nucleus. The shell is demarcated by zones of very light enkephalin staining. **C**. Photomicrograph showing the differential distribution of DA-immunoreactivity in the ventral striatum. Note the dark, cone-shaped area in the shell of the nucleus accumbens and the light patches in the border region between the caudate-putamen (C-P) and the nucleus accumbens. **D**. Low-power photomicrograph of the patchy distribution of DA-immunoreactivity in the dorsolateral part of the caudate-putamen. ac, anterior commissure; ICjM, major island of Calleja; OT, olfactory tubercle

accumbens roughly shows three different intensities. Rostrolaterally, relatively large patches of strong immunoreactivity, closely associated with the anterior commissure, stand out against an otherwise moderately stained matrix of uneven intensity (Figure 5A). These patches extend dorsally into the caudate-putamen complex. More caudally, in the border region between the nucleus accumbens and the caudate-putamen complex, the dark patches of enkephalin-immunoreactivity are smaller in size (Figure 5B). Caudomedially, in the nucleus accumbens, regions virtually non-immunoreactive for enkephalin stand out against a cone-shaped area in the shell of moderate staining intensity. This area extends ventrally and laterally, where it becomes less clearly demarcated. A distinct relationship between the cell clusters and the distribution of enkephalin exists. Virtually all cell clusters are in register with regions of low enkephalin-immunoreactivity, whereas moderate staining for enkephalin overlies relatively cell-poor regions (Figures 5 and 6; Berendse and Groenewegen, 1990).

The distribution of DA, substance P, CaBP and ChAT was studied in relation to the enkephalin compartments in the nucleus accumbens. Rostrolaterally, patches of intense enkephalin-immunoreactivity overlie similarly shaped areas of weak DA-, ChAT- and substance P-immunoreactivity and strong CaBP-immunoreactivity. In the matrix, all these neurochemical markers are present in moderate, but slightly varying, intensity. In the caudomedial part of the nucleus accumbens, the cone-shaped area of moderate enkephalin-staining matches densely DA-, ChAT- and substance P-labeled areas, whereas CaBP-immunoreactivity is absent from the entire shell region. The relatively small strong enkephalin-positive patches in the border region between the caudate-putamen complex and the nucleus accumbens coincide with similarly shaped areas that stain darkly for substance P and lightly for DA and CaBP (Figure 6). The distribution of ChAT-immunoreactivity is homogeneous in this region.

The heterogeneous pattern of ChAT-stained neuropil correlates well with the distribution of perikarya that are positive for the same marker (Phelps and Vaughn, 1986; Meredith et al., 1989). Thus, most neuronal cell bodies and their dendrites are confined to darkly or moderately stained zones. In material double-labeled for ChAT and enkephalin, it appears that most ChAT-positive neurons lie outside dark enkephalin-positive patches. A small number of ChAT-labeled neurons are located close to the borders of these patches and these cells have processes that usually follow the edge of the patch. Only occasionally do they cross over into the patch (Meredith et al., 1989).

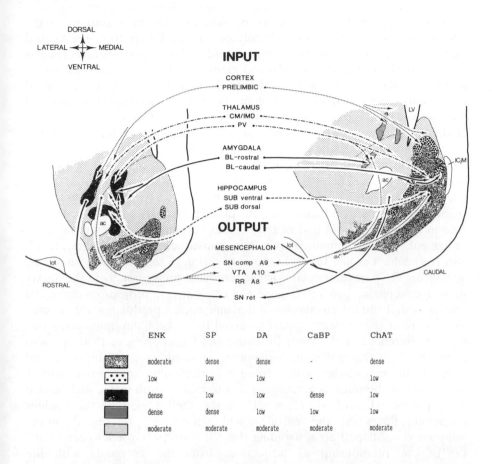

Figure 6. Two levels of the nucleus accumbens showing the compartmental distribution of various neuroactive substances and the relationship of some afferent and efferent fiber systems with this compartmental structure. Note that the prelimbic cortex and the amygdala project to different compartments within a certain region of the ventral striatum but that, as indicated by individual arrows, these projections most probably stem from distinct neuronal populations within these areas. Further, note the difference between the shell and the core of the nucleus accumbens. ac, anterior commissure; BL, basolateral amygdaloid nucleus; CaBP, calcium-binding protein; ChAT, choline acetyltransferase; CM, central medial thalamic nucleus; ENK, enkephalin; ICjM, major island of Calleja; IMD, intermediodorsal thalamic nucleus; lot, lateral olfactory tract; LV, lateral ventricle; RR, retrorubral area (A8); PV, paraventricular thalamic nucleus; SN comp, substantia nigra, pars compacta (A9); SN ret, substantia nigra, pars reticulata; SP, substance P; SUB, subiculum; VTA, ventral tegmental area (A10)

Connectivity Patterns

As can be appreciated from Figure 6, most afferent fiber systems of the nucleus accumbens are topographically organized. Fibers from the ventral subiculum, the caudal basolateral amygdaloid nucleus and the paraventricular thalamic nucleus project to caudal and medial parts of the nucleus, whereas more laterally and rostrally in the nucleus there is a convergence of projections from the dorsal subiculum, the rostral basolateral amygdaloid nucleus, and the parataenial and central medial thalamic nuclei (Groenewegen et al., 1987; Berendse and Groenewegen, 1990; Groenewegen et al., 1990a).

The extent to which the distribution of the afferent systems of the ventral striatum concurs with its compartmental structure depends on the site of origin of the fibers. The projections of the thalamic midline and intralaminar nuclei have a distinct relationship with the ventral striatal compartments (Figure 6). The paraventricular nucleus projects strongly to the cone-shaped area in the caudomedial part of the nucleus accumbens, avoiding the areas of low enkephalin-immunoreactivity and, consequently, the cell clusters (*cf.* also Herkenham et al., 1984). In the core region of the nucleus accumbens, fibers from the paraventricular nucleus terminate preferentially in the darkly stained enkephalin patches (Figure 6). By contrast, projections from the central medial and intermediodorsal thalamic nuclei, predominantly directed to the core of the nucleus, appear to avoid the enkephalin-immunoreactive patches (Berendse et al., 1988; Berendse and Groenewegen, 1990; see also Figure 6). Hippocampal inputs originating primarily in the subiculum tend to ignore the boundaries of the strong enkephalin-immunoreactive patches in the core of the nucleus accumbens and terminate both inside and outside these patches (Figure 6). However, in the shell region of the nucleus accumbens, fibers from the ventral subiculum terminate preferentially in the cell-poor cone-shaped area, avoiding the cell clusters (Groenewegen et al., 1987). The relationship of projections from the amygdala with the compartments in the ventral striatum appears to be quite complicated (Wolters, Lohman and Groenewegen, unpublished observations). Depending on the location of the PHA-L injections in the amygdala, fibers are found in the caudal and ventral parts of the nucleus accumbens, inside or outside the cell clusters, and in the rostrolateral part of the nucleus inside or outside the dark enkephalin patches (Figure 6). On the basis of the results of retrograde tracing experiments, it may be assumed that the majority of the amygdaloid projections to the striatum stem from neurons in the basolateral nucleus, and that only small contributions arise from the basomedial and other amygdaloid nuclei (Kelley et al., 1982). Although there appear to be distinct relationships between the amygdaloid input and the compartments in the ventral striatum in individual experiments, until now it has been extremely difficult to relate these patterns precisely to the nucleus or subnucleus of origin in the amygdala (Figure 6; *cf.* also Ragsdale and Graybiel, 1988).

The output of the nucleus accumbens is also organized in a compartmental fashion. The overall distribution of ventral striatal projections in the mesencephalon, as found in our experiments with small injections of PHA-L in the nucleus accumbens, concurs with the pattern described by Nauta et al. in 1978. However, our results reveal two different labeling patterns in the substantia nigra that may be related to different populations of neurons in the ventral striatum. One pattern consists of terminations predominantly in the dorsomedial part of the pars reticulata of the substantia nigra, with little labeling in the adjacent A9 cell group. The second pattern is characterized by extensive terminal labeling in the ventral tegmental area (A10), the substantia nigra pars compacta (A9), and the retrorubral cell group (A8). Injections of the retrograde tracers Fluoro-Gold (Fluorochrome Inc., USA) or Choleratoxin subunit B (List Biochemical Laboratories, USA) in the ventral mesencephalon support the idea that at least two populations of ventral striatal projection neurons exist, one of which projects preferentially to the DA cell groups. Following injections of either of the two retrograde tracers in the ventral tegmental area, clusters of retrogradely labeled neurons are found in the ventral striatum (Groenewegen et al., 1990a). These cell clusters avoid the dark enkephalin patches in the rostrolateral part of the nucleus accumbens, overlie the small patches in the border region of the caudate-putamen complex and the nucleus accumbens, and fill the cone-shaped area in the caudomedial part of the nucleus (Figure 6). More experiments are needed to understand the precise organization of the ventral striatonigral pathways.

Definition and Function of Compartments

The prevailing notion in the literature is that the striatum has a bicompartmental structure: island/matrix, striosome/matrix or patch/matrix. The differential distribution of AChE activity initially led to the distinction between striosomes (striosomal bodies), as defined on the basis of a regional low AChE activity, and the surrounding matrix (Graybiel and Ragsdale, 1978, see above). Many subsequent studies have compared the AChE pattern with the distribution of other neurochemical substances, receptors or afferents and efferents of the striatum. Although striosomes are apparent in most species studied, e.g. cat, monkey and human, they are only clearly present in certain parts of the striatum, in particular in the head of the caudate nucleus (Graybiel, 1984c). In the rat, in which AChE activity is less clearly compartmentalized, the distribution of opioid receptors or that of CaBP is advocated as compartmental marking (Herkenham and Pert, 1981; Gerfen et al, 1985). In the literature, the relationship of the immunoreactivity pattern of a particular substance (or the distribution of a receptor) with AChE-poor striosomes (or opioid receptor-rich patches) in a certain region of the striatum is often generalized to hold for the entire striatal domain. In view of observations mentioned below, which suggest that the structural organization of the striatum is more complex and diverse than a simple bimodal compartmentation, such generalizations may not be justified. These data will be discussed first. Concomitantly, evidence is accumulating from anatomical and developmental studies that the compartments have a structural cellular basis. These latter findings provide a framework for a functional interpretation of the striatal compartmentation, and will be discussed subsequently.

First, as noted by Graybiel et al. (1981), the specific interrelationships between the patterns of different neuroactive substances are not constant throughout the entire striatum. For example, substance P-immunoreactive areas in the dorsal part of the caudate nucleus of the cat correspond to AChE-poor striosomes, whereas in more ventral regions of the nucleus they appear to avoid the striosomes. Our data on the ventral striatum of the rat (discussed in the previous section) confirm these observations. For example, the immunoreactivity for DA, enkephalin and substance P differs in the various patches of the ventral striatum (Figure 6). In general, it may be stated that the interrelations between different receptors or neurochemical markers, and also the relationship of inputs and outputs with the compartments, are constant in a specific part of the striatum across individual animals of the same species. However, such interrelations vary from one region in the striatum to another in a certain species and, in addition, from species to species in a specific part of the striatum.

Second, it has recently been suggested by Faull et al. (1989) that a third compartment is present in the striatum of the human. These authors describe AChE-poor striosomes in the caudate nucleus that are surrounded by annular regions which are AChE-negative. Neurotensin receptor binding appears to be high within these annular regions, low in the AChE-poor striosomes, and moderate in the AChE-rich matrix. Annular regions, but now surrounding enkephalin-rich patches, have also been observed in the ventral striatum of the rat (Voorn et al., 1989). These annular regions appear to be observed by the inputs from the midline and intralaminar thalamic nuclei: fibers from the paraventricular thalamic nucleus terminate in both the patches and their surrounding annular regions, whereas fibers from thalamic nuclei that project primarily to the matrix avoid the annular regions (Berendse and Groenewegen, 1990).

Third, the distribution of many neurochemical substances, receptors, and afferents and efferents in the matrix compartment of the striatum is far from homogeneous (Malach and Graybiel, 1986; Ragsdale and Graybiel, 1988; Voorn et al., 1989; Desban et al., 1989). A clear example is the patchy distribution of striatal afferents from sensory cortical areas in the caudate nucleus of the cat conveying submodality-specific sensory information. Within the matrix, these patches form an interdigitating pattern (Malach and Graybiel, 1986).

Finally, in the putamen of the monkey, functionally distinct, microexcitable zones can be defined on the basis of physiological experiments (Alexander and DeLong, 1985a, b). Histochemical or cellular counterparts for these physiologically distinct zones have as yet not been identified.

The above-mentioned findings may indicate that the striatum is composed of a multitude of different compartments, precluding an unequivocal definition of a striatal compartment. However, primarily on the basis of findings in the developing striatum, it may be argued that there are basically two compartments in the striatum. According to this view, a single compartment does not necessarily have the same neurochemical composition and connectional characteristics throughout the striatum. In other words, either of the two compartments, i.e. striosomes/patches or matrix, may attain different phenotypes in different parts of the striatum and in different species, but throughout the striatum they maintain the same basic structure and the same functional role. This supposes a cellular, morphological basis for the striatal compartmentation. The results of developmental studies seem to be in favor of this (Graybiel, 1984b, c; Van der Kooy and Fishell, 1987). In the rat, neurons born before embryonic day 15 primarily aggregate to form patches, whereas later-born neurons preferentially take part in the formation of the matrix (Van der Kooy and Fishell, 1987; Krushel et al., 1989). Likewise, in the cat, early-born subpopulations of cells align with striosomes, whereas later-born neurons are distributed in a more scattered way (Graybiel, 1984b, c). It has been suggested that the early developing dopaminergic nigrostriatal system plays an important role in this pattern formation of the striatum (Graybiel, 1984b). In the rat, lesions of the ascending dopaminergic system, but not of the corticostriatal system, interfere with the development of the patchy distribution of opiate receptors (Lança et al., 1986). It further appears that the reciprocal relationship between the patch neurons and the ventrally located, CaBP-negative dopaminergic neurons is established prenatally, whereas the matrix projection to the pars reticulata of the substantia nigra and the dopaminergic projections from the CaBP-positive, dorsally located dopaminergic neurons are established postnatally (Fishell and Van der Kooy, 1989; Gerfen et al., 1987b). The results of our own studies on the developing dopaminergic system do not fully support the idea of a developmental dissociation in the dopaminergic innervation of the patch and matrix compartments. Using immunohistochemical methods to detect dopaminergic neurons and fibers, it was found that, both at the level of the striatum and of the substantia nigra, patch and matrix innervating systems develop simultaneously during embryogenesis and in the early postnatal period (Voorn et al., 1988). Therefore, the exact role of the dopaminergic system in the development of the striatal compartmental structure is still unclear.

A cytoarchitectonic basis for the neurochemical compartments is further supported by the results of experiments in the rat in which intracellular injections of horseradish peroxidase in the dorsal striatum were combined with enkephalin staining (Penny et al., 1988). Medium-size spiny neurons were found to retain their dendritic arborizations and their recurrent axon collaterals within the compartments in which the perikarya reside. In the same study, the dendrites of a large neuron were seen to ignore the neurochemically defined boundaries of the compartments. However, in a study in the cat and the ferret, it was observed that a considerable proportion of Golgi-impregnated medium-size spiny neurons possess dendrites that ignore the borders between striosomes and matrix (Bolam et al., 1988). In contrast, the dendritic arborizations of other neurons were influenced by the compartmental boundaries. The discrepancy between the results of these two studies could be due to species differences, but more important might be the fact that compartments cannot be defined unambiguously in the striatum by means of (immuno)histochemical markers (see discussion above). Nevertheless, the above-cited data suggest that there are populations of striatal neurons that, by virtue of their geometry and the orientation of their dendrites (and possibly also of their recurrent collaterals; Penny et al., 1988; Chang et al., 1982), form the basis for 'private territories', i.e. patch versus matrix compartments. The compartmentation of (immuno)histochemical markers would then, at least in part, be a reflection of this ordered distribution of the striatal neurons and their dendrites (see also Groenewegen et al., 1990b). Neurons of which the dendrites or the local axons do not obey the boundaries between the so-defined compartments may constitute the anatomical basis for intercompartmental communication. Somatostatin-immunoreactive neurons have been considered to play such a role (Gerfen, 1985; *cf*. also Meredith et al., 1989).

The question can be raised as to whether the data discussed above justify the conclusion that the striatum as a whole is bicompartmentally organized. A definite answer to this question cannot be given at present. In particular, the available knowledge of the developmental and cytoarchitectonic compart-mentation of the ventral striatum is too scarce to draw the conclusion that the structure of this part of the striatum is fully comparable to that of the dorsal striatum. In this context, it is important to note that the time and pattern of development both of the neurons of the ventral striatum (Bayer, 1981) and of its dopaminergic innervation (Voorn et al., 1988) differ from those of the dorsal striatum. The subdivision of the nucleus accumbens in a shell and a core region, the presence of cell clusters in the shell and of patch/matrix configurations in the core, all suggest that the basic structure of the ventral striatum is more complex than that of the dorsal striatum.

Previously, the compartmental organization of the striatum has been compared with the laminar and columnar structure of the cortex (Graybiel, 1983). As noted in the rat by Van der Kooy and Fishell (1987), both the deep layers of the cortex and the striatal patches are the first to appear in embryonic development, whereas more superficial cortical layers and the striatal matrix compartment develop later. Interestingly, Gerfen (1989) has shown recently that the compartmental distribution of corticostriatal fibers is related to their laminar origin. Thus, as already discussed above, deep layers of the prelimbic, cingulate and motor cortices project to striatal patches, whereas more superficial layers of the same cortical areas send fibers to the matrix. This contrasts with an earlier notion of a functional dissociation of the striatum into a 'limbic' patch and a 'non-limbic' matrix compartment that was based on connectional criteria (Gerfen, 1984). The above-mentioned dichotomy in the corticostriatal projections would support the bicompartmental structure of the striatum. Furthermore, these data allow for an intriguing comparison between the cortical and striatal functional–anatomical structure. In both telencephalic structures, different levels of structural–functional organization can be recognized.

First, as discussed above, the striatum may be subdivided into functionally different sectors on the basis of the organization of the corticostriatal projections. Such a level of functional organization is directly comparable with the subdivision of the cortex in functionally different areas on the basis of its relationships with different thalamic nuclei. Second, just as the cytoarchitectonic lamination of the cortex is a prominent morphological feature throughout the cortical mantle, the patch/matrix compartmental organization appears to be a general characteristic of the striatum. However, the laminar organization of the cortex merely defines the input and output laminae of a certain cortical area and, as such, provides only limited insight into the functional organization of the cortex. Likewise, the compartmental structure of the striatum may provide the basis for a segregation of different input/output channels through this structure (Graybiel, 1984a). However, the morphological substrates of functional subunits in the cortex are thought to be organized orthogonally to its horizontal, laminar organization, and, in various cortical regions, are defined as cortical columns. This columnar organization was demonstrated most elegantly, both anatomically and physiologically, for the primary visual cortex (*cf.* Braitenberg, 1985) but appears to be a general organizational principle for other neocortical areas as well (*cf.* Eccles, 1984). Considering the functions of the striatal compartments, we might speculate, in analogy with the laminar and columnar organization of the cortex, that the functional subunits in the striatum are not formed by the different compartments per se. Rather, the morphological substrate of striatal functional subunits appears to be constituted by the anatomical combination of a subregion of the matrix and an adjacent patch region. At present, little is known about the communication between different, adjacent striatal compartments. Therefore, studies of the anatomical and physiological interactions of anatomically adjacent patch and matrix regions are needed to determine the functional significance of striatal compartmentation. Third, a further level of structural–functional organization in both the cortex and the striatum is the specific arrangement of input–output relationships at the cellular level, as will be briefly discussed for the striatum immediately below.

SYNAPTIC ORGANIZATION

At least seven types of neurons have been identified in the mammalian striatum, mainly on the basis of Golgi studies (Graybiel and Ragsdale, 1983; Parent, 1986). The medium-size, densely spiny neuron constitutes the most frequent neuronal cell type with over 90 per cent of the total cell population (Kemp and Powell, 1971). Other well-known types of striatal neurons are the large, aspinous cholinergic interneurons (Bolam et al., 1984; Phelps et al., 1985; Graybiel and Ragsdale, 1983; Parent, 1986) and the medium-size aspinous GABAergic and somatostatinergic interneurons (Bolam et al., 1983a; DiFiglia and Aronin, 1982). It is now generally accepted on the basis of results of intracellular injections (Chang et al., 1981; Chang and Kitai, 1985) and retrograde tracing studies (Grofova, 1975; Bolam et al., 1981a, b) that the medium-size, densely spiny neurons form the main projection neurons of the striatum. Moreover, by virtue of their number and morphology, these neurons receive the greatest proportion of the extrinsic and intrinsic fibers, and may therefore be considered as the central neuronal elements in the striatal circuitry. Most of the medium-size spiny neurons use GABA as a neurotransmitter (Kita and Kitai, 1988). A large proportion of these neurons probably also contain either substance P or enkephalin (Gerfen and Young, 1988).

Bolam and co-workers have elucidated important aspects of the synaptic organization of the dorsal striatum by employing a combination of Golgi impregnation, tract-tracing and immunocytochemical techniques. This combination of methods allowed the authors to establish immunohistochemically, or connectionally, characterized synaptic inputs on neurons which were identified on the basis of their morphology (Golgi technique) and/or their efferent connections (retrograde tracing). As argued by Bolam and Izzo (1987), there is a large number of possible interactions in the striatum between neuronal elements of different extrinsic or intrinsic origin. Therefore, the following summary of the synaptic organization of the dorsal and the ventral striatum (Figures 7A and B, respectively) provides only a limited impression of the real complexity of the ultrastructural anatomy of these regions.

It has been demonstrated in the dorsal striatum of the rat that terminals immunoreactive for tyrosine hydroxylase make symmetrical synaptic contacts with medium-size spiny neurons that project to the substantia nigra (Freund et al., 1984). More than half of these presumptive DA inputs contact the necks of dendritic spines, whereas most of the remaining terminals make synaptic contacts with dendritic shafts, often close to a dendritic spine. Apart from the symmetrical tyrosine hydroxylase-positive contacts, a large proportion of the heads of the spines are contacted by unlabeled asymmetrical synapses. In this way triads are formed, i.e. arrangements of two extrinsic structures and the dendritic element of a striatal neuron (Figure 7). By means of degeneration experiments, Bouyer et al. (1984b) have shown that the unlabeled terminals, at least in part, are derived from the cortex (*cf.* Somogyi et al., 1981a). These cortical inputs are thought to use glutamate as a transmitter (Fonnum et al., 1981; Christie et al., 1987; Fuller et al., 1987). Freund et al. (1984) hypothesized that thalamic inputs may also take part in the formation of the earlier-mentioned triads. However, Dubé et al. (1988) have recently shown that the fibers from the parafascicular thalamic nucleus make contact primarily with the shafts of sparsely spiny medium-size cells (Figure 7A). Moreover, the axons of medium-size densely spiny neurons presumably contact other striatal neurons by means of symmetrical synapses that occur predominantly on the shafts of proximal dendrites and, to a lesser degree, on somata (Bolam et al., 1983b, 1985; Bolam and Izzo, 1988). Thus, as Bolam and Izzo (1987, 1988) concluded, extrinsic inputs from the substantia nigra and the cortex terminate on the distal parts of the dendrites of projection neurons, whereas inputs from intrinsic origin, i.e. from their companion medium-size spiny neurons, terminate predominantly on the proximal parts of the dendrites and on the somata of the projection neurons (Figure 7A).

The role of the cholinergic neurons in the striatal circuitry is far from clear. These interneurons are contacted by different types of synapses (Phelps et al., 1985). For instance, substance P-positive terminals, presumably stemming from medium-size spiny neurons, have been shown to contact the cholinergic neurons (Bolam et al., 1986), and other inputs may be derived from the cortex or the thalamus (Phelps et al., 1985). Morphological evidence for a DA input to cholinergic neurons is scarce (*cf.* Lehman and Langer, 1983). Recently, Chang (1988) has shown close appositions of tyrosine hydroxylase-immunoreactive boutons with ChAT-positive dendrites and somata, but these appositions lack synaptic specializations.

The cholinergic interneurons give rise to an extensive plexus of fibers and terminals in the striatum (Phelps et al, 1985; Phelps and Vaughn, 1986;

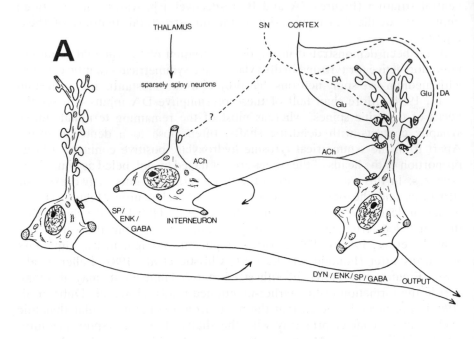

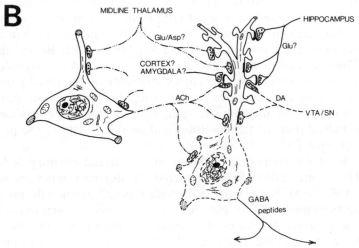

Figure 7. A number of aspects of the presumptive synaptic contacts of the medium-size, densely spiny neurons and the cholinergic neurons in the dorsal (**A**) and the ventral striatum (**B**). ACh, acetylcholine; Asp, aspartate; DA, dopamine; DYN, dynorphin; ENK, enkephalin; GABA, gamma-amino butyric acid; Glu, glutamate; SN, substantia nigra; SP, substance P; VTA, ventral tegmental area

Meredith et al., 1989). Izzo and Bolam (1988) have demonstrated that identified striatonigral neurons are the postsynaptic targets of some cholinergic terminals. The distribution of the terminals over the medium-size spiny neurons is comparable to that of DA terminals on these cells, i.e. predominantly with symmetrical specializations on dendritic shafts and spines (Freund et al., 1984; Izzo and Bolam, 1988). As a result of their particular position on the spiny neurons, intermediate between the cortical input on the heads of spines and the local input on the proximal dendrites, the DA and cholinergic terminals may affect these output neurons of the dorsal striatum in a similar way (Izzo and Bolam, 1988).

An important issue is whether the synaptic organization that has been demonstrated in the dorsal striatum can be generalized for the entire striatum. As shown by Voorn et al. (1986), the ultrastructural characteristics of the DA innervation of the ventral striatum in the rat are quite similar to those of the dorsal striatum (*cf.* Arluison et al., 1984; Bouyer et al., 1984a). In particular, spines postsynaptic to DA terminals are simultaneously contacted by unlabeled axons. Recently, in agreement with the findings of Totterdell and Smith (1989), experiments in our laboratory have shown that, in the nucleus accumbens, fibers from the hippocampus and DA inputs may converge on dendrites or spines of the same neurons, in some cases forming triads as described above (Figure 8). Meredith et al. (1990), employing a combination of glutamate decarboxylase (GAD) immunocytochemistry and degeneration following fornix/fimbria lesions, demonstrated that the spines postsynaptic to hippocampal afferents are glutamic acid decarboxylase (GAD)-immunoreactive and thus most probably GABAergic (Figures 7B and 9B).

The synaptic relations of thalamic inputs to the dorsal and the ventral striatum may differ in some respects. Dubé et al. (1988) found that, in the dorsal striatum, fibers from the parafascicular thalamic nucleus predominantly form synaptic contact with sparsely spiny, medium-size neurons. According to recent data from our laboratory, fibers from the midline thalamic nuclei contact not only the dendritic shafts and spines of as yet unidentified neurons but also establish synaptic relations with the dendrites and somata of ChAT-positive neurons (Figure 9A; Meredith and Wouterlood, 1990). In the same study, contacts between degenerating terminals following lesions of the fornix/fimbria and cholinergic neurons were rarely observed. Most probably, these terminals contact almost exclusively the spiny appendages of dendrites.

There may be further differences between the organization of the cholinergic systems in the dorsal and the ventral striatum (Phelps and Vaughn, 1986; Meredith et al., 1989), although in both regions the relationship of cholinergic terminals with the dendritic shafts and the spines of output neurons is most probably comparable (Phelps and Vaughn, 1986; Izzo and Bolam, 1988). Therefore, the 'parallel dopamine/acetylcholine

48

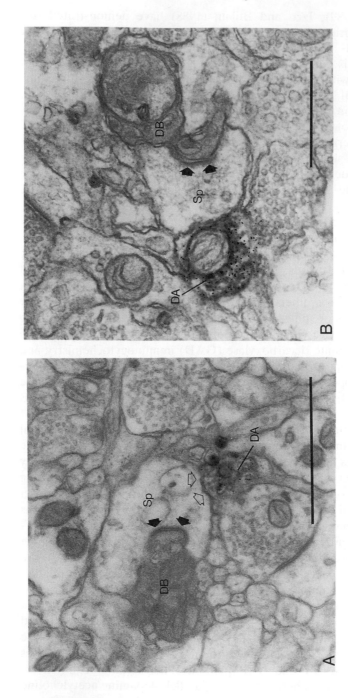

Figure 8. Electron micrographs which show two examples of a 'triad' of a hippocampal input, a dopaminergic terminal and a dendritic spine belonging to a ventral striatal neuron. The hippocampal boutons show signs of degeneration following a lesion of the fimbria/fornix 3 days before sacrifice. The dopaminergic terminals are immunocytochemically visualized using an antibody against dopamine (*cf.* Voorn et al., 1986); the immunoreaction product is gold-intensified (small particles) by means of the procedure of VandenPol and Gorcs (1986). In (**A**) both the hippocampal bouton and the DA bouton show synaptic specializations with the spine (arrows). In (**B**) the DA-immunoreactive profile is closely apposed to the spine, but no membrane specializations are visible. The degenerating hippocampal bouton forms a synapse with the spine (arrows). DB, degenerating bouton; Sp, spine. Bars 1 μm

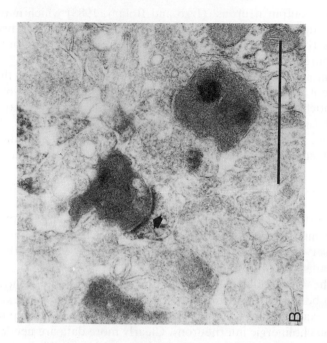

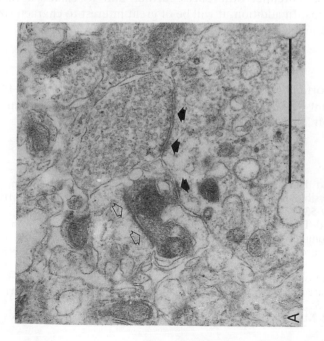

Figure 9. Electron micrographs which show two examples of synaptic relationships in the medial part of the nucleus accumbens. **A.** Thalamostriatal degenerating bouton making an asymmetrical synaptic contact with a ChAT-labeled dendrite (single filled arrow). The same dendrite receives input also from an unlabeled symmetrical synaptic junction (two filled arrows). In addition, the degenerated terminal establishes an asymmetrical synaptic contact with an unlabeled profile (two open arrows). Bar 1 μm. **B.** Degenerating boutons in the nucleus accumbens following a lesion of the fimbria/fornix. One of the boutons makes an asymmetrical contact with a presumptive GABAergic spine (GAD-positive; filled arrow). Bar 1 μm

input to striatal spiny output neurons' (Izzo and Bolam, 1988) which may, at least in part, account for the well-known interactions between these two transmitter systems (*cf.* Lehman and Langer, 1983) might hold for both striatal regions (Figure 7).

An important characteristic of the ventral striatum is its input from the amygdala. At present, nothing is known about the synaptic specializations and the postsynaptic relationships of amygdaloid inputs to the ventral striatum. On the basis of physiological and pharmacological experiments (Yim and Mogenson, 1988), it seems likely that inputs from the amygdala establish direct contact with output neurons and that they may be modulated by DA inputs. This would suggest that the amygdaloid inputs and the hippocampal inputs have similar relationships with DA afferents and output neurons. However, on the basis of the results of pharmacobehavioral and physiological studies (Cools et al., Chapter 6; Mogenson and Yim, Chapter 4 this volume), the question may be raised as to whether these two inputs contact the same set of neurons in the ventral striatum or whether they reach different populations of output neurons.

In conclusion, the basic cellular design of the dorsal and the ventral striatum appears to be directly comparable. However, differences may exist with respect to, for example, the synaptic organization of the thalamic inputs and the inputs to the cholinergic interneurons. Clearly more data are needed to substantiate these potential differences further and to establish their functional implications. In addition, it will be of great interest to characterize ultrastructurally the amygdaloid afferents of the striatum.

ACKNOWLEDGEMENTS

This work was supported by Medigon/NWO Program Grant No. 900–550–093 and by NATO-Grant 87/229. Our thanks to Mrs Joan Hage for secretarial assistance and to Mr Dirk de Jong for the photography.

REFERENCES

Alexander, G.E. and DeLong, M.R. (1985a) Microstimulation of the primate neostriatum. I. Physiological properties of striatal microexcitable zones. *Journal of Neurophysiology* **53**, 1401–1416.

Alexander, G.E. and DeLong, M.R. (1985b) Microstimulation of the primate neostriatum. II. Somatotopic organization of striatal microexcitable zones and their relation to neuronal response properties. *Journal of Neurophysiology* **53**, 1417–1430.

Alexander, G.E., DeLong, M.R. and Strick, P.L. (1986) Parallel organization of functionally segregated circuits linking basal ganglia and cortex. *Annual Review of Neuroscience* **9**, 357–381.

Arluison, M., Dietl, M. and Thibault, J. (1984) Ultrastructural morphology of dopaminergic nerve terminals and synapses in the striatum of the rat using tyrosine hydroxylase immunocytochemistry: a topographical study. *Brain Research Bulletin* **13**, 269–285.

Bayer, S.A. (1981) A correlated study of neurogenesis, morphogenesis and cytodifferentiation in the rat nucleus accumbens. In: Chronister, R.B. and deFrance, J.F. (eds) *The Neurobiology of the Nucleus Accumbens.* Brunswick, Maine, USA: Haer Institute, pp. 173–197.

Beckstead, R.M. (1979) An autoradiographic examination of corticocortical and subcortical projections of the mediodorsal-projection (prefrontal) cortex in the rat. *Journal of Comparative Neurology* **184**, 43–62.

Beckstead, R.M., Wooten, G.F. and Trugman, J.M. (1988) Distribution of D1 and D2 dopamine receptors in the basal ganglia of the cat determined by quantitative autoradiography. *Journal of Comparative Neurology* **268**, 131–145.

Berendse, H.W. and Groenewegen, H.J. (1990) The organization of the thalamostriatal projections in the rat, with special emphasis on the ventral striatum. *Journal of Comparative Neurology* **299**, 187–228.

Berendse, H.W. and Groenewegen, H.J. (1991) Restricted cortical termination fields of the midline and intralaminar thalamic nuclei in the rat. *Neuroscience* (in press).

Berendse, H.W., Voorn, P., te Kortschot, A. and Groenewegen, H.J. (1988) Nuclear origin of thalamic afferents of the ventral striatum determines their relation to patch/matrix configurations in enkephalin-immunoreactivity in the rat. *Journal of Chemical Neuroanatomy* **1**, 3–10.

Besson, M.-J., Graybiel, A.M. and Nastuk, M.A. (1988) [^{3}H]SCH 23390 binding to D1 dopamine receptors in the basal ganglia of the cat and primate: delineation of striosomal compartments and pallidal and nigral subdivisions. *Neuroscience* **26**, 101–119.

Bolam, J.P. and Izzo, P.N. (1987) Possible sites of transmitter interaction in the neostriatum: an anatomical approach. In: Sandler, M., Feuerstein, C. and Scatton, B. (eds) *Neurotransmitter Interactions in the Basal Ganglia.* New York: Raven Press, pp. 47–58.

Bolam, J.P. and Izzo, P.N. (1988) The postsynaptic targets of substance P-immunoreactive terminals in the rat neostriatum with particular reference to identified spiny striatonigral neurons. *Experimental Brain Research* **70**, 361–377.

Bolam, J.P., Powell, J.F., Totterdell, S. and Smith, A.D. (1981a) The proportion of neurons in the rat neostriatum that project to the substantia nigra demonstrated using horseradish peroxidase conjugated with wheatgerm agglutinin. *Brain Research* **220**, 339–343.

Bolam, J.P., Somogyi, P., Totterdell, S. and Smith, A.D. (1981b) A second type of striatonigral neuron: a comparison between retrogradely labelled and Golgi-stained neurons at the light and electron microscopic levels. *Neuroscience* **6**, 2141–2157.

Bolam, J.P., Clarke, D.J., Smith, A.D. and Somogyi, P. (1983a) A type of aspiny neuron in the rat neostriatum accumulates [^{3}H]τ-aminobutyric acid: combination of Golgi-staining, autoradiography, and electron microscopy. *Journal of Comparative Neurology* **213**, 121–134.

Bolam, J.P., Somogyi, P., Takagi, H., Fodor, I. and Smith, A.D. (1983b) Localization of substance P-like immunoreactivity in neurons and nerve terminals in the neostriatum of the rat: a correlated light and electron microscopic study. *Journal of Neurocytology* **12**, 325–344.

Bolam, J.P., Wainer, B.H. and Smith, A.D. (1984) Characterization of cholinergic neurons in the rat neostriatum. A combination of choline acetyltransferase immunocytochemistry, Golgi-impregnation and electron microscopy. *Neuroscience* **12**, 711–718.

Bolam, J.P., Powell, J.F., Wu, J.-Y. and Smith, A.D. (1985) Glutamate decarboxy-lase-immunoreactive structures in the rat neostriatum: a correlated light and electron microscopic study including a combination of Golgi impregnation with immunocytochemistry. *Journal of Comparative Neurology* **237**, 1–20.

Bolam, J.P., Ingham, C.A., Izzo, P.N., Levey, A.I., Rye, D.B., Smith, A.D. and Wainer, B.H. (1986) Substance P-containing terminals in synaptic contact with cholinergic neurons in the neostriatum and basal forebrain: a double immunocytochemical study in the rat. *Brain Research* **397**, 279–289.

Bolam, J.P., Izzo, P.N. and Graybiel, A.M. (1988) Cellular substrate of the histochemically defined striosome/matrix system of the caudate nucleus: a combined Golgi and immunocytochemical study in cat and ferret. *Neuroscience* **24**, 853–875.

Bouyer, J.J., Joh, T.H. and Pickel, V.M. (1984a) Ultrastructural localization of tyrosine hydroxylase in the rat nucleus accumbens. *Journal of Comparative Neurology* **227**, 92–103.

Bouyer, J.J., Park, D.H., Joh, T.H. and Pickel, V.M. (1984b) Chemical and structural analysis of the relation between cortical inputs and tyrosine hydroxylase-containing terminals in rat neostriatum. *Brain Research* **302**, 267–275.

Braitenberg, V. (1985) Charting the visual cortex. In: Jones, E.G. and Peters, A. (eds) *Cerebral Cortex, Vol. 3, Visual Cortex*. New York: Plenum Press, pp. 379–414.

Butcher, L.L. and Hodge, G.K. (1976) Postnatal development of acetylcholinesterase in the caudate-putamen and substantia nigra of rats. *Brain Research* **106**, 223–240.

Carlsen, J., Zaborszky, L. and Heimer, L. (1985) Cholinergic projections from the basal forebrain to the basolateral amygdaloid complex: a combined retrograde fluorescent and immunohistochemical study. *Journal of Comparative Neurology* **234**, 155–167.

Chang, H.T. (1988) Dopamine-acetylcholine interaction in the rat striatum: a dual-labeling immunocytochemical study. *Brain Research Bulletin* **21**, 295–304.

Chang, H.T. and Kitai, S.T. (1985) Projection neurons of the nucleus accumbens: an intracellular labeling study. *Brain Research* **347**, 112–116.

Chang, H.T., Wilson, C.J. and Kitai, S.T. (1981) Single neostriatal efferent axons in the globus pallidus: a light and electron microscopic study. *Science* **213**, 915–918.

Chang, H.T., Wilson, C.J. and Kitai, S.T. (1982) A Golgi study of rat neostriatal neurons: light microscopic analysis. *Journal of Comparative Neurology* **208**, 107–126.

Chesselet, M.F. and Graybiel, A.M. (1986) Striatal neurons expressing somatostatin-like immunoreactivity: evidence for a peptidergic interneuronal system in the cat. *Neuroscience* **17**, 547–571.

Christie, M.J., Summers, R.J., Stephenson, J.A., Cook, C.J. and Beart, P.M. (1987) Excitatory amino acid projections to the nucleus accumbens septi in the rat: a retrograde transport study utilizing D[³H]aspartate and [³H]GABA. *Neuroscience* **22**, 425–439.

DeLong, M.R. and Georgopoulos, A.P. (1981) Motor functions of the basal ganglia. In: Brookhart, J.M., Mountcastle V.B. and Brooks V.B. (eds) *Handbook of Physiology, Section 1, The Nervous System, Vol. II, Part 2*. Bethesda: American Physiological Society, pp. 1017–1061.

Desban, M., Gauchy, C., Kemel, M.L., Besson, M.J. and Glowinski, J. (1989) Three-dimensional organization of the striosomal compartment and patchy distribution of striatonigral projections in the matrix of the cat caudate nucleus. *Neuroscience* **29**, 551–566.

DiFiglia, M. and Aronin, N. (1982) Ultrastructural features of immunoreactive somatostatin neurons in the rat caudate-nucleus. *Journal of Neuroscience* **2**, 1267–1274.

Domesick, V.B. (1981) Further observations on the anatomy of nucleus accumbens and caudatoputamen in the rat: similarities and contrasts. In: Chronister, R.B. and deFrance, J.F. (eds). *The Neurobiology of the Nucleus Accumbens*. Brunswick, Maine, USA: Haer Institute, pp. 7–41.

Dubé, L., Smith, A.D. and Bolam, J.P. (1988) Identification of synaptic terminals of thalamic or cortical origin in contact with distinct medium-size spiny neurons in the rat neostriatum. *Journal of Comparative Neurology* **267**, 455–471.

Eccles, J.C. (1984) The cerebral cortex: a theory of its operation. In: Jones, E.G. and Peters, A. (eds) *Cerebral Cortex, Vol. 2, Functional Properties of Cortical Cells*. New York: Plenum Press, pp. 1–38.

Faull, R.L.M. and Villiger, J.W. (1986) Heterogeneous distribution of benzodiazepine receptors in the human striatum: a quantitative autoradiographic study comparing the pattern of receptor labelling with the distribution of acetylcholinesterase staining. *Brain Research* **381**, 153–158.

Faull, R.L.M., Dragunow, M. and Villiger, J.W. (1989) The distribution of neurotensin receptors and acetylcholinesterase in the human caudate nucleus: evidence for the existence of a third neurochemical compartment. *Brain Research* **488**, 381–386.

Feigenbaum-Langer, L. and Graybiel, A.M. (1989) Distinct nigrostriatal projections systems innervate striosomes and matrix in the primate striatum. *Brain Research* **498**, 344–350.

Fishell, G. and Van der Kooy, D. (1989) Pattern formation in the striatum: developmental changes in the distribution of striatonigral projections. *Developmental Brain Research* **45**, 239–255.

Fonnum, F., Storm-Mathisen, J. and Divac, I. (1981) Biochemical evidence for glutamate as neurotransmitter in corticostriatal and corticothalamic fibres in the rat brain. *Neuroscience* **6**, 863–875.

Freund, T.F., Powell, J.F. and Smith, A.D. (1984) Tyrosine hydroxylase-immunoreactive boutons in synaptic contact with identified striatonigral neurons, with particular reference to dendritic spines. *Neuroscience* **13**, 1189–1215.

Fuller, T.A., Russchen, F.T. and Price, J.L. (1987) Sources of presumptive glutamatergic/aspartergic afferents to the rat ventral striatopallidal region. *Journal of Comparative Neurology* **258**, 317–338.

Gerfen, C.R. (1984) The neostriatal mosaic: compartmentalization of corticostriatal input and striatonigral output systems. *Nature* **311**, 461–464.

Gerfen, C.R. (1985) The neostriatal mosaic. I. Compartmental organization of projections from the striatum to the substantia nigra in the rat. *Journal of Comparative Neurology* **236**, 454–476.

Gerfen, C.R. (1989) The neostriatal mosaic: striatal patch-matrix organization is related to cortical lamination. *Science* **246**, 385–388.

Gerfen, C.R. and Young III, W.S. (1988) Distribution of striatonigral and striatopallidal peptidergic neurons in both patch and matrix compartments: an *in situ* hybridization histochemistry and fluorescent retrograde tracing study. *Brain Research* **460**, 161–167.

Gerfen, C.R., Baimbridge, K.G. and Miller, J.J. (1985) The neostriatal mosaic:

compartmental distribution of calcium-binding protein and parvalbumin in the basal ganglia of the rat and monkey. *Proceedings of the National Academy of Science, USA* **82**, 8780–8784.

Gerfen, C.R., Herkenham, M. and Thibault, J. (1987a) The neostriatal mosaic: II. Patch- and matrix-directed mesostriatal dopaminergic and non-dopaminergic systems. *Journal of Neuroscience* **7**, 3915–3934.

Gerfen, C.R., Baimbridge, K.G. and Thibault, J. (1987b) The neostriatal mosaic: III. Biochemical and developmental dissociation of patch-matrix mesostriatal systems. *Journal of Neuroscience* **7**, 3935–3944.

Goldman, P.S. and Nauta, W.J.H. (1977) An intricately patterned prefrontocaudate projection in the Rhesus monkey. *Journal of Comparative Neurology* **171**, 369–386.

Goldman-Rakic, P.S. (1982) Cytoarchitectonic heterogeneity of the primate neostriatum: subdivision into island and matrix cellular compartments. *Journal of Comparative Neurology* **205**, 398–413.

Goldman-Rakic, P.S. (1988) Changing concepts of cortical connectivity: parallel distributed cortical networks. In: Rakic, P. and Singer, W. (eds) *Neurobiology of Neocortex*. Chichester: Wiley, pp. 177–202.

Goldman-Rakic, P.S. and Porrino, L.J. (1985) The primate mediodorsal (MD) nucleus and its projection to the frontal lobe. *Journal of Comparative Neurology* **242**, 535–560.

Goldman-Rakic, P.S. and Selemon, L.D. (1986) Topography of corticostriatal projections in nonhuman primates and implications for functional parcellation of the neostriatum. In: Jones, E.G. and Peters, A. (eds) *Cerebral Cortex, Vol 5*. New York: Plenum, pp. 447–466.

Graybiel, A.M. (1983) Compartmental organization of the mammalian striatum. In: Changeux, J.-P., Glowinski, J., Imbert, M. and Bloom, F.E. (eds) *Molecular and Cellular Interactions Underlying Higher Brain Functions, Progress in Brain Research, Vol. 58*. Amsterdam: Elsevier, pp. 247–256.

Graybiel, A.M. (1984a) Neurochemically specified subsystems in the basal ganglia. In: Evered, D. and O'Connor, M. (eds) *Functions of the Basal Ganglia*. London: Pitman, pp. 114–149.

Graybiel, A.M. (1984b) Correspondence between the dopamine islands and striosomes of the mammalian striatum. *Neuroscience* **13**, 1157–1187.

Graybiel, A.M. (1984c) Modular patterning in the development of the striatum. In: Reinoso-Suarez, F. and Ajmone-Marsan, C. (eds) *Cortical Integration*. New York: Raven Press, pp. 223–235.

Graybiel, A.M. and Ragsdale Jr, C.W. (1978) Histochemically distinct compartments in the striatum of human monkey, and cat demonstrated by acetylthiocholinesterase staining. *Proceedings of the National Academy of Science, USA* **75**, 5723–5726.

Graybiel, A.M. and Ragsdale Jr, C.W. (1983) Biochemical anatomy of the striatum. In: Emson, P.C. (ed.) *Chemical Neuroanatomy*. New York: Raven Press, pp. 427–504.

Graybiel, A.M., Ragsdale Jr, C.W., Yoneoka, E.S. and Elde, R.P. (1981) An immunohistochemical study of enkephalin and other neuropeptides in the striatum of the cat with evidence that the opiate peptides are arranged to form mosaic patterns in register with the striosomal compartments visible by acetylcholinesterase staining. *Neuroscience* **6**, 377–397.

Groenewegen, H.J. (1988) Organization of the afferent connections of the mediodorsal thalamic nucleus in the rat, related to the mediodorsal-prefrontal topography. *Neuroscience* **24**, 379–431.

Groenewegen, H.J. and Berendse, H.W. (1990) Connections of the subthalamic nucleus with ventral striatopallidal parts of the basal ganglia in the rat. *Journal of Comparative Neurology* **294**, 607–622.

Groenewegen, H.J., Vermeulen-Van der Zee, E., Te Kortschot, A. and Witter, M.P. (1987) Organization of the projections from the subiculum to the ventral striatum in the rat. A study using anterograde transport of *Phaseolus vulgaris*-leucoagglutinin. *Neuroscience* **23**, 103–120.

Groenewegen, H.J., Meredith, G.E., Berendse, H.W., Voorn, P. and Wolters, J.G. (1989) The compartmental organization of the ventral striatum in the rat. In: Crossman, A.R. and Sambrook, M.A. (eds) *Neural Mechanisms in Disorders of Movement*. London: John Libbey, pp. 45–54.

Groenewegen, H.J., Berendse, H.W., Wolters, J.G., Witter, M.P. and Lohman, A.H.M. (1990a) The anatomical relationship of the prefrontal cortex with the striatopallidal system, the thalamus and the amygdala: evidence for a parallel organization. In: Uylings, H.B.M., Van Eden, C.G., De Bruin, J.P.C., Corner, M.A. and Feenstra, M.P.G. (eds) *Progress in Brain Research, Vol. 85*, Amsterdam: Elsevier, pp. 95–118.

Groenewegen, H.J., Arts, M.P.M. and Berendse, H.W. (1990b) A cellular basis for the compartmental structure of the ventral striatum in the rat. *European Journal of Neuroscience*, Suppl. **3**, 294.

Grofova, I. (1975) The identification of striatal and pallidal neurons projecting to the substantia nigra. An experimental study by means of retrograde axonal transport of horseradish peroxidase. *Brain Research* **91**, 286–291.

Grove, E.A. (1988) Efferent connections of the substantia innominata in the rat. *Journal of Comparative Neurology* **277**, 347–364.

Grove, E.A., Haber, S.N., Domesick, V.B. and Nauta, W.J.H. (1983) Differential projections from AChE-positive and AChE-negative ventral pallidum cells in the rat. *Society for Neuroscience Abstracts* **10**, 16.

Groves, P.M., Martone, M., Young, S.J. and Armstrong, D.M. (1988) Three-dimensional pattern of enkephalin-like immunoreactivity in the caudate nucleus of the cat. *Journal of Neuroscience* **8**, 892–900.

Haber, S.N. and Nauta, W.J.H. (1983) Ramifications of the globus pallidus in the rat as indicated by patterns of immunohistochemistry. *Neuroscience* **9**, 245–260.

Haber, S.N., Groenewegen, H.J., Grove, E.A. and Nauta, W.J.H. (1985) Efferent connections of the ventral pallidum: evidence of a dual striato pallidofugal pathway. *Journal of Comparative Neurology* **235**, 322–335.

Haber, S.N., Lynd, E., Klein, C. and Groenewegen, H.J. (1990) Topographic organization of the ventral striatal efferent projections in the Rhesus monkey: an anterograde tracing study. *Journal of Comparative Neurology* **293**, 282–298.

Heimer, L. and Wilson, R.D. (1975) The subcortical projections of the allocortex: similarities in the neural associations of the hippocampus, the piriform cortex, and the neocortex. In: Santini, M. (ed.) *Golgi Centennial Symposium*. New York: Raven Press, pp. 177–193.

Heimer, L., Zaborszky, L., Zahm, D.S. and Alheid, G.F. (1987) The ventral striatopallidothalamic projection: I. The striatopallidal link originating in the striatal parts of the olfactory tubercle. *Journal of Comparative Neurology* **255**, 571–591.

Herkenham, M. and Nauta, W.J.H. (1977) Afferent connections of the habenular nuclei in the rat. A horseradish peroxidase study, with a note on the fiber-of-passage problem. *Journal of Comparative Neurology* **173**, 123–146.

Herkenham, M. and Pert, C.B. (1981) Mosaic distribution of opiate receptors, parafascicular projections and acetylcholinesterase in rat striatum. *Nature* **291**, 415–418.

Herkenham, M., Moon Edley, S. and Stuart, J. (1984) Cell clusters in the nucleus accumbens of the rat, and the mosaic relationship of opiate receptors, acetylcholinesterase and subcortical afferent terminations. *Neuroscience* **11**, 561–593.

Izzo, P.N. and Bolam, J.P. (1988) Cholinergic synaptic input to different parts of spiny striatonigral neurons in the rat. *Journal of Comparative Neurology* **269**, 219–234.

Jimenez-Castellanos, J. and Graybiel, A.M. (1987) Subdivisions of the dopamine-containing A8–A9–A10 complex identified by their differential mesostriatal innervation of striosomes and extrastriosomal matrix. *Neuroscience* **23**, 223–242.

Jimenez-Castellanos, J. and Graybiel, A.M. (1989) Compartmental origins of striatal efferent projections in the cat. *Neuroscience* **32**, 297–321.

Kelley, A.E., Domesick, V.B. and Nauta, W.J.H. (1982) The amygdalostriatal projection in the rat — an anatomical study by anterograde and retrograde tracing methods. *Neuroscience* **7**, 615–630.

Kemp, J.M. and Powell, T.P.S. (1971) The structure of the caudate nucleus of the cat: light and electron microscopy. *Philosophical Transactions of the Royal Society, London* **262**, 383–401.

Kita, H. and Kitai, S.T. (1988) Glutamate decarboxylase immunoreactive neurons in rat neostriatum: their morphological types and populations. *Brain Research* **447**, 346–352.

Krushel, L.A., Connolly, J.A. and Van der Kooy, D. (1989) Pattern formation in the mammalian forebrain: patch neurons from the rat striatum selectively reassociate in vitro. *Developmental Brain Research* **47**, 137–142.

Künzle, H. (1975) Bilateral projections from precentral motor cortex to the putamen and other parts of the basal ganglia. An autoradiographic study in *Macaca fascicularis*. *Brain Research* **88**, 195–209.

Lança, A.J., Boyd, S., Kolb, B.E. and Van der Kooy, D. (1986) The development of a patchy organization of the rat striatum. *Developmental Brain Research* **27**, 1–10.

Lehman, J. and Langer, S.Z. (1983) The striatal cholinergic interneuron: synaptic target of dopaminergic terminals? *Neuroscience* **10**, 1105–1120.

Loopuyt, L.D. (1989) Distribution of dopamine D-2 receptors in the rat striatal complex and its comparison with acetylcholinesterase. *Brain Research Bulletin* **22**, 805–817.

Malach, R. and Graybiel, A.M. (1986) Mosaic architecture of the somatic sensory-recipient sector of the cat's striatum. *Journal of Neuroscience* **6**, 3426–3458.

McGeorge, A.J. and Faull, R.L.M. (1989) The organization of the projection from the cerebral cortex to the striatum in the rat. *Neuroscience* **29**, 503–537.

Meredith, G.E. and Wouterlood, F.G. (1990) The relationship of fibers and terminals from the hippocampus and thalamus to choline acetyltransferase-immunoreactive neurons in nucleus accumbens of the rat. *Journal of Comparative Neurology* **296**, 204–221.

Meredith, G.E., Blank, B. and Groenewegen, H.J. (1989) The distribution and compartmental organization of the cholinergic neurons in nucleus accumbens of the rat. *Neuroscience* **31**, 327–345.

Meredith, G.E., Wouterlood, F.G. and Pattiselanno, A. (1990) Hippocampal fibers make synaptic contacts with glutamate decarboxylase immunoreactive neurons in the rat nucleus accumbens. *Brain Research* **513**, 329–334.

Nastuk, M.A. and Graybiel, A.M. (1988) Autoradiographic localization and biochemical characteristics of M1 and M2 muscarinic binding sites in the striatum of the cat, monkey, and human. *Journal of Neuroscience* **8**, 1052–1062.

Nauta, H.J.W. (1979) A proposed conceptual reorganization of the basal ganglia and telencephalon. *Neuroscience* **4**, 1875–1881.

Nauta, H.J.W. (1986a) A simplified perspective on the basal ganglia and their relation to the limbic system. In: Doane, B.K. and Livingston, K.E. (eds) *The Limbic System: Functional Organization and Clinical Disorders*. New York: Raven Press, pp. 67–77.

Nauta, W.J.H. (1986b) Circuitous connections linking cerebral cortex, limbic system, and corpus striatum. In: Doane, B.K. and Livingston, K.E. (eds) *The Limbic System: Functional Organization and Clinical Disorders*. New York: Raven Press, pp. 43–54.

Nauta, W.J.H. and Domesick, V.B. (1979) The anatomy of the extrapyramidal system. In: Fuxe, K. and Calne, D.B. (eds) *Dopaminergic Ergot Derivates and Motor Function*. Oxford: Pergamon Press, pp. 3–22.

Nauta, W.J.H. and Domesick, V.B. (1984) Afferent and efferent relationships of the basal ganglia. In: Evered, D. and O'Connor, M. (eds) *Functions of the Basal Ganglia*. London: Pitman, pp. 3–23.

Nauta, W.J.H., Smith, G.P., Faull, R.L.M. and Domesick, V.B. (1978) Efferent connections and nigral afferents of the nucleus accumbens septi in the rat. *Neuroscience* **3**, 385–401.

Olson, L., Seiger, A. and Fuxe, K. (1972) Heterogeneity of striatal and limbic dopamine innervation: highly fluorescent islands in developing and adult rats. *Brain Research* **44**, 283–288.

Parent, A. (1986) *Comparative Neurobiology of the Basal Ganglia*. Chichester: Wiley.

Penny, G.R., Wilson, C.J. and Kitai, S.T. (1988) Relationship of the axonal and dendritic geometry of spiny projection neurons to the compartmental organization of the neostriatum. *Journal of Comparative Neurology* **269**, 275–289.

Phelps, P.E. and Vaughn, J.E. (1986) Immunocytochemical localization of choline acetyltransferase in rat ventral striatum: a light and electron microscopic study. *Journal of Neurocytology* **15**, 595–617.

Phelps, P.E., Houser, C.R. and Vaughn, J.E. (1985) Immunocytochemical localization of choline acetyltransferase within the rat neostriatum: a correlated light and electron microscopic study of cholinergic neurons and synapses. *Journal of Comparative Neurology* **238**, 286–307.

Poletti, C.E. and Creswell, G. (1977) Fornix system efferent projections in the Squirrel monkey: an experimental degeneration study. *Journal of Comparative Neurology* **175**, 101–108.

Ragsdale Jr, C.W. and Graybiel, A.M. (1981) The fronto-striatal projection in the cat and monkey and its relationship to inhomogeneities established by acetylcholinesterase histochemistry. *Brain Research* **208**, 259–266.

Ragsdale Jr, C.W. and Graybiel, A.M. (1988) Fibers from the basolateral nucleus of the amygdala selectively innervate striosomes in the caudate nucleus of the cat. *Journal of Comparative Neurology* **269**, 506–522.

Reep, R.L. and Winans, S.S. (1982) Efferent connections of dorsal and ventral agranular insular cortex in the hamster, *Mesocricetus auratus*. *Neuroscience* **7**, 2609–2635.

Russchen, F.T. and Price, D.L. (1984) Amygdalostriatal projections in the rat. Topographical organization and fiber morphology shown using the lectin PHA-L as an anterograde tracer. *Neuroscience Letters* **47**, 15–22.

Russchen, F.T., Bakst, I., Amaral, D.G. and Price, J.L. (1985) The amygdalostriatal projections in the monkey. An anterograde tracing study. *Brain Research* **329**, 241–257.

Russchen, F.T., Amaral, D.G. and Price, J.L. (1987) The afferent input to magnocellular division of the mediodorsal thalamic nucleus in the monkey, *Macaca fascicularis*. *Journal of Comparative Neurology* **256**, 175–210.

Schneider, J.S. (1987) Functions of the basal ganglia: an overview. In: Schneider, J.S. and Lidsky, T. I. (eds) *Basal Ganglia and Behavior: Sensory Aspects of Motor Functioning*. Toronto: Huber, pp. 1–8.

Selemon, L.D. and Goldman-Rakic, P.S. (1985) Longitudinal topography and interdigitation of corticostriatal projections in the Rhesus monkey. *Journal of Neuroscience* **5**, 776–794.

Selemon, L.D. and Goldman-Rakic, P.S. (1988) Common cortical and subcortical targets of the dorsolateral prefrontal and posterior parietal cortices in the rhesus monkey: evidence for a distributed neural network subserving spatially guided behavior. *Journal of Neuroscience* **8**, 4049–4068.

Sesack, S.R., Deutch, A.Y., Roth, R.H. and Bunney, B.S. (1989) Topographical organization of the efferent projections of the medial prefrontal cortex in the rat: an anterograde tract-tracing study with *Phaseolus vulgaris*-leucoagglutinin. *Journal of Comparative Neurology* **290**, 213–240.

Somogyi, P., Bolam, J.P. and Smith, A.D. (1981a) Monosynaptic cortical input and local axon collaterals of identified striatonigral neurons. A light and electron microscopic study using the Golgi-peroxidase transport-degeneration procedure. *Journal of Comparative Neurology* **195**, 567–584.

Somogyi, P., Bolam, J.P., Totterdell, S. and Smith, A.D. (1981b) Monosynaptic input from the nucleus accumbens-ventral striatum region to retrogradely labelled nigrostriatal neurones. *Brain Research* **217**, 245–263.

Swerdlow, N.R. and Koob, G.F. (1987) Dopamine, schizophrenia, mania, and depression: toward a unified hypothesis of cortico-striato-pallido-thalamic function. *Behavioral and Brain Sciences* **10**, 197–245.

Totterdell, S. and Smith, A.D. (1989) Convergence of hippocampal and dopaminergic input onto identified neurons in the nucleus accumbens of the rat. *Journal of Chemical Neuroanatomy* **2**, 285–298.

VandenPol, A.N. and Gorcs, T. (1986) Synaptic relations between neurons containing vasopressin, gastrin-releasing peptide, vasoactive intestinal polypeptide, and glutamate decarboxylase immunoreactivity in the suprachiasmatic nucleus: dual ultrastructural immunocytochemistry with gold-substituted silver peroxidase. *Journal of Comparative Neurology* **252**, 507–521.

Van der Kooy, D. and Fishell, G. (1987) Neuronal birthdate underlies the development of striatal compartments. *Brain Research* **401**, 155–161.

Voorn, P., Jorritsma-Byham, B., Van Dijk, C. and Buijs, R.M. (1986) The dopaminergic innervation of the ventral striatum in the rat: a light- and electron-microscopical study with antibodies against dopamine. *Journal of Comparative Neurology* **251**, 84–99.

Voorn, P., Kalsbeek, A., Jorritsma-Byham, B. and Groenewegen, H.J. (1988) The pre- and postnatal development of the dopaminergic cell groups in the ventral mesencephalon and the dopaminergic innervation of the striatum of the rat. *Neuroscience* **25**, 857–887.

Voorn, P., Gerfen, C.R. and Groenewegen, H.J. (1989) The compartmental organization of the ventral striatum of the rat: immunohistochemical distribution of enkephalin, substance P, dopamine, and calcium binding protein. *Journal of Comparative Neurology* **289**, 189–201.

Walker, R.H., Arbuthnott, G.W. and Wright, A.K. (1989) Electrophysiological and anatomical observations concerning the pallidostriatal pathway in the rat. *Experimental Brain Research* **74**, 303–310.

Willner, P. (1983) Dopamine and depression: a review of recent evidence. I. Empirical studies. *Brain Research Reviews* **6**, 211–224.

Witter, M.P., Groenewegen, H.J., Lopes da Silva, F.H. and Lohman, A.H.M. (1989) Functional organization of the extrinsic and intrinsic circuitry of the parahippocampal region. *Progress in Neurobiology* **33**, 161–253.

Yeterian, E.H. and VanHoesen, G.W. (1978) Cortico-striate projections in the Rhesus monkey: the organization of certain cortico-caudate connections. *Brain Research* **139**, 43–63.

Yim, C.Y. and Mogenson, G.J. (1988) Neuromodulatory action of dopamine in the nucleus accumbens: an *in vivo* intracellular study. *Neuroscience* **26**, 403–415.

Young III, W.S., Alheid, G.F. and Heimer, L. (1984) The ventral pallidal projection to the mediodorsal thalamus: a study with fluorescent retrograde tracers and immunohistofluorescence. *Journal of Neuroscience* **4**, 1626–1638.

Zaborszky, L., Alheid, G.F., Beinfeld, M.C., Eiden, L.E., Heimer, L. and Palkovits, M. (1985) Cholecystokinin innervation of the ventral striatum: a morphological and radioimmunological study. *Neuroscience* **14**, 427–453.

Zahm, D.S. (1989) The ventral striatopallidal parts of the basal ganglia in the rat. II. Compartmentation of ventral pallidal efferents. *Neuroscience* **30**, 33–50.

Zahm, D.S. and Heimer, L. (1987) The ventral striatopallidothalamic projection. III. Striatal cells of the olfactory tubercle establish direct synaptic contact with ventral pallidal cells projecting to mediodorsal thalamus. *Brain Research* **404**, 327–331.

Zahm, D.S. and Heimer, L. (1988) Ventral striatopallidal parts of the basal ganglia in the rat: I. Neurochemical compartmentation as reflected by the distributions of neurotensin and substance P immunoreactivity. *Journal of Comparative Neurology* **272**, 516–535.

Zahm, D.S., Zaborszky, L., Alheid, G.F. and Heimer, L. (1987) The ventral striatopallidothalamic projection: II. The ventral pallidothalamic link. *Journal of Comparative Neurology* **255**, 592–605.

3

Neurotransmission in the Mesoaccumbens Dopamine System

FRANCIS J. WHITE
Wayne State University School of Medicine, Department of Psychiatry,
Cellular and Clinical Neurobiology Program, Neuropsychopharmacology
Laboratory, Lafayette Clinic, 951 E. Lafayette, Detroit MI 48207, USA

INTRODUCTION

Despite increasing knowledge of the anatomical distribution of dopamine (DA) within the central nervous system, the original definition of DA-containing systems has been largely maintained. The DA neurons of the mesencephalon were originally divided into three groups, labeled A8, A9 and A10, which form a continuous band from the lateral- and caudal-most extent of the substantia nigra pars lateralis (A8), rostromedially through the substantia nigra pars compacta (A9), to the ventral tegmental area (VTA) (A10) along the midline ventral to the red nucleus, and surrounding the interpeduncular nucleus (Carlsson et al., 1962; Dahlström and Fuxe, 1964; Andén et al., 1966; Ungerstedt, 1971). Historically, the terminal projections of these cell groups have provided the terminology of the DA neuronal systems: the nigrostriatal system, originating in the A9 cells and projecting to the striatum, and the 'mesolimbic' system, originating in the A10 cells and projecting to structures closely associated with the limbic system. The most prominent recipient of A10 DA projections is the nucleus accumbens (NAc); additional terminations occur in the surrounding olfactory tubercle, lateral septum and bed nucleus of stria terminalis.

During the early 1970s, the development of more sensitive fluorescence histochemical techniques allowed the identification of mesocortical DA systems (Berger et al., 1974; Hökfelt et al., 1974; Lindvall et al., 1974).

The Mesolimbic Dopamine System: From Motivation to Action.
Edited by P. Willner and J. Scheel-Krüger
© 1991 John Wiley & Sons Ltd

During the 1980s, several other ascending A10 DA pathways to such areas as the hippocampus, habenula, amygdala and entorhinal cortex have been described (Phillipson and Griffith, 1980; Scatton et al., 1980). Accordingly, some anatomists have proposed a modified terminology to describe the ascending DA pathways (Björklund and Lindvall, 1985) which incorporates the view that the caudate-putamen, NAc and olfactory tubercle form a continuous striatal complex (Heimer and Wilson, 1975), and that the DA projections to this area should therefore be subsumed under the term mesostriatal DA system. The DA projections to the more classical limbic areas (amygdala, hippocampus, septum and prefrontal cortex) would be referred to as the mesolimbocortical DA system (Björklund and Lindvall, 1985). Nevertheless, the term mesolimbic DA system is still conventionally used to refer to the mesoaccumbens DA projection. In recognition of the proposed new terminology and the need for descriptive accuracy, the present chapter will use the term mesoaccumbens DA system. The great majority of electrophysiological studies to be described were performed on this specific system.

The aim of this chapter is to review current knowledge regarding regulation of mesoaccumbens DA neurons, and the mechanisms underlying transmission from these neurons to their targets within the NAc. Throughout the discussion, comparisons will be made to the more extensively characterized nigrostriatal DA system to point out similarities and differences between the regulation of these two important dopaminergic neuronal systems.

ELECTROPHYSIOLOGICAL CHARACTERISTICS OF MESOACCUMBENS DA NEURONS

Early Studies

The initial demonstration that both A9 and A10 DA neurons could be identified by their distinctive electrophysiological 'signature', when monitored with extracellular single unit recording techniques, was provided by the classical studies of Bunney and colleagues (1973a, b). Midbrain DA neurons are distinguishable from non-DA neurons within the mesencephalon by their long duration action potentials (greater than 2.5 ms), which often display a distinctive initial segment notch, and slow (1–10 Hz) irregular or slow bursting firing patterns (Figure 1). Midbrain DA neurons are highly sensitive to systemic (IV) administration of DA agonists such as apomorphine (Bunney et al., 1973a, b) which suppress spontaneous activity by acting on DA autoreceptors along the somatodendritic extent of the neurons, as evidenced by the similar inhibitory effects produced by iontophoretic administration of DA (Aghajanian and Bunney, 1977).

During the 1970s, most electrophysiological studies of DA neurons dealt

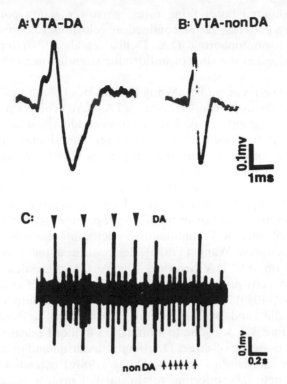

Figure 1. Oscilloscope tracings comparing wave forms (**A** and **B**) and firing patterns (**C**) of A10 DA neurons and non-DA, reticulata-like neurons in the VTA

exclusively with the substantia nigra. Antidromic stimulation and collision testing techniques identified nigrostriatal A9 DA neurons as slow conducting (0.5 m/s), consistent with earlier observations that DA neurons possess thin, unmyelinated axons (Hökfelt and Ungerstedt, 1973), and projecting to the striatum in a topographically defined manner (Guyenet and Aghajanian, 1978).

Mesoaccumbens DA Neurons—Identification and Characterization

In 1980, several investigators focused their attention on the physiological attributes of DA neurons within the A10 cell group. German et al. (1980) reported that antidromically identified mesoaccumbens neurons possessed physiological and pharmacological properties identical to those of nigrostriatal A9 DA cells. Yim and Mogenson (1980) reported that stimulation of the NAc identified distinguishable subtypes of VTA neurons: Type A neurons exhibited characteristics identical to those of A9 DA neurons whereas Type

B neurons exhibited faster firing rates, narrower action potentials, more rhythmic firing patterns, faster conduction velocities (2.5 m/s), and a lack of sensitivity to iontophoretic DA. Deniau et al. (1980) reported similar results and extended the sites of antidromic stimulation to the septum and frontal cortex.

In a detailed series of studies, Wang (1981a, b, c) confirmed and extended these findings. As in previous reports, VTA–NAc projection neurons were divided into two groups. Type I neurons were identified as A10 DA cells whereas Type II neurons exhibited characteristics similar to those of the Type B cells reported by Yim and Mogenson (1980). Wang (1981a) also provided histochemical evidence for both DA and non-DA VTA–NAc projection neurons, and demonstrated that the antidromic response to NAc stimulation of Type I, but not Type II, VTA neurons was blocked by the catecholamine neurotoxin 6-hydroxydopamine (6-OHDA). Using a combination of electrical stimulation, microiontophoresis and selective lesioning procedures, Wang (1981b) demonstrated the existence of DA autoreceptors on A10 DA neurons. The current-dependent inhibition of many A10 DA cells produced by NAc stimulation (Wolf et al., 1978; Yim and Mogenson, 1980) was attenuated by 6-OHDA lesions of the median forebrain bundle, and by DA receptor antagonists, indicating that this suppression of activity was due to stimulation-induced release of DA in the VTA and the presence of direct DA dendrodendritic and/or axon collateral autoregulatory mechanisms. Finally, Wang (1981c) extended his studies to the A10 DA neurons projecting to the medial prefrontal cortex (mPFC) and anterior cingulate cortex (aCC). As previously suggested by Deniau et al. (1980), the mesocortical DA neurons displayed physiological characteristics similar to those of mesoaccumbens and nigrostriatal DA neurons. Both mesoaccumbens and mesocortical DA neurons were inhibited by amphetamine, an effect not altered by destruction of forebrain feedback pathways. This latter finding was quite different from that previously reported for nigrostriatal DA neurons since the effects of amphetamine on A9 neurons are attenuated by such lesion procedures.

AUTORECEPTOR REGULATION OF A10 DA NEURONAL ACTIVITY

Of all the potential regulators of A10 DA neuronal activity, the one most thoroughly studied is autoregulation provided by impulse-regulating somatodendritic DA autoreceptors on mesoaccumbens A10 DA neurons. The following sections will discuss evidence for the existence of these autoreceptors, their pharmacological characterization and functional relevance.

Evidence for Somatodendritic Autoreceptors

As discussed above, the original identification of somatodendritic autoreceptors came from electrophysiological studies indicating that iontophoretic administration of DA inhibits the firing of DA neurons, including those in A10, and that this effect is reversed by DA antagonists (Aghajanian and Bunney, 1977). Electrical stimulation of the NAc also inhibits DA cells and, in some cases, this effect can be blocked by DA antagonists (Wang, 1981b), suggesting dendritic release of DA following antidromic stimulation of VTA–NAc fibers (Korf et al., 1976). In addition, this effect of NAc stimulation can be potentiated by DA uptake inhibitors such as cocaine (Einhorn et al., 1988). Recently, intracellular recordings obtained from A10 DA neurons in an *in vitro* VTA slice preparation revealed that DA, applied in the superfusion medium, readily suppressed the firing of A10 DA neurons (Mueller and Brodie, 1989), as had previously been demonstrated for A9 DA neurons in a nigral slice preparation with both extracellular (Pinnock, 1983) and intracellular recordings (Lacey et al., 1987; Silva and Bunney, 1988).

In addition to functional evidence for DA autoreceptors, anatomical evidence for their presence has been provided by ligand-binding techniques. Gundlach et al. (1982) first demonstrated the presence of [^{3}H]spiperone binding sites in homogenates of rat VTA, and suggested that they may be DA autoreceptors. Evidence confirming the presence of DA receptors on A10 DA neurons has come from the demonstration of reductions in the autoradiographic localization of DA receptor-binding following 6-OHDA lesions of A10 DA cells (Bouthenet et al., 1987; Morelli et al., 1988).

Pharmacological Characterization of Somatodendritic Autoreceptors

During the late 1970s, considerable evidence accumulated to indicate the presence of more than one DA receptor. Current evidence indicates that central nervous system DA receptors exist as two distinct subtypes, D1 and D2 (Kebabian and Calne, 1979), defined on the basis of a stimulatory association with a DA-sensitive adenylate cyclase or the lack of such an association, respectively. In subsequent studies, D2 receptors which inhibit adenylate cyclase were also identified (Onali et al., 1985; Stoof and Kebabian, 1981).

White and Wang (1984e) first demonstrated that somatodendritic DA autoreceptors were of the D2 subtype. Thus, A10 DA neurons were readily inhibited by iontophoresis of the dopaminergic ergots, including lisuride, pergolide, bromocriptine and LY 141865 (White and Wang, 1984e), which stimulate D2 DA receptors (Kebabian and Calne, 1979; Tsuruta et al., 1981). In contrast, iontophoresis of the D1-selective agonist SKF 38393 (Setler et al., 1978; Sibley et al., 1982) exerted no effect on A10 DA unit activity (White and Wang, 1984e). Antagonism studies also supported the exclusive existence of D2 autoreceptors since iontophoretic ejection of the D2 selective blocker sulpiride, but not the D1 selective antagonist SCH 23390 (Hytell, 1983; Iorio et al., 1983), attenuated the inhibitory effects of DA and D2 agonists on A10 DA cells (White and Wang, 1984e). Intracellular recordings from nigral DA neurons maintained *in vitro* have also identified only D2 autoreceptors (Lacey et al., 1987). Both DA and the selective D2 agonist quinpirole, the active enantiomer of LY 141865 (Titus et al., 1983), but not SKF 38393, prevented action potential generation and hyperpolarized DA neurons, effects which were antagonized by sulpiride, but not by SCH 23390. Additional experimental manipulation revealed that DA acts on D2 autoreceptors to increase membrane K^+ conductance (Lacey et al., 1987; Silva and Bunney, 1988) and, as with many receptors coupled to K^+ channels, the D2 autoreceptor appears to act via an inhibitory guanine nucleotide regulatory protein, probably G_i, since intranigral pretreatment with pertussin toxin greatly attenuated the inhibitory effects of intravenous apomorphine and iontophoretic DA on A9 DA neurons (Innis and Aghajanian, 1987).

Subsequent autoradiographic studies have also demonstrated that D2 receptors are present at relatively high densities within the VTA (Bouthenet et al., 1987; Charuchinda et al., 1987), whereas D1 receptors are extremely sparse (Dawson et al., 1986; Dubois et al., 1986; Savasta et al., 1986) or absent (Altar and Hauser, 1987). Similarly, the VTA appears to lack both DA-stimulated cyclic adenosine monophosphate (cAMP; Lorez and Burkard, 1979; Beart and McDonald, 1980) and the DA and adenylate cyclase-related phosphoprotein DARPP-32 (Walaas and Greengard, 1984), which are markers for D1 receptors.

Physiological Relevance of Somatodendritic Autoreceptors

Although impulse-regulating somatodendritic autoreceptors are of considerable relevance from a pharmacological perspective, questions exist as to their relevance as normal physiological regulators of neuronal activity. Although systemic administration of DA receptor antagonists increases the firing of A9 DA neurons, the extent to which this reflects actions at autoreceptors, as opposed to activation of striatonigral loops, has been openly debated. Lesions of the striatonigral pathway prevent the increase in A9 DA cell firing normally produced by DA receptor blockers (Kondo and Iwatsubo, 1980; Hand et al., 1987), and intrastriatal injection of haloperidol has been reported to increase nigral DA cell activity (Iwatsubo and Clouet, 1977), although others have found the opposite effect (Groves et al., 1975). Microiontophoretic application of the DA antagonist trifluoperazine fails to increase the activity of A9 DA cells (Aghajanian and

Bunney, 1977; Chiodo and Bunney, 1984). Similarly, bath application of DA receptor blockers fails to increase activity recorded from nigral DA neurons in slice preparations (Pinnock, 1984b). However, local microinjection of DA antagonists into the nigra does increase the activity of DA cells (Groves et al., 1975; Last and Greenfield, 1987). No clear consensus exists regarding the extent to which somatodendritic DA autoreceptors on A9 DA cells are tonically involved in regulating neuronal activity.

Early studies of A10 DA neurons found that, like A9 DA cells, iontophoretic application of trifluoperazine failed to produce increases in firing (Aghajanian and Bunney, 1977; Wang, 1981b). In contrast, similar application of the selective D2 DA antagonist (−)sulpiride increased the firing of many A10 DA neurons, particularly those with slower basal firing rates (White and Wang, 1984e). Although not mentioned in the text, close examination of the rate histograms in Hand et al. (1987) indicates that iontophoretic administation of both haloperidol and clozapine accelerated the firing of some A10 DA cells. These investigators also reported that, whereas the effects of systemic haloperidol on A9 DA cells were eliminated by hemitransections rostral to the midbrain, effects on A10 DA cells were spared, suggesting tighter autoregulation of A10 as compared to A9 DA cells (Hand et al., 1987).

Additional evidence suggesting that somatodendritic DA autoreceptors tonically regulate A10 unit activity comes from studies regarding the effects of repeated amphetamine or cocaine administration on A10 DA cells, in which the sensitivity of impulse-regulating A10 DA autoreceptors is greatly reduced, and both the number of spontaneously active DA cells and their average firing rate is increased (White and Wang, 1984b; Henry et al., 1989). Furthermore, there is a tight negative correlation between basal firing rate and sensitivity of impulse-regulating autoreceptors to DA and DA agonists (Tepper et al., 1982; White and Wang, 1984a). The increase in firing rate is a result of the decrease in autoreceptor sensitivity (not vice versa) as evidenced by the fact that, when normally slow DA cells are accelerated by iontophoretic glutamate, there is no alteration in the inhibitory efficacy of iontophoretic DA (White and Wang, 1984a).

Mesoaccumbens versus Mesocortical DA Cells

One of the most important findings regarding autoreceptor regulation of DA neuronal activity was the report that DA cells projecting to the mPFC and aCC lacked impulse-regulating somatodendritic autoreceptors, as well as synthesis-modulating nerve-terminal autoreceptors (Bannon and Roth, 1983; Chiodo et al., 1984). Antidromically identified mesoprefrontal DA neurons were reported to exhibit extraordinarily fast basal firing rates (9.3 spikes/s) and considerable bursting activity (54 per cent of spikes occurring in bursts) as compared to nigrostriatal DA cells; similar, albeit less dramatic (5.9 spikes/s; 38 per cent burst spikes) effects were reported for mesocingulate DA cells (Chiodo et al., 1984). In addition, mesocortical DA cells were completely insensitive to the inhibitory effects of IV apomorphine or iontophoretic DA (Chiodo et al., 1984). White and Wang (1984a) also reported that mesocortical DA cells (both mPFC and aCC) fired significantly faster (6.4 spikes/s) than mesoaccumbens DA cells (3.7 spikes/s), and were less sensitive to IV apomorphine and iontophoretic DA. These latter investigators concluded that mesocortical DA systems differed from other DA cell systems in that they contain a higher proportion of DA neurons which are characterized by relatively low density (or sensitivity) of somatodendritic autoreceptors, i.e. they differed quantitatively rather than qualitatively. However, other studies have failed to suppport these findings. Shepard and German (1984) reported that a subpopulation of mesocortical DA cells possess autoreceptors and fire at rates comparable to mesoaccumbens DA cells. More recently, Groves and colleagues (Gariano et al., 1989) reported that antidromically identified mesocortical DA cells exhibited firing rates and agonist sensitivity similar to those of nigrostriatal and mesoaccumbens DA cells. In addition, at least two other studies have reported the existence of mesocortical DA neurons exhibiting relatively slow (2–3 spikes/s) firing rates (Wang, 1981c; Mantz et al., 1989). The reasons for these discrepancies are currently unknown, but may reflect differences in levels of anesthesia since mesocortical DA cells are particularly affected by general anesthesia (Galloway et al., 1986).

NON-DOPAMINERGIC REGULATION OF A10 DA NEURONAL ACTIVITY

Given the potential importance of understanding afferent regulation of DA neuronal activity, it is surprising that so few electrophysiological reports have appeared regarding the possible inputs to A10 DA neurons and the means by which such inputs influence mesoaccumbens DA activity. In this section, studies regarding non-dopaminergic regulation of A10 unit activity will be reviewed and comparisons to the A9 DA system will be emphasized.

Long-Loop Feedback Regulation of Mesoaccumbens DA Neurons

Anatomical evidence clearly indicates that the striatonigral feedback pathway is more extensive than the corresponding NAc–VTA projection (Swanson and Cowan, 1975; Nauta et al., 1978; Phillipson, 1979). It now appears that both autoreceptor and striatonigral feedback systems are involved in the effects of systemic amphetamine on A9 DA neurons (Bunney and Aghajanian, 1978), whereas only autoreceptor mechanisms appear to be involved in such effects on A10 DA neurons (Wang, 1981c; White et al., 1987). Although these findings support the notion that A10 DA neurons are more tightly regulated by autoreceptors than A9 DA cells (Anden et al., 1983; Kehr, 1974; Wang, 1981c), A10 DA autoreceptors do not appear to be more sensitive to DA agonists than A9 DA autoreceptors (Clark and Chiodo, 1988).

Biochemical evidence indicates that the NAc–VTA projection, like the striatonigral system, appears to be primarily GABAergic (Waddington and Cross, 1978; Walaas and Fonnum, 1980). Electrophysiological studies have also identified a GABAergic NAc–VTA system since the rate-suppressant effects of NAc stimulation on many (unidentified) VTA neurons were blocked by the GABA antagonist bicuculline (Wolf et al., 1978). In more extensive studies, Mogenson and colleagues demonstrated that nearly half of the A10 DA neurons tested were inhibited by NAc stimulation at short (less than 10 ms) latencies, and that this effect was potentiated by nipecotic acid, an inhibitor of GABA uptake, and blocked by picrotoxin (Maeda and Mogenson, 1980; Yim and Mogenson, 1980), which blocks the Cl^- channel associated with the GABA/benzodiazepine receptor complex. These studies also identified A10 DA neurons which were excited by NAc stimulation as well as neurons exhibiting complex patterns of inhibition and excitation. In addition, many non-DA VTA neurons are also inhibited by NAc stimulation (Maeda and Mogenson, 1980). Thus, it appears that a NAc–VTA GABAergic feedback system may affect A10 DA neurons both directly and indirectly via local GABAergic interneurons and/or collaterals of GABA efferents.

Additional evidence for a functional NAc–VTA feedback system has been obtained from recent pharmacological studies of A10 DA neurons. For example, the inactivation (depolarization block) of A10 DA neurons produced by repeated administration of haloperidol is greatly attenuated if rats first receive ibotenic acid lesions of the NAc (White and Wang, 1983a). In addition, lesions of the NAc–VTA pathway, produced either by ibotenic acid or acute hemitransections, significantly attenuate the inhibitory effects of systemic cocaine, but not amphetamine, on A10 DA neurons (Einhorn et al., 1988; White et al., 1987). The difference between amphetamine and cocaine in this regard is probably due to differences in their mechanisms of action, i.e. the enhancement of dendritic release by amphetamine should produce significantly greater extracellular concentrations of DA within the VTA (Kalivas et al., 1989) than would blockade of DA uptake by cocaine (Bradberry and Roth, 1989). Since the inhibitory effects of cocaine on NAc neurons are considerably greater than those on A10 DA cells, which are only partial (Einhorn et al., 1988), it seems likely that NAc–VTA feedback regulatory mechanisms are only apparent when autoreceptor-induced inhibition is insufficient to compensate for enhanced activation of postsynaptic DA receptors (White et al., 1987). In other words, long-loop feedback inhibition in the mesoaccumbens DA system is largely redundant because of the tight regulation of activity by DA autoreceptors.

There also appear to be feedback projections from cortical terminations of A10 DA cells. Retrograde tracing studies identified cortical–VTA projections emanating from exactly those deep cortical regions (mPFC, aCC) which receive A10 DA terminals (Beckstead, 1979; Phillipson, 1979). Electrophysiological studies have identified antidromic responses of mPFC neurons to VTA stimulation (Thierry et al., 1983; Peterson et al., 1987) as well as an excitatory effect on A10 DA neurons produced by electrical stimulation of the mPFC (Thierry et al., 1979). Lesion studies, indicating a decrease in the high affinity uptake of d-[^{3}H]aspartate following excitotoxin injections into the mPFC, suggest that this mPFC–VTA excitatory system may be aspartatergic (Christie et al., 1985).

GABAergic Regulation and the Role of VTA Neurons

There is abundant evidence for regulation of A9 DA neurons by presumed GABAergic interneurons within the substantia nigra pars reticulata (SNr). In addition to direct inhibitory influences of GABAergic striatonigral neurons on A9 DA cell firing, these GABAergic afferents also terminate on non-DA SNr neurons. A first clue to the possibility of inhibitory interneurons regulating nigral DA activity was that IV administration of the GABA-agonist muscimol increased the firing of A9 DA cells (Grace and Bunney, 1979; Waszczak et al., 1980) in direct contrast to iontophoretic muscimol which inhibits DA neurons (Waszczak et al., 1980). This paradoxical finding led to the suggestion that muscimol inhibits GABA-containing neurons and thereby disinhibits DA neurons. This concept was supported by the finding that SNr neurons were approximately 20 times more sensitive to the inhibitory effects of iontophoretic GABA than were A9 DA neurons (Grace and Bunney, 1979; Waszczak et al., 1980). In addition, iontophoresis of GABA into the SNr caused a picrotoxin-reversible increase in the activity of A9 DA neurons (Grace and Bunney, 1979). Because systemic muscimol increased the activity of A9 DA neurons at the same doses which inhibited SNr cells (Grace and Bunney, 1979), and these effects were not diminished by kainic acid lesions of the striatum (Waszczak et al., 1980), it seems likely that GABA agonists increase DA cell firing by preferential inhibitory effects on SNr neurons rather than on striatonigral projection cells.

Intracellular recordings obtained from A9 DA cells *in vivo* provided further support for a GABA–GABA-DA striatonigral system (Grace and Bunney, 1985). Stimulation of the caudate elicits a short latency inhibitory postsynaptic potential (IPSP) in DA neurons which is followed by a rebound depolarization. This IPSP appears to be mediated by GABA for three reasons: first, its reversal potential is similar to that predicted for the reversal of GABAergic effects mediated by Cl^- conductances; second, intracellular injections of Cl^- reverse this IPSP; and third, the reversal potential for depolarization of A9 DA cells by the GABA-antagonist picrotoxin is similar to the reversal potential of the IPSP. In addition, low-intensity pulses delivered to the striatum inhibit SNr cells while enhancing the activity of A9 DA cells, unless muscimol is used to suppress SNr cells, in which case a direct inhibition of A9 neurons is observed (Grace and Bunney, 1985).

These findings suggest that GABAergic striatonigral feedback pathways exert two opposing influences on A9 DA neuronal activity. An inhibitory influence is mediated via a direct GABAergic striatonigral input, while an indirect excitatory influence is mediated by GABA-mediated inhibition of inhibitory GABA interneurons within the SNr. Since GABA receptors on SNr neurons are more sensitive than those on the DA neurons, the disinhibition of DA neurons may be the dominant effect of the striatonigral feedback loop (Grace and Bunney, 1985).

The VTA does not possess an organizational analog to the SNr and there are no reported studies of possible GABA–GABA-DA NAc–VTA feedback loops similar to those conducted in the striatonigral system. Nevertheless, there is pharmacological evidence suggestive of such an anatomical arrangement within the VTA. First, as for A9 DA cells, systemic administration of GABA agonists excites A10 DA cells (Waszczak and Walters, 1980). Second, as demonstrated for SNr and A9 DA neurons (Ross et al., 1982), systemic administration of benzodiazepines inhibits the firing of non-DA VTA neurons, which exhibit electrophysiological properties similar to SNr cells, and enhances the firing of A10 DA cells (O'Brien and White, 1987). Additionally, iontophoretic application of benzodiazepines inhibits non-DA VTA cells and fails to excite A10 DA cells (O'Brien and White, 1987). Finally, as also reported for the nigra (Iwatsubo and Clouet, 1977), systemic morphine inhibits non-DA VTA cells while exciting A10 DA neurons (Gysling and Wang, 1983; Matthews and German, 1984). These findings are all consistent with the disinhibition hypothesis and the presence of a relationship between reticulata-like non-DA and A10 DA VTA neurons similar to that observed within the nigra (O'Brien and White, 1987).

Intracellular recordings obtained from both nigral (Pinnock, 1984a; Lacey et al., 1988) and VTA slices (Mueller and Brodie, 1989) indicate that midbrain DA neurons possess $GABA_B$ receptors. The selective $GABA_B$-agonist baclofen inhibits DA neurons in these slice preparations, an effect typically accompanied by membrane hyperpolarization. $GABA_B$ and the D2 receptor are linked to the same K^+ conductance on midbrain DA neurons, probably via G_i (Innis and Aghajanian, 1987; Lacey et al., 1988).

Serotonin

Despite anatomical evidence indicating that serotonin (5-HT) neurons within the raphe nuclei are the source of a dense projection to the VTA (Phillipson, 1979; Steinbusch, 1981), almost nothing is known about the influence of 5-HT on A10 DA cell activity. While it has been reported that electrical stimulation of the dorsal raphe inhibits unidentified nigral neurons (Fibiger and Miller, 1977; Dray et al., 1976), no such studies have been reported for A10 DA cells. Biochemical studies suggest that 5-HT increases DA release from A10 DA dendrites as studied in brain slices (Beart and McDonald, 1982).

Intravenous administration of the 5-HT agonist 5-methoxydimethyltryptamine increases the firing of A10 DA neurons (White and Wang, 1983b; White, 1986a). Because this effect is not influenced by lesions of the raphe–VTA pathway, it is unlikely that the enhanced firing results from a loss of tonic inhibition by 5-HT neurons.

Microiontophoretic administration of 5-HT does not directly affect A9 DA neuronal activity (Aghajanian and Bunney, 1974; Collingridge and Davies, 1981), but may affect it indirectly by attenuating the ability of glutamate to produce excitation (Aghajanian and Bunney, 1974). These findings suggest that 5-HT may influence DA cell activity indirectly by modulating other excitatory inputs. Although electrophysiological effects of 5-HT on VTA neurons have not been reported, anatomical studies indicate that 5-HT terminals innervate both DA and non-DA neurons within the VTA and, thus, are in a position to produce both direct and indirect effects on A10 DA neuronal activity (Hervé et al., 1987).

Recently, 5-HT_3 antagonists have been reported to antagonize increases in DA release within the NAc produced by systemic administration of morphine and nicotine, but not amphetamine (Carboni et al., 1989; Imperato and Angelucci, 1989). Since the effect of the 5-HT_3 antagonist ICS 205-930 was observed following its administration into the VTA (Imperato and Angelucci, 1989), and since morphine and nicotine, but not amphetamine, increase DA release via impulse-dependent processes, it appears that 5-HT_3 antagonists exert an action on neuronal activity within the VTA. To date, there are no reports regarding the effects of 5-HT_3 antagonists on A10 DA neuronal firing rates. Repeated administration of the selective 5-HT_3 antagonist MDL 73,147EF has been reported to decrease the number of spontaneously active A10 DA neurons (Sorenson et al., 1989).

Noradrenaline (Norepinephrine)

As with 5-HT, little is currently known about the possible regulation of A10 cell activity by noradrenaline (NA). Iontophoretic administration of NA inhibits A10 DA cells, an effect blocked by both the D2 antagonist sulpiride and the α-2 antagonist piperoxane (White and Wang, 1984e). However, similar administration of either α or β agonists fails to influence A10 DA neurons (White and Wang, 1984e). Nigral DA cells *in vitro* are hyperpolarized by NA, an effect blocked by sulpiride but not by the selective α-2 antagonist idazoxan (Lacey et al., 1987). Since piperoxane, unlike idazoxan, also blocks D2 receptors (Waldmeier et al., 1982), the ability of piperoxane to block the inhibitory effects of iontophoretic NA may represent an action at the D2 autoreceptor; however, piperoxane was reported not to block the effects of iontophoretic DA on A9 DA cells (Aghajanian and Bunney, 1977).

Recently, it was reported that although the α-2 agonist clonidine (IV) failed to affect either A9 or A10 DA cell firing rates, it did 'regularize' the activity of these cells (defined as a decrease in the variation coefficient of the interspike intervals around their mean), converting irregular and bursting firing patterns to regular, pacemaker-like activity (Grenhoff and Svensson, 1988, 1989), similar to that observed in slice preparations. However, without iontophoretic experiments it is impossible to know the location of the α-2 receptors responsible for this effect.

Acetylcholine

To date, there have been no reported studies of the effects of acetylcholine (ACh) on A10 DA neurons. Within the nigra, iontophoretic administration of ACh was first reported to excite non-DA SNr cells, but not A9 DA cells (Aghajanian and Bunney, 1974; Collingridge and Davies, 1981; Pinnock and Dray, 1982; Scarnati et al., 1986). A secondary inhibition of nigral DA cells following ACh iontophoresis into the SNr was observed by Aghajanian and Bunney (1974) and attibuted to enhanced firing of GABAergic interneurons. In contrast, other investigators have reported excitatory effects of iontophoretic ACh on A9 DA cells (Dray and Straughan, 1976; Lichtensteiger et al., 1982).

Nicotine applied either systemically or iontophoretically activates A10 DA cells, apparently via a nicotinic ACh receptor (Grenhoff et al., 1986; Mereu et al., 1987). The effect of IV nicotine has been reported to be greater on A10 than on A9 DA cells (Mereu et al., 1987). Recent intracellular recordings from A10 DA cells *in vitro* indicate that ACh and nicotine depolarize and excite most of these neurons through direct actions on nicotinic receptors; A9 neurons in nigral slices were observed to respond in the same manner (Calabresi et al., 1989). Therefore, it appears that most DA neurons possess nicotinic cholinergic receptors which are directly responsive to ACh.

The source of possible cholinergic innervation of midbrain DA neurons has not yet been firmly established. Several recent reports have concentrated on an excitatory projection from the pedunculopontine nucleus to the nigra

(Beninato and Spencer, 1988; Niijima and Yoshida, 1988), and a cholinergic pathway synapsing onto nicotinic receptors, presumably located on A9 DA cells, has been suggested (Clarke et al., 1987; but see Scarnati et al., 1986). Similar studies of the VTA have not been reported.

Cholecystokinin

The discovery of the coexistence of cholecystokinin octapeptide (CCK) and DA within a subset of rat midbrain DA cells, predominantly within the VTA (Hökfelt et al., 1980), led to considerable interest in the possible regulation of DA cell activity by this peptide. Although much of the work has been focused on CCK/DA interactions within the target areas of the A10 DA cells, primarily the NAc (Wang et al., 1984; White and Wang, 1984d), additional interest was generated by the finding that CCK could excite a subpopulation of A10 DA neurons when given IV and nearly all DA neurons when applied iontophoretically (Skirboll et al., 1981). CCK was also shown to potentiate the inhibitory effects of apomorphine on DA neurons, suggesting a modulatory effect at DA autoreceptors (Hommer and Skirboll, 1983). Direct demonstration of such modulation was provided when it was shown that iontophoretic administration of CCK enhances the inhibitory effects of both DA and GABA on DA cells (Chiodo et al., 1987). However, this effect has not always been observed (White and Wang, 1985), perhaps owing to the sampling of different populations of DA neurons. Recently, Brodie and Dunwiddie (1987) reported that CCK increased the firing of most A10 DA cells in an *in vitro* slice preparation and enhanced DA-induced inhibition in about half of the neurons tested. Thus, it appears that CCK can modulate the ability of DA agonists to inhibit cellular activity in a subpopulation of DA neurons (for review see Freeman and Chiodo, 1987).

Opioid Systems

Studies with morphine have provided further evidence that A9 and A10 cells can be differentially regulated. Iwatsubo and Clouet (1977) first demonstrated the excitatory effects of systemic morphine on nigral DA neurons and reported that such effects could also be produced by direct injection of morphine into the caudate nucleus, implying a feedback pathway-mediated effect. This suggestion was supported by the finding that kainic acid lesions of the striatum attenuated the excitatory effects of morphine on A9 DA cells (Kondo and Iwatsubo, 1980). Other studies supported the notion that morphine activates nigral DA cells via indirect mechanisms, since local application of morphine failed to increase A9 cell firing; in fact, direct administration of morphine potently inhibited the firing of SNr neurons, suggesting that morphine activated nigral DA neurons via inhibition of GABAergic interneurons (Finnerty and Chan, 1979; Hommer and Pert, 1983).

Direct comparisons of A9 and A10 DA cells indicated differential regulation of activity by morphine. Activation of A10 DA cells by morphine was demonstrated by Gysling and Wang (1983), and Matthews and German (1984). In the latter report, morphine was found to be two to three times more effective at stimulating A10 as compared to A9 DA cells. Unlike previous studies, both Matthews and German (1984) and Gysling and Wang (1983) reported that iontophoretic morphine activated both A9 and A10 DA neurons. Nevertheless, the more potent effect of iontophoretic morphine was an inhibition of non-DA cells within the SNr and VTA (Gysling and Wang, 1983), again suggesting disinhibition as a mechanism for the increase in DA cell activity produced by systemic morphine. These investigators also demonstrated that hemitransections abolished the excitatory effects of morphine on A9, but not A10, DA cells (Gysling and Wang, 1983), a differential effect similar to that recently reported for DA receptor blockers (see above). Recent intracellular recordings from DA and non-DA neurons in a nigral slice indicated that non-DA cells, but not DA cells, possessed μ-opioid receptors, supporting the possible role of interneurons in morphine-induced activation of A9 DA cells (Lacey et al., 1989).

Recently, it was reported that IV injections of the κ-opioid agonist U50, 488 produced effects on nigral DA cells that were opposite to those observed with the μ-opioid agonist morphine (Walker et al., 1987). Thus, U50,488 partially inhibited the firing of most A9 DA cells. Direct injection of this compound into the striatum also inhibited a few A9 DA cells, implicating feedback pathways as mediators of the effect observed during systemic administration. Our laboratory has recently extended studies of U50,488 to A10 DA cells (Jeziorski and White, 1989). As in the nigra, U50,488 partially inhibited the firing of A10 DA cells. Less pronounced inhibitory effects were observed with iontophoretic administration of this κ-agonist. Whether this represents a difference between A9 and A10 DA cells is yet to be determined.

Other Regulatory Influences on A10 DA Neurons

Among the other pathways which may regulate A10 DA cells is an inhibitory projection from the lateral habenula. Electrical stimulation of the lateral habenula, but not the surrounding structures, inhibits the vast majority of both A9 and A10 DA neurons (Christoph et al., 1986). This inhibitory pathway descends via the fasciculus retroflexus since electrolytic lesions of this fiber system abolished the effect. In addition, the inhibition was initiated by neurons within the lateral habenula rather than by fibers of passage, since kainic acid lesions also abolished the effect. Because the habenula receives a variety of afferents from limbic, cortical and basal ganglia sources (Herkenham and Nauta, 1977; Graetrex and Phillipson, 1982), it was speculated that this nucleus may constitute an important relay station between these forebrain structures and midbrain DA neurons. Unfortunately, pharmacological identification of the transmitter involved in this pathway has not yet been reported.

Similar studies using electrical stimulation have also identified projection systems from the amygdala, lateral septum and lateral hypothalamus to the VTA (Maeda and Mogenson, 1981a, b). Both monosynaptic and polysynaptic inhibitions and excitations of presumed A10 DA neurons were reported but, again, no evidence for the neurochemical composition of such pathways was presented.

DIFFERENCES IN DA NEURONAL FIRING PATTERNS

Although antidromically identified nigrostriatal and mesoaccumbens DA cells appear quite similar in many aspects, comparative studies have recently identified potentially important differences. One of the most interesting aspects of DA neurons is their ability to fire action potentials in bursts in which a series of two to ten spikes with progressively decreasing amplitude and increasing duration typically occur. Burst onsets are usually defined as two to three spikes occurring within 80 ms of one another, while burst terminations are defined as an interspike interval of greater than 160 ms (Grace and Bunney, 1984b). In a recent comparison of nigrostriatal and mesoaccumbens DA neurons, Clark and Chiodo (1988) classified bursting DA neurons as those exhibiting at least two three-spike bursts out of 500 recorded action potentials. Whereas only 32 per cent of A9 nigrostrial DA neurons exhibited burst-firing activity, about half (51 per cent) of A10 mesoaccumbens DA neurons fired in bursts. In addition, the average length of the post-burst inhibitory phase (time between last burst spike and subsequent non-burst spike) was significantly longer for mesoaccumbens A10 DA cells. Clark and Chiodo (1988) speculated that this longer post-burst inhibition may be due to a greater amount of dendritic DA released by A10 as compared to A9 neurons following spike discharge. This may result in a greater degree of membrane hyperpolarization, possibly via a Ca^{++}-activated K^+ current (Grace and Bunney, 1984a, b; Shepard and Bunney, 1988). Whether this finding is related to the greater autoregulation of A10 DA neurons awaits investigation.

Gariano and Groves (1988) recently reported that a subpopulation (approximately 5 per cent) of DA neurons within the VTA and medial nigra exhibited burst firing following electrical stimulation of the mPFC. The cortically evoked burst firing was similar to that observed for spontaneous bursts with respect to the number of spikes within the burst, the average interspike interval, and the presence of decreased spike amplitude and increased interspike intervals within each burst. Thus, it is possible that corticomesencephalic projections play a role in the control of firing patterns within midbrain DA neurons.

Speculation about the significance of burst firing in DA neurons has centered on the possibility of greater release of DA from terminals during burst activity (Gonon, 1988) or of preferential release of one co-transmitter, such as CCK versus DA (Grace and Bunney, 1984b; Gonon, 1988). Interestingly, Freeman and Bunney (1987) have reported that over 90 per cent of A10 DA neurons recorded from unanesthetized, freely-moving rats exhibited burst firing, and that electrically coupled discharges of more than one A10 DA neuron could frequently be observed. Moreover, stroking of the vibrissae and auditory stimuli produced reliable trains of burst firing, indicating that this mode of activity is important in the animal's orientation and response to the environment.

REGULATION OF ACCUMBENS NEURONS BY A10 DA CELLS

Once released from the nerve terminals of A10 DA neurons, DA appears to act through D1 and D2 receptors to influence the activity of its neuronal targets. The purpose of the remainder of this chapter is to review recent evidence regarding the effects of DA on the NAc target cells of A10 DA neurons, to demonstrate the roles of D1 and D2 DA receptors in regulating the neuronal activity of NAc (and striatal) neurons, and to discuss the ways in which such DA receptor activations may be related to behavior.

Multiple DA Receptors within the NAc

Perhaps the most important recent development in our understanding of DA receptors has been the discovery of behaviorally relevant interactions between D1 and D2 receptors. Although once thought not to be involved in DA related functions, the D1 receptor is now known to participate in many aspects of DA neurotransmission and their behavioral sequelae (Clark and White, 1987). Our laboratory has been particularly concerned with electrophysiological characterizations of the pharmacological properties of DA receptors within the rat NAc. In our first study (White and Wang, 1986), we tested the effects of iontophoretic administration of D1 and D2 agonists on both spontaneously active NAc neurons and on neurons made to fire by the iontophoretic administration of glutamate. We reported that microiontophoretic administration of the D2 agonist LY 141865 inhibited the activity of 30 of the 40 NAc neurons tested (Table 1). In addition, we

Table 1. Responsiveness of Nucleus Accumbens Neurons to
D1 and D2 Agonists

Agonist	Number of NAc neurons Responding/Total	Percentage
SKF 38393	17/45	38
LY 141865	30/40	75
SKF 38393 + LY 141865	9/30	30

observed that 17 out of 45 NAc neurons were inhibited by similar administration of the D1 agonist SKF 38393. Selectivity of these effects at the two receptors was demonstrated during antagonism tests. Thus, the D2 antagonist sulpiride selectively blocked the effects of LY 141865 (Figure 2A), whereas the D1 antagonist SCH 23390 completely blocked the effects of SKF 38393 while partially attenuating the effects of LY 141865 (Figure 2B).

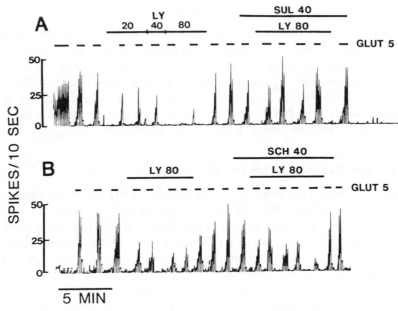

Figure 2. Cumulative rate histograms illustrating the inhibitory effects of iontophoretically ejected LY 141865 (0.01 M) on the glutamate-induced firing of two NAc neurons. **A,** Sulpiride (0.05 M) significantly attenuated the inhibitory effects of LY 141865. **B,** Failure of SCH 23390 (0.05 M) to block the inhibitory effects of LY 141865. Horizontal bars indicate the length of iontophoretic ejection and numbers indicate current in nanoamperes (nA). From White and Wang (1986) with permission

Following the discovery of both D1- and D2-receptive NAc neurons, we determined that a subpopulation of neurons was inhibited by both agonists (Table 1). More importantly, on those cells which were inhibited by both SKF 38393 and LY 141865, co-administration of the two drugs produced synergistic (supra-additive) inhibition (Figure 3). These findings indicated that certain NAc neurons may possess both D1 and D2 receptors, and that these receptors may play a synergistic role at regulating activity (White and Wang, 1986).

Interactions Between D1 and D2 DA Receptors

Our initial finding suggesting a cooperative effect of co-activation of D1 and D2 receptors on NAc neuronal activity was somewhat surprising in view of the prevailing idea that these two DA receptors exert opposing roles in a variety of biochemical models. When we first reported these results (White and Wang, 1984c), only one behavioral finding could be considered as

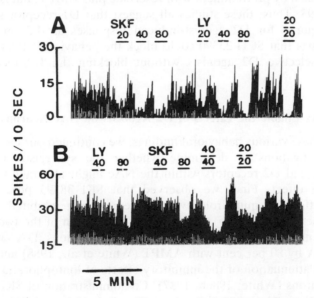

Figure 3. Cumulative rate histograms illustrating the inhibitory effects of iontophoretically ejected SKF 38393 and LY 141865 (both at 0.01 M) simultaneously applied on spontaneously active NAc neurons. **A,** A cell inhibited by both LY 141865 and SKF 38393, and the apparent supra-additive effects of co-administration of these two agonists. **B,** Another cell inhibited by both LY 141865 and SKF 38393. Note the more pronounced extent and duration of the inhibition caused by the co-application of the two agonists as compared to either one administered alone. Horizontal bars indicate the length of iontophoretic ejection and numbers indicate current in nanoamperes (nA). Adapted from White and Wang (1986) with permission

consistent with a synergistic interaction between D1 and D2 receptors. Gershanik et al. (1983) had demonstrated that both SKF 38393 and LY 141865 were required to reverse the akinesia observed in reserpinized mice. Subsequently, other reports have shown similar behavioral effects. Braun and Chase (1986) reported that, in rats acutely depleted of DA with the tyrosine hydroxylase-inhibitor α-methylparatyrosine (AMPT), stereotyped behaviors were produced only by the combined administration of D1 and D2 selective agonists, suggesting that concurrent activation of both D1 and D2 receptors was necessary for the expression of DA-mediated behaviors. Subsequently, this group demonstrated that SKF 38393 can potentiate the circling response induced by quinpirole in rats with excitotoxin-induced lesions of the caudate nucleus, a rotational model in which DA receptors remain normosensitive. Moreover, when AMPT was used to deplete DA in these rats, the quinpirole response was markedly reduced, but was reinstated by SKF 38393 (Barone et al., 1986). Jackson and Hashizume (1986) reported that the locomotor stimulant effect of bromocriptine is abolished by pretreatment with reserpine plus AMPT, but is reinstated by SKF 38393. Thus, these studies all suggest that D1 receptor stimulation may be required for D2 agonist-induced responses as did, in hindsight, earlier findings that SCH 23390 could block the behavioral effects of mixed D1/D2 or selective D2 agonists without blocking the D2 receptor (see below).

D1 Receptors Enable the Effects of D2 Agonists on NAc Neurons

In view of these various behavioral findings, we continued our electrophysiological investigations to determine whether the synergistic interactions between D1 and D2 receptors within the NAc might also take the form of an enabling effect. First, we observed that SKF 38393 potentiated the inhibitory effects of quinpirole even on neurons not inhibited by the D1 agonist alone (White, 1986b). To study the interaction of the two receptors in the absence of receptor occupation by endogenous DA, we acutely depleted DA by 80 per cent with AMPT (White et al., 1988) and observed a significant attenuation of the inhibitory effects of iontophoretic quinpirole on NAc neurons (White, 1986b, 1987). Co-administration of SKF 38393 (at currents producing little inhibition) and quinpirole 'reinstated' the inhibitory response to quinpirole (Figure 4). Thus, activation of D1 receptors by SKF 38393 in rats acutely depleted of DA enables D2 receptor occupation by quinpirole to produce an inhibition of neuronal activity, suggesting that endogenous DA may act as D1 receptors to enable D2-mediated events in the intact rat (White, 1986b, 1987).

We have recently confirmed and extended these original observations (Wachtel et al., 1989). First, we demonstrated that the inhibitory effects of

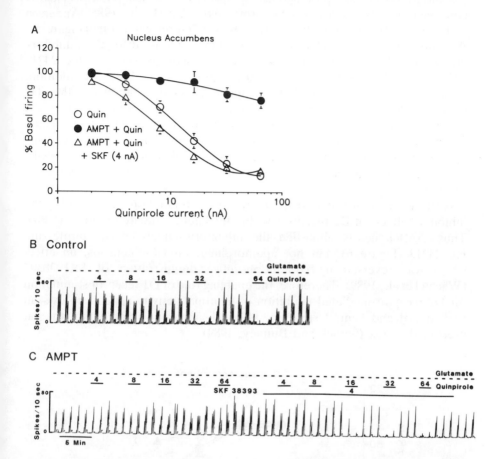

Figure 4. Inhibition of the firing of nucleus accumbens (NAc) neurons by iontophoretic administration of the D2 agonist, quinpirole (QUIN). **A,** Current-response curves illustrating the attenuation of the inhibitory effect of QUIN by pretreatment with alpha-methylparatyrosine (AMPT) and the reinstatement of the QUIN-induced inhibition on the same neurons with co-iontophoresis of SKF 38393 (4 nA). Each point represents the mean ± SEM (QUIN control, $n = 11$; AMPT, $n = 12$; AMPT and SKF 38393, $n = 11$). **B,** Cumulative rate histogram illustrating the typical inhibitory effect of iontophoretic QUIN on a glutamate-driven NAc neuron in an untreated control rat. **C,** Cumulative rate histogram illustrating the attenuation of the QUIN-induced inhibition of a glutamate-driven NAc neuron in an AMPT-pretreated rat and the restoration of inhibition during co-iontophoresis of SKF 38393. Note that the 4 nA current of SKF 38393 alone slightly potentiated the excitatory effect of glutamate on this cell. Bars indicate the duration of iontophoretic current and numbers represent the current, in nanoamperes (nA). From Wachtel et al., 1989, with permission

the mixed D1/D2 receptor agonist apomorphine, which possesses nearly equivalent affinity for the two receptors (Arnt and Hyttel, 1985; Andersen and Nielsen, 1986), were still evident in AMPT-pretreated rats (Figure 5). We also reported that D1 receptor activation is required for the inhibitory effects of other selective D2 DA receptor agonists such as RU 24213 (Wachtel et al., 1989) and B-HT 920 (Johansen et al., 1988). In addition, we have recently observed that iontophoretic administration of other D1 agonists, SKF 75670 and SKF 81297 (Andersen et al., 1987; Arnt et al., 1988), also enabled the inhibitory effects of quinpirole in AMPT-pretreated rats (Johansen and White, 1988). Thus, the requirement of D1 receptor activation for D2 receptor-mediated inhibition of NAc neurons is not specific to the particular agonists employed but appears to be a general phenomenon of D1/D2 receptor interaction.

Next, we demonstrated that D1 receptor stimulation also enables the inhibitory effects of D2 receptors within the lateral caudate-putamen (CPu). Thus, AMPT nearly abolished the inhibitory effects of quinpirole and RU 24213 (Figure 6), but not apomorphine, on CPu neurons, an effect which was reversed by co-iontophoretic administration of SKF 38393 (Wachtel et al., 1989). Therefore, the enabling role of D1 receptor stimulation for D2 receptor-mediated inhibition of neuronal activity appears to exist in both dorsal and ventral striatum, although apparently not within the rat prefrontal cortex (Sesack and Bunney, 1989).

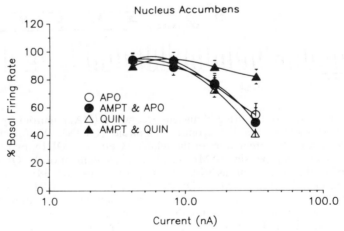

Figure 5. Inhibition of NAc neurons by iontophoretically administered apomorphine (APO) and quinpirole (QUIN). Current-response curves illustrating the inability of AMPT pretreatment to alter the inhibitory effect of APO, whereas the effect of QUIN was attenuated. Each point represents the mean ± SEM (APO control, $n = 10$; AMPT and APO, $n = 15$; QUIN control, $n = 9$; AMPT and QUIN, $n = 8$). From Wachtel et al., 1989, with permission

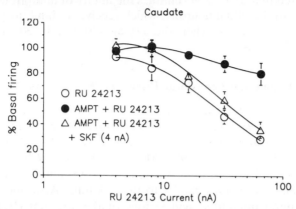

Figure 6. Inhibition of CPu neurons by iontophoretic administration of RU 24213 Current-response curves illustrating the attenuation of the RU 24213-induced inhibitory effect on CPu neurons in AMPT-pretreated rats, and the ability of SKF 38393 (4 nA) to restore the inhibition produced by RU 24213. Points represent the mean $\pm$ SEM ($n = 10$ for each group). From Wachtel et al., 1989, with permission

In a series of elegant studies, Walters and colleagues demonstrated D1/D2 interactions on rat globus pallidus neurons following IV injections of selective D1 and D2 receptor agonists (Carlson et al., 1987a; Walters et al., 1987) which are strikingly similar to those that we observed during the iontophoretic administration of these agonists onto NAc and CPu cells. Acute depletion of DA with AMPT attenuated the partial (as compared to apomorphine) excitatory effects of quinpirole, but not the marked excitatory effects of apomorphine. Subsequent administration of SKF 38393 to AMPT-pretreated rats which had received quinpirole produced marked increases in pallidal firing equivalent to those produced by apomorphine or by the combination of SKF 38393 and quinpirole in normal rats (Walters et al., 1987). Recently, this group has also demonstrated that the excitatory effects of IV apomorphine on pallidal neurons are attenuated by ipsilateral quinolinic acid lesions of the rostral striatum (Pan et al., 1987; Pan and Walters, 1988). Therefore, it seems likely that the excitatory effects of apomorphine on pallidal neurons results from disinhibition subsequent to inhibition of striatopallidal CPu neurons, which are thought to be GABAergic (Fonnum et al., 1978; Nagy et al., 1978; Staines et al., 1980). Our findings within the CPu suggest that the permissive role of D1 receptor stimulation for D2 agonist-induced excitation previously observed within the globus pallidus (Walters et al., 1987) may be the result of direct enabling actions in the CPu occurring on striatopallidal GABAergic neurons. Similarly, Yang and Mogenson (1989) recently reported that SKF 38393 enables the ability of quinpirole to increase the firing of ventral pallidal neurons, which receive an inhibitory input from NAc GABAergic neurons, when the D1 agonist is infused into the NAc prior to the D2 agonist.

D1 Receptors Enable the Behavioral Effects of D2 Agonists

Behavioral evidence for D1/D2 synergism has been reported for locomotion (Braun and Chase, 1986; Jackson and Hashizume, 1986; Starr et al., 1987), stereotyped licking and gnawing (Braun and Chase, 1986; Mashurano and Waddington, 1986; Arnt et al., 1987; Meller et al., 1988; White et al., 1988), climbing (Moore and Axton, 1988; Vasse et al., 1988) and ipsilateral rotation in rats with hemitransections caudal to the striatum (Arnt and Perregaard, 1987) or unilateral quinolinic acid lesions of the striatum (Barone et al., 1986). Synergistic behavioral interactions are also evident in rats with supersensitive DA receptors, such as contralateral rotation observed in rats with unilateral 6-hydroxydopamine (6-OHDA) lesions of the nigrostriatal DA system (Robertson and Robertson, 1986; Sonsalla et al., 1988).

The first indication of a specific enabling relationship in behavioral studies was that the selective D1 receptor antagonist SCH 23390 could block stereotyped behaviors produced either by mixed DA agonists (Mailman et al., 1984; Arnt, 1985) or by selective D2 agonists (Arnt, 1985; Breese and Meuller, 1985; Molloy and Waddington, 1985; Pugh et al., 1985; Longoni et al., 1987b). More direct support came from many recent reports indicating that acute DA depletions produced by AMPT and/or reserpine abolished the locomotor activation and low-component stereotyped behaviors (repetitive sniffing) produced by selective D2 receptor agonists (Braun and Chase, 1986; Jackson and Hashizume, 1986; Longoni et al., 1987b; Meller et al., 1988; White et al., 1988). Similar interactions have also been reported for D2 agonist-induced yawning (Longoni et al., 1987a; Ushijima et al., 1988) and circling in rats with quinolinic acid lesions of the striatum (Barone et al., 1986). However, as in our electrophysiological experiments, acute DA depletion failed to alter apomorphine-induced stereotyped gnawing, presumably because apomorphine supplies the necessary D1 stimulation (White et al., 1988).

D2 Receptor Stimulation is Unnecessary for D1 Agonist Effects

One of the remaining questions as to the enabling role of D1 receptor stimulation for D2 receptor-mediated functional effects is the extent to which this relationship is reciprocal. Our studies suggest that this is not the case (White et al., 1987, 1988; Wachtel et al., 1989). The inhibitory effects of the D1 receptor agonist SKF 38393 on both NAc (Figure 7) and CPu cells are not altered by acute DA depletion. In addition, the characteristic grooming responses produced by the D1 agonist SKF 38393 (Molloy and Waddington, 1984, 1987a, b; Starr and Starr, 1986a, b) are still evident in rats acutely depleted of DA (greater than 99.5 per cent reductions in striatal DA) by pretreatment with reserpine plus AMPT (Figure 8). More indirectly, it has been reported that blockade of D2 receptors unmasks apomorphine-induced grooming responses, suggesting that D1 stimulation produced grooming in the absence of D2 tone (Molloy and Waddington, 1984; Starr and Starr, 1986a; Starr et al., 1987). Although some (not all) D2 selective antagonists have been reported to attenuate SKF 38393-induced grooming (Molloy and Waddington, 1987b), this may be due to competing behavioral effects of the antagonist, e.g. catalepsy.

Mechanisms of Enabling

Although it has been suggested that the behavioral reflections of D1/D2 receptor interactions are due to actions at D1 and D2 receptors located on different neurons (Longoni et al., 1987b; Waddington and O'Boyle, 1987), perhaps within separate brain sites (Robertson and Robertson, 1987; Waddington and O'Boyle, 1987; Barone et al., 1986), or participating in parallel neural circuits (Creese, 1987), the demonstration of D1 receptor enabling of D2 function on individual neurons using microiontophoresis

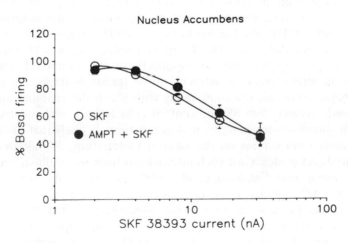

Figure 7. Inhibition of NAc neurons by iontophoretic administration of the D_1 agonist, SKF 38393. Current-response curves illustrating the failure of AMPT pretreatment to affect the inhibition of NAc neurons by SKF 38393. Each point represents the mean ± SEM (SKF 38393) control, $n = 10$; AMPT and SKF 38393, $n = 11$). From Wachtel et al., 1989, with permission

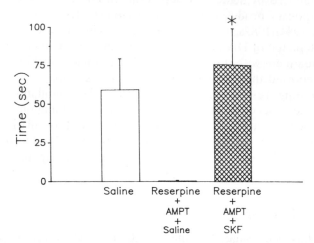

Figure 8. Grooming behavior induced by a 16 mg/kg dose of SKF 38393 ($n = 8$) as compared to saline ($n = 5$) in rats pretreated with a combination of reserpine (5 mg/kg) and AMPT (250 mg/kg) and in non-treated controls ($n = 8$). In rats that received reserpine/AMPT, SKF 38393 induced a significant increase in grooming as compared to saline ($P < 0.001$). From White et al., 1988, with permission

suggests that such behavioral effects could be mediated by D1 and D2 receptors located on the same striatal cells. Others have also speculated that both D1 and D2 receptors may exist on the same striatal neurons, based on the effects of D1 and D2 agonists on cAMP formation both in brain slices (Stoof and Kebabian, 1981) and in primary cultures (Chneiweiss et al., 1988). Although our microiontophoretic results do not rule out effects of drugs on interneurons or afferent nerve terminals impinging upon the neuron being recorded, the consistency with which the enabling interaction is observed (greater than 85 per cent of cells tested), and the fact that it occurs on glutamate-driven units, makes it extremely likely that the observed effects result from actions on the neuron under study. Although there is, as yet, no direct evidence for such interactions from intracellular recordings, it is interesting that Calabresi et al. (1987) observed inhibitory effects of D1, but not D2, agonists on striatal neurons recorded intracellularly from an *in vitro* slice preparation. Our results would suggest that this observation might have resulted from a removal of D1 receptor tone (decreased DA release) during slice preparation, rendering D2 agonists ineffective.

The mechanisms underlying the enabling phenomenon remain unknown. Given that D1 and D2 receptors are defined by their actions on adenylate cyclase, it might be reasoned that enhanced cAMP production is the consequence of D1 stimulation necessary for the expression of D2 receptor effects. Yet, in contrast to the synergistic effects of combined D1/D2 receptor stimulation on many functional measures the effects of D2 receptor stimulation on cAMP production in dorsal striatal membranes oppose those of D1 receptors (Stoof and Kebabian, 1981; Onali et al., 1985; Kelly and Nahorski, 1986). Interestingly, this effect is not observed with NAc membrane preparations (Stoof and Verheijden, 1986; Kelly and Nahorski, 1987). Therefore, despite different relationships between D1 and D2 receptors with respect to adenylate cyclase within these areas, the enabling phenomenon appears identical. It is still possible that enhanced cAMP production activates other intracellular events (e.g. phosphorylation of proteins involved in channel gating) which are required for D2 receptor-mediated alterations in membrane conductance. Alternatively, D1 and D2 receptors may influence other transduction mechanisms within striatal cells or jointly regulate ligand-gated conductance channels. It has recently been suggested that both D1 and D2 receptors may decrease a voltage-dependent, tetrodotoxin-sensitive inward conductance (presumably Na^+) in striatal cells *in vitro* (Calabresi et al., 1987, 1988), although the D2 effect was evident only in rats chronically depleted of DA with reserpine or nigrostriatal DA lesions (Calabresi et al., 1988). Using whole cell patch recordings from acutely dissociated striatal cells, Freedman and Weight (1988) reported that quinpirole, but not SKF 38393, activated K^+ channels when the agonist was present in the patch pipette. The lack of D1 receptor function in this preparation may be due to a number of factors, including alteration of D1 receptors during the dissociation process, the removal of dendritic processes, perhaps possessing the majority of D1 (and D2) receptors (Freund et al., 1984), during dissociation, and the possibility that D1 and D2 receptors may act on other types of ion channels.

D2 DA Autoreceptors do not Require Enabling

Unlike postsynaptic D2 DA receptors in the NAc and CPu, impulse-regulating somatodendritic autoreceptors on DA neurons in the VTA and substantia nigra zona compacta (SNc) do not appear to be responsive to D1 receptor activation. For both A10 (White and Wang, 1984e) and A9 (Carlson et al., 1987b) DA neurons, autoreceptor-mediated inhibition of DA cells occurs in response to D2 agonists, but not to SKF 38393. The inability of SKF 38393 to alter DA cell activity is not due to the partial agonist characteristic of this drug since the full D1 agonist SKF 81297 (Andersen et al., 1987) produced similar results on midbrain DA neurons (Wachtel and White, unpublished findings). Since SKF 38393 can potentiate quinpirole-induced inhibition of NAc cells which are not directly inhibited by the D1 agonist (White, 1986b, 1987), it is possible that such 'silent' effects of D1 receptor stimulation might occur on DA neurons to modulate the effects of

D2 agonists at impulse-regulating autoreceptors. This does not appear to be the case. SCH 23390 fails to alter the inhibitory effects of IV quinpirole on either A9 or A10 DA cells (Carlson et al., 1986; Wachtel et al., 1989). Acute DA depletion does not diminish the effects of quinpirole. Neither IV nor iontophoretic administration of SKF 38393 alters quinpirole-induced inhibitions of midbrain DA cells (Figure 9). These findings are consistent with the notion that impulse-regulating somatodendritic DA autoreceptors are exclusively of the D2 subtype (White and Wang, 1984e). Similar manipulations of nerve-terminal, synthesis-modulating receptors also reveal a lack of D1 receptor involvement in (or enabling of) D2 receptor-mediated inhibition of DA synthesis (Wachtel et al., 1989).

CONCLUSIONS

Given the speculated involvement of mesoaccumbens A10 DA neurons in psychiatric disease and reinforcement mechanisms, it is surprising that we know so little about the factors which regulate their activity. Electrophysiological analyses have clearly demonstrated the existence of D2, $GABA_B$ and nicotinic cholinergic receptors on A10 DA neurons. However, little is known about other receptors which may be located on A10 DA neurons or the possible sources of afferents to these cells which might utilize such receptors. The fact that DA neurons recorded from brain slices spontaneously exhibit only pacemaker potentials, failing to fire in the irregular or bursting patterns observed *in vivo*, clearly indicates that important afferents are lost during slice preparation. Recent intracellular studies have shown that DA cells *in vitro* maintain the necessary conductances to fire in irregular and bursting patterns. Administration of apamin, which specifically inhibits Ca^{++}-activated K^+ channels and thereby reduces afterhyperpolarizations observed in DA cells following action potential generation, results in the emergence of these patterns of activity (Shepard and Bunney, 1988). However, we do not presently know what types of mechanism normally override the regulation of firing by CA^{++}-activated K^+ channels *in vivo*.

The finding that clonidine causes regular, 'pacemaker-like' activity *in vivo* suggests that NA may be important in producing irregular and bursting patterns. Such an effect is unlikely to be due to α-2 adrenoceptors on DA neurons since iontophoretic clonidine does not affect DA cells. It seems more likely that this effect of clonidine is due to a loss of NA innervation subsequent to clonidine-induced suppression of NA-containing neurons within the locus ceruleus (Svensson et al., 1975). In fact, reserpine pretreatment abolished the regularizing effect of clonidine. Given the postulated role of locus ceruleus NA systems in the control of vigilance and adaptive behavioral responses (Aston-Jones, 1985), it is interesting to consider the findings of Freeman and Bunney (1987) that A10 DA cells in

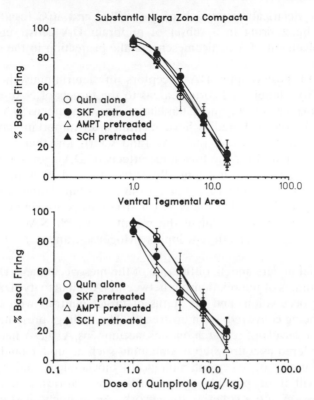

Figure 9. Cumulative dose-response curves illustrating inhibition of substantia nigra (A9, top) and ventral tegmental area (A10, bottom) DA neurons by IV administration of quinpriole (QUIN) after either pretreatment with the D1 agonist SKF 38393, the D1 antagonist SCH 23390 or AMPT. None of these D1 receptor manipulations altered the inhibitory effects of QUIN at somatodentric D2 DA autoreceptors. Each point represents the mean ± SEM (A9: n = 10,9,9,8; A10: n = 14,10,7,10 for control, SKF 38393, AMPT and SCH 23390 pretreatments, respectively). From Wachtel et al., 1989, with permission

unanesthetized rats switch to a burst firing mode upon presentation of certain stimuli requiring an orientating response of the animal. Since such stimuli also increase NA unit firing within the locus ceruleus (Aston-Jones, 1985), whereas α-2 agonists 'regularize' DA activity patterns, it may be that enhanced NA activity is related to bursting in DA cells, whereas a loss of NA tone is related to a loss of burst activity. Iontophoretic and lesion studies are needed to test this possibility. In addition, similar studies of other possible afferents will be required before we can achieve a thorough understanding of the regulatory factors which influence rates and patterns of A10 DA firing. In this regard, Gariano and Groves (1988)·recently reported that electrical stimulation of the mPFC and aCC resulted in the initiation of burst firing in a subset of midbrain DA cells, suggesting a possible involvement of a corticomesencephalic projection in the control of firing pattern.

The role of postsynaptic DA receptors in determining the flow of information from limbic and cortical areas to the targets of NAc neurons is of equal importance to our understanding of mesoaccumbens DA function. Our electrophysiological studies have identified an important principle of DA receptor function within the NAc (and CPu), i.e. that D1 receptor stimulation is required for the functional effects of DA agonists. However, NAc neurons typically are not tonically active. Instead, they fire in phasic patterns which reflect excitatory inputs from important limbic and cortical areas. The role of DA within the NAc (or striatum) is not simply to inhibit neuronal activity but to modulate the extent to which NAc neurons are responsive to these other afferent inputs (Mogenson and Yim, Chapter 4, this volume).

Our eventual understanding of the role of the mesoaccumbens DA system will require studies of the relationship between DA cell activity, DA release, DA receptor occupation, and the status of target neurons with respect to information being conveyed 'from upstream'. The findings presented herein, representing a decade of research on mesoaccumbens A10 DA neurons, can only be considered as a first step to obtaining such an understanding. Only with combinations of electrophysiological, biochemical and behavioral approaches will it be possible to synthesize the various aspects of DA neurotransmission into a cohesive framework. Accordingly, it is imperative that DA systems be studied at various levels of analysis, from single channels studied in isolated cell preparations to awake, intact animals behaving in the environment. Just as the effects of intracerebral drug injections on behavior are more meaningful with an understanding of the receptor and transduction mechanisms affected by such drugs, so studies of single ion channels affected by DA are more meaningful when the cell types possessing those channels are identified, and the roles of those cells in controlling behaviorally relevant messages are appreciated. With the increasing sophistication of applicable technologies, the next decade should witness considerable advancement in our understanding of mesolimbic DA and its role in normal and aberrant behavior.

ACKNOWLEDGEMENTS

I thank Stephen Wachtel, Dr Xiu-Ti Hu, Patricia Johansen, Rich Brooderson, Dr Matthew P. Galloway, Dr David Clark and Dr Stephan Hjorth for their valuable scientific contributions to the experimental results presented herein. This work was supported by United States Public Health Service Grants

MH-40832 and DA-04093 and by the American Parkinson's Disease Association.

REFERENCES

Aghajanian, G.K. and Bunney, B.S. (1974) Dopaminergic and non-dopaminergic neurons of the substantia nigra: differential responses to putative transmitters. In: Boissier, J.R., Hippius, H. and Pichot, P. (eds) *Proceedings: 9th International Congress, Collegium Internationale Neuropsychopharmacologicum, Vol. 359.* Amsterdam: Excerpta Medica, pp. 444-452.

Aghajanian, G.K. and Bunney, B.S. (1977) Dopamine 'autoreceptors': pharmacological characterization by microiontophoretic single cell recording studies. *Naunyn-Schmiedeberg's Archives de Pharmacologie* **297**, 1–7.

Altar, C.A. and Hauser, K. (1987) Topography of substantia nigra innervation by D_1 receptor-containing striatal neurons. *Brain Research* **410**, 1–11.

Andén, N.-E., Dahlström, A., Fuxe, K., Larsson, K., Olson, L. and Ungerstedt, U. (1966) Ascending monoamine neurons to telencephalon and diencephalon. *Acta Physiologica Scandinavica* **67**, 313–326.

Andén, N.E., Grabowska-Andén, M., Lindgren, S. and Thornström, U. (1983) Synthesis rate of dopamine: difference between corpus striatum and limbic system as a possible explanation of variations in reactions to drugs. *Naunyn-Schmiedeberg's Archives de Pharmacologie* **323**, 193–198.

Andersen, P.H. and Nielsen, E.B. (1986) The dopamine D_1 receptor: biochemical and behavioral aspects. In: Breese, G.R. and Creese, I. (eds) *Neurobiology of Central D_1 Dopamine Receptors.* New York: Plenum Press, pp. 73–91.

Andersen, P.H., Nielsen, E.B., Scheel-Krüger, J., Jansen, J.A. and Hohlweg, R. (1987) Thienopyridine derivatives as the first selective, full efficacy, dopamine D1 receptor agonists. *European Journal of Pharmacology* **137**, 291–292.

Arnt, J. (1985) Behavioral stimulation is induced by separate dopamine D-1 and D-2 receptor sites in reserpine-pretreated but not in normal rats. *European Journal of Pharmacology* **113**, 79–88.

Arnt, J. and Hyttel, J. (1985) Differential involvement of dopamine D-1 and D-2 receptors in the circling behavior induced by apomorphine, SK&F 38393, pergolide and LY 171555 in 6-hydroxydopamine-lesioned rats. *Psychopharmacology* **85**, 346–352.

Arnt, J. and Perregaard, J. (1987) Synergistic interaction between D-1 and D-2 receptor agonists: circling behavior of rats with hemitransection. *European Journal of Pharmacology* **143**, 45–53.

Arnt, J., Hytell, J. and Meier, E. (1987) Dopamine D-1 receptor agonists combined with the selective D-2 agonist quinpirole facilitate the expression of oral stereotyped behaviour in rats. *European Journal of Pharmacology* **133**, 137–145.

Arnt, J., Hyttel, J. and Meier, E. (1988) Inactivation of dopamine D-1 or D-2 receptors differentially inhibits stereotypies induced by dopamine agonists in rats. *European Journal of Pharmacology* **155**, 37–47.

Aston-Jones, G. (1985) Behavioral functions of locus coeruleus derived from cellular attributes. *Physiological Psychology* **13**, 118–126.

Bannon, M.J. and Roth, R.H. (1983) Pharmacology of mesocortical dopamine neurons. *Pharmacological Reviews* **35**, 53–68.

Barone, P., Davis, T.A., Braun, A.R. and Chase, T.N. (1986) Dopaminergic mechanisms and motor function: characterization of D-1 and D-2 dopamine receptor interactions. *European Journal of Pharmacology* **123**, 109–114.

Beart, P.M. and McDonald, D. (1980) Neurochemical studies of the mesolimbic dopaminergic pathway: somatodendritic mechanisms and GABAergic neurones in the rat ventral tegmentum. *Journal of Neurochemistry* **34**, 1622–1629.

Beart, P.M. and McDonald, D. (1982) 5-Hydroxytryptamine and 5-hydroxytryptamin-ergic-dopaminergic interactions in the ventral tegmental area of rat brain. *Journal of Pharmacy and Pharmacology* **34**, 591–593.

Beckstead, R.M. (1979) An autoradiographic examination of corticocortical and subcortical projections of the medialdorsal-projection (prefrontal) cortex in the rat. *Journal of Comparative Neurology* **184**, 43–62.

Beninato, M. and Spencer, R.F. (1988) The cholinergic innervation of the rat substantia nigra: a light and electron microscopic immunohistochemical study. *Experimental Brain Research* **72**, 178–184.

Berger, B., Tassin, J.P., Blanc, F., Moyne, M.A. and Thierry, A.M. (1974) Histochemical confirmation for dopaminergic innervation of the rat cerebral cortex after destruction of the noradrenergic ascending pathway. *Brain Research* **81**, 332–337.

Björklund, A. and Lindvall, O. (1985) Dopamine-containing systems in the CNS. In: Björklund, A. and Hökfelt, T. (eds) *Handbook of Chemical Neuroanatomy Vol. 2, Part 1.* Amsterdam: Elsevier, pp. 55–122.

Bouthenet, M.-L., Martres, M.-P., Sales, N. and Schwartz, J.-C. (1987) A detailed mapping of dopamine D-2 receptors in rat central nervous system by autoradiography with [^{125}I]Iodosulpiride. *Neuroscience* **20**, 117–155.

Bradberry, C.W. and Roth, R.H. (1989) Cocaine increases extracellular dopamine in rat nucleus accumbens and ventral tegmental area as shown by *in vivo* microdialysis. *Neuroscience Letters* **103**, 97–102.

Braun, A.R. and Chase, T.N. (1986) Obligatory D1-D2 receptor coactivation and the generation of dopamine agonist related behaviors. *European Journal of Pharmacology* **131**, 301–306.

Breese, G.R. and Mueller, R.A. (1985) SCH 23390 antagonism of a D-2 agonist depends upon catecholaminergic neurons. *European Journal of Pharmacology* **113**, 109–114.

Brodie, M.S. and Dunwiddie, T.V. (1987) Cholecystokinin potentiates dopamine inhibition of mesenchephalic dopamine neurons in vitro. *Brain Research* **425**, 106–113.

Bunney, B.S. and Aghajanian, G.K. (1978) d-Amphetamine-induced depression of central dopamine neurons: evidence for mediation by both autoreceptors and a striatal-nigral feedback pathway. *Naunyn-Schmiedeberg's Archives de Pharmacologie* **304**, 255–261.

Bunney, B.S., Aghajanian, G.K. and Roth, R.H. (1973a) Comparison of effects of L-DOPA, amphetamine and apomorphine on firing rate of rat dopaminergic neurons. *Nature New Biology* **245**, 123–125.

Bunney, B.S., Walters, J.R., Roth, R.H. and Aghajanian, G.K. (1973b) Dopaminergic neurons: effect of antipsychotic drugs and amphetamine on single cell activity. *Journal of Pharmacology and Experimental Therapeutics* **185**, 560–571.

Calabresi, P., Mercuri, N., Stanzione, P., Stefani, A. and Bernardi, G. (1987) Intracellular studies on the dopamine-induced firing inhibition of neostriatal neurons *in vitro*: evidence for D1 receptor involvement. *Neuroscience* **20**, 757–771.

Calabresi, P., Benedetti, M., Mercuri, N.B. and Bernardi, G. (1988) Endogenous dopamine and dopaminergic agonists modulate synaptic excitation in neostriatum:

intracellular studies from naive and catecholamine-depleted rats. *Neuroscience* **27**, 145–157.

Calabresi, P., Lacey, M.G. and North, R.A. (1989) Nicotinic excitation of rat ventral tegmental neurones in vitro studied by intracellular recording. *British Journal of Pharmacology* **98**, 135–140.

Carboni, E., Acquas, E. and Di Chiara, G. (1989) Evidence for a 5-HT-DA interaction in the mesolimbic system. *Behavioural Pharmacology* **1**, 8 (suppl).

Carlson, J.H., Bergstrom, D.A. and Walters, J.R. (1986) Neurophysiological evidence that D-1 dopamine receptor blockade attenuates postsynaptic but not autoreceptor-mediated effects of dopamine agonists. *European Journal of Pharmacology* **23**, 237–251.

Carlson, J.H., Bergstrom, D.A. and Walters, J.R. (1987a) Stimulation of both D-1 and D-2 dopamine receptors appears necessary for full expression of postsynaptic effects of dopamine agonists: a neurophysiological study. *Brain Research* **400**, 205–218.

Carlson, J.H., Bergstrom, D.A., Weick, B.G. and Walters, J.R. (1987b) Neurophysiological investigation of effects of the D-1 agonist SKF 38393 on tonic activity of subtantia nigra dopamine neurons. *Synapse* **1**, 411–416.

Carlsson, A., Falck, B. and Hillarp, N.-Å. (1962) Cellular localization of brain monoamines. *Acta Physiologica Scandinavica* 1–27 (suppl) **196**.

Charuchinda, C., Supavilai, P., Karobath, M. and Palacios, J.M. (1987) Dopamine D_2 receptors in the rat brain: autoradiographic visualization using a high-affinity selective agonist ligand. *Journal of Neuroscience* **7**, 1352–1360.

Chiodo, L.A. and Bunney, B.S. (1984) Effects of dopamine antagonists on midbrain dopamine cell activity. In: Usdin, E., Carlsson, A., Dahlström, A. and Engel, J. (eds) *Catecholamines: Neuropharmacology and Central Nervous System—Theoretical Aspects*. New York: Alan R. Liss Inc., pp. 369–391.

Chiodo, L.A., Bannon, M.J., Grace, A.A., Roth, R.H. and Bunney, B.S. (1984) Evidence for the absence of impulse-regulating somatodendritic and synthesis-modulating nerve terminal autoreceptors on subpopulations of mesocortical dopamine neurons. *Neuroscience* **12**, 1–16.

Chiodo, L.A., Freeman, A.S. and Bunney, B.S. (1987) Electrophysiological studies on the specificity of the cholecystokinin receptor antagonist proglumide. *Brain Research* **410**, 205–211.

Chneiweiss, H., Glowinski, J. and Premont, J. (1988) Mu and delta opiate receptors coupled negatively to adenylate cyclase on embryonic neurons from the mouse striatum in primary cultures. *Journal of Neuroscience* **8**, 3376–3382.

Christie, M.J., Bridge, S., James, L.B. and Bear, P.M. (1985) Excitotoxin lesions suggest an aspartatergic projection from rat medial prefrontal cortex to ventral tegmental area. *Brain Research* **333**, 169–172.

Christoph, G.R., Leonzio, R.J. and Wilcox, K.S. (1986) Stimulation of the lateral habenula inhibits dopamine-containing neurons in the substantia nigra and ventral tegmental area of the rat. *Journal of Neuroscience* **6**, 613–619.

Clark, D. and Chiodo, L.A. (1988) Electrophysiological and pharmacological characterization of identified nigrostriatal and mesoaccumbens dopamine neurons in the rat. *Synapse* **2**, 474–485.

Clark, D. and White, F.J. (1987) Review: D1 dopamine receptor—the search for a function: a critical evaluation of the D1/D2 dopamine receptor classification and its functional implications. *Synapse* **1**, 347–388.

Clarke, P.B.S., Hommer, D.W., Pert, A. and Skirboll, L.R. (1987) Innervation of substantia nigra neurons by cholinergic afferents from pedunculopontine nucleus in the rat: neuroanatomical and electrophysiological evidence. *Neuroscience* **23**, 1011–1019.

Collingridge, G.L. and Davies, J. (1981) The influence of striatal stimulation and putative neurotransmitters on identified neurons in rat substantia nigra. *Brain Research* **212**, 345–360.

Creese, I. (1987) Biochemical properties of CNS dopamine receptors. In: Meltzer, H.Y. (ed.) *Psychopharmacology: The Third Generation of Progress.* New York: Raven Press, pp. 257–264.

Dahlström, A. and Fuxe, K. (1964) Evidence for the existence of monoamine containing neurons in the central nervous system. I. Demonstration of monoamines in the cell bodies of brain stem neurons. *Acta Physiologica Scandinavica* **232**, 1–55 (suppl 62).

Dawson, T.M., Gehlert, D.R., McCabe, R.T., Barnett, A. and Wamsley, J.K. (1986) D-1 dopamine receptors in the rat brain: a quantitative autoradiographic analysis. *Journal of Neuroscience* **6**, 2352–2365.

Deniau, J.M., Thierry, A.M. and Feger, J. (1980) Electrophysiological identification of mesencephalic ventromedial tegmental (VMT) neurons projecting to the frontal cortex, septum and nucleus accumbens. *Brain Research* **189**, 315–326.

Dray, A. and Straughan, D.W. (1976) Synaptic mechanisms in the substantia nigra. *Journal of Pharmacy and Pharmacology* **28**, 400–405.

Dray, A., Goyne, T.J., Oakley, N.R. and Tanner, T. (1976) Evidence for the existence of a raphe projection to the substantia nigra in the rat. *Brain Research* **113**, 45–47.

Dubois, A., Savasta, M., Curet, O. and Scatton, B. (1986) Autoradiographic distribution of the D_1 agonist [^{3}H]SKF 38393, in the rat brain and spinal cord. Comparison with the distribution of D_2 dopamine receptors. *Neuroscience* **19**, 125–137.

Einhorn, L.C., Johansen, P.A. and White, F.J. (1988) Electrophysiological effects of cocaine in the mesoaccumbens dopamine system: studies in the ventral tegmental area. *Journal of Neuroscience* **8**, 100–112.

Fibiger, H.C. and Miller, J.J. (1977) An anatomical and electrophysiological investigation of the serotonergic projection from the dorsal raphe nucleus to the substantia nigra in the rat. *Neuroscience* **2**, 975–987.

Finnerty, E.P. and Chan, S.H.H. (1979) Morphine suppression of substantia nigra zona reticulata neurons in the rat: implicated role for a novel striatonigral feedback mechanism. *European Journal of Pharmacology* **59**, 307–310.

Fonnum, F., Gottesfeld, Z. and Grofová, I. (1978) Distribution of glutamate decarboxylase, choline acetyl-transferase, and aromatic amino acid decarboxylase in the basal ganglia of normal and operated rats. Evidence for striatopallidal, striatoentopeduncular and striatonigral gabaergic fibers. *Brain Research* **143**, 125–138.

Freedman, J.E. and Weight, F.F. (1988) Single K^+ channels activated by D2 dopamine receptors in acutely dissociated neurons form rat corpus striatum. *Proceedings of the National Academy of Science* **85**, 3618–3622.

Freeman, A.S. and Bunney, B.S. (1987) Activity of A9 and A10 dopaminergic neurons in unrestrained rats: further characterization and effects of apomorphine and cholecystokinin. *Brain Research* **405**, 46–55.

Freeman, A.S. and Chiodo, L.A. (1987) Electrophysiological aspects of cholecystokin-in/dopamine interactions in the central nervous system. In: Chiodo, L.A. and Freeman, A.S. (eds) *Neurophysiology of Dopaminergic Systems—Current Status and Clinical Perspectives.* Detroit: Lakeshore Publishing Co., 205–236.

Freund, T.F., Powell, J.F. and Smith, A.D. (1984) Tyrosine hydroxylase-immunoreactive boutons in synaptic contact with identified striatonigral neurons, with particular reference to dendritic spines. *Neuroscience* **13**, 1189–1215.

Galloway, M.P., Wolf, M.E. and Roth, R.H. (1986) Regulation of dopamine synthesis in the medial prefrontal cortex is mediated by release nodulating autoreceptors: studies in vivo. *Journal of Pharmacology and Experimental Therapeutics* **236**, 689–698.

Gariano, R.F. and Groves, P.M. (1988) Burst firing induced in midbrain dopamine neurons by stimulation of the medial prefrontal and anterior cingulate cortices. *Brain Research* **462**, 194–198.

Gariano, R.F., Tepper, J.M., Sawyer, S.F., Young, S.J. and Groves, P.M. (1989) Mesocortical dopamine neurons. 1. Electrophysiological properties and evidence for soma-dentritic autoreceptors. *Brain Research Bulletin* **22**, 511–516.

German, D.C., Dalsass, M. and Kiser, R.S. (1980) Electrophysiological examination of the ventral tegmental (A10) area in the rat. *Brain Research* **181**, 191–197.

Gershanik, O., Heikkila, R.E. and Duvoisin, R.C. (1983) Behavioral correlates of dopamine receptor activation. *Neurology* **33**, 1489–1492.

Gonon, F.G. (1988) Nonlinear relationship between impulse flow and dopamine released by rat midbrain dopaminergic neurons as studied by in vivo electrochemistry. *Neuroscience* **24**, 19–28.

Grace, A.A. and Bunney, B.S. (1979) Paradoxical GABA excitation of nigral dopaminergic cells: indirect mediation through reticulata inhibitory neurons. *European Journal of Pharmacology* **59**, 211–219.

Grace, A.A. and Bunney, B.S. (1984a) The control of firing pattern in nigral dopamine neurons: single spike firing. *Journal of Neuroscience* **4**, 2866–2876.

Grace, A.A. and Bunney, B.S. (1984b) The control of firing pattern in nigral dopamine neurons: burst firing. *Journal of Neuroscience* **4**, 2877–2890.

Grace, A.A. and Bunney, B.S. (1985) Opposing effects of striatonigral feedback pathways on midbrain dopamine cell activity. *Brain Research* **333**, 271–284.

Graetrex, R.M. and Phillipson, O.T. (1982) Demonstration of synaptic input from prefrontal cortex to the habenula in the rat. *Brain Research* **238**, 192–197.

Grenhoff, J. and Svensson, T.H. (1988) The alpha-2 agonist clonidine regularizes substantia nigra dopamine cell firing. *Life Science* **42**, 2003–2008.

Grenhoff, J. and Svensson, T.H. (1989) Clonidine modulates dopamine cell firing in rat ventral tegmental area. *European Journal of Pharmacology* **165**, 11–18.

Grenhoff, J., Aston-Jones, G. and Svensson, T.H. (1986) Nicotinic effects on the firing pattern of midbrain dopamine neurons. *Acta Physiologica Scandinavica* **128**, 351–358.

Groves, P.M., Wilson, C.J., Young, S.J. and Rebec, G.V. (1975) Self-inhibition by dopaminergic neurons. *Science* **210**, 654–656.

Gundlach, A.L., McDonald, D. and Beart, P.M. (1982) [³H]Spiperone labels non-cyclase-linked dopamine receptors in the ventral tegmental area of rat brain. *Journal of Neurochemistry* **39**, 890–894.

Guyenet, P.G. and Aghajanian, G.K. (1978) Antidromic identification of dopaminergic and other output neurons of the rat substantia nigra. *Brain Research* **150**, 69–84.

Gysling, K. and Wang, R.Y. (1983) Morphine-induced activation of A10 dopamine neurons in the rat. *Brain Research* **277**, 119–127.

Hand, T.H., Hu, X.-T. and Wang, R.Y. (1987) Differential effects of acute clozapine and haloperidol on the activity of ventral tegmental (A10) and nigrostriatal (A9) dopamine neurons. *Brain Research* **415**, 257–269.

Heimer, L. and Wilson, R.D. (1975) The subcortical projections of the allocortex: similarities in the neural associations of the hippocampus, the piriform cortex and the neocortex. In: Santini, M. (ed.) *Golgi Centennial Symposium Proceedings.* New York: Raven, pp. 177–193.

Henry, D.J., Greene, M.A. and White, F.J. (1989) Electrophysiological effects of cocaine in the mesoaccumbens dopamine system: repeated administration. *Journal of Pharmacology and Experimental Therapeutics* **251**, 833–839.

Herkenham, M. and Nauta, W.J. (1977) Efferent connections of the habenular nuclei in the rat. *Journal of Comparative Neurology* **187**, 19–48.

Hervé, D., Pickel, V.M., Joh, T.H. and Beaudet, A. (1987) Serotonin axon terminals in the ventral tegmental area of the rat: fine structure and synaptic input to dopaminergic neurons. *Brain Research* **435**, 71–83.

Hökfelt, T.A. and Ungerstedt, U. (1973) Specificity of 6-hydroxydopamine induced degeneration of central monoamine neurons: an electron and fluorescence microscopic study with special reference to intracerebral injection on the nigro-striatal dopamine system. *Brain Research* **60**, 269–297.

Hökfelt, T., Ljungdahl, A., Fuxe, K. and Johansson, O. (1974) Dopamine nerve terminals in the limbic cortex: aspects of the dopamine hypothesis of schizophrenia. *Science* **184**, 177–179.

Hökfelt, T., Skirboll, L., Rehfeld, J.F., Goldstein, M., Markey, K. and Dann, O. (1980) A subpopulation of mesenchephalic dopamine neurons projecting to limbic area contains a cholecystokinin-like peptide: evidence from immunohistochemistry combined with retrograde tracing. *Neuroscience* **5**, 2093–2124.

Hommer, D.W. and Pert, A. (1983) The actions of opioids in the rat substantia nigra: an electrophysiological analysis. *Peptides* **4**, 603–608.

Hommer, D.W. and Skirboll, L.R. (1983) Cholecystokinin-like peptides potentiate apomorphine-induced inhibition of dopamine neurons. *European Journal of Pharmacology* **91**, 151–152.

Hytell, J. (1983) SCH-23390—The first selective dopamine D-1 antagonist. *European Journal of Pharmacology* **91**, 153–154.

Imperato, A. and Angelucci, L. (1989) 5-HT$_3$ receptors control dopamine release in the nucleus accumbens of freely moving rats. *Neuroscience Letters* **101**, 214–217.

Innis, R.B. and Aghajanian, G.K. (1987) Pertussis toxin blocks autoreceptor-mediated inhibition of dopaminergic neurons in rat substantia nigra. *Brain Research* **411**, 139–143.

Iorio, L.C., Barnett, A., Leitz, F.H., Houser, V.P. and Korduba, C.A. (1983) SCH 23390, a potential benzazepine antipsychotic with unique interactions on dopaminergic systems. *Journal of Pharmacology and Experimental Therapeutics* **226**, 462–468.

Iwatsubo, K. and Clouet, D.H. (1977) Effects of morphine and haloperidol on the electrical activity of rat nigrostriatal neurons. *Journal of Pharmacology and Experimental Therapeutics* **202**, 429–436.

Jackson, D.M. and Hashizume, M. (1986) Bromocriptine induces marked locomotor stimulation in dopamine-depleted mice when D-1 dopamine receptors are stimulated with SKF38393. *Psychopharmacology* **90**, 147–149.

Jeziorski, M. and White, F.J. (1989) Electrophysiological effects of selective opiate receptor agonists on A10 dopamine (DA) neurons. *Society for Neuroscience Abstracts* **15**, 1001.

Johansen, P.A. and White, F.J. (1988) D1/D2 dopamine receptor interactions in the nucleus accumbens: the role of cAMP in electrophysiological responses. *Society for Neuroscience Abstracts* **14**, 931.

Johansen, P.A., Clark, D. and White, F.J. (1988) B-HT 920 stimulates postsynaptic D2 dopamine receptors in the normal rat: electrophysiological and behavioral evidence. *Life Science* **43**, 515–524.

Kalivas, P.W., Bourdelais, A., Abhold, R. and Abbott, L. (1989) Somatodendritic release of endogenous dopamine: in vivo dialysis in the A10 dopamine region. *Neuroscience Letters* **100**, 215–220.

Kebabian, J.W. and Calne, D.B. (1979) Multiple receptors for dopamine. *Nature* **277**, 93–96.

Kehr, W. (1974) Temporal changes in catecholamine synthesis of rat forebrain structures following axotomy. *Journal of Neural Transmission* **35**, 307–317.

Kelly, E. and Nahorski, S.R. (1986) Specific inhibition of dopamine D-1 mediated cyclic AMP formation by dopamine D-2, muscarinic cholinergic, and opiate receptor stimulation in striatal slices. *Journal of Neurochemistry* **47**, 1512–1516.

Kelly, E. and Nahorski, S.R. (1987) Dopamine D-2 receptors inhibit D-1 stimulated cyclic AMP accumulation in striatum but not limbic forebrain. *Naunyn-Schmiedeberg's Archives de Pharmacologie* **335**, 508–512.

Kondo, Y. and Iwatsubo, K. (1980) Diminished responses of nigral dopaminergic neurons to haloperidol and morphine following lesions of the striatum. *Brain Research* **181**, 237–240.

Korf, J., Zieleman, M. and Westerink, B.H.C. (1976) Dopamine release in the substantia nigra? *Nature* **260**, 257–258.

Lacey, M.G., Mercuri, N.B. and North, R.A. (1987) Dopamine acts of D_2 receptors to increase potassium conductance in neurones of the rat substantia nigra zona compacta. *Journal of Physiology (Lond.)* **392**, 397–416.

Lacey, M.G., Mercuri, N.B. and North, R.A. (1988) On the potassium conductance increase activated by $GABA_B$ and dopamine D2 receptors in rat substantia nigra neurons. *Journal of Physiology (Lond.)* **410**, 437–453.

Lacey, M.G., Mercuri, N.B. and North, R.A. (1989) Two cell types in rat substantia nigra zona compacta distinguished by membrane properties and the actions of dopamine and opioids. *Journal of Neuroscience* **9**, 1233–1241.

Last, A.T.J. and Greenfield, S.A. (1987) Neuroleptic-induced changes in the firing pattern of guinea pig nigrostriatal neurons. *Experimental Brain Research* **66**, 394–400.

Lichtensteiger, W., Hefti, F., Felix, D., Huwyler, T., Melamed, E. and Schlumpf, M. (1982) Stimulation of nigrostriatal dopamine neurones by nicotine. *Neuropharmacology* **21**, 963–968.

Lindvall, O., Björkland, A., Moore, R.Y. and Stenevi, U. (1974) Mesencephalic dopamine neurons projecting to neocortex. *Brain Research* **81**, 325–331.

Longoni, R., Spina, L. and Di Chiara, G. (1987a) Permissive role of D-1 receptor stimulation by endogenous dopamine for the expression of postsynaptic D-2-mediated behavioural responses. Yawning in rats. *European Journal of Pharmacology* **134**, 163–173.

Longoni, R., Spina, L. and Di Chiara, G. (1987b) Permissive role of D-1 receptor stimulation for the expression of D-2 mediated behavioral responses: a quantitative phenomenological study in rats. *Life Science* **41**, 2135–2145.

Lorez, H.P. and Burkard, W.P (1979) Absence of dopamine sensitive adenylate cyclase in the A10 region, the origin of mesolimbic dopamine neurons. *Experientia* **35**, 744–746.

Maeda, H. and Mogenson, G.J. (1980) An electrophysiological study of inputs to neurons of the ventral tegmental area from the nucleus accumbens and medial preoptic-anterior hypothalamic areas. *Brain Research* **197**, 365–377.

Maeda, H. and Mogenson, G.J. (1981a) A comparison of the effects of electrical stimulation of the lateral and ventromedial hypothalamus on the activity of neurons in ventral tegmental area and substantia nigra. *Brain Research Bulletin* **7**, 283–291.

Maeda, H. and Mogenson, G.J. (1981b) Electrophysiological responses of neurons of the ventral tegmental area to electrical stimulation of amygdala and lateral septum. *Neuroscience* **6**, 367–376.

Mailman, R.B., Schultz, D.W., Lewis, M.H., Staples, L., Rollema, H. and Dehaven, D.L. (1984) SCH 23390: a selective D1 dopamine antagonist with potent D2 behavioural actions. *European Journal of Pharmacology* **101**, 159–160.

Mantz, J., Thierry, A.M. and Glowinski, J. (1989) Effect of noxious tail pinch on the discharge rate of mesocortical and mesolimbic dopamine neurons: selective activation of the mesocortical system. *Brain Research* **476**, 377–381.

Mashurano, M. and Waddington, J.L. (1986) Stereotyped behavior in response to the selective D-2 dopamine receptor agonist RU 24213 is enhanced by pretreatment with the selective D-1 agonist SKF 38393. *Neuropharmacology* **25**, 947–949.

Matthews, R.T. and German, D.C. (1984) Electrophysiological evidence for excitation of rat ventral tegmental area dopamine neurons by morphine. *Neuroscience* **11**, 617–625.

Meller, E., Bordi, F. and Bohmaker, K. (1988) Enhancement by the D1 dopamine agonist SKF 38393 of specific components of stereotypy elicited by the D2 agonists LY 171555 and RU 24213. *Life Science* **42**, 2561–2567.

Mereu, G., Yoon, K.-W.P., Boi, V., Gessa, G.L., Naes, L. and Westfall, T.C. (1987) Preferential stimulation of ventral tegmental area dopaminergic neurons by nicotine. *European Journal of Pharmacology* **141**, 395–399.

Molloy, A.G. and Waddington, J.L. (1984) Dopaminergic behavior stereospecifically promoted by the D-1 agonist R-SKF-38393 and selectively blocked by the D-1 antagonist SCH-23390. *Psychopharmacology* **82**, 409–410.

Molloy, A.G. and Waddington, J.L. (1985) The enantiomers of SKF 83556, a new selective D-1 dopamine receptor antagonist, stereospecifically block stereotyped behavior induced by apomorphine and by the selective D-2 agonist RU 24213. *European Journal of Pharmacology* **116**, 183–186.

Molloy, A.G. and Waddington, J.L. (1987a) Assessment of grooming and other behavioural responses to the D-1 dopamine receptor agonist SK & F 38393 and its R- and S-enantiomers in the intact adult rat. *Psychopharmacology* **92**, 164–168.

Molloy, A.G. and Waddington, J.L. (1987b) Pharmacological characterization in the rat of grooming and other behavioural responses to the D1 dopamine receptor agonist R-SK&F 38393. *Journal of Psychopharmacology* **1**, 177–183.

Moore, N.A. and Axton, M.S. (1988) Production of climbing behavior in mice requires both D1 and D2 receptor activation. *Psychopharmacology* **94**, 263–266.

Morelli, M., Mennini, T. and Di Chiara, G. (1988) Nigral dopamine autoreceptors are exclusively of the D_2 type: quantitative autoradiography of $[^{125}I]$Iodosulpiride and $[^{125}I]$SCH 23982 in adjacent brain sections. *Neuroscience* **27**, 865–870.

Mueller, A.L. and Brodie, M.S. (1989) Intracellular recording from putative dopamine-containing neurons in the ventral tegmental area of Tsai in a brain slice preparation. *Journal of Neuroscience Methods* **28**, 15–22.

Nagy, J.I., Vincent, S.R., Lehmann, J., Fibiger, H.C. and McGeer, E.G. (1978) The use of kainic acid in the localization of enzymes in the substantia nigra. *Brain Research* **149**, 431–441.

Nauta, W.J.H., Smith, G.P., Faull, R.L.M. and Domesick, V.B. (1978) Efferent connections and nigral afferents of the nucleus accumbens septi in the rat. *Neuroscience* **3**, 385–401.

Niijima, K. and Yoshida, M. (1988) Activation of mesenchephalic dopamine neurons by chemical stimulation of the nucleus tegmenti pedunculopontinus pars compacta. *Brain Research* **451**, 163–171.

O'Brien, D.P. and White, F.J. (1987) Inhibition of non-dopamine cells in the ventral tegmental area by benzodiazepines: relationship to A10 dopamine cell activity. *European Journal of Pharmacology* **142**, 343–354.

Onali, P., Olianas, M.C. and Gessa, G.L. (1985) Characterization of dopamine receptors mediating inhibition of adenylate cyclase activity in rat striatum. *Molecular Pharmacology* **28**, 138–145.

Pan, H.S. and Walters, J.R. (1988) Unilateral lesion of the nigrostriatal pathway decreases the firing rate of globus pallidus neurons in the rat. *Synapse* **2**, 650–656.

Pan, H.S., Bergstrom, D.A., Carlson, J.H., Engber, T.M., Chase, T.N. and Walters, J.R. (1987) Apomorphine's effects on the activity of globus pallidus neurons are related to rotational behavior in rats with unilateral quinolinic acid lesions of the striatum. *Society for Neuroscience Abstracts* **13**, 489.

Peterson, S.L., St. Mary, J.S. and Harding, N.R. (1987) Cis-flupenthixol antagonism of the rat prefrontal cortex neuronal response to apomorphine and ventral tegmental area input. *Brain Research Bulletin* **18**, 723–729.

Phillipson, O.T. (1979) Afferent projections to the ventral tegmental area of Tsai and interfascicular nucleus: a horseradish peroxidase study in the rat. *Journal of Comparative Neurology* **187**, 117–144.

Phillipson, O.T. and Griffith, A.C. (1980) The neurones of origin for the mesohabenular dopamine pathway. *Brain Research* **197**, 213–218.

Pinnock, R.D. (1983) Sensitivity of compacta neurones in the rat substantia nigra slice to dopamine agonists. *European Journal of Pharmacology* **96**, 269–276.

Pinnock, R.D. (1984a) Hyperpolarizing action of baclofen on neurons in the rat substantia nigra slice. *Brain Research* **322**, 337–340.

Pinnock, R.D. (1984b) The actions of antipsychotic drugs on dopamine receptors in the rat substantia nigra. *British Journal of Pharmacology* **81**, 631–635.

Pinnock, R.D. and Dray, A. (1982) Differential sensitivity of presumed dopaminergic and non-dopaminergic neurones in rat substantia nigra to electrophoretically applied substance P. *Neuroscience Letters* **29**, 153–158.

Pugh, M.T., O'Boyle, K.M., Molloy, A.G. and Waddington, J.L. (1985) Effects of the putative D-1 antagonist SCH 23390 on stereotyped behaviour induced by the D-2 agonist RU24213. *Psychopharmacology* **87**, 308–312.

Robertson, G.S. and Robertson, H.A. (1986) Synergistic effects of D1 and D2 dopamine agonists on turning behaviour in rats. *Brain Research* **384**, 387–390.

Robertson, G.S. and Robertson, H.A. (1987) D1 and D2 dopamine agonist synergism: separate sites of action? *Trends in Pharmacological Sciences* **8**, 295–299.

Ross, R.J., Waszczak, B.L., Lee, E.K. and Walters, J.R. (1982) Effects of benzodiazepines on single unit activity in the substantia nigra pars reticulata. *Life Science* **31**, 1025–1033.

Savasta, M., Dubois, A. and Scatton, B. (1986) Autoradiographic localization of D1 dopamine receptors in rat brain with [^{3}H]SCH 23390. *Brain Research* **375**, 291–301.

Scarnati, E., Proia, A., Campana, E. and Pacitti, C. (1986) A microiontophoretic study on the nature of the putative synaptic transmitter involved in the pedunculopontine-substantia nigra pars compacta excitatory pathway of the rat. *Experimental Brain Research* **62**, 470–478.

Scatton, B., Simon, H., Le Moal, M. and Bischoff, S. (1980) Origin of dopaminergic innervation of the rat hippocampal formation. *Neuroscience Letters* **18**, 125–131.

Sesack, S.R. and Bunney, B.S. (1989) Pharmacological characterization of the receptor mediating electrophysiological responses to dopamine in the rat medial prefrontal cortex: a microiontophoretic study. *Journal of Pharmacology and Experimental Therapeutics* **248**, 1323–1333.

Setler, P.E., Saran, H.M., Zirkle, C.L. and Saunders, H.L. (1978) The central effects of a novel dopamine agonist. *European Journal of Pharmacology* **50**, 419–430.

Shepard, P.D. and Bunney, B.S. (1988) Effects of apamin on the discharge properties of putative dopamine-containing neurons in vitro. *Brain Research* **463**, 380–384.

Shepard, P.D. and German, D.C. (1984) A subpopulation of mesocortical dopamine neurons possess autoreceptors. *European Journal of Pharmacology* **114**, 401–402.

Sibley, D.R., Leff, S.D. and Creese, I. (1982) Interactions of novel dopaminergic ligands with D-1 and D-2 dopamine receptors. *Life Science* **31**, 637–645.

Silva, N.L. and Bunney, B.S. (1988) Intracellular studies of dopamine neurons in vitro: pacemakers modulated by dopamine. *European Journal of Pharmacology* **149**, 307–315.

Skirboll, L.R., Grace, A.A., Hommer, D.W., Rehfeld, J., Goldstein, M., Hökfelt, T. and Bunney, B.S. (1981) Peptide-monoamine coexistence: studies of the actions of cholecystokinin-like peptide on the electrical activity of midbrain dopamine neurons. *Neuroscience* **6**, 2111–2124.

Sonsalla, P.K., Manzino, L. and Heikkila, R.E. (1988) Interactions of D1 and D2 dopamine receptors on the ipsilateral *vs.* contralateral side in rats with unilateral lesions of the dopaminergic nigrostriatal pathway. *Journal of Pharmacology and Experimental Therapeutics* **247**, 180–185.

Sorenson, S.M., Humphreys, T.M. and Palfreyman, M.G. (1989) Effect of acute and chronic MDL 73,147EF, a 5-HT$_3$ receptor antagonist, on A9 and A10 dopamine neurons. *European Journal of Pharmacology* **163**, 115–118.

Staines, W.A., Nagy, J.I., Vincent, S.R. and Fibiger, H.C. (1980) Neurotransmitters contained in efferents of the striatum. *Brain Research* **194**, 391–402.

Starr, B.S. and Starr, M.S. (1986a) Differential effects of dopamine D1 and D2 agonists and antagonists on velocity of movement, rearing and grooming in the mouse. *Neuropharmacology* **25**, 455–463.

Starr, B.S. and Starr, M.S. (1986b) Grooming in the mouse is stimulated by the dopamine D1 agonist SKF 38393 and by low doses of the D1 antagonist SCH 23390, but is inhibited by dopamine D2 agonists, D2 antagonists and high doses of SCH 23390. *Pharmacology Biochemistry and Behavior* **24**, 837–839.

Starr, B.S., Starr, M.S. and Kilpatrick, I.C. (1987) Behavioral role of dopamine D$_1$ receptors in the reserpine-treated mouse. *Neuroscience* **22**, 179–188.

Steinbusch, H.W.M. (1981) Distribution of serotonin-immunoreactivity in the central nervous system of the rat. Cell bodies and terminals. *Neuroscience* **6**, 557–618.

Stoof, J.C. and Kebabian, J.W. (1981) Opposing roles for D-1 and D-2 domamine receptors in efflux of cyclic AMP from rat neostriatum. *Nature* **294**, 366–368.

Stoof, J.C. and Verheijden, P.F.H.M. (1986) D-2 receptor stimulation inhibits cyclic AMP formation brought about by D-1 receptor stimulation in rat neostriatum but not nucleus accumbens. *European Journal of Pharmacology* **129**, 205–206.

Svensson, T.H., Bunney, B.S. and Aghajanian, G.K. (1975) Inhibition of both noradrenergic and serotonergic neurons in brain by the α-adrenergic agonist clonidine. *Brain Research* **92**, 291–306.

Swanson, L.W. and Cowan, W.M. (1975) A note on the connections and development of the nucleus accumbens. *Brain Research* **92**, 324–330.

Tepper, J.M., Nakamura, S., Spanis, C.W., Squire, L.R. and Groves, P.M. (1982)

Subsensitivity of catecholaminergic neurons to direct acting agonists after single or repeated electroconvulsive shock. *Biological Psychiatry* **17**, 1059–1070.

Thierry, A.M., Deniau, J.M. and Feger, J. (1979) Effects of stimulation of the frontal cortex on identified output VMT cells in the rat. *Neuroscience Letters* **15**, 103–107.

Thierry, A.M., Chevalier, G., Ferron, A. and Glowinski, J. (1983) Dienchephalic and mesenchephalic efferents of the medial prefrontal cortex in the rat: electrophysiological evidence for the existence of branched neurons. *Experimental Brain Research* **50**, 275–282.

Titus, R.D., Kornfeld, E.C., Jones, N.D., Clemens, J.A., Fuller, R.W., Hahn, R.A., Hynes, M.D., Mason, N.R., Wong, D.T. and Foreman, M.M. (1983) Resolution and absolute configuration of an ergoline-related dopamine agonist trans-4,4a,5,6,7,8,8a,9-octahydro-5-propyl-iH(or2H)pyrazolo(3,4-g)quinoline. *Journal of Medical Chemistry* **26**, 1112–1116.

Tsuruta, K., Frey, E.A., Grewe, C.W., Cote, T.E., Eskay, R.L. and Kebabian, J.W. (1981) Evidence that LY-141865 specifically stimulates the D-2 dopamine receptor. *Nature* **292**, 463–465.

Ungerstedt, U. (1971) Stereotaxic mapping of the monoamine pathways in the rat brain. *Acta Physiologica Scandinavica* **367**, 1–48 (suppl).

Ushijima, I., Mizuki, Y. and Yamada, M. (1988) The mode of action of bromocriptine following pretreatment with reserpine and α-methyl-p-tryosine in rat. *Psychopharmacology* **95**, 29–33.

Vasse, M., Chagraoui, A. and Protrais, P. (1988) Climbing and stereotyped behaviours in mice require the sitmulation of D-1 dopamine receptors. *European Journal of Pharmacology* **148**, 221–229.

Wachtel, S.R., Hu, X.-T., Galloway, M.P. and White, F.J. (1989) D1 dopamine receptor stimulation enables the postsynaptic, but not autoreceptor, effects of D2 dopamine agonists in nigrostriatal and mesoaccumbens dopamine systems. *Synapse* **4**, 327–346.

Waddington, J.L. and Cross, A.L. (1978) Neurochemical changes following kainic acid lesions of the nucleus accumbens: implications for a GABAergic accumbal-ventral tegmental pathway. *Life Science* **22**, 1011–1014.

Waddington, J.L. and O'Boyle, K.M. (1987) The D-1 dopamine receptor and the search for its functional role: from neurochemistry to behavior. *Reviews in Neuroscience* **1**, 157–184.

Walaas, I. and Fonnum, F. (1980) Biochemical evidence for gamma-aminobutyrate containing fibers from the nucleus accumbens to the substantia nigra and ventral tegmental area in the rat. *Neuroscience* **5**, 63–72.

Walaas, S.I. and Greengard, P. (1984) DARPP-32, a dopamine- and adenosine 3':5'-monophosphate-regulated phosphoprotein enriched in dopamine-innervated brain regions. I. Regional and cellular distribution in the rat brain. *Journal of Neuroscience* **4**, 84–98.

Waldmeier, P.C., Ortmann, R. and Bischoff, S. (1982) Modulation of dopaminergic transmission by alpha-noradrenergic agonists and antagonists: evidence for antidopaminergic properties of some alpha antagonists. *Experientia* **38**, 1168–1176.

Walker, J.M., Thompson, L.A., Frascella, J. and Friedrich, M.W. (1987) Opposite effects of μ and κ opiates on the firing-rate of dopamine cells in the substantia nigra of the rat. *European Journal of Pharmacology* **134**, 53–59.

Walters, J.R., Bergstrom, D.A., Carlson, J.H., Chase, T.N. and Braun, A.R. (1987) D1 dopamine receptor activation required for postsynaptic expression of D2 agonist effects. *Science* **236**, 719–722.

Wang, R.Y. (1981a) Dopaminergic neurons in the rat ventral tegmental area. I. Identification and characterization. *Brain Research Reviews* **3**, 123–140.

Wang, R.Y. (1981b) Dopaminergic neurons in the rat ventral tegmental area. II. Evidence for autoregulation. *Brain Research Reviews* **3**, 141–151.

Wang, R.Y. (1981c) Dopaminergic neurons in the rat ventral tegmental area. III. Effects of d- and l-amphetamine. *Brain Research Reviews* **3**, 153–165.

Wang, R.Y., White, F.J. and Voigt, M.M. (1984) Cholecystokinin, dopamine and schizophrenia. *Trends in Pharmacological Sciences* **5**, 436–438.

Waszczak, B.L. and Walters, J.R. (1980) Intravenous GABA agonist administration stimulates firing of A10 dopaminergic neurons. *European Journal of Pharmacology* **66**, 141–144.

Waszczak, B.L., Eng, N. and Walters, J.R. (1980) Effects of muscimol and picrotoxin on single-unit activity of substantia nigra neurons. *Brain Research* **188**, 185–197.

White, F.J. (1986a) Comparative effects of LSD and lisuride: clues to specific hallucinogenic drug actions. *Pharmacology Biochemistry and Behavior* **24**, 364–379.

White, F.J. (1986b) Electrophysiological investigations of the D-1 dopamine receptor. *Clinical Neuropharmacology* **9**, 29–31.

White, F.J. (1987) D1 dopamine receptor stimulation enables the inhibition of nucleus accumbens neurons by a D2 receptor agonist. *European Journal of Pharmacology* **135**, 101–105.

White, F.J. and Wang, R.Y. (1983a) Comparison of the effects of chronic haloperidol treatment on A9 and A10 dopamine neurons in the rat. *Life Science* **32**, 983–993.

White, F.J. and Wang, R.Y. (1983b) Comparison of the effects of LSD and lisuride on A10 dopamine neurons in the rat. *Neuropharmacology* **22**, 669–676.

White, F.J. and Wang, R.Y. (1984a) A10 dopamine neurons: role of autoreceptors in determining firing rate and sensitivity to dopamine agonists. *Life Science* **34**, 1161–1170.

White, F.J. and Wang, R.Y. (1984b) Electrophysiological evidence for A10 dopamine autoreceptor subsensitivity following chronic d-amphetamine treatment. *Brain Research* **309**, 283–292.

White, F.J. and Wang, R.Y. (1984c) Electrophysiological evidence for both D-1 and D-2 dopamine receptors in the nucleus accumbens of the rat. *Abstracts of the Collegium International Neuropsychopharacologicum* **14**, 270.

White, F.J. and Wang, R.Y. (1984d) Interactions of cholecystokinin octapeptide and dopamine on nucleus accumbens neurons. *Brain Research* **300**, 161–166.

White, F.J. and Wang, R.Y. (1984e) Pharmacological characterization of dopamine autoreceptors in the rat ventral tegmental area: microiontophoretic studies. *Journal of Pharmacology and Experimental Therapeutics* **231**, 275–280.

White, F.J. and Wang, R.Y. (1985) Effects of chronic treatment with cholecystokinin (CCK) on midbrain dopamine neurons. *Annals of the New York Academy of Science* **448**, 682–685.

White, F.J. and Wang, R.Y. (1986) Electrophysiological evidence for the existence of both D-1 and D-2 dopamine receptors in the rat nucleus accumbens. *Journal of Neuroscience* **6**, 274–280.

White, F.J., Wachtel, S.R. Johansen, P.A. and Einhorn, L.C. (1987) Electrophysiological studies of the rat mesoaccumbens dopamine system: focus on dopamine receptor subtypes, interactions, and the effects of cocaine. In: Chiodo, L.A. and Freeman A.S. (eds) *Neurophysiology of Dopaminergic Systems—Current Status and Clinical Perspectives*. Detroit: Lakeshore Publishing Co., pp. 317–365.

White, F.J., Bednarz, L.M., Wachtel, S.R., Hjorth, S. and Brooderson, R.J. (1988) Is stimulation of both D1 and D2 receptors necessary for the expression of dopamine-mediated behaviors? *Pharmacology Biochemistry and Behavior* **30**, 189–193.

Wolf, P., Olpe, H.R., Avrith, D. and Haas, H.L. (1978) GABAergic inhibition of neurons in the ventral tegmental area. *Experientia* **34**, 73–74.

Yang, C.R. and Mogenson, G.J. (1989) Ventral pallidal neuronal responses to dopamine receptor stimulation in the nucleus accumbens. *Brain Research* **489**, 237–246.

Yim, C.Y. and Mogenson, G.J. (1980) Effect of picrotoxin and nipécotic acid on inhibitory response of dopaminergic neurons in the ventral tegmental area to stimulation of the nucleus accumbens. *Brain Research* **199**, 466–472.

4

Neuromodulatory Functions of the Mesolimbic Dopamine System: Electrophysiological and Behavioural Studies

GORDON J. MOGENSON AND CONRAD C. YIM
Department of Physiology, The University of Western Ontario, London, Ontario, Canada N6A 5C1

INTRODUCTION

Since its discovery in the mid 1960s, brain dopamine (DA) has been a focus of intense interest. Initially attention was directed to the nigrostriatal DA system, implicated in Parkinson's disease, but in recent years there has been an increasing number of studies of the mesolimbic and mesocortical DA systems. Major reasons are their possible role in affect and mood, in schizophrenia and, more generally, in limbic–motor integration. Progress in the investigation of both nigrostriatal and mesolimbic DA systems has been very much enhanced by the mapping of DA neurons and their neural projections, and by the development of chemical compounds that are relatively specific DA agonists and antagonists (Fibiger and Phillips, 1986; Hoebel, 1988).

Much of the inital research on dopaminergic function was based on the hypothesis that DA is a neuromediating transmitter, similar in action to a classical transmitter such as GABA or glutamic acid. Early electrophysiological and pharmacological findings provided good evidence that DA is such a transmitter: DA is released by terminal depolarization, there are specific postsynaptic receptors for DA, and iontophoretic application of DA, or

The Mesolimbic Dopamine System: From Motivation to Action.
Edited by P. Willner and J. Scheel-Krüger

© 1991 John Wiley & Sons Ltd

stimulation of dopaminergic neurons, produces postsynaptic responses that can be blocked by specific DA antagonists (McLennan and York, 1967; Feltz, 1969; Connor, 1970; Kitai et al., 1976). Indeed, there is still an ongoing debate as to whether DA is an inhibitory or excitatory neurotransmitter. However, extensive research findings over the last few years have provided insights which suggest a neuromodulatory role for DA.

The term neuromodulation is rather loosely defined. Kupfermann (1979) defined a neuromediating transmitter as one that binds to receptors of ligand-mediated ion channels and directly produces membrane depolarization or hyperpolarization. A neuromodulator, on the other hand, does not produce such changes in membrane potential by itself, but acts, either directly or indirectly, via second messenger systems to modify the postsynaptic effects brought about by neuromediating transmitters. Kaczmarek and Levitan (1987), in their monograph on the subject, define neuromodulation as 'the ability of neurons to alter their electrical properties in response to intracellular biochemical changes resulting from synaptic or hormonal stimulation' and a neuromodulator as a substance that brings about such actions. These authors suggested that neuromodulation is one of the most important aspects of nervous function, for it allows plastic changes in neuronal activity and thus the choice of different patterns of behaviour at different times.

The classification of DA as a neuromediating transmitter or neuromodulator is not clear-cut. Since there is a good deal of empirical evidence showing that DA produces a direct postsynaptic action, it cannot be strictly classified as a neuromodulator. Nevertheless, as indicated in Kupfermann's review, very few compounds can be considered as pure neuromodulators; however, much of the new information about the actions of DA in the central nervous system in the past few years suggest that it is more likely to be a neuromodulator than a neuromediating transmitter. In an earlier review (Mogenson and Yim, 1981), we implicitly suggested such a function for DA when we described the mesolimbic DA projection as a 'gating' pathway which modulates the limbic–motor interphase. A number of other investigators have proposed similar concepts, and have suggested that the mesolimbic DA system influences the 'throughput' of the ventral striatum, and that mesolimbic DA projections have a selective influence on limbic inputs and a 'focusing' or 'enabling' influence on limbic–motor integration (Simon and Le Moal, 1988; see Table 1).

Given that the mesolimbic DA projection may have a neuromodulatory function rather than a neuromediating one, an understanding of the functional significance of DA in the ventral striatum will come predominantly from investigation of the interaction of DA with inputs to the nucleus accumbens (for example, from amygdala and hippocampus), and with neurotransmitters that mediate these inputs (such as glutamate and GABA).

This has been our approach in the past 7 or 8 years of research, and we have also followed a strategy of using a combination of complementary electrophysiological and behavioural techniques. Since this is a distinctive approach it is of interest to review some of our earlier findings.

EXPERIMENTAL EVIDENCE OF A NEUROMODULATORY FUNCTIONAL ROLE OF THE MESOLIMBIC DA PROJECTION

Electrophysiological Experiments

Initial evidence of a neuromodulatory function for DA came from electrophysiological experiments. We were interested in determining the synaptic action of DA in the accumbens and undertook a series of extracellular single unit recording experiments to determine the response of accumbens neurons to stimulation of the ventral tegmental area (VTA), where the cell bodies of the mesolimbic DA projection are located. Although both excitatory and inhibitory responses were observed, none was blocked by DA antagonists (Mogenson and Yim, 1981). It was initially puzzling that the endogenous release of DA was not associated with an electrophysiological response. Subsequently, it was shown that accumbens neurons were strongly activated by stimulation of the basolateral nucleus of the amygdala and this excitatory response was attenuated by concurrent stimulation of the VTA at 10 Hz (Figure 1). It should be noted that, while the excitatory response to amygdala stimulation was substantially attenuated, the baseline activity of the accumbens neuron was not significantly altered and individual VTA stimulus pulses did not produce direct synaptic responses (Yim and Mogenson, 1982). This selective gating effect of VTA stimulation on an afferent input to the accumbens was shown to be due to the endogenous release of DA and was the first evidence of a neuromodulatory action of DA. In later experiments, we have demonstrated similar modulatory action of DA on hippocampal input to the accumbens (Yang and Mogenson, 1984) and cortical input to the caudate nucleus (Hirata et al., 1984; Vives and Mogenson, 1986). Investigators from other laboratories have confirmed and extended these observations (Bergstrom and Walters, 1984; Ferron et al., 1984; Abercrombie and Jacobs, 1985; Thierry et al., 1988).

The cellular mechanism of this neuromodulatory action of DA remains to be clearly elucidated. Evidence from our intracellular recording experiments (Yim and Mogenson, 1986, 1988) and terminal excitability tests (Yang and Mogenson, 1987) suggest a presynaptic action, possibly mediated by D2 receptors (Vives and Mogenson, 1986; Yang and Mogenson, 1987). There is good evidence to suggest that the attenuation of responses to afferent inputs is due to a reduction in transmitter release caused by a

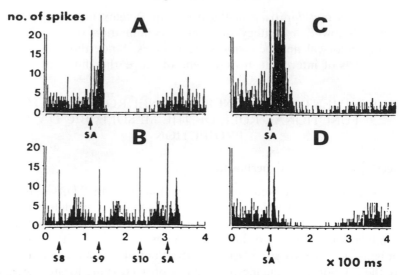

Figure 1. Excitatory responses of two accumbens neurons to single pulse stimulation of the basolateral amygdala (SA) are shown in panels **A** and **C**. The excitatory response was reduced when the amygdala stimulation was preceded by conditioning VTA stimulation (panel **B**, train of 10 pulses, 300 μA for 0.15 ms at 10 Hz, pulses 8, 9, and 10 are shown). For the second accumbens neuron the excitatory response to amygdala stimulation was reduced by the iontophoretic application of 10 nA of DA (see panel **D**). With low iontophoretic current, DA has little or no effect on the spontaneous activity of accumbens neurons consistent with a neuromodulatory action of DA. (Modified from Yim and Mogenson, 1982)

synaptic action of DA on these afferent terminals (Schwarcz et al., 1978; Theodorou et al., 1981; Mitchell and Doggett, 1980; Rowland and Roberts, 1980; Godukhin et al., 1984). The mechanism by which DA attenuates transmitter release remains speculative (Mogenson and Yang, 1987). Other investigators have reported neuromodulatory action of DA in other brain areas (Waszczak and Walters, 1986; Bernardi et al., 1984), and different mechanisms have been proposed. It remains to be determined whether DA has multiple neuromodulatory actions at different sites or a common mechanism of action.

Behavioural Experiments

Pijnenburg and co-workers, in classical experiments in 1973, suggested a functional role for DA in the accumbens; they showed that the administration of DA to the nucleus accumbens increased locomotor activity in rats. We extended those observations and demonstrated for the first time that endogenous DA produced similar hyperlocomotor effects. Since mesolimbic

DA neurons receive GABA afferents (Yim and Mogenson, 1980), injections of picrotoxin, a GABA antagonist, into the VTA were expected to cause the endogenous release of DA into the nucleus accumbens. A significant increase in locomotor activity in an open field test was indeed observed, and was attenuated by injecting the DA antagonist, spiroperidol, into the nucleus accumbens (Figure 2). These observations suggest that mesolimbic DA projection to the accumbens may be involved in the initiation of locomotor activity. This suggestion is supported by experiments in which the release of DA from the accumbens has been shown to be associated with locomotion (O'Neill and Fillenz, 1985; Louilot et al., 1986; Hernandez and Hoebel, 1988; Phillips et al., 1988).

While these early experiments indicate that DA may be associated with the initiation of locomotor activity, and locomotion has been used as a behavioural model in the investigation of dopaminergic function in numerous studies, it is not clear whether or not this is the physiological action of endogenous DA. Since our electrophysiological findings demonstrated that a major functional

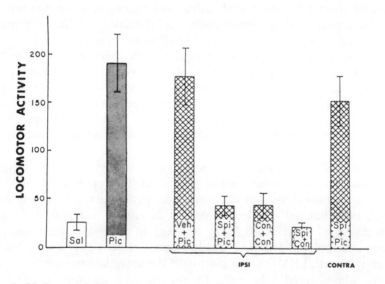

Figure 2. Unilateral injections of picrotoxin (Pic, 0.15 μg in 0.2 μl) into the VTA increased locomotor activity in an open field test more than fivefold as compared to control injections of isotonic saline. Measurements are for a period of 30 minutes. Pretreating the ipsilateral (IPSI) accumbens with spiroperidol (Spi, 1.0 μg in 1.0 μl) reversed this increase, while pretreating the contralateral accumbens (Contra) had little or no effect. Control (Con) procedures also included unilateral injections of the vehicle for spiroperidol (Veh) into the accumbens and no injections into the accumbens and into the VTA (where the treatments are shown the treatment above was administered to the accumbens and the treatment below was administered to the VTA). (After Mogenson et al. 1979)

role of DA in the accumbens was likely to be neuromodulatory, it was important to obtain complementary evidence in behavioural experiments.

The amygdala and hippocampus are two major limbic structures that provide robust inputs to the nucleus accumbens. As indicated in the previous section, these inputs are modified by DA, either released endogenously or applied by microiontophoresis. The amygdala and hippocampus contribute to a number of adaptive behaviours (Mogenson, 1977) and presumably to limbic–motor integration (Mogenson, 1987). Locomotor activity is an important component of a number of these behaviours, such as 'fight and flight' reactions, food procurement and mating.

Locomotor activity is reliably altered by injecting N-methyl-D-aspartate (NMDA), an excitatory amino acid, into the amygdala and hippocampus: locomotion is decreased when NMDA is administered to the basolateral amygdala and increased by administering NMDA to the ventral subiculum of the hippocampus. Presumably these behavioural responses are mediated by the glutamatergic projections to the nucleus accumbens from the amygdala and from the hippocampus (see below; Mogenson and Nielsen, 1984a).

Arrest of locomotion associated with an orientating reaction was reported in classical experiments involving electrical stimulation of the amygdala of cats (Ursin and Kaada, 1960). These investigators suggested that the effects of chronic amygdala stimulation are similar to the early phase of the 'fight and flight' reaction. In contrast, lesions of the amygdala have been reported to increase exploratory behaviour and locomotion (Robinson, 1963; White and Weingarten, 1976). The results of our experiments, presented here, support the view that DA has modulatory effects on amygdala inputs to the accumbens that mediate the locomotor component of these behavioural reactions.

To have a steady baseline of locomotor activity for the amygdala experiments, wooden panels were placed in the open field apparatus equipped with photocells and counters. The panels resulted in a doubling of locomotion that did not decline over a 20-minute test period. Bilateral administration of NMDA (0.2 and 0.4 µg) to the basolateral amygdala produced a dose-dependent decrease in locomotor activity (Figure 3A). This attenuating effect of NMDA stimulation of the amygdala was reversed when DA was administered bilaterally to the nucleus accumbens (Yim and

---

Figure 3. The effects of injections of DA and of L-glutamic diethyl ester HCL (GDEE) on reduction of locomotor activity from injections of NMDA into the basolateral amygdala. **A.** Control levels of locomotor activity measured in an open field apparatus are shown in the left columns at the left block (for saline injections into the amygdala and no saline injections the activity scores were approximately 330 photobeam interruptions). This spontaneous locomotor activity was reduced to 275 when 0.2 µg of NMDA was administered to the basolateral amygdala (shown in middle columns, left block) and to 210 when 0.4 µg of NMDA was administered

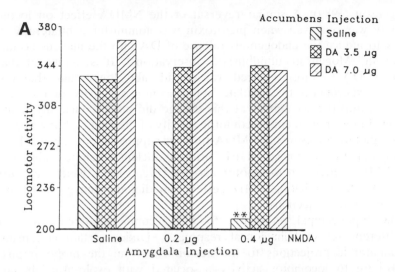

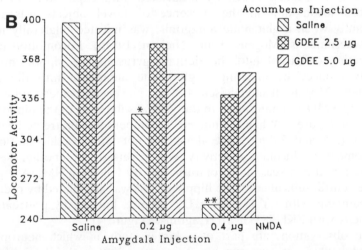

to the basolateral amygdala (shown in right columns, left block). This suppression of activity from NMDA was completely reversed when DA (3.5 μg and 7.0 μg) was injected into the nucleus accumbens (see middle and right blocks, all columns). As shown in the columns at the left, these relatively low doses of DA had no effect on locomotor activity. These behavioural results provide a functional demonstration of the neuromodulatory action of DA shown previously in electrophysiological experiments. **B**. Control levels of locomotor activity are shown in the left blocks of the columns as in **A**. This spontaneous locomotor activity was reduced in a dose-dependent manner when NMDA (0.2 and 0.4 μg) was injected into the basolateral amygdala. This reduction of locomotor activity was reversed when the glutamate antagonist, GDEE (2.5 and 5.0 μg), was injected into the nucleus accumbens (see middle and right blocks of all columns). (After Yim and Mogenson, 1989)

Mogenson, 1989). A similar reversal of the NMDA effect on locomotor activity was observed when picrotoxin was administered bilaterally to the VTA to induce the endogenous release of DA into the nucleus accumbens (Yim and Mogenson, unpublished observations). It is significant that the dose of DA (3.5 μg) required was considerably lower than that used in similar experiments to stimulate hyperlocomotor activity in the rat. DA injected into the accumbens at this dosage did not produce any significant change in the spontaneous locomotor activity of the animal, but was effective in completely reversing the NMDA-induced suppression of activity. Injection of a glutamate antagonist, GDEE, into the nucleus accumbens also reversed the NMDA effect on locomotor activity (Figure 3B), which supports the earlier suggestion that the NMDA effect is mediated by amygdala–accumbens glutamatergic projections.

The hippocampal projection to the accumbens appears to mediate a different set of behavioural responses. Under certain circumstances, glutamatergic projections to the accumbens from the hippocampus also contribute to locomotor activity associated with exploratory behaviour. Enhanced locomotion in the presence of novel objects was reduced significantly when a glutamate antagonist was injected bilaterally into the nucleus accumbens (Mogenson and Nielsen, 1984b). Locomotion initiated by injecting carbachol into the dentate gyrus of the hippocampus was similarly reduced by injecting a glutamate antagonist into the nucleus accumbens (Mogenson and Nielsen, 1984a). The enchancement of locomotor activity by NMDA administered to the ventral subiculum of the hippocampus is shown in Figure 4. When the nucleus accumbens was pretreated with DA, in doses (3.5 and 7.0 μg) that alone did not influence locomotion, this enhancement of locomotor activity was reversed. In another series of experiments, the increase in locomotor activity following NMDA injections into the ventral subiculum of the hippocampus was attenuated by pretreating the accumbens with LY 171555, a D2 agonist, but not by pretreating the accumbens with SKF 38393, a D1 agonist (Figure 4).

These observations are part of a larger study in which neuropharma-cological–behavioural experiments demonstrated that signals, initiated by injecting NMDA into the ventral subiculum of the hippocampus to enhance locomotor activity, were transmitted via the nucleus accumbens and subpallidal region to the mesencephalic locomotor region (MLR) (Yang and Mogenson, 1987). This study included electrophysiological recording experiments which demonstrated that ventral pallidal neurons inhibited by electrical stimulation of the ventral subiculum of the hippocampus had this inhibitory response reversed by injections of the D2 agonist, LY171555, into the accumbens (Figure 5). The D1 agonist SKF 38393 had no effect, although in other experiments this D1 agonist had an enabling influence on the action of the D2 agonist (see White, Chapter 3, this volume). A large

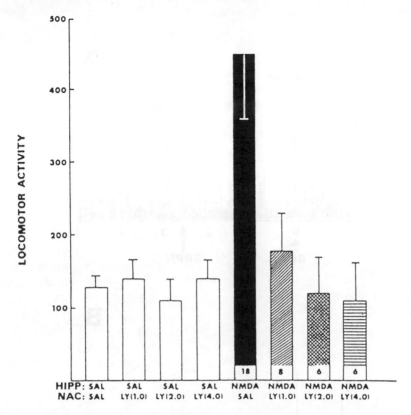

Figure 4. Unilateral microinjection of NMDA (0.5 µg) into the ventral subiculum of the hippocampus resulted in a fourfold increase in locomotor activity as compared to control microinjections of isotonic saline. This locomotor response was reduced significantly when the ipsilateral nucleus accumbens was pretreated with the D2 agonist LY 171555 (1.0, 2.0 and 4.0 µg). (After Yang and Mogenson, 1987)

number of the ventral pallidal neurons were shown to be activated antidromically by electrical stimulation of the pedunculopontine nucleus of the MLR, indicating that they were ventral pallidal output neurons to the MLR. Taken together, the results of these neuropharmacological–behavioural and electrophysiological experiments suggest that a D2-mediated mechanism in the accumbens modulates signals transmitted along the hippocampus–accumbens–ventral pallidal circuit that subserves locomotor activity. There is evidence to suggest that the D2 receptor mechanism that modulates excitatory hippocampal inputs to the accumbens is presynaptic (White, Chapter 3, this volume; Yang and Mogenson, 1986).

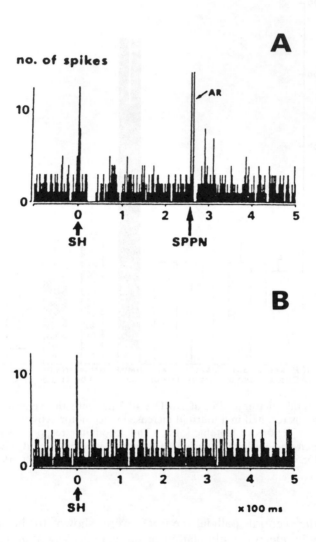

Figure 5. Peristimulus time histograms showing the activity of a subpallidal neuron that was inhibited by single pulse stimulation (500 μA, 0.15 ms duration) of the ventral subiculum of the hippocampus (SH) and antidromically activated (AR) by single pulse stimulation of the pedunculopontine nucleus (SPPN). In **B**, the inhibitory response to hippocampal stimulation (SH) was reduced markedly 5 minutes after the D2 agonist, LY 171555 (2 μg/0.2 μl) was injected into the medial nucleus accumbens. (After Yang and Mogenson, 1987)

Theoretical Implications

The neuromodulatory action of DA is likely to be of considerable functional significance. This is indicated by the suggestions of a number of investigators in recent years that appear in Table 1. The quotations from Willner (1983), Oades (1985) and Toan and Schultz (1985) are especially relevant. More recently we have elaborated on these earlier suggestions by proposing that the focusing or selective influence on limbic–motor integration is exerted by a D2-mediated mechanism that acts presynaptically. The proposal is as follows.

According to the environmental demands, signals which initiate locomotor components of these behaviours (such as food and water procurement and retrieval of pups for maternal care) can be inhibited presynaptically by D2 dopaminergic mechanisms (exerted by the VTA mesolimbic dopaminergic afferents) onto the axonal terminals of hippocampal–accumbens neurons (Yang and Mogenson, 1986). In the nucleus accumbens where multiple limbic afferent

Table 1. The Functional Significance of DA

Cortex → dorsal striatum → dorsal pallidum
      DA⟋

Amygdala → ventral striatum → ventral pallidum
      DA⟋

DA modulates the responsiveness of dorsal and ventral striatal neurons to afferent stimulation (Yim and Mogenson, 1982; Abercrombie and Jacobs, 1985; Vives and Mogenson, 1986)

DA modulates the influence that various sensory events have on motor output (Beninger, 1983)

. . . biologically significant stimuli converge on the VTA and influence the firing of the meso-limbic DA system; activity in this system modulates the transfer of information through the nucleus accumbens, which acts as a 'limbic motor interface', receiving inputs from the amygdala and other structures traditionally implicated in emotional and motivational behaviours, and sending its output to the motor system (Willner, 1983)

. . . the nucleus accumbens may be important for the release of locomotion involved in goal-directed behavior. (Kelley and Stinus, 1984)

. . . an increase of dopamine activity promotes the likelihood of switching between alternative sources of information. The act of switching may increase the probability of a new input to a given brain region influencing the output and/or resulting in an ongoing input being shut off from influencing the input (Oades, 1985)

Dopamine contributes to a 'focussing' mechanism by which information from the strongest cortical and limbic inputs pass to the pallidum and less prominent activity is lost (Toan and Schultz, 1985)

inputs converge (Groenewegen et al., 1982; Phillipson and Griffiths, 1985), a dopaminergic regulating mechanism which involved presynaptic inhibition can selectively inhibit one incoming input without inhibiting the accumbens neuron completely by postsynaptic inhibition. Thus, presynaptic inhibition still enables the same accumbens neuron to be activated by other inputs. Furthermore, in view of the recent finding that low levels of dopamine present in striatal synapses also act postsynaptically to increase signal to noise ratio of striatal neurons (Chiodo and Berger, 1986; Rolls et al., 1984), it is conceivable that while this postsynaptic mechanism facilitates the transfer of converging input signals from one limbic structure, e.g. the amygdala, via the accumbens output neurons to the subpallidal sites, the incoming signals to the accumbens from the other limbic structures, e.g. the hippocampus, are inhibited presynaptically. Accordingly, a more appropriate set of adaptive behaviours mediated by the non-hippocampal limbic input can be expressed by the animal (Yang and Mogenson, 1987).

As the concept of the neuromodulatory action of DA was gaining acceptance, it was demonstrated that peptides are present in the brain (Hökfelt et al., 1980). One of these peptides, cholecystokinin (CCK), is of special interest because of its relatively high concentration in the nucleus accumbens and its co-existence with DA in the mesolimbic projection. In the following section, we will consider the possibility that the modulating action of DA on accumbens inputs and throughputs involves interaction with CCK.

INTERACTIONS BETWEEN DA AND CCK IN THE ACCUMBENS: A CO-MODULATORY ACTION?

Background

CCK has long been recognized as an intestinal hormone. Most recently it was identified in the brain (Vanderhaeghen, 1975; Innis et al., 1979) and subsequently considered a putative neurotransmitter (Pinget et al., 1979; Emson et al., 1980). Following its identification in the brain, extensive research has been conducted to determine its physiological function in the central nervous system. While it has been shown that CCK either inhibits or excites a variety of central nervous system neurons (Ishibashi et al., 1979; Phillis and Kirkpatrick, 1980; Dodd and Kelly, 1981; Skirboll et al., 1981; Morin et al., 1983; Chiodo and Bunney, 1983), a number of studies have suggested a putative interaction between DA and CCK. There is good evidence that CCK modulates DA release in the accumbens (Fuxe et al., 1980; Markstein and Hökfelt, 1984; Voigt and Wang, 1984; Voigt et al., 1986; Lane et al., 1986; Phillips et al., 1988) and perhaps vice versa as well (Meyer and Krauss, 1983; Martin et al., 1986; Hutchison et al., 1986; Altar and Boyar, 1989). Behaviourally, CCK was initially shown to potentiate DA in the accumbens (Crawley et al., 1985; Worms et al., 1986; Morency et al., 1987), but more recent reports suggest an antagonist effect (Takeda et al., 1986; Weiss et al., 1988; Dauge et al., 1989a).

Since DA appears to function as a neuromodulator in the striatum, the observation that DA and CCK have significant interactions suggests the interesting possibility that the two transmitters may act either separately or jointly to modulate the action of a third. We investigated this possibility following the same approach used in investigating the neuromodulatory action of DA. Experiments were designed to determine the effect of CCK, either singly or combined with DA, on another transmitter system. Many of the results described below are from current on-going projects and are preliminary.

Electrophysiological Investigations

To investigate whether or not there is a modulatory type of interaction between DA and CCK, we extended the electrophysiological experiments on the modulatory action of DA on amygdala inputs to accumbens neurons, to include the combined application of DA and CCK. In an initial series of experiments, recordings were made extracellularly from neurons in the nucleus accumbens of rats. Accumbens neurons showed a strong excitatory response to amygdala stimulation. Concurrent stimulation of the VTA at 10 Hz produced significant attentuation of the excitatory response, as shown previously. Iontophoretic application of proglumide, a specific CCK antagonist, enhanced this effect of VTA stimulation by an average of 250 per cent in approximately one-half of accumbens neurons tested (Figures 6A and B). These results suggest that endogenous DA was released during VTA stimulation, and that this modulated the excitatory response, but in a subpopulation of the mesolimbic DA cells, CCK was co-released with DA and acted as a functional DA antagonist. With iontophoresis of proglumide, the antagonistic effect of CCK was blocked, and DA produced an enhanced effect. Results from these experiments do not provide information as to whether the antagonistic effect of CCK was mediated via its action on DA release, as shown in a number of pharmacological studies, or via an interaction at the postsynaptic level. To distinguish between these two alternative mechanisms, a second series of experiments was performed.

The responses of accumbens neurons were monitored on-line in horizontal raster plots as shown in Figure 7. A vertical raster plot displays unit activities following a trigger to the computer along the vertical axis. Successive sweeps were displayed along the horizontal axis. A stimulus pulse was delivered to the amygdala 40 ms after the start of the sweep, and responses of the accumbens neuron to the stimulation were recorded as a series of dots plotted along the vertical axis. The first 100 sweeps of the raster plot shown in Figure 7 represent the control excitatory response of the accumbens

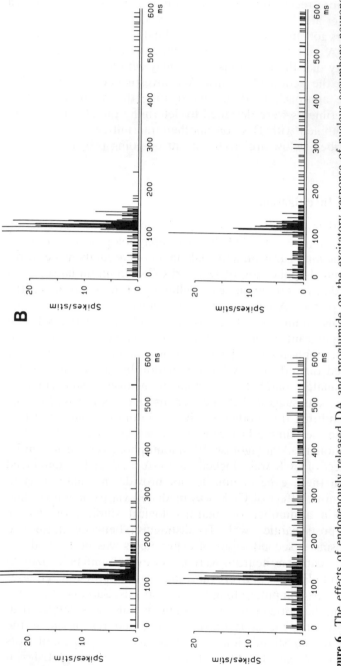

Figure 6. The effects of endogenously released DA and proglumide on the excitatory response of nucleus accumbens neurons to electrical stimulation of the basolateral amygdala. **A.** Peristimulus time histogram to show the excitatory response of an accumbens neuron to amygdala stimulation (550 μA, 0.15 ms) and the effect of VTA stimulation on the response. The upper panel shows the control response, while the lower panel shows the response to identical amygdala stimulations, except that each stimulation was preceded by 10 pulses of stimulation to the VTA (400 μA, 0.15 ms). The response was attenuated by 24 per cent (a reduction from 5.55 spikes/stim to 4.11 spikes/stim). A relatively low current was used to stimulate the VTA to produce only a marginal suppression. **B.** The same tests as shown in **A** were repeated following iontophoretic application of proglumide, a specific CCK antagonist, to the accumbens neurons. The response to amygdala stimulation was slightly enhanced (from 5.55 spikes/stim to 5.88 spikes/stim). However, the effect of superimposed VTA stimulation was significantly enhanced (62 per cent attenuation, a reduction from 5.88 spikes/stim to 2.23 spikes/stim), and see Yin and Mogenson (1991)

neuron to amygdala stimulation. Starting at sweep 100, DA (30 nA) was applied iontophoretically. DA produced a significant suppression of the excitatory response as illustrated by the reduction in the cluster of dots above the stimulus artifact. Upon termination of the iontophoretic application, the response recovered gradually over 20–30 seconds. Iontophoretic application of CCK at currents in excess of 75 nA produced an increase in spontaneous activity in about 60 per cent of accumbens neurons as well as an enhancement of the excitatory response to amygdala stimulation. At lower iontophoretic currents (less than 50 nA), CCK did not produce any significant effect on accumbens neurons. However, the same dose of CCK, when applied simultaneously with DA, completely reversed the inhibitory effect of DA. These observations suggest that the postsynaptic response to DA was modulated by CCK. This interaction between CCK and DA does not appear to be a simple algebraic summation of an excitatory and an inhibitory response since the dose of CCK was carefully titrated not to produce any significant effect on the accumbens neuron by itself. The effect of CCK was blocked by simultaneous iontophoresis of proglumide. GABA, an inhibitory transmitter, produced similar suppression of the excitatory response, but, unlike the suppression produced by DA, it was not reversed by CCK (Figure 8).

Behavioural Investigations

These electrophysiological observations suggest that CCK may function as an endogenous DA antagonist in the accumbens. To determine whether or not these observations have behavioural relevance, two series of experiments investigating possible interaction between DA and CCK were conducted in the behaving animal.

In the first series, animals were injected with picrotoxin into the VTA to increase locomotor activity. Previous experiments have shown that picrotoxin disinhibits dopaminergic neurons in the VTA and releases DA in the accumbens which stimulates locomotor activity (Mogenson et al., 1979; Yim and Mogenson, 1980). If CCK is co-released with DA in a subpopulation of the mesolimbic DA neurons when VTA is stimulated, an injection of proglumide, a specific CCK antagonist, into the accumbens should block potential interactions between CCK and DA, and modify the locomotor activity induced by picrotoxin. Results from these experiments showed that proglumide had a biphasic effect on DA-stimulated locomotor activity depending on the initial activity level. When a low dose of picrotoxin (0.0125 μg) was injected, which increased the locomotor activity by 6 per cent compared to the control concurrent injection of proglumide into the accumbens further enhanced the locomotor activity by 20 per cent (Figure 9A) in a dose-dependent manner. However, at a higher dose of picrotoxin

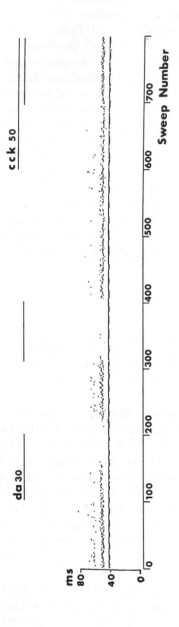

Figure 7. A vertical raster plot to show the response of an accumbens neuron to amygdala stimulation, and the effects of iontophoretic application of DA and CCK on the response. Individual spikes are plotted as single dots on the raster plot. Activities recorded from the neuron following a trigger to the computer are displayed along the vertical axis and successive sweeps are displayed along the horizontal axis. The line of dots along the 40 ms time mark represents stimulus artifacts from the amygdala stimulation delivered at that time. The cluster of dots is the responses of the neuron to the stimulations. The horizontal bars mark iontophoretic application of drugs. Note that the first application of DA (30 nA) gradually brought on a strong suppression of the excitatory response. The second application had a shorter onset latency owing to priming of the electrode. Application of CCK at 50 nA did not produce significant changes in the control response, but completely reversed the effect of DA

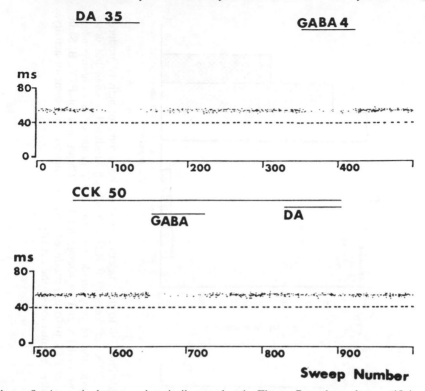

Figure 8. A vertical raster plot similar to that in Figure 7 to show the specificity of the antagonistic interaction between CCK and DA. DA and GABA were iontophoretically applied at currents titrated to produce equivalent inhibition of the response to amygdala stimulation. CCK applied at 50 nA completely reversed the attenuation produced by DA, but not that produced by GABA. (After Yin and Mogenson, 1991)

(0.05 μg), injection of proglumide into the accumbens significantly attenuated the stimulated locomotor activity (Figures 9A and B). This biphasic action is difficult to interpret. The enhancement of proglumide at low doses of picrotoxin is consistent with electrophysiological observations and the hypothesis that endogenous CCK acts as a functional DA antagonist. Whether the effects of higher doses of picrotoxin indicate that CCK enhances the effect of DA, as suggested by Crawley et al. (1985), or that proglumide has non-specific blocking effects, remains to be investigated.

A second series of behavioural experiments investigated the possible effects of CCK on the modulatory action of DA. As indicated earlier, injection of NMDA into the amygdala produces a dose-dependent suppression of spontaneous locomotor activity, which is completely reversed by low

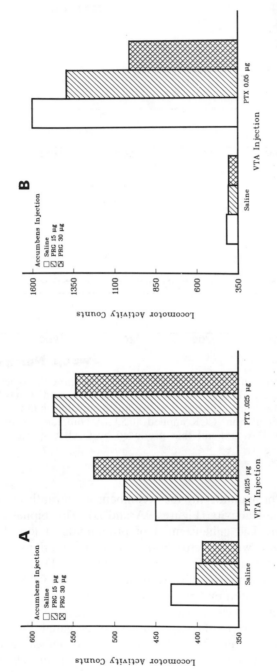

Figure 9. Dose-dependent effects of proglumide (PRG) administered to the nucleus accumbens on locomotor activity produced by injections of picrotoxin into the VTA. A. Picrotoxin (PTX) at doses of 0.0125 to 0.025 μg produced a small but dose-dependent increase in locomotor activity. Concurrent injection of proglumide into the VTA produced a dose-dependent enhancement of locomotor activity for the 0.0125 μg dose of PTX and no change for the 0.025 μg dose of PTX. **B**. Same experimental paradigm as in A, except that a higher dose of PTX (0.05 μg) produced a fivefold increase in locomotor activity. At this activity level, proglumide produced a dose-dependent attenuation of the activity

doses (3.5–5.0 µg) of DA injected into the accumbens. Since the low dose of DA did not enhance locomotor activity by itself, this is probably an example of neuromodulatory action. Preliminary results show that CCK (40 ng), when injected into the accumbens along with DA, attenuated this neuromodulatory action of DA.

Theoretical Implications

On consideration of the evidence that has been accumulated on the actions of CCK in the accumbens, it seems reasonable to suggest that the compound may have a function similar to that of DA. There is evidence that CCK acts like a neuromediating transmitter; a subpopulation of the CCK projection from the midbrain to the ventral striatum may well function as a signal transmission line. On the other hand, other CCK neurons, as well as CCK contained in DA neurons, appear to have a primarily neuromodulatory function.

The modulatory actions of CCK seem to be inextricably coupled to the actions of DA, itself a neuromodulator. For this reason, the term co-modulation, first proposed by Agnati and Fuxe (1983), is used to describe its relation to DA. More and more evidence, from pharmacological, electrophysiological, as well as behavioural, experiments, suggests that the co-modulatory action is one of functional antagonism (Bunney and Shi, 1988; Dauge et al., 1989b; Wang, 1988).

Although possible synaptic effects of CCK have been investigated in central nervous system dopaminergic as well as non-dopaminergic neurons (Ishibashi et al., 1979; Phillis and Kirkpatrick, 1980; Dodd and Kelly, 1981; Skirboll et al., 1981; Morin et al., 1983; Chiodo and Bunney, 1983), surprisingly little has been reported on its electrophysiological action on accumbens neurons. The only reports were those of DeFrance and co-workers (1984), who showed that CCK attenuated hippocampal evoked population spikes in the accumbens and potentiated the actions of DA and acetylcholine; and of Wang and Hu (1986), who demonstrated a primarily excitatory action of CCK on accumbens neurons. Our own experiments, designed specifically to investigate interaction between transmitters, showed that CCK, at doses which did not produce direct postsynaptic action, reversed the inhibitory modulatory action of DA. CCK did not modulate the postsynaptic action of other transmitters, but specifically attenuated the actions of DA. The inhibitory effect of GABA, which was equivalent to that of DA, was not reversed by CCK. Moreover, since iontophoretically applied exogenous DA and CCK were used, the antagonistic interaction could not be explained in terms of the attenuation of DA release that has been repeatedly demonstrated in pharmacological experiments (Fuxe et al., 1980; Markstein and Hökfelt, 1984; Voigt and Wang, 1984; Voigt et al.,

1986; Lane et al., 1986; Phillips et al., 1988). It should be noted, however, that although the term antagonism is used to describe the interaction between CCK and DA, it does not necessarily imply competition at the same receptor sites. The term is used rather to describe a form of functional interaction. However, there is good evidence of specific CCK binding receptors in the accumbens (Beinfeld et al., 1981) and the receptor–receptor interaction described by Fuxe et al. (1983) may account for the electrophysiological responses we observed.

Results from our behavioural experiments are in general agreement with those from electrophysiological experiments, though less consistent. Similar functional antagonism between CCK and DA in the accumbens was demonstrated. Our observations are opposite to those of Crawley et al. (1985; Crawley, 1988), but other studies have reported results similar to ours (Katsuura and Itoh, 1982; Cohen et al., 1982; Van Ree et al., 1983; Takeda et al., 1986). Two recent reports, however, suggest a possible explanation of the contrasting observations. Weiss and co-workers (1988) showed that CCK potentiated amphetamine–induced stereotypy but antagonized locomotor activity, and Vaccarino and Vaccarino (1989) reported that proglumide antagonized self-stimulation when it was injected into the caudal area of the accumbens, but mildly facilitated the same behaviour when it was injected into the rostral regions. The clarification of behavioural functions of accumbens CCK remains a continuing research objective.

The well-established fact that DA autoregulates its own release presents a theoretical challenge of the notion that CCK co-existing with DA in the same neuron also regulates its release. One hypothesis is that the release of CCK, and hence its feedback inhibition on DA release, is only prominent at high activity levels of DA neurons (Phillips et al., 1986; Wang, 1988). Wang indeed proposed an integrated model of the interdependent regulation of DA and CCK release in the accumbens which forms a focal point of his group's research. Agnati and Fuxe (1983; Fuxe et al., 1983), on the other hand, proposed that 'the presence of dopamine co-modulators such as CCK in the DA synapse makes possible a heterostatic regulation of the synapse. By means of receptor–receptor interactions, peptide comodulators may change the set point of the main transmission line without inducing homeostatic feedback responses on synthesis and release of the main transmitter, opening up a new way to modulate chemical transmission in general'. Our own electrophysiological observations are in favour of this suggestion.

The evidence that CCK may be an endogenous DA antagonist was of considerable interest because of the possibility of modifying clinical treatment of psychotic disorders with CCK or its analogue as an adjunct to conventional neuroleptics (Bissette and Nemeroff, 1985; Nair et al., 1986; Phillips et al., 1986; Wang, 1988). The advantage of such treatment is obvious, since CCK is primarily localized in the ventral striatum and, notably absent in the dorsal striatum, a CCK-based antipsychotic would have few of the Parkinsonian side-effects associated with DA antagonist. A number of clinical trials have been attempted. Although results are mixed (Montgomery and Green, 1988), the potential of substantial advances in our treatment of psychotic disorders derived from the basic research on CCK and DA functions cannot be underestimated.

REFERENCES

Abercrombie, E.D. and Jacobs, B.L. (1985) Dopaminergic modulation of sensory response of striatal neurons: single unit studies. *Brain Research* **358**, 27–33.

Agnati, L.F. and Fuxe, K. (1983) Subcortical limbic 3H-N-propylnorapomorphine binding sites are markedly modulated by cholecystokinin-8 in vitro, *Bioscience Reports* **3**, 1101–1105.

Altar, C.A. and Boyar, W.C. (1989) Brain CCK-8 receptors mediate the suppression of dopamine release by cholecystokinin. *Brain Research* **483**, 321–326.

Beinfeld, M.C., Meyer, D.K., Eskay, R.L., Jensen, R.T. and Brownstein, M.J. (1981) The distribution of cholecystokinin immunoreactivity in the central nervous system of the rat as determined by radioimmunoassay. *Brain Research* **212**, 51–57.

Beninger, R.J. (1983) The role of dopamine in locomotor activity and learning. *Brain Research Reviews* **6**, 173–196.

Bergstrom, D.A. and Walters, J.R. (1984) Dopamine attenates the effects of GABA on single unit activity in the globus pallidus. *Brain Research* **310**, 23–33.

Bernardi, G., Calabresi, P., Mercuri, N. and Stanzione, P. (1984) Evidence for a neuromodulatory role of dopamine in rat striatal neurons. *Clinical Neuropharmacology* **7**, 66–67 (suppl 1).

Bissette, G. and Nemeroff, C.B. (1985) Do neuropeptide systems mediate some of the effects of antipsychotic drugs. *Progress in Clinical and Biological Research* **192**, 349–353.

Bunney, B.S. and Shi, W. (1988) Cholecystokinin and neurotensin: comparison of their effects on midbrain dopamine neurons. In: Wang, R.Y. and Schoenfeld, R. (eds) *Cholecystokinin Antagonists*. New York: Alan R. Liss, Inc., pp. 165–180.

Chiodo, L.A. and Berger, T.W. (1986) Interactions between dopamine and amino acid-induced excitation and inhibition in the striatum. *Brain Research* **375**, 198–203.

Chiodo, L.A. and Bunney, B.S. (1983) Proglumide: selective antagonism of excitatory effects of cholecystokinin in central nervous system. *Science* **219**, 1449–1451.

Cohen, S.L., Knight, M., Tamminga, C.A. and Chase, T.N. (1982) Cholecystokinin effects on conditioned avoidance behaviour, stereotypy and catalepsy. *European Journal of Pharmacology* **83**, 213–222.

Connor, J.D. (1970) Caudate nucleus neurones: correlation of the effects of substantia nigra stimulation with iontophoretic dopamine. *Journal of Physiology (Lond.)* **208**, 691–703.

Crawley, J.N. (1988) Modulation of mesolimbic dopaminergic behaviors by cholecystokinin. *Annals of the New York Academy of Science* **537**, 380–396.

Crawley, J.N., Stivers, J.A., Blumstein, L.K. and Paul, S.M. (1985) Cholecystokinin potentiates dopamine-mediated behaviors: evidence for modulation specific to a site of coexistence. *Journal of Neuroscience* **5**, 1972–1983.

Dauge, V., Dor, A., Feger, J. and Roques, B.P. (1989a) The behavioral effects of

CCK-8 injected into the medial nucleus accumbens are dependent on the motivational state of the rat. *European Journal of Pharmacology* **163**, 25–32.

Dauge, V., Durieux, D., Derrien, F., Corringer, P-J, Rogues, B.P. and Feger, J. (1989b) New evidence for heterogeneity within the nucleus accumbens: behavioral and biochemical studies with CCK-8 and analogues. *Behavioural Pharmacology* **1**, 32 (suppl. 1).

DeFrance, J.F., Sikes, R.W. and Chronister, R.B. (1984) Effects of CCK-8 in the nucleus accumbens. *Peptides* **5**, 1–6.

Dodd, J. and Kelly, J.S. (1981) The actions of cholecystokinin and related peptides on pyramidal neurons of the mammalian hippocampus. *Brain Research* **205**, 337–350.

Emson, P.C., Lee, C.M. and Rehfeld, J.F. (1980) Cholecystokinin octapeptide: vesicular localization and calcium dependent release from rat brain in vitro. *Life Science* **26**, 2157–2163.

Feltz, P. (1969) Dopamine, amino acids and caudate unitary responses to nigral stimulation. *Journal of Physiology (Lond.)* **205**, 8–9P.

Ferron, A., Thierry, A.M., LeDouarin, C. and Glowinski, J. (1984) Inhibitory influence of the mesocortical dopaminergic system on spontaneous activity or excitatory response induced from the thalamic mediodorsal nucleus in the rat medial prefrontal cortex. *Brain Research* **302**, 257–265.

Fibiger, H.C. and Phillips, A.G. (1986) Reward, motivation and cognition: psychobiology of mesotelencephalic dopamine systems. In: Bloom, F.E. and Geiger, S.R. (eds) *Handbook of Physiology: The Nervous System. Volume 4, Intrinsic Regulatory Systems of the Brain.* Bethesda: American Physiological Society, pp. 647–675.

Fuxe, K., Andersson, K., Locatelli, V., Agnati, L.F., Hokfelt, T., Skirboll, L. and Mutt, V. (1980) Cholecystokinin peptides produce marked reduction of dopamine turnover in discrete areas in the rat brain following intraventricular injection. *European Journal of Pharmacology* **67**, 325–331.

Fuxe, K., Agnati, L.F., Benfenati, F., Celani, M., Zini, I., Zoli, M. and Mutt, V. (1983) Evidence for the existence of receptor–receptor interactions in the central nervous system. Studies on the regulation of monoamine receptors by neuropetides. *Journal of Neural Transmission* **18**, 165–179 (suppl).

Godukhin, O.V., Zharikova, A.D. and Budantsev, A.Yu. (1984) Role of presynaptic dopamine receptors in regulation of the glutamatergic neurotransmission in rat neostriatum. *Neuroscience* **12**, 377–383.

Groenewegen, H.J., Room, P., Witter, M.P. and Lohman, H.M. (1982) Cortical afferents of the nucleus accumbens in the cat, studied with anterograde and retrograde transport techniques. *Neuroscience* **7**, 977–995.

Hernandez, L. and Hoebel, B.G. (1988) Feeding and hypothalamic stimulation increase dopamine turnover in the accumbens. *Physiology and Behavior* **44**, 599–606.

Hoebel, B.G. (1988) Neuroscience and motivation: pathways and peptides that define motivational systems. In: Atkinson, R.C., Hernstein, R.J., Lindzey, G. and Luce, R.D. (eds) *Steven's Handbook of Experimental Psychology, Second Edition, Volume 1: Perception and Motivation.* New York: John Wiley and Sons Inc., pp. 547–625.

Hirata, K., Yim, C.Y. and Mogenson, G.J. (1984) Excitatory input from sensory motor cortex to neostriatum and its modification by conditioning stimulation of the substantia nigra. *Brain Research* **321**, 1–8.

Hökfelt, T., Skirboll, L., Rehfeld, J.F., Goldstein, M., Markey, K. and Dann, O.

(1980) A subpopulation of mesencephalic dopamine neurons projecting to limbic areas contains a cholecystokinin-like peptide: evidence from immunohistochemistry combined with retrograde tracing. *Neuroscience* 5, 2093–2124.

Hutchison, J.B., Strupish, J. and Nahorski, S.R. (1986) Release of endogenous dopamine and cholecystokinin from rat striatal slices: effects of amphetamine and dopamine antagonists. *Brain Research* 370, 310–314.

Innis, R.B., Correa, F.M.A., Uhl, G.R., Schneider, B. and Snyder, S.H. (1979) Cholecystokinin octapeptide-like immunoreactivity: histochemical localization in rat brain. *Proceedings of the National Academy of Science* 76, 521–525.

Ishibashi, S., Oomura, Y., Okajima, T. and Shibata, S. (1979) Cholecystokinin, motilin and secretin effects on the central nervous system. *Physiology and Behavior* 23, 401–403.

Kaczmarek, L.K. and Levitan, I.B. (1987) *Neuromodulation*. New York: Oxford University Press.

Katsuura, G. and Itoh, S. (1982) Sedative action of cholecystokinin octapeptide on behavioral excitation by thyrotropin releasing hormone and methamphetamine in the rat. *Japanese Journal of Physiology* 32, 83–91.

Kelley, A.E. and Stinus, L. (1984) Neuroanatomical and neurochemical substrates of affective behavior. In: Fox, N.A. and Davidson, R.J. (eds) *The Psychobiology of Affective Development*. Hillsdale, New Jersey: Lawrence Erlbaum Associates, pp. 1–75.

Kitai, S.T., Sugimori, M. and Kocsis, J.D. (1976) Excitatory nature of dopamine in the nigro-caudate pathway. *Brain Research* 24, 351–363.

Kupfermann, I. (1979) Modulatory actions of neurotransmitters. *Annual Review of Neuroscience* 2, 447–465.

Lane, R.F., Blaha, C.D. and Phillips, A.G. (1986) In vivo electrochemical analysis of cholecystokinin-induced inhibition of dopamine release in the nucleus accumbens. *Brain Research* 397, 200–204.

Louilot, A., Le Moal, M. and Simon, H. (1986) Differential reactivity of dopaminergic neurons in the nucleus accumbens in response to different behavioral situations. An in vivo voltammetric study in free moving rats. *Brain Research* 397, 395–400.

Markstein, R. and Hökfelt, T. (1984) Effect of cholecystokinin-octapeptide on dopamine release from slices of cat caudate nucleus. *Journal of Neuroscience* 4, 570–575.

Martin, J.R., Beinfeld, M.C. and Wang, R.Y. (1986) Modulation of cholecystokinin release from posterior nucleus accumbens by D-2 dopamine receptor. *Brain Research* 397, 253–258.

McLennan, H. and York, D.H. (1967) The action of dopamine on neurones of the caudate nucleus. *Journal of Physiology (Lond.)* 189, 393–402.

Meyer, D.K. and Krauss, J. (1983) Dopamine modulates cholecystokinin release in neostriatum. *Nature* 301, 338–340.

Mitchell, P.R. and Doggett, N.S. (1980) Modulation of striatal [3H]-glutamic acid release by dopaminergic drugs. *Life Science* 26, 2073–2081.

Mogenson, G.J. (1977) *The Neurobiology of Behavior: An Introduction*. Hillsdale, New Jersey: Lawrence Erlbaum Associates.

Mogenson, G.J. (1987) Limbic-motor integration. In: Epstein, A.N. (ed.) *Progress in Psychobiology and Physiological Psychology*. New York: Academic Press Inc., pp. 117–170.

Mogenson, G.J. and Nielsen, M. (1984a) Neuropharmacological evidence to suggest that the nucleus accumbens and subpallidal region contribute to exploratory locomotion. *Behavioral and Neural Biology* 42, 52–60.

128 *Mogenson and Yim*

Mogenson, G.J. and Nielsen, M. (1984b) A study of the contribution of hippocampal-accumbens-subpallidal projections to locomotor activity. *Behavioral and Neural Biology* **42**, 38–51.

Mogenson, G.J. and Yang, C.R. (1987) Dopamine modulation of limbic and cortical inputs to striatal neurons. In: Chiodo, L.A. and Freeman, A.S. (eds) *Neurophysiology of Dopaminergic Systems—Current Status and Clinical Perspectives.* Detroit: Lakeshore Publishing Company, pp. 237–251.

Mogenson, G.J. and Yim, C.Y. (1981) Electrophysiological and neuropharmacological behavioral studies of the nucleus accumbens and implications for its role as a limbic-motor interface. In: Chronister, R.B. and DeFrance, J.F. (eds) *The Neurobiology of the Nucleus Accumbens.* Brunswick: Haer Institute of Electrophysiological Research, pp. 210–229.

Mogenson, G.J., Wu, M. and Manchanda, S.K. (1979) Locomotor activity initiated by microinfusions of picrotoxin into the ventral tegmental area. *Brain Research* **161**, 311–319.

Montgomery, S.A. and Green, M.C. (1988) The use of cholecystokinin in schizophrenia: a review. *Psychological Medicine* **18**, 593–603.

Morency, M.A., Ross, G.M., Hesketh, D. and Mishra, R.K. (1987) Effects of unilateral intracerebroventricular microinjections of cholecystokinin (CCK) on circling behavior of rats. *Peptides* **8**, 989–995.

Morin, M.P., De Marchi, P., Champagnat, J., Vanderhaeghen, J.J., Rossier, J. and Denavit-Saubie, M. (1983) Inhibitory effect of cholecystokinin octapeptide on neurons in the nucleus tractus solitarius. *Brain Research* **265**, 333–338.

Nair, N.P., Lal, S. and Bloom, D.M. (1986) Cholecystokinin and schizophrenia. *Progress in Brain Research* **65**, 237–258.

Oades, R.D. (1985) The role of noradrenaline in turning and dopamine in switching between signals in the central nervous system. *Neuroscience and Biobehavioral Reviews* **9**, 261–282.

O'Neill, R.D. and Fillenz, M. (1985) Simultaneous monitoring of dopamine release in rat frontal cortex, nucleus accumbens and striatem: effect of drugs, circadian changes and correlations with motor activity. *Neuroscience* **16**, 49–55.

Phillips, A.G., Lane, R.F. and Blaha, C.D. (1986) Inhibition of dopamine release by cholecystokinin: relevance to schizophrenia. *Trends in Pharmacological Sciences* **7**, 126–129.

Phillips, A.G., Blaha, C.D., Fibiger, H.C. and Lane, R.F. (1988) Interactions between mesolimbic dopamine neurons, cholecystokinin, and neurotensin: evidence using in vivo voltammetry. *Annals of the New York Academy of Science* **537**, 347–361.

Phillipson, O.T. and Griffiths, A.C. (1985) The topographic order of inputs to nucleus accumbens in the rat. *Neuroscience* **16**, 275–296.

Phillis, J.W. and Kirkpatrick, J.R. (1980) The actions of motilin, cholecystokinin, somatostatin, vasoactive intestinal peptide, and other peptides on rat cerebral cortical neurons. *Canadian Journal of Physiology* **58**, 612–623.

Pijnenburg, A.J.J., Woodruff, G.N. and Van Rossum, J.M. (1973) Ergometrine-induced locomotor activity following intracerebral injection into the nucleus accumbens. *Brain Research* **59**, 289–302.

Pinget, M., Straus, E. and Yalow, R.S. (1979) Release of cholecystokinin peptides from a synaptosome-enriched fraction of rat cerebral cortex. *Life Science* **25**, 339–342.

Robinson, E. (1963) Effect of amygdalectomy on fear-motivated behaviour of rats. *Journal of Comparative Physiology Psychology* **56**, 814–820.

Rolls, E.T., Thorpe, S.J., Boytin, M., Szabo, I. and Perrett, D.I. (1984) Responses of striatal neurons in the behaving monkey. 3. Effects of iontophoretically applied dopamine on normal responsiveness. *Neuroscience* **12**, 1201–1212.

Rowland, G.J. and Roberts, P.J. (1980) Activation of dopamine receptors inhibits calcium dependent glutamate release from cortico-striatal terminals in vitro. *European Journal of Pharmacology* **62**, 241–242.

Schwarcz, R., Creese, I., Coyle, J.T. and Snyder, S.H. (1978) Dopamine receptors localised on cerebral cortical afferents in rat corpus striatum. *Nature* **271**, 766–768.

Simon, H. and Le Moal, M. (1988) Mesencephalic dopaminergic neurons: role in the general economy of the brain. In: Kalivas, P.W. and Nemeroff, C.B. (eds) *The Mesocorticolimbic Dopamine System*. New York: The New York Academy of Sciences, pp. 235–253.

Skirboll, L.R., Grace, A.A., Hommer, D.W., Rehfeld, J., Goldstein, M., Hokfelt, T. and Bunney, B.S. (1981) Peptide-monoamine coexistence: studies of the actions of cholecystokinin-like peptides on the electrical activity of midbrain dopamine neurons. *Neuroscience* **6**, 2111–2124.

Takeda, Y., Kamiya, Y., Honda, K., Takano, Y. and Kamiya, H. (1986) Effect of injection of CCK-8 into the nucleus caudatus on the behavior of rats. *Japanese Journal of Pharmacology* **40**, 569–575.

Theodorou, A., Reavill, C., Jenner, P. and Marsden, C.D. (1981) Kainic acid lesions of striatum and decortication reduce specific 3-H-sulpiride binding in rats, so D-2 receptors exist postsynaptically on corticostriate afferents and striatal neurones. *Journal of Pharmacy and Pharmacology* **33**, 439–444.

Thierry, A.M., Mantz, J., Milla, C. and Glowinski, J. (1988) Influence of the mesocortical prefrontal dopamine neurons on their target cells. In: Kalivas, P.W. and Nemeroff, C.B. (eds) *The Mesocorticolimbic Dopamine System*. New York: The New York Academy of Sciences, pp. 101–111.

Toan, I.L. and Schultz, W. (1985) Responses of rat pallidum cells to cortex stimulation and effects of altered dopaminergic activity. *Neuroscience* **15**, 683–694.

Ursin, H. and Kaada, B.R. (1960) Subcortical structures mediating the attention response induced by amygdala stimulation. *Experimental Neurology* **2**, 109–122.

Vaccarino, F.J. and Vaccarino, A.L. (1989) Antagonism of cholecystokinin function in the rostral and caudal nucleus accumbens: differential effects on brain stimulation reward. *Neuroscience Letters* **97**, 151–156.

Vanderhaeghen, J.J., Signeau, J.C. and Gept, W. (1975) New peptide in the vertebrate CNS reacting with gastrin antibodies. *Nature* **257**, 604–605.

Van Ree, J.M., Gaffori, O. and De Wied, D. (1983) In rats the behavioral profile of CCK-8-related peptides resembles that of antipsychotic agents. *European Journal of Pharmacology* **93**, 65–78.

Vives, F. and Mogenson, G.J. (1986) Electrophysiological study of the effects of D-1 and D-2 dopamine antagonists on the interactions of converging inputs from the sensory-motor cortex and substantia nigra neurons in the rat. *Neuroscience* **17**, 349–359.

Voigt, M.M. and Wang, R.Y. (1984) In vivo release of dopamine in the nucleus accumbens of the rat: modulation by cholecystokinin. *Brain Research* **296**, 189–193.

Voigt, M., Wang, R.Y. and Westfall, T.C. (1986) Cholecystokinin octapeptides alter the release of endogenous dopamine from the rat nucleus accumbens in vitro. *Journal of Pharmacology and Experimental Therapeutics* **237**, 147–153.

Wang, R.Y. (1988) Cholecystokinin, dopamine, and schizophrenia: recent progress and current problems. In: Kalivas, P.W. and Nemeroff, C.B. (eds) *The Mesocorticolimbic Dopamine System*. New York: The New York Academy of Sciences, pp. 362–379.

Wang, R.Y. and Hu, X.T. (1986) Does cholecystokinin potentiate dopamine action in the nucleus accumbens? *Brain Research* **380**, 363–367.

Waszczak, B.L. and Walters, J.R. (1986) Endogenous dopamine can modulate inhibition of substantia nigra pars reticulata neurons elicited by GABA iontophoresis or striatal stimulation. *Journal of Neuroscience* **6**, 120–126.

Weiss, F., Tanzer, D.J. and Ettenberg, A. (1988) Opposite actions of CCK-8 on amphetamine-induced hyperlocomotion and stereotype following intracerebroventricular and intra-accumbens injections in rats. *Pharmacology Biochemistry and Behavior* **30**, 309–317.

White, N. and Weingarten, H. (1976) Effects of amygdaloid lesions on exploration by rats. *Physiology and Behavior* **17**, 73–79.

Willner, P. (1983) Dopamine and depression: a review of recent evidence: II. Theoretical approaches. *Brain Research Reviews* **6**, 225–236.

Worms, P., Martinez, J., Briet, C., Castro, B. and Biziere, K. (1986) Evidence for dopaminomimetic effect of intrastriatally injected cholecystokinin octapeptide in mice. *European Journal of Pharmacology* **121**, 395–401.

Yang, C.R. and Mogenson, G.J. (1984) Electrophysiological responses of neurones in the nucleus accumbens to hippocampal stimulation and the attenuation of the excitatory responses by the mesolimbic dopaminergic system. *Brain Research* **324**, 69–84.

Yang, C.R. and Mogenson, G.J. (1986) Dopamine enhances terminal excitability of hippocampal-accumbens neurons via D-2 receptor: role of dopamine in presynaptic inhibition. *Journal of Neuroscience* **6**, 2470–2478.

Yang, C.R. and Mogenson, G.J. (1987) Hippocampal signal transmission to the pedunculopontine nucleus and its regulation by dopamine D2 receptors in the nucleus accumbens: an electrophysiological and behavioural study. *Neuroscience* **23**, 1041–1055.

Yim, C.Y. and Mogenson, G.J. (1980) Effect of picrotoxin and nipecotic acid on inhibitory response of dopaminergic neurons in the ventral tegmental area to stimulation of the nucleus accumbens. *Brain Research* **199**, 466–472.

Yim, C.Y. and Mogenson, G.J. (1982) Response of nucleus accumbens neurons to amygdala stimulation and its modification by dopamine. *Brain Research* **239**, 401–415.

Yim, C.Y. and Mogenson, G.J. (1986) Mesolimbic dopamine projection modulates amygdala-evoked EPSP in nucleus accumbens neurons: an in vivo study. *Brain Research* **369**, 347–352.

Yim, C.Y. and Mogenson, G.J. (1988) Neuromodulatory action of dopamine in the nucleus accumbens: an in vivo intracellular study. *Neuroscience* **26**, 403–415.

Yim, C.Y. and Mogenson, G.J. (1989) Low doses of accumbens dopamine modulate amygdala suppression of spontaneous exploratory activity in rats. *Brain Research* **477**, 202–210.

Yim, C.Y. and Mogenson, G.J. (1991) Electrophysiological evidence of modulatory interaction between dopamine and cholecystokinin in the nucleus accumbens. *Brain Research* (in press).

5

The Role of Limbic–Accumbens–Pallidal Circuitry in the Activating and Reinforcing Properties of Psychostimulant Drugs

LUIGI PULVIRENTI, NEAL R. SWERDLOW, CAROL B. HUBNER AND GEORGE F. KOOB

Department of Neuropharmacology, Research Institute of Scripps Clinic, 10666 No. Torrey Pines Road, La Jolla CA 92037, USA

INTRODUCTION

It is known that psychomotor stimulant drugs produce a variety of behavioral effects in humans and animals. The understanding of the neuroanatomical and neurochemical elements involved in the action of these drugs has been the target of much research over the past few years. Administration to naive animals of sympathomimetic drugs such as amphetamine and cocaine, or opiate drugs such as heroin, induces a state of behavioral activation that resembles a state of high motivation in normal individuals (Lyon and Robbins, 1975; Seiden et al., 1975). The fact that stimulant drugs are also drugs of abuse in humans (Jaffe, 1985) suggests the intriguing possibility that the understanding of the neural substrates of motor activation may provide insight into the neural determinants of motivation.

It is known that the nucleus accumbens of the ventral striatum is a critical structure for the expression of hyperactivity induced by various activating drugs (Swerdlow et al., 1986). The functional connections of the nucleus accumbens have been extensively studied (Swerdlow et al., 1986; Swerdlow and Koob, 1987a), and it has been hypothesized that a striato-pallido-

The Mesolimbic Dopamine System: From Motivation to Action.
Edited by P. Willner and J. Scheel-Krüger

© 1991 John Wiley & Sons Ltd

thalamic circuit may be responsible for many of the effects produced by psychomotor stimulants. In addition, the availability of an animal model of intravenous drug self-administration in the rat has allowed a parallel approach to the study of the neurochemical mechanisms underlying the rewarding effects of psychostimulant and opiate drugs. As will be elaborated, similar neural circuit dynamics appear to underlie drug-induced states of arousal and motivational activation.

THE NEURAL SUBSTRATE FOR THE MOTOR ACTIVATING PROPERTIES OF PSYCHOSTIMULANTS

The pharmacological profile of the sympathomimetic agents cocaine and amphetamine reveals that their mechanism of action primarily involves catecholamine transmission in the brain. Cocaine is known to block monoamine re-uptake, while amphetamine induces release of catecholamines from nerve terminals (Iversen and Fray, 1982). Behavioral evidence, however, suggests that the activating properties of these drugs actually depend upon activation of the dopamine (DA) system in the brain. Administration of DA receptor blockers reduces cocaine- and amphetamine-induced locomotion, and destruction of DA terminals within the nucleus accumbens using the selective neurotoxin 6-hydroxydopamine (6-OHDA) prevents the expression of hyperlocomotion induced by these agents (Kelly et al., 1975). These studies indicate that activation of DA transmission within the nucleus accumbens is a critical component of the activating properties of amphetamine and cocaine.

To study the neural efferents from the nucleus accumbens that mediate this DA-dependent behavior, an experimental model of exaggeration of function was developed. One of the consequences of destruction of pre-synaptic DA terminals in the nucleus accumbens is the development of a postsynaptic DA receptor supersensitivity (Staunton et al., 1982). If animals receiving 6-OHDA lesions of the nucleus accumbens are challenged with a small dose of the direct DA agonist apomorphine, they show a greatly enhanced locomotor stimulation relative to controls (Kelly et al., 1975). Therefore, the study of this 'supersensitive' response has the advantage of a functional quantification of an exaggerated DA receptor activation within the nucleus accumbens, thus allowing the investigation of the output of the DA system alone.

Efferents from the nucleus accumbens are known to innervate the substantia innominata, lateral preoptic area, globus pallidus and thalamus (Swanson, 1967; Swanson and Cowan, 1975; Williams et al., 1977; Nauta et al., 1978; Mogenson et al., 1983). Since a region of the ventral pallidum (VP) that includes the substantia innominata and lateral preoptic area receives the densest input from the nucleus accumbens (Swanson, 1967;

Swanson and Cowan, 1975; Nauta et al., 1978; Mogenson et al., 1983), lesions and pharmacological studies of this structure were performed. Both electrolytic and ibotenic acid (Swerdlow et al., 1984a, b) lesions of the ventral pallidum (VP) reduced the 'supersensitive' locomotor response to apomorphine, thus suggesting that the output of DA activation within the nucleus accumbens requires integrity of the VP. The fact that the fiber-sparing lesion obtained with ibotenic acid reduced the locomotor response also suggests that the efferent projections from the nucleus accumbens translate DA receptor activation to activation of spinal motoneurons by synapsing first onto cells within the VP.

Neurochemical studies have suggested that first-order efferents projections from the nucleus accumbens may be GABAergic in nature (Jones and Mogenson, 1980). Also, it has been suggested that the action of DA may be the inhibition of GABA transmission in the VP (Mogenson and Nielsen, 1984a). To test the hypothesis of a GABA link, the effect of intra-VP injections of muscimol, a GABA agonist, on apomorphine-stimulated locomotion was studied. If the net effect of nucleus accumbens DA was a reduction of GABA transmission within the VP, then activation of GABA receptors by muscimol would oppose the apomorphine effect. Indeed, intra-VP administration of 1, 2 and 5 ng of muscimol reduced apomorphine-induced locomotion in a dose-dependent manner (Swerdlow and Koob, 1984). Similarly, infusion of picrotoxin, a GABA antagonist, into the VP induced locomotor hyperactivity (Swerdlow and Koob, 1987b). These data suggest that GABA transmission within the VP is a critical substrate for the expression of locomotor activity and is an important link in the DA-mediated output of the nucleus accumbens.

At this point it was of interest to determine whether any one of the several efferent pathways originating from the VP would be responsible for the expression of this 'supersensitive' locomotor response. Projections from the VP that might constitute the next link in the efferent circuitry included: first, fibers directed rostrally towards the medial prefrontal cortex (MPFC), cholinergic in nature (Divac et al., 1978; Saper, 1984); second, fibers innervating the dorsomedial nucleus of the thalamus (DMT) (Vives and Mogenson, 1985); and third, projections to the pedunculopontine nucleus (PPN), which is the rat homolog of the mesencephalic locomotor region (Grillner and Shik, 1973; Swanson et al., 1984). The approach used to investigate the possible contribution of each single structure to the functional output of the nucleus accumbens–VP circuit was to perform selective lesions of these regions in rats which had received 6-OHDA lesions of the nucleus accumbens, and to challenge the animals with apomorphine.

Electrolytic lesion of the MPFC did not alter the locomotor response induced by 0.1 mg/kg of apomorphine (Swerdlow and Koob, 1987b). This indicates that large areas of VP terminal fields within the MPFC are not critical for the behavioral expression of nucleus accumbens dopaminergic activation. Similarly, lesions of the PPN do not affect the 'supersensitive' locomotor response (Swerdlow and Koob, 1987b). The main finding of this study was, however, that destruction of the DMT significantly reduced this nucleus accumbens DA-dependent locomotor activation (Swerdlow and Koob, 1987b). These results suggest that the third 'critical link' in the locomotion sequence originating from stimulation of DA receptors within the nucleus accumbens is activation of a neural pathway projecting from the VP to the DMT.

The picture that emerges from these studies delineates the neural connections that constitute the functional output of the DA synapses within the nucleus accumbens, and indicates that the nucleus accumbens (Figure 1) is involved in locomotor response and in goal-directed behavior. Given the similarity between the state of behavioral activation induced by psychostimulant drugs and the state of motivational arousal experienced by normal subjects, it is conceivable that activation of the nucleus accumbens may constitute a common neural substrate of these behavioral activities. The availability of techniques of drug self-administration in animals has proven to be a valid experimental approach to address this issue. The question is whether the same circuit responsible for the psychomotor activating properties of cocaine and amphetamine is also involved in the reinforcing properties of these drugs.

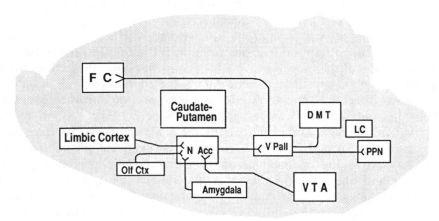

Figure 1. Brain interconnecting circuitry participating in the reinforcing and activating properties of psychostimulant drugs. VTA, Ventral tegmental area; V Pall, ventral pallidum; LC, locus coeruleus; PPN, pedunculopontine nucleus; DMT, dorsal medial thalamus; NAcc, nucleus accumbens; Olf Ctx, olfactory cortex; FC, frontal cortex

THE NEURAL SUBSTRATES FOR THE REINFORCING
PROPERTIES OF PSYCHOSTIMULANTS

As stated above, amphetamine and cocaine are self-administered by rats through the intravenous route. The first indication that the brain DA system was involved came from the observation that pharmacological manipulation of the noradrenergic system did not modify cocaine self-administration (Roberts et al., 1977; DeWit and Wise, 1977), while the DA receptor antagonists, haloperidol, chlorpromazine, sulpiride, thioridazine and others, reduced the rewarding value of cocaine (Roberts and Vickers, 1984). In these tests, rats are exposed for a limited time daily to the self-administration sessions and, in these conditions, the animals self-administer a constant quantity of drug over time, without showing signs of tolerance or dependence. A treatment that reduces the rewarding value of the drug (such as a DA receptor antagonist for cocaine or an opiate antagonist for heroin) causes an increase in drug intake: this is thought to be a compensatory mechanism for the animal to restore the original rewarding properties of cocaine, reduced by competitive antagonism at the receptor site (Koob and Goeders, 1989).

Later studies focused on the identification of the critical regional site, within the dopaminergic system, responsible for cocaine reward. Neurotoxic lesions of the nucleus accumbens using 6-OHDA abolished cocaine self-administration, while similar lesions of the caudate-putamen were ineffective (Roberts et al., 1980; Koob and Goeders, 1989). Further evidence for an involvement of the nucleus accumbens came from studies using the progressive ratio paradigm. In this procedure, the response requirement (lever pressing) to obtain a single i.v. injection of cocaine is progressively increased after each reinforcement is achieved. Eventually, animals reach a so-called breaking point (maximum number of presses each animal is willing to perform to obtain the drug): this is considered a measure of the relative reinforcing value of cocaine. Lesions of the nucleus accumbens, but not of the caudate-putamen, reduce the breaking point for i.v. cocaine self-administration, thus suggesting a loss of 'interest' in the animal towards the drug (Koob and Goeders, 1989).

The fact that the DA system within the nucleus accumbens appears to be the critical substrate, not only for the locomotor activating properties but also for the rewarding properties of cocaine, raises the question as to whether the same output system from the nucleus accumbens that was described for locomotion also subserves cocaine self-administration. This hypothesis is further supported by studies from the literature suggesting that lesion of the cell bodies within the nucleus accumbens using kainic acid reduces cocaine self-administration (Zito et al., 1985). In an attempt to identify a critical 'second link' of the nucleus accumbens output, ibotenic acid lesions of the VP were performed in animals trained to self-administer cocaine. Compared to sham controls, rats receiving a lesion within the VP showed a decrease in cocaine intake and a decrease in the 'interest' for cocaine, as measured in the progressive ratio paradigm (Hubner and Koob, 1990). These results suggest that the same accumbens–pallidal circuitry may be responsible for the expression of the psychomotor activating properties of cocaine, and may be critical for the maintenance of cocaine self-administration in rats.

LIMBIC MODULATION OF ACCUMBENS FUNCTION

It appears from all the studies discussed above that the nucleus accumbens and its neuronal output system are at least part of a circuit underlying the expression of the stimulatory and reinforcing effects of psychostimulant drugs. It is of interest, however, to determine if and how inputs of corticolimbic origin play any role in the modulation of the accumbens function. The nucleus accumbens is an important relay structure that lies between the motor and the limbic system. It is known that a large contingent of afferents to the nucleus accumbens arise from allocortical structures. Indeed, neuroanatomical studies have shown that these fibers arise mainly from the amygdaloid complex and the hippocampal formation, and appear to be glutamatergic in nature (Kelley and Domesick, 1982; Kelley et al., 1982; Fuller et al., 1987). Furthermore, several studies by Mogenson and colleagues have suggested that this glutamatergic projection may be the functional interface between the limbic and the motor system (Mogenson, 1984, 1987; Mogenson and Nielsen, 1984b).

Some anatomical evidence about the ultrastructural connection between glutamate and DA terminals within the nucleus accumbens suggests that the two systems may lie in close apposition (Sesack and Pickel, 1989; Totterdell and Smith, 1990), while a possible reciprocal functional connection between the two neurotransmitters has been suggested on the basis of electrophysiological, biochemical and behavioral studies. Electrophysiological evidence indicates that a large percentage of accumbens neurons respond to stimulation of the basolateral amygdala or the ventral subiculum of the hippocampus, and that this activation of nucleus accumbens neurons may be mediated by glutamatergic fibers (Yang and Mogenson, 1985). Moreover, behavioral studies suggest that this pathway may mediate locomotor activity. In fact, locomotion induced by novelty or by microinjections of carbachol in the dentate gyrus of the hippocampus is reduced by concomitant pharmacological blockade of glutamate receptors within the nucleus accumbens (Mogenson and Nielsen, 1984a, b). Other indirect evidence for a possible glutamate-DA interaction comes from neurochemical and behavioral studies suggesting that injection of the glutamate agonist N-methyl-D-aspartate (NMDA) within the nucleus accumbens stimulates locomotor activity (Donzanti and Uretsky, 1983), and that this critically depends upon facilitation of endogenous nucleus accumbens DA transmission (Boldry and Uretsky, 1988; Payson and Donzanti, 1989).

Following these observations, studies were initiated to determine whether endogenous nucleus accumbens glutamate transmission could modulate the activating properties of cocaine. Previous results indicate that, indeed, pharmacological blockade of nucleus accumbens glutamate receptors reduced the hyperactivity induced by systemic injection of cocaine and amphetamine, but not caffeine (Pulvirenti et al., 1989a, 1990). Thus it seems that endogenous glutamate function within the nucleus accumbens modulates DA-mediated locomotion, possibly at a presynaptic level within the DA synapse. This finding is further supported by the preliminary observations from our group that in rats trained to self-administer cocaine, blockade of accumbens NMDA receptors using 2-amino-5-phosphonovaleric acid (AP5) reduces the rewarding properties of the drug, as measured by an increase in cocaine intake (Pulvirenti et al., 1989b).

Taken together, these findings suggest that endogenous glutamatergic transmission at the level of the nucleus accumbens plays a 'permissive' role on the DA-dependent activating effect of psychostimulant drugs (Figure 2). According to this hypothesis, glutamate tone may reflect the modulating effect of allocortical structures such as the amygdala and the hippocampus, and it is tempting to speculate that this glutamate–DA interaction within the nucleus accumbens may be at least one of the neurochemical bases of limbic–motor integrative mechanisms. The possibility then that the processing of sensory (amygdala) and mnemonic (hippocampus) information finds its

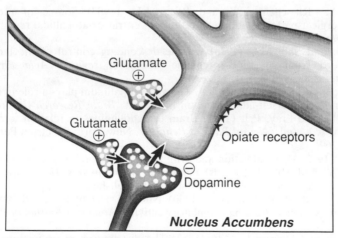

Figure 2. Schematic representation of putative glutamate–DA interaction within the nucleus accumbens

access to the motor effectors of the mesocorticolimbic system via the DA gating mechanism of the nucleus accumbens remains a fascinating hypothesis worthy of test.

ACKNOWLEDGEMENTS

This is publication number 6290-NP of the Research Institute of Scripps Clinic. This work was partially supported by NIDA grants DA 04043 and DA 04398. L. Pulvirenti is a Visiting Scientist from the III Department of Neurology, University of Pavia, Italy.

REFERENCES

Boldry, R.C. and Uretsky, N.J. (1988) The importance of dopaminergic neurotransmission in the hypermotility response produced by the administration of N-methyl-D-aspartic acid into the nucleus accumbens. *Neuropharmacology* **27**, 569–577.

DeWit, H. and Wise, R.A. (1977) Blockade of cocaine reinforcement in rats with the dopamine blocker pimozide, but not with the noradrenergic blockers phentolamine and phenoxybenzamine. *Canadian Journal of Psychology* **31**, 195–203.

Divac, I., Bjorklund, A., Lindvall, O. and Passingham, R.E. (1978) Converging projections from the medio-dorsal nucleus and mesencephalic dopaminergic neurons to the neocortex in three species. *Journal of Comparative Neurology* **180**, 59–72.

Donzanti, B.A. and Uretsky, N.J. (1983) Effects of excitatory amino acids on locomotor activity after bilateral microinjections into the rat nucleus accumbens: possible dependence on dopaminergic mechanisms. *Neuropharmacology* **22**, 971–981.

Fuller, T.A., Russchen, F.T. and Price, J.L. (1987) Source of presumptive glutamatergic/aspartergic afferents to the rat ventral striatopallidal region. *Journal of Comparative Neurology* **258**, 317–338.

Grillner, S. and Shik M.I. (1973) On the descending control of the lumbosacral spinal cord from the 'mesencephalic locomotor region'. *Acta Physiologica Scandinavica* **87**, 320–333.

Hubner, C.B. and Koob, G.F. (1990). The ventral pallidum plays a role in mediating heroin and cocaine self-administration in the rat. *Brain Research* (in press).

Iversen, S.D. and Fray, P.J. (1982) Brain catecholamines in relation to affect. In: Beckman, A.L. (ed.) *Neural Basis of Behavior*. New York: Spectrum Publications, pp. 229–269.

Jaffe, J.H. (1985) Drug addiction and drug abuse. In: Goodman, L.S., Gilman, A., Rall, T.W. and Murad, F. (eds) *Goodman and Gilman's The Pharmacological Basis of Therapeutics*. New York: Macmillan Publishing Co., pp. 532–580.

Jones, D.L. and Mogenson, G.J. (1980) Nucleus accumbens to globus pallidus GABA projection subserving ambulatory activity. *American Journal of Physiology* **238**, R63–R69.

Kelley, A.E. and Domesick, V.B. (1982) The distribution of projections from the hippocampal formation to the nucleus accumbens in the rat: an anterograde and retrograde horseradish peroxidase study. *Neuroscience* **7**, 2321–2335.

Kelley, A.E., Domesick, V.B. and Nauta, W.J.H. (1982) The amygdalostriatal projections in the rat—an anatomical study by anterograde and retrograde tracing methods. *Neuroscience* **7**, 615–630.

Kelly, P.H., Seviour, P. and Iversen, S.D. (1975) Amphetamine and apomorphine responses in the rat following 6-OHDA lesions of the nucleus accumbens septi and corpus striatum. *Brain Research* **94**, 507–522.

Koob, G.F. and Goeders, N.E. (1989) Neuroanatomical substrates of drug self-administration. In: Liebman, J. and Cooper, S. (eds) *The Neuropharmacological Basis of Reward*. Oxford: Oxford University Press, pp. 214–263.

Lyon, M. and Robbins, T. (1975) The action of central nervous system stimulant drugs: a general theory concerning amphetamine effects. In: Essman, W.B. and Vatzelli L. (eds) *Current Developments in Psychopharmacology*. New York: Spectrum Publications, 80–162.

Mogenson, G.J. (1984) Limbic-motor integration with emphasis on initiation of exploratory and goal directed behavior. In: Bandler, R. (ed) *Modulation of Sensorimotor Activity During Alteration in Behavioral States*. New York: Alan R. Liss Inc., pp. 121–137.

Mogenson, G.J. (1987) Limbic-motor integration. In: Epstein, A.N. (ed.) *Progress in Psychobiology and Physiological Psychology, Vol. 12*. New York: Academic Press, pp. 117–170.

Mogenson, G.J. and Nielsen, M. (1984a) Neuropharmacological evidence that the nucleus accumbens and subpallidal region contribute to exploratory locomotion. *Behavioral and Neural Biology*, **42**, 52–60.

Mogenson, G.J. and Nielsen, M. (1984b) A study of the contribution of the hippocampal-accumbens-subpallidal projections to locomotor activity. *Behavioral and Neural Biology*, **42**, 38–51.

Mogenson, G.J., Swanson, C.W. and Wu, M. (1983) Neural projections from the nucleus accumbens to globus pallidus, substantia innominata and lateral preoptic area: an anatomical and electrophysiological investigation in the rat. *Journal of Neuroscience* **3**, 189–202.

Nauta, W.J.H., Smith, J.P., Faull, R.L.M. and Domesick, V.B. (1978) Efferent connections and nigral afferents of the nucleus accumbens septi in the rat. *Neuroscience* **3**, 385–410.

Payson, M.M. and Donzanti, B.A. (1989) Effect of excitatory amino acids on 'in vivo' dopamine release and metabolism in the nucleus accumbens. *Society for Neuroscience Abstracts* **15**, 584.

Pulvirenti, L., Swerdlow, N.R. and Koob, G.F. (1989a) Microinjection of a glutamate antagonist into the nucleus accumbens reduces psychostimulant locomotion in rats. *Neuroscience Letters* **103**, 213–218.

Pulvirenti, L., Sung, R. and Koob, G.F. (1989b) Microinjection of NMDA, but not quisqualate receptor antagonists into the nucleus accumbens modulates intravenous cocaine self-administration in rats. *Society for Neuroscience Abstracts* **15**, 1098.

Pulvirenti, L., Swerdlow, N.R. and Koob, G.F. (1990) in preparation.

Roberts, D.C.S. and Vickers, G. (1984) Atypical neuroleptics increase self-administration of cocaine: an evaluation of a behavioral screen for antipsychotic activity. *Psychopharmacology* **82**, 135–139.

Roberts, D.C.S., Corcoran, M.E. and Fibiger, H.C. (1977) On the role of ascending noradrenergic systems in intravenous self-administration of cocaine. *Pharmacology Biochemistry and Behavior* **6**, 615–620.

Roberts, D.C.S., Koob, G.F., Klonoff, P. and Fibiger H.C. (1980) Extinction and recovery of cocaine self-administration following 6-hydroxydopamine lesions of the nucleus accumbens. *Pharmacology Biochemistry and Behaviour* **12**, 781–787.

Saper, C.B. (1984) Organization of cerebral cortical afferent systems in the rat. II. Magnocellular basal nucleus. *Journal of Comparative Neurology* **222**, 313–321.

Seiden, L.S., MacPhail, R.C. and Emmett-Oglesby, M.W. (1975) Catecholamines and drug-behavior interactions. *Federation Proceedings* **34**, 1823–1831.

Sesack, S.R. and Pickel, V.M. (1989) Ultrastructural basis for modulatory interactions between hippocampal and dopaminergic afferents to the rat nucleus accumbens. *Society for Neuroscience Abstracts* **15**, 1229.

Staunton, D., Magistretti, P., Koob, G.F., Shoemaker, W. and Bloom F.E. (1982) Dopaminergic supersensitivity induced by denervation and chronic receptor blockade is additive. *Nature* **229**, 72–74.

Swanson, L.W. (1967) An autoradiographic study of the efferent connections of the preoptic region in the rat. *Journal of Comparative Neurology* **167**, 227–256.

Swanson, L.W. and Cowan, W.M. (1975) A note on the connections and development of the nucleus accumbens. *Brain Research* **92**, 324–330.

Swanson, L.W., Mogenson, G.J., Gerfen, C.R. and Robinson, P. (1984) Evidence for a projection from the lateral preoptic area and substantia innominata to the 'mesencephalic locomotor region' in the rat. *Brain Research* **295**, 161–178.

Swerdlow, N.R. and Koob, G.F. (1984) The neural substrate of apomorphine-stimulated locomotor activity following denervation of the nucleus accumbens. *Life Science* **33**, 2537–2544.

Swerdlow, N.R. and Koob, G.F. (1987a) Dopamine, schizophrenia, mania and depression: toward a unified hypothesis of cortico-striato-pallido-thalamic function. *Behavioral and Brain Sciences* **10**, 197–245.

Swerdlow, N.R. and Koob, G.F. (1987b) Lesions of the dorsomedial nucleus of the thalamus, medial prefrontal cortex and pedunculopontine nucleus: effect on locomotor activity mediated by nucleus accumbens-ventral pallidal circuitry. *Brain Research* **412**, 233–243.

Swerdlow, N.R., Swanson, L.W. and Koob, G.F. (1984a) Electrolytic lesions of the substantia innominata and lateral preoptic area attenuate the 'supersensitive' locomotor response to apomorphine resulting from denervation of the nucleus accumbens. *Brain Research* **306**, 141–148.

Swerdlow, N.R., Swanson, L.W. and Koob, G.F. (1984b) Substantia innominata: critical link in the behavioral expression of mesolimbic dopamine stimulation in the rat. *Neuroscience Letters* **50**, 19–24.

Swerdlow, N.R., Vaccarino, F.J., Amalric, M. and Koob, G.F. (1986) The neural substrate for the motor-activating properties of psychostimulants: a review of recent findings. *Pharmacology, Biochemistry and Behavior* **25**, 233–248.

Totterdell, S. and Smith, A.D. (1990) Convergence of hippocampal and dopaminergic input onto identified neurons in the nucleus accumbens of rats. *Journal of Chemical Neuroanatomy* (in press).

Vives, F. and Mogenson, G.J. (1985) Electrophysiological evidence that the mediodorsal nucleus of the thalamus is a relay between the ventral pallidum and the medial prefrontal cortex in the rat. *Brain Research* **334**, 329–337.

Williams, D.J., Crossman, A.R. and Slater, P. (1977) The efferent projections of the nucleus accumbens in the rat. *Brain Research* **130**, 217–227.

Yang, C.R. and Mogenson, G.J. (1985) An electrophysiological study of the neural projections from the hippocampus to the ventral pallidum and the subpallidal areas by way of the nucleus accumbens. *Neuroscience* **15**, 1015–1024.

Zito, K.A., Vickers, G. and Roberts, D.C.S. (1985) Disruption of cocaine and heroin self-administration following kainic acid lesions of the nucleus accumbens. *Pharmacology, Biochemistry and Behavior* **23**, 1029–36.

6

Gating Function of Noradrenaline in the Ventral Striatum: Its Role in Behavioural Responses to Environmental and Pharmacological Challenges

A.R. COOLS, R. VAN DEN BOS, G. PLOEGER AND
B.A. ELLENBROEK

Department of Pharmacology, University of Nijmegen, PO Box 9101, 6500
HB Nijmegen, The Netherlands

SYNOPSIS

Many studies have shown that the ventral striatum (nucleus accumbens) contains, among others, noradrenaline (NA) and dopamine (DA) (Palmer and Chronister, 1980; Allin et al., 1988). Today, several authors prefer to describe both catecholamines as modulators of synaptic transmission rather than as agents which transmit specific details of moment-to-moment information. Thus, mesolimbic DA is believed to play a permissive role (Simon and LeMoal, 1984), whereas NA is believed to have a 'gating' action (Waterhouse et al., 1988). Thus, both catecholamines are believed to modulate information that arrives at the ventral striatum (Mogenson and Yim, 1980). Owing to the fact that the possible role of mesolimbic NA in this respect is largely overlooked and underestimated by most researchers, the present survey focuses attention upon this neuroactive compound, especially in relation to its control of hippocampal and amygdaloid inputs of the ventral striatum.

The Mesolimbic Dopamine System: From Motivation to Action.
Edited by P. Willner and J. Scheel-Krüger   © 1991 John Wiley & Sons Ltd

This chapter consists of two parts. In the first part, evidence is accumulated in favour of the new concept that there are two fundamentally distinct types of NA–DA interaction within the ventral striatum, each having its own role in modulating the hippocampal and amygdaloid inputs of the ventral striatum: the interaction between β-receptors and D2 receptors modulating the hippocampal inputs of the ventral striatum, and the interaction between α-receptors and the non-classic DA$_i$ receptors modulating the amygdaloid inputs of the ventral striatum. It is suggested that activation of mesolimbic β-receptors, which belong to the dorsal noradrenergic bundle, produces an enhanced DA activity at the level of D2 receptors, which, in turn, inhibits the excitatory action of hippocampal inputs on neurons in the ventral striatum; and that inhibition of mesolimbic α-receptors, which appear to belong to the ventral noradrenergic bundle, produces an enhanced DA activity at the level of so-called DA$_i$ receptors, which, in turn, inhibits the excitatory action of amygdaloid inputs on neurons in the ventral striatum.

We also provide data in favour of the hypothesis that these distinct NA–DA interactions direct the nature of the seesaw between the hippocampal and amygdaloid inputs in a highly characteristic manner. It is suggested that 'opening of the hippocampal gate' by means of β-receptors or D2 antagonists prevents a 'closed amygdaloid gate' from being opened. Conversely, 'closing of the hippocampal gate' by means of β-receptors or D2 agonists facilitates the 'opening of the amygdaloid gate'. For convenience, the former and latter states are labelled as seesaw I and seesaw II, respectively.

The second part of this chapter presents experimental data showing that α-receptors located in the ventral striatum play a highly specific role in the control of behaviour. Our data show that these receptors are only behaviourally active when animals are challenged by environmental and/or pharmacological stimuli. In this part we also present original data showing that the well-known sensitization of dexamphetamine-induced hyperactivity is due to changes at the level of these α-receptors, which are believed to be presynaptically localized upon dopaminergic terminals within the ventral striatum; the same mechanism appears to underlie the sensitization induced by the psychostimulants cocaine, methylphenidate, pipradrol and phencyclidine.

On the basis of the available data we reach the conclusion that the dexamphetamine-induced change in mesolimbic α-receptors is due to the ability of dexamphetamine to accelerate ultimately the transition from seesaw II to seesaw I: this transition is a mechanism to compensate for the original dexamphetamine-induced transition from seesaw I to seesaw II, which is itself the consequence of the ability of dexamphetamine to enhance NA activity at the level of the α-receptors within the ventral striatum.

Finally, we put forward the hypothesis that the α-receptors within the ventral striatum are critically involved in the mechanisms by which the transition between seesaw II and seesaw I comes to control behavioural responses to a single stressful event, be it environmental or pharmacological.

DISTINCT TYPES OF NA–DA INTERACTIONS WITHIN THE VENTRAL STRIATUM

Interaction Between Mesolimbic β-Receptors and D2 Receptors

The ventral striatum contains both α- and β-receptors (Sawaya et al., 1977; Nurse et al., 1985). The β-receptors are known to control the hippocampal input of the ventral striatum: activation of these receptors has been found to inhibit the excitatory action of the hippocampal input on neurons in the ventral striatum (Unemoto et al., 1985a, b). Since stimulation of the locus coeruleus produces a similar effect, which can be blocked by a selective β-receptor (but not by an α-receptor) antagonist (Unemoto et al., 1985a, b), it appears that the dorsal NA bundle modulates the hippocampal input via β-receptors. Given the fact that activation of β-receptors within the ventral striatum enhances the release of DA (Nurse et al., 1985), it cannot be excluded that this NA modulation is indirect. DA itself is known to exert a similar 'gating' action on the hippocampal input of the ventral striatum; the latter effect is direct and mediated via D2, but not D1, receptors (DeFrance et al., 1985; Yang and Mogenson, 1986, 1987). These data together strongly suggest that stimulation of the dorsal NA bundle activates β-receptors; this indirectly results in an enhanced activation of D2 receptors, which inhibits the excitatory action of the hippocampal input on neurons in the ventral striatum. In other words, activation of intra-accumbens β-receptors belonging to the dorsal NA bundle directly or indirectly blocks the arrival of hippocampal inputs at the level of the ventral striatum and, accordingly, closes the hippocampal gate, whereas inhibition of these β-receptors opens this gate. α-Receptors are known to play no role in this respect (Unemoto et al., 1985a, b).

Interaction between Mesolimbic α-NA and Non-Classical DA Receptors

Although mesolimbic α-receptors are unable to modify hippocampal inputs of the ventral striatum (see above), activation of intra-accumbens α-receptors has been found to suppress the release of DA within the ventral striatum (Nurse et al., 1985). This recent biochemical finding provides direct evidence in favour of our earlier hypothesis that activation of intra-accumbens α-receptors inhibits dopaminergic activity within the ventral striatum (Cools et al., 1979; Cools, 1980). The DA receptors involved in this effect differ from the classical D2 and D1 receptors (Cools, 1977; Cools and van Rossum, 1980; Cools and Oosterloo, 1983). The receptors in question, which are labelled DA_i receptors, are characterized by the following properties: (1) they are stimulated by DA and (3,4-dihydroxyphenyl)-2-imidazoline (DPI) (the mixed D1/D2 agonist apomorphine, the selective D2 agonist LY 171555, the selective, but partial, D1 agonist SKF 38393, and NA are inactive in this respect); (2) they are inhibited by ergometrine (the mixed D1/D2 antagonist haloperidol, the selective D2 antagonist raclopride, the selective D1 antagonist SCH 23390, the α-receptor antagonist phentolamine, and the $5HT_2$-antagonist ritanserin are ineffective in this respect); (3) they are concentrated in brain areas innervated by dopaminergic A8 and A10 fibres; and (4) they mediate sedation and orofacial dyskinesias in rats and cats, as well as inhibition of spontaneously firing DA cells in the *Helix aspersa* (DA_i receptors are among other properties stimulated by DA and apomorphine, inhibited by haloperidol, concentrated in brain areas innervated by dopaminergic A9 fibres, and mediate typical striatal functions in rats and cats as well as excitation of spontaneously firing DA cells in the *Helix aspersa*. For similarities and dissimilarities between the DA_i/DA_e concept and D1/D2 concept see Cools et al., 1988a).

Since the mesolimbic α-receptors, which control the activity at the level of DA_i receptors, play no role in the modulation of hippocampal inputs of the ventral striatum (see above), the above-mentioned data indicates that there must exist an additional, intra-accumbens circuitry, in which the latter α-NA/DA_i interaction takes place. It is known that the ventral striatum is innervated not only by the dorsal bundle, but also by the ventral bundle which arises in the A1, A2 and A5 cells (Cedarbaum and Aghajanian, 1978; Lindvall and Bjorklund, 1978; Speciale et al., 1978; O'Donohue et al., 1979). Lesioning this ventral bundle reduces the amount of NA within the ventral striatum (O'Donohue et al., 1979) and produces a transition from sniffing to licking in dexamphetamine-treated rats (Braestrup, 1977). The lesion-induced transition from sniffing to licking is mimicked by systemic or intraventricular administration of α-noradrenergic, but not β-noradrenergic, antagonists (Mogilnicka and Braestrup, 1976; Zebrowska-Lupina et al., 1978); lesions of the dorsal noradrenergic bundle are ineffective in this respect (Pycock, 1977). The display of DA-dependent licking requires an enhanced dopaminergic activity at the level of the DA_i receptors within the ventral striatum, which are under the inhibitory control of α-receptors (Cools, 1977).

Together, these data lay the foundation for the hypothesis that both the transition from sniffing to licking which occurs after lesioning the ventral NA bundle, and the transition from sniffing to licking which occurs after administration of α-blockers, are actually due to the enhanced DA_i activity within the ventral striatum, being the immediate consequence of the experimentally induced decrease in the α-adrenergic activity within the ventral striatum. Since mesolimbic α-receptors do not control the hippocampal inputs (see above), the possibility that the DA_i receptors which are involved in this α-NA/DA_i interaction exert a 'gating' action on hippocampal inputs can be excluded. In this context, it is relevant to recall that intra-accumbens DA not only modulates hippocampal inputs, but also inhibits the excitatory input from the basolateral region of the amygdala (Yim and Mogenson, 1986, 1988). The nature of the dopaminergic receptors involved in the latter effect is not yet delineated. However, it is not unlikely that the DA_i receptors may be involved (see below). If so, it will be evident that activation of α-receptors, which results in an inhibition of the DA_i activity, can open the amygdaloid gate in the ventral striatum, whereas inhibition of these receptors can close this gate.

Dexamphetamine and its Possible Ability to Open the Amygdaloid Gate within the Ventral Striatum

The suggestion that activation of mesolimbic α-receptors may open the amygdaloid gate implies that compounds which directly or indirectly increase activity at the level of intra-accumbens α-receptors, and/or directly or indirectly decrease the activity at the level of intra-accumbens DA_i receptors, can also open the amygdaloid gate. In this context it is relevant to consider the mechanisms underlying dexamphetamine-induced behavioural responses. There is now abundant evidence that the dexamphetamine-induced increase in central α-noradrenergic activity plays an important modulatory role in behavioural responses such as locomotor hyperactivity. Apart from the fact that dexamphetamine increases noradrenergic activity (Taylor and Snyder, 1971), most studies agree that decreasing noraderenergic activity, or inhibiting α-receptors, attenuates these dexamphetamine-induced responses (Rolinski and Scheel-Krüger, 1973; Dickinson et al., 1988). The conventional view that dexamphetamine leads to an increased DA activity within the ventral striatum is well established (Hernandez et al., 1987; Carboni et al., 1989; Kolta et al., 1989; Kuczenski and Segal, 1989). Local application of dexamphetamine in the ventral striatum is highly effective in producing hyperactivity (Pijnenburg, 1976), and lesioning the ventral striatum with 6-hydroxydopamine (6-OHDA) suppresses the locomotor response following systemic administration of dexamphetamine (Costall et al., 1977; Clarke et al., 1988). However, there is actually little evidence to support the conventional view that dexamphetamine-induced hyperactivity requires an *enhanced* DA activity within this brain structure. Although both the mixed D2/D1 antagonist haloperidol and the pure D2 antagonist raclopride suppress the dexamphetamine response (Pijnenburg, 1976; van den Bos et al., 1988), intra-accumbens administration of the mixed D2/D1 agonist apomorphine produces exactly the same effect (Costall and Naylor, 1976). Second, the finding that intra-accumbens administration of 6-OHDA suppresses the dexamphetamine response (Gold et al., 1988) does not prove that intra-accumbens DA is essential, as this treatment also destroys non-dopaminergic elements, particularly noradrenergic elements (Taghzouti et al., 1985). Third, the finding that dexamphetamine enhances the release of DA within the ventral striatum only provides valid evidence in favour of the conventional hypothesis if hyperactivity correlates with the DA release. As has been shown recently, this is not the case: in fact, the dexamphetamine-induced behavioural activity disappears long before the drug-induced release of DA returns to baseline levels (cf. Robinson et al., 1988; Figures 2 and 3). Indeed, an earlier study found that the maximum increase in intra-accumbens 3,4-dihydroxy-phenylacetic acid (DOPAC) release was seen in animals which display immobility (Louilot et al., 1986).

The available data concerning the involvement of DA receptor subtypes in hyperactivity are even more complex. Neither intra-accumbens application of the selective D2 agonist LY 171555 nor that of the selective, but partial, D1 agonist SKF 38393 elicits hyperactivity in naive animals; the same holds true for combined injections of both compounds, although there are some contradictory findings in this respect (Fletcher and Starr, 1987; Dreher and Jackson, 1989). Extensive replications of these studies have been performed in our laboratory. Using our conventional procedure in well-habituated and well-handled rats (Cools, 1986), we have found direct evidence that intra-accumbens injections of the D2 agonist LY 171555, the D1 agonist SKF 38393, or combinations of these agents (1.0–10.0 μg/0.5 μl; eight or nine rats per treatment), are completely ineffective in naive rats (Cools et al., 1988b). On the other hand, there is evidence that DA, DPI (a selective, but not specific, agonist of DA_i receptors), and L-DOPA (in combination with the L-amino acid decarboxylase inhibitor Ro 4-4602) actually inhibit hyperactivity elicited from the ventral striatum, and that the depleting agent reserpine, in combination with the tyrosine hydroxylase inhibitor α-methylparatyrosine, enhances the hyperactivity elicited from the ventral striatum (Cools and Van Rossum, 1980). The latter data have led us to postulate that this hyperactivity is due to a reduction of intra-accumbens DA at the level of the DA_i receptors (Cools, 1986). Although the suppression of hyperactivity by intra-accumbens DPI may be abolished by lesions of the medial raphe nuclei, a role for serotonin in this phenomenon (Costall et al., 1979) appears unlikely in view of the fact that the ventral striatum is primarily innervated by the dorsal raphe nuclei, but not by the medial raphe nuclei (Steinbusch, 1981).

Taking all these data together, it appears that systemic administration of dexamphetamine increases locomotor activity by enhancing activity at the level of intra-accumbens α-receptors, and decreasing activity at the level of the DA_i receptors. If so, dexamphetamine opens the amygdaloid gate by preventing the DA_i receptors from exerting their inhibitory action upon the amygdaloid input of the ventral striatum. Although there is no doubt that dexamphetamine can exert additional actions on other neurotransmitter systems inside and outside the ventral striatum, it is relevant to point out that this view fits nicely with the recent finding that intra-accumbens application of dexamphetamine ameliorates the impairment of instrumental behaviour maintained by a conditioned reinforcer, which followed lesions in the basolateral region of the amygdala (Everitt et al., 1989; see also Cador et al., Chapter 9, this volume). These data imply, then, that intra-accumbens administration of dexamphetamine mimics the effects characteristic of an open amygdaloid gate. It remains to be seen whether those dexamphetamine-induced behavioural responses which require an intact ventral striatum and which are attenuated by α-noradrenergic antagonists are actually the consequences of such an opened amygdaloid gate. For the moment, it is sufficient to mention that active neural elements of the basolateral region of the amygdala are necessary if application of dexamphetamine into the ventral striatum is to facilitate the acquisition of conditioned reinforcement (Cador et al., 1989; Everitt et al., 1989). Thus, it appears that compounds such as dexamphetamine, which increases the activity at the level of the intra-accumbens α-receptors and, indirectly, decreases the activity at the level of the intra-accumbens DA_i receptors, can indeed open the amygdaloid gate.

Mesolimbic Interaction between Hippocampal and Amygdaloid Inputs of the Ventral Striatum

The data summarized above lay the foundation for the concept that there are at least two distinct types of intra-accumbens NA–DA interaction, each having its own role in 'gating' hippocampal and amygdaloid inputs of the ventral striatum (Figures 1 and 2). Thus, activation of mesolimbic β-receptors belonging to the dorsal noradrenergic bundle, and/or activation of mesolimbic D2 receptors, is suggested to close the hippocampal gate, whereas inhibition of these β-receptors and/or D2 receptors is suggested to open this gate. Alternatively, inhibition of mesolimbic α-receptors, which appear to belong to the ventral noradrenergic bundle and/or activation of mesolimbic DA_i receptors, is suggested to close the amygdaloid gate, whereas activation of these α-receptors and/or inhibition of the DA_i receptors is suggested to open the latter gate. Since outputs of the ventral subiculum of the hippocampus converge heavily with outputs of the basolateral region of the amygdala in the anteromedial region of the ventral striatum (Phillipson and Griffiths, 1985; Groenewegen et al., 1987; Oades and Halliday, 1987), spontaneously occurring or experimentally induced changes in the hippocampal input may have direct consequences for the functioning of the amygdaloid input, and vice versa. Thus, pharmacological manipulations of one type of NA–DA interaction may have direct consequences for the expression of the function of the other type of NA–DA interaction.

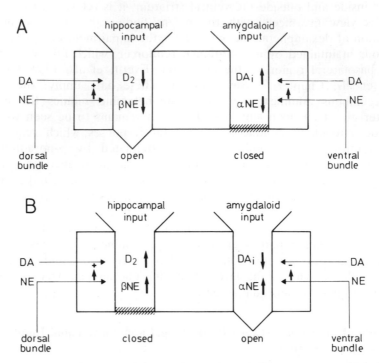

Figure 1. Site and function of β-noradrenergic and D2 receptors modulating the hippocampal inputs of the ventral striatum, and α-noradrenergic and DA_i receptors modulating the amygdaloid inputs to the ventral striatum. A, seesaw I; B, seesaw II; NE, noradrenaline

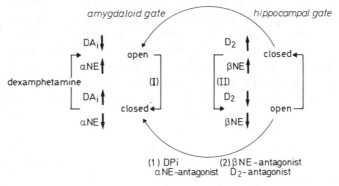

Figure 2. Main characteristics of the relationship between so-called seesaw I (open hippocampal gate and closed amygdaloid gate), and so-called seesaw II (closed hippocampal gate and open amygdaloid gate) within the ventral striatum. NE, noradrenaline

Coupling between an Open Hippocampal Gate and a Closed
Amygdaloid Gate within the Ventral Striatum

Since both systemic administration of α-noradrenergic antagonists and the intra-accumbens injection of the DA_i agonist DPI, namely manipulations which close the amygdaloid gate, suppress the hyperactivity induced by systemic administration of dexamphetamine (see above), it is evident that the dexamphetamine response requires an open amygdaloid gate. However, both β-noradrenergic antagonists and D2 antagonists, namely manipulations which open the hippocampal gate (see above), are also effective in attenuating this dexamphetamine-induced hyperactivity (Weinstock and Speiser, 1974; Pijnenburg, 1976; van den Bos et al., 1988). These data clearly reveal that closure of the amygdaloid gate and opening of the hippocampal gate produce identical effects; however, they do not indicate whether or not these phenomena are causally coupled to one another. However, β-adrenergic antagonists, which open the hippocampal gate, only inhibit the dexamphetamine-induced hyperactivity when given before, but not after, the dexamphetamine treatment (Weinstock and Speiser, 1974). This finding reveals two important aspects of the hippocampal–amygdaloid interaction within the ventral striatum. First, it shows that opening of the hippocampal gate prevents manipulations which normally open the amygdaloid gate from doing so. Second, it shows that this prevention only occurs when the amygdaloid gate is not yet opened.

This insight may explain why D2 antagonists prevent the acquisition of incentive motivational learning, but do not suppress the maintenance of incentive motivational learning (Beninger, 1983). The basolateral region of the amygdala and its projection to the ventral striatum (see above) are critically involved in the mechanisms by which conditioned, or secondary, reinforcers come to control behaviour by association with primary reinforcers (Cador et al., 1989; Everitt et al., 1989). The acquisition of incentive motivational learning requires an open amygdaloid gate in the ventral striatum. Since D2 antagonists, like α-noradrenergic antagonists, open the hippocampal gate and, consequently, prevent the amygdaloid gate from being opened (see above), it is evident that D2 antagonists prevent the acquisition of incentive motivational learning. It is, however, clear that animals well-trained in operant tasks involving reinforcement already have an open amygdaloid gate, implying that manipulations which open the hippocampal gate can no longer hinder the opening of the amygdaloid gate: accordingly, D2 antagonists are unable to interrupt the maintenance of incentive motivational learning.

Coupling between a Closed Hippocampal Gate and an Open
Amygdaloid Gate within the Ventral Striatum

Since opening of the hippocampal gate appears to prevent opening of the amygdaloid gate, it is reasonable to expect that closing of the hippocampal gate might result in the opening of the amygdaloid gate. In this context, it is useful to consider the hyperactivity which follows hippocampal damage (Reinstein et al., 1982).

If one accepts the conventional view that the hippocampal accumbens neurons are glutamatergic (Walaas and Fonnum, 1979; Christie et al., 1987), one might predict that intra-accumbens administration of glutamate antagonists would also elicit hyperactivity. In practice, however, intra-accumbens administration of glutamate agonists elicits hyperactivity, while glutamate antagonists suppress locomotor activity (Arnt, 1981; Mogenson and Nielsen, 1984; Hamilton et al., 1986). However, the amygdala–accumbens fibres are also glutamatergic (Christie et al., 1987; Robinson and Beart, 1988), so these results are difficult to interpret.

It is more relevant to note that intra-accumbens application of the DA_i agonist DPI, which closes the amygdaloid gate (see above), reverses behavioural deficits in animals with hippocampal damage (particularly hyperactivity and decreased grooming frequency and rearing bout duration), whereas intra-accumbens application of the mixed D2/D1 antagonist haloperidol, which opens the hippocampal gate, remains ineffective in this respect (Reinstein et al., 1982; Springer and Isaacson, 1982; Hannigan et al., 1984). The effects of DPI provide direct evidence that an open amygdaloid gate is an essential prerequisite for the display of behavioural responses triggered by hippocampal damage. It has already been discussed that an open hippocampal gate is accompanied by a closed amygdaloid gate. It has now become evident that closure of the hippocampal gate by means of hippocampal damage opens the amygdaloid gate, and that this effect seems responsible for the hyperactivity which follows hippocampal damage. As mentioned above, the same appears to hold true for the hyperactivity elicited by dexamphetamine.

Factors Directing the Mesolimbic Interaction between Hippocampal
and Amygdaloid Inputs of the Ventral Striatum

The above discussion of the interplay between the hippocampal and amygdaloid inputs of the ventral striatum has formed the foundation for the concept that there exists a real seesaw between the two inputs. An open hippocampal gate prevents a closed amygdaloid gate from being opened: it maintains a seesaw state marked by an open hippocampal gate and a closed amygdaloid gate (seesaw I). A closed hippocampal gate facilitates the opening of the amygdaloid gate: it maintains an opposite seesaw state which is marked by a closed hippocampal gate and an open amygdaloid gate (seesaw II). Each seesaw state should correspond to a particular neurochemical state within the ventral striatum. Hence animals marked by seesaw I must have a low α- and β-adrenergic activity, a low D2 activity, and a high DA_i activity, whereas animals marked by seesaw II must have a high α- and β-adrenergic activity, a high D2 activity, and a low DA_i activity. This forms the foundation for the notion that animals marked by seesaw I have a susceptibility for agonists and antagonists of the receptors involved, which is opposite to that of animals marked by seesaw II. Although both pharmacological and environmental stimuli can alter the neurochemical state and, accordingly, determine the nature of the seesaw (see below), genetic factors are also important in this respect. In fact, pharmacogenetic selection of apomorphine-susceptible and apomorphine-unsusceptible rats from a normal outbred Wistar strain has enabled us to develop two lines of rats which vary greatly in the amount of NA within their ventral striatum as well as their susceptibility to intra-accumbens injection of selective α-adrenergic and dopaminergic agents (Sutanto et al., 1989; Cools et al., 1990). Because these differences are at least partly genetically determined (Segal et al., 1975), these lines allow us to perform precisely those experiments required to provide direct evidence in favour of the concepts described above.

The seesaw concept also results in the clear-cut notion that mesolimbic noradrenergic mechanisms play a critical role in modulating the opening and closing of the hippocampal and amygdaloid gates. For that reason, it is relevant to recall two main features of the central noradrenergic processes.

First, a great variety of environmental challenges varying from a short-term confrontation with novelty to long-term individual housing are known to enhance central noradrenergic activity (Oades, 1985). Such challenges can be predicted to 'produce' animals marked by seesaw II: such animals will have a closed hippocampal gate and an open amygdaloid gate, as soon as challenges such as lack of habituation, lack of handling, food-deprivation, social isolation, etcetera start to increase the release of NA. It will also be clear that well-habituated and well-handled animals which are not challenged by any stressor will be marked by seesaw I, implying that they have an open hippocampal gate and a closed amygdaloid gate. This insight has far reaching consequences for understanding the behaviour shown by animals in different situations. It also suggests that the ability of catecholaminergic agents to change behaviour varies according to the neurochemical alterations produced by environmental challenges. For example, it can be predicted that D2 agonists, for instance, will be differentially effective in habituated, well-handled and socially housed rats which remain devoid of the confrontation with any stressor, and non-habituated, non-handled, individually housed or otherwise stressed animals.

Second, noradrenergic processes, especially α- and β-receptors within mesolimbic structures, have an enormous capacity to maintain homeostasis: these noradrenergic receptors have been found to adapt their sensitivity in the manner inversely related to the degree of their stimulation by NA (Reisine, 1981): an increased NA release makes postsynaptic binding sites sensitive to antagonists but insensitive to agonists, whereas a decreased NA release makes postsynaptic binding sites sensitive to agonists but insensitive to antagonists. In fact, noradrenergic binding sites change 'states' or 'configurations' upon excessive exposure to agonists or antagonists in such a way as to favour the counterpart ligand (U'Prichard et al., 1977; Greenberg et al., 1978; Hata et al., 1980). Furthermore, an increased NA release is known to enhance the potency of noradrenergic agonists to inhibit its presynaptic release on the one hand, and to reduce the potency of noradrenergic antagonists to enhance its presynaptic release on the other hand, and vice versa (Starke, 1979).

These, and related data, have led us to the conclusion that the noradrenergic synapses can occur in two different states (Figure 3): synapses

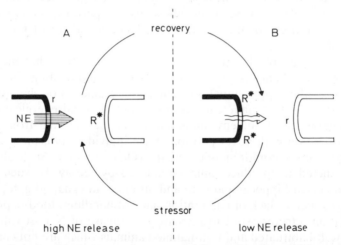

Figure 3. Relationship between the amount of noradrenaline (NE) released in the synaptic cleft and the functional state of postsynaptic and presynaptic noradrenergic receptors. Synapses with a high NE release (left side) have postsynaptic noradrenergic receptors in the 'antagonist' state, i.e. receptors that are sensitive to noradrenergic antagonists and insensitive to noradrenergic agonists (R*), and presynaptic noradrenergic receptors in the 'agonist' state, i.e. receptors that are sensitive to noradrenergic agonists and insensitive to noradrenergic antagonists (r). The mirror image holds true for synapses with a low NE release (right side). As discussed in the text, the latter state (right side) is characteristic for well-habituated and well-handled animals which are not challenged by any environmental and/or pharmacological stimulus, whereas the state depicted at the left side is characteristic for animals which are challenged by one or another stressor

with a high NA release have postsynaptic adrenergic receptors in the 'antagonist' state and presynaptic adrenergic receptors in the 'agonist' state, whereas synapses with a low NA release have postsynaptic adrenergic receptors in the 'agonist' state and presynaptic adrenergic receptors in the 'antagonist' state. Short-term environmental or pharmacological challenges can produce rapid (minutes–hours) transitions between the two states of the NA synapses in the ventral striatum, whereas the persistence of the challenge-induced state varies according to the nature and strength of the challenge (Cools et al., 1987; Cools, 1988; Cools, unpublished data). In fact, the above-mentioned features of the NA synapses within the ventral striatum are identical to those originally discovered by Antelman and his colleagues as being essential features of the overall NA system (Antelman et al., 1980, 1989; Antelman and Chiodo, 1983; Antelman, 1988). Given these properties of the noradrenergic processes, it will be clear that spontaneously occurring and environmentally or pharmacologically induced changes in the mesolimbic noradrenergic activity may cause rapid transitions between seesaw I and seesaw II, as long as these homeostatic mechanisms are operational. Accordingly, genetic, internal or external factors which alter the properties of these homeostatic mechanisms within the ventral striatum will have far reaching consequences for the ability of animals to respond adequately to a changing internal or external environment. This is indeed the case: in advanced age, for instance, these homeostatic mechanisms are deficient with the consequence that aged animals have a reduced ability to adapt behaviourally and phsysiologically to their environment (Weiss, 1988).

EXPERIMENTAL STUDIES: STRESS AND SENSITIZATION

Behavioural Role of Mesolimbic α-Receptors in Non-Stressed Animals

The available literature suggests that intra-accumbens application of noradrenergic agents only influences behaviour when animals are challenged by environmental or drug-induced changes (see below). In this context it should be noted that studies using injection volumes larger than 1 μl and/or more than 10 μg provide no valid information because of the non-selectivity and non-specificity of these methods. Using small volumes and doses, we have carefully re-investigated the (in)ability of intra-accumbens injections of the selective α-noradrenergic agonist phenylephrine to alter behaviour. As mentioned above, well-habituated animals should be marked by seesaw I, and should have a relatively low noradrenergic activity in the ventral striatum and, accordingly, postsynaptic receptors susceptible to agonists. In view of these considerations, we analysed the effects of intra-accumbens injections of phenylephrine in rats which were both thoroughly familarized with the injection procedure (by administration of two dummy injections and one injection with the solvent on 3 successive days preceding the test-day) and thoroughly habituated to the experimental cage for three periods, each of 6 hours. The experiments showed that otherwise naive, male rats belonging to our outbred Wistar strain, weighing 200 ± 20 g, and equipped with intracerebral cannulae according to previously described procedures (Cools, 1986) did not show any sign of behavioural change after bilateral injections of varying doses of phenylephrine (0.5–10.0 μg/0.5 μl per side; eight or nine rats per treatment) into the anterodorsal part of the medial region of the ventral striatum. Detailed analysis of the data, which were collected for a period of 240 minutes after the injection and which were analysed in terms of frequencies/minute, revealed that the behavioural activity was neither increased nor decreased during any period after the injection, not even during the initial 1–15 minutes after the injection (see Figure 6). Thus, selective and specific activation of α-receptors within the ventral striatum of otherwise undisturbed rats remains devoid of any effect. As shown below, this does not hold true for rats challenged by internal or external stimuli.

Behavioural Role of Mesolimbic α-Receptors in Stressed Animals

Environmental Challenges

At least three studies show that activation of noradrenergic receptors in the ventral striatum does alter the behaviour of rats challenged by environmental stimuli. First, rats tested in the so-called forced-swim test show an α-adrenergic-specific increase in swimming movements following intra-accumbens application of NA and noradrenergic agents (Plaznik et al., 1985). Second, recent studies in our laboratory have shown that selective activation of α-receptors within the ventral striatum (by means of intra-accumbens application of 750 ng/0.5 μl phenylephrine) inhibits switching to cue-directed behaviours without affecting the ability to switch to non cue-directed behaviours in the so-called 'swimming without escape' test (van den Bos et al., unpublished data). Finally, in non-habituated rats put in a novel environment, intra-accumbens NA (but not DA) decreased exploratory behaviour (Svensson and Ahlenius, 1983). All three sets of data indicate that exposure to a new environment, a challenging event sometimes labelled as a stressor, changes the neurochemical state within the brain in such a way that activation of the postsynaptic α-receptors within the ventral striatum produces specific behavioural changes that do not occur in well-habituated and well-handled animals.

In an attempt to understand this phenomenon, it is useful to recall that: (*1*) environmental challenges enhance central noradrenergic activity, which subsides during coping with, or habituation to, these challenges; and that

(2) spontaneously or experimentally induced changes in central noradrenergic activity are immediately followed by adaptations of the neurochemical state within central NA synapses (see above).

In this context it is relevant to note that the processing of information via the amygdaloid gate must precede the processing of information via the hippocampal gate (see Scheel-Krüger and Willner, Chapter 22, this volume). Thus, under natural circumstances in which environmental changes challenge or stress the organism and, accordingly, enhance the release of noradrenaline, the initially closed amygdaloid gate, which is at that time accompanied by an open hippocampal gate (Figure 1: seesaw I), opens. Subsequently, the hippocampal gate closes, with the ultimate result that the organism will be marked by an open amygdaloid gate and a closed hippocampal gate (Figure 1: seesaw II). When recovering from the challenge or stressor, noradrenaline release returns to baseline levels; consequently, seesaw I (Figure 1) is reintroduced. Both the nature (pharmacological or environmental) and the rate of transitions between the distinct seesaw states are determined by the magnitude of the challenge.

Thus, environmental challenges of non-stressed animals which are marked by seesaw I (open hippocampal gate and closed amygdaloid gate) produce a transition to seesaw II (closed hippocampal gate and open amygdaloid gate). This state is in turn followed by a transition to seesaw I as soon as the animal starts to cope with, or habituate to, these challenges. Given the notion (see above) that seesaw II is marked by postsynaptic noradrenergic receptors in the 'antagonist' state and presynaptic noradrenergic receptors in the 'agonist' state (see above), it will be evident that, in animals challenged by environmental stimuli, noradrenergic agonists can only activate presynaptic receptors, with the result that the release of NA is inhibited. The resulting decrease in the release of NA immediately creates a new situation within the synapse, marked by the presence of postsynaptic adrenergic receptors in the 'agonist' state and presynaptic adrenergic receptors in the 'antagonist' state (see above). Thus, NA agonists given in such a situation actually promote effects characteristic of a return to a low baseline activity within NA synapses (Antelman and Caggiula, 1977). The finding that intra-accumbens application of NA decreases exploratory behaviour fits in with this notion. Both a decreasing α-adrenergic activity and/or a decreasing β-adrenergic activity within the ventral striatum should attenuate exploratory behaviour: a decrease in postsynaptic α-adrenergic activity enhances the release of DA at the level of DA_i receptors, which in turn is known to suppress locomotor activity (see above); a decrease in β-adrenergic activity within the ventral striatum as a consequence of lesioning the dorsal NA bundle (see above), inhibits exploratory behaviour (Pisa et al., 1988). The most intriguing aspect of this mechanism of action, however, is the notion that NA agonists given in such a situation actually facilitate the transition from seesaw II to seesaw I. Consequently, these agents accelerate the process of coping with, or habituation to, environmental challenges.

Although this explanation of these phenomena is speculative and, accordingly, requires extensive research to be (in)validated, the available data unequivocally show that environmental challenges alter the neurochemical state within the brain in such a way that behavioural responses can be elicited by selective activation of α-adrenergic receptors in the ventral striatum. This does not occur in animals which are not challenged by environmental stimuli.

Drug-Induced Challenges

There are at least three studies showing that drug-induced challenges also alter the neurochemical state within the brain in such a way that behavioural responses can be elicited by selective activation of α-receptors in the ventral striatum. First, intra-accumbens administration of α-adrenergic agonists is known to elicit explosive motor behaviour in rats pretreated with a behaviourally ineffective dose of picrotoxin injected into the deeper layers of the superior colliculus; the latter effect has been found to be specific for α-receptors within the ventral striatum (Cools et al., 1987). Second, intra-accumbens application of the α-adrenergic agonist phenylephrine is found to counteract the tonic EMG activity of the triceps muscle elicited by intra-accumbens administration of haloperidol (Ellenbroek et al., 1988). Finally, intra-accumbens application of the α-adrenergic agonist phenylephrine becomes effective in rats sensitized by systemic or intra-accumbens injections of dexamphetamine. Since the latter information is not only new, but also highly relevant for understanding at least some aspects of the function of α-receptors within the ventral striatum, we present the latter data in more detail (see below).

All three sets of data clearly reveal that drug treatments, like environmental stimuli, can alter the neurochemical state within the ventral striatum in such a way that behavioural responses can be elicited by selective activation of α-receptors in the ventral striatum, a phenomenon which does not occur in well-habituated and well-handled animals which are not challenged by any additional stimulus. The fact that both pharmacological and environmental challenges produce similar effects would suggest that the drugs act as stressors. In other words, the drug treatments may, directly (dexamphetamine: see below) or indirectly, as a consequence of the stressful event (the picrotoxin- and haloperidol-induced changes), have produced a transition from seesaw I to seesaw II, followed subsequently by a transition from seesaw II to seesaw I to counteract the original transition. This implies that intra-accumbens injections of phenylephrine produce behavioural effects by activating presynaptic NA receptors, thereby promoting the transition from seesaw II to seesaw I. We will return to this hypothesis after having discussed the role of mesolimbic α-receptors in dexamphetamine-induced sensitization.

Role of Mesolimbic α-Receptors in Dexamphetamine-Induced Sensitization

Methods

In principle, all experiments were performed according to previously described procedures using similar techniques, methods and locomotor cages (Cools, 1986). Male Wistar rats weighing 200 ± 20 g were equipped with cannulae directed at the anterodorsal part of the medial region of the ventral striatum. After recovery from anaesthesia they were habituated to their locomotor cage for three periods, each of 6 hours, starting 7 days after the operation. To adapt the rats to the injection procedure, they received dummy injections at the beginning of the first two habituation sessions and a single treatment with distilled water at the beginning of the last habituation session, according to the time schedule used in the actual experiments (see below). On each test-day the rats were rehabituated to the cage for a period of 45 minutes: bilateral injections of the drugs dissolved in distilled water (0.5 µl per side) were always given during the light period around 10.00 am (standard light/dark periodicity: light from 6.00 am to 6.00 pm). When the rats received a combined treatment of an antagonist and an agonist, the antagonist was given 3 minutes before the agonist. When priming injections were given, the subsequent test was performed precisely 24 hours later. The data were analysed with a two-way fixed ANOVA, and Newman–Keuls test comparisons were calculated where appropriate, unless otherwise indicated. Each experiment was performed with nine rats.

Dexamphetamine-Induced Sensitization to Dexamphetamine-Induced Hyperactivity

As shown in the left part of Figure 4, intra-accumbens injections of 10.0 µg of dexamphetamine sulphate which elicited an increased locomotor activity on the priming day induced a clear-cut and significant sensitization to a subsequent, similar treatment on the test-day. In additional experiments we found that this single exposure to dexamphetamine caused persistent, cascading sensitization to subsequent intra-accumbens injections of dexamphetamine (data not shown). The right part of Figure 4 shows that intra-accumbens injections of the α-adrenergic antagonist phentolamine (0.5 µg) given 3 minutes prior to the dexamphetamine injection on the test-day attenuated this sensitizing effect; lower doses of phentolamine (0.1 µg) were ineffective in this respect (data not shown). Higher doses of phentolamine

158

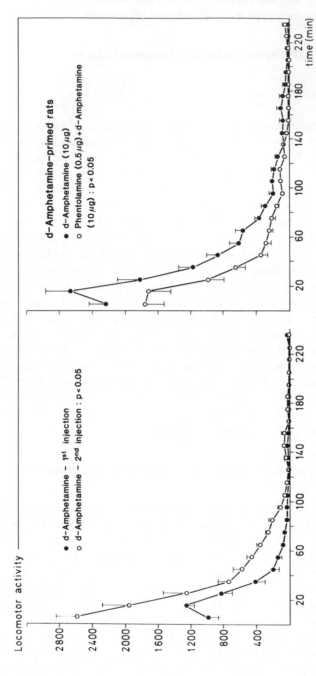

Figure 4. Dexamphetamine-induced sensitization to a subsequent exposure to intra-accumbens injections of 10.0 µg dexamphetamine: the locomotor activity, elicited by intra-accumbens injections of 10.0 µg dexamphetamine 24 hours after a similar treatment on the priming day, was significantly greater than that found on the priming day (n = 9) (left panel). Inhibition of the dexamphetamine-induced sensitized locomotor activity by intra-accumbens injections of 0.5 µg phentolamine given 3 minutes prior to intra-accumbens injections of 10.0 µg dexamphetamine on the test-day in animals (n = 9) which were pretreated with intra-accumbens injections of 10.0 µg dexamphetamine on the priming day (right panel)

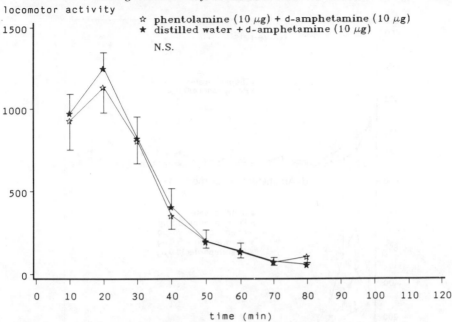

Figure 5. Lack of any effect of intra-accumbens injections of 10.0 μg phentolamine given 3 minutes prior to intra-accumbens injections of 10.0 μg dexamphetamine in naive animals ($n = 9$): the dexamphetamine-induced hyperactivity remained unaffected

(up to 10.0 μg) fully inhibited the sensitizing effect, but never reduced locomotor activity below that elicited by the priming injection. Phentolamine alone (10.0 μg) was completely unable to attenuate the dexamphetamine-induced response on the priming day (Figure 5). These data strongly suggest that α-receptors within the ventral striatum are involved in the sensitization of dexamphetamine-induced hyperactivity, but not in the hyperactivity response itself.

The next four experiments provide direct evidence in favour of this hypothesis.

Critical Role of Mesolimbic α-Receptors in the Sensitization of Dexamphetamine-Induced Hyperactivity

A single intra-accumbens exposure to 10.0 μg of dexamphetamine (Figure 6) altered the neurochemical state within the ventral striatum in such a way that the originally behaviourally ineffective α-receptors became highly susceptible to the α-noradrenergic agonist phenylephrine: intra-accumbens injections of phenylephrine (0.5–10.0 μg) produced a dose-dependent

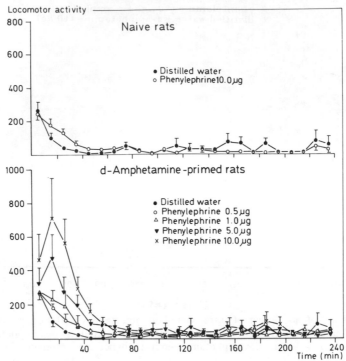

Figure 6. Locomotor activity elicited by intra-accumbens injections of phenylephrine (0.5–10.0 µg) in naive animals (top) and in animals which were pretreated with intra-accumbens injections of 10.0 µg dexamphetamine 24 hours earlier (bottom): dexamphetamine-induced sensitization to a subsequent exposure to phenylephrine ($n = 9$/test-group)

increase in the locomotor activity in rats primed 24 hours earlier with 10.0 µg dexamphetamine. This phenylephrine effect appeared to be dependent on the dose of the priming injections of dexamphetamine given 24 hours earlier: Figure 7 shows that administration of dexamphetamine (1.0–10.0 µg) on the priming day produced an increasing degree of sensitization of hyperactivity induced by 10.0 µg phenylephrine on the test-day. The effect of phenylephrine (10.0 µg) was inhibited by phentolamine (5.0 µg) given 3 minutes prior to phenylephrine on the test-day (Figure 8). Finally, the dexamphetamine-induced sensitization of phenylephrine-induced hyperactivity was indeed mediated by the α-receptors themselves: phentolamine (10.0 µg) given 3 minutes prior to the priming injections of dexamphetamine (10.0 µg) did not attenuate the dexamphetamine-induced hyperactivity on the priming day

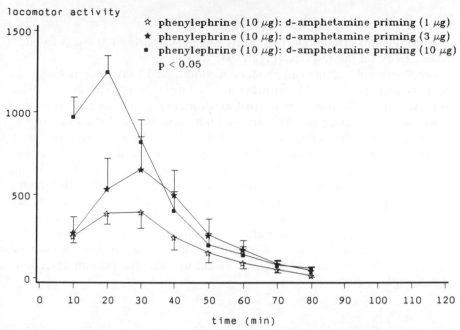

Figure 7. Dose-dependency of the sensitizing effect of intra-accumbens injections of dexamphetamine (1.0–10 μg) to intra-accumbens injections of 10.0 μg phenylephrine given 24 hours after the dexamphetamine treatment (n = 9/test-group)

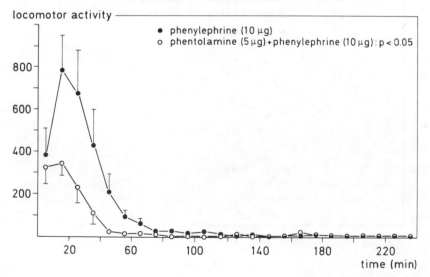

Figure 8. Effect of intra-accumbens injections of 5.0 μg phentolamine given 3 minutes prior to intra-accumbens injections of 10.0 μg phenylephrine in animals (n = 9) which were pretreated with intra-accumbens injections of 10.0 μg dexamphetamine 24 hours earlier: suppression of the dexamphetamine-induced sensitization to phenylephrine

(Figure 5), but did suppress the ability of phenylephrine (10.0 µg) to elicit hyperactivity on the test-day (Figure 9).

Since dexamphetamine can produce a conditioned locomotor response in the environment if it has been previously administered (Gold et al., 1988; also see below), the following control experiment was included. Two groups of animals were equipped with intra-accumbens cannulae, habituated to the experimental locomotor cages, and familiarized with the injection procedures as described above. Animals in the first group received dexamphetamine (10.0 µg/0.5 µl per side) and were immediately returned to their home cages, whereas animals in the second group received the same treatment but were tested in the experimental cages, to which they were already habituated. On the test-day both groups received phenylephrine (10.0 µg/0.5 µl per side) and were tested in the experimental locomotor cages. As shown in Figure 10, dexamphetamine sensitized the mesolimbic α-receptors independent of the environment in which the priming injections of dexamphetamine were given.

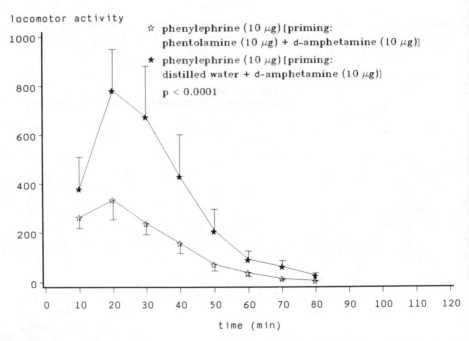

Figure 9. After-effect of intra-accumbens injections of 10.0 µg phentolamine given 3 minutes prior to intra-accumbens injections of 10.0 µg dexamphetamine in naive animals (*n* = 9) upon locomotor activity elicited by intra-accumbens injections of 10.0 µg phenylephrine given 24 hours later: suppression of the dexamphetamine-induced sensitization to phenylephrine

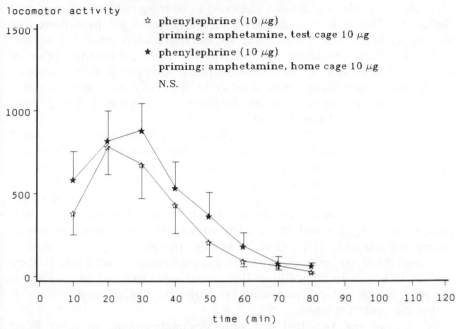

locomotor activity

☆ phenylephrine (10 μg)
priming: amphetamine, test cage 10 μg

★ phenylephrine (10 μg)
priming: amphetamine, home cage 10 μg

N.S.

time (min)

Figure 10. Lack of environmental conditioning of the sensitization (induced by intra-accumbens injections of 10.0 μg dexamphetamine) to a subsequent exposure to intra-accumbens injections of 10.0 μg phenylephrine: the effect of phenylephrine injections was independent of the environment in which the priming injections were given (*n* = 9/test-group)

In conclusion, it is clear that dexamphetamine alters the neurochemical state within the ventral striatum in such a way that behavioural responses can be elicited by selective activation of α-receptors within the ventral striatum. Given the notion that dexamphetamine enhances the activity at the level of mesolimbic α-receptors which in turn results in a reduced activity at the level of the mesolimbic DA_i receptors (see above), it is clear that dexamphetamine initially produces a transition from seesaw I to seesaw II. As mentioned above, this effect is believed to underlie the display of dexamphetamine-induced hyperactivity. Given the adaptational properties of the mesolimbic noradrenergic processes (see above), this transition in turn promotes a shift from seesaw II to seesaw I, thereby creating a situation within NA synapses which is marked by the presence of postsynaptic receptors in the 'agonist' state, and presynaptic receptors in the 'antagonist' state (Figure 3). Thus, a priming injection of dexamphetamine makes the postsynaptic α-receptors within the ventral striatum highly susceptible to α-adrenergic agonists. These findings show that dexamphetamine produces precisely those effects which are suggested to be triggered by environmental challenges. This is fully in line with the earlier reported hypothesis that dexamphetamine, and at least some stressors, are interchangeable in their ability to induce sensitization (Antelman et al., 1980). From this point of view, one can predict that environmental or pharmacological interventions which induce sensitization will directly or indirectly alter noradrenergic activity within the ventral striatum: future research is required to provide evidence in favour of this suggestion.

To date, the vast majority of studies of dexamphetamine-induced sensitization of dexamphetamine-induced hyperactivity have provided evidence that DA synapses in the ventral striatum play a critical role in this phenomenon (Robinson and Becker, 1986). In fact, there is evidence that presynaptic receptors modulating the release of DA from dopaminergic terminals in the ventral striatum are necessary (Gold et al., 1988). The present data, together with the fact that mesolimbic α-receptors are able to control the release of DA within the ventral striatum (see above), allow us to extend this hypothesis as follows. Dexamphetamine-induced sensitization appears to be due to the ability of dexamphetamine to affect mesolimbic α-receptors which are presynaptically localized on dopaminergic terminals within the ventral striatum.

In view of the fact that not only dexamphetamine but also other psychostimulants can sensitize animals (Peris and Zahniser, 1989), the question arises whether other psychostimulants are also able to sensitize mesolimbic α-receptors. As shown in Figures 11 and 12, we found that intra-accumbens injections of cocaine, methylphenidate, pipradrol and phencyclidine (10.0 µg/0.5 µl per side), given on the priming day, also made the pretreated animals susceptible to intra-accumbens injections of phenylephrine (10.0 µg/0.5 µl per side) given on the test-day. In other words, other psychostimulants, like dexamphetamine, also sensitize mesolimbic α-receptors. These data allow the conclusion that the α-receptors within the ventral striatum play a fundamental role in sensitization.

Critical Role of Mesolimbic α-Receptors in Conditioned Hyperactivity Produced by Systemic Dexamphetamine

Psychostimulant-induced hyperactivity can be classically conditioned through the repeated pairing of the unconditioned locomotor drug effect with a previously neutral testing environment (Robinson and Becker, 1986). Recently, it has been shown that mesolimbic DA released from intact DA terminals within the ventral striatum is critically involved in the development and expression of conditioned locomotor responses (Gold et al., 1988). The evidence that mesolimbic α-receptors which control the release of DA within the ventral striatum, are sensitized by dexamphetamine suggests that

165

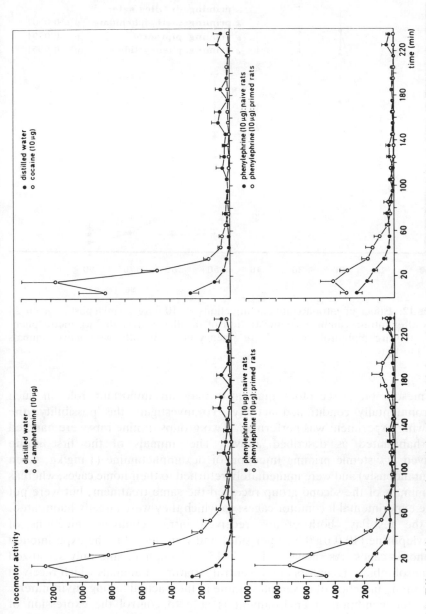

Figure 11. Effect of intra-accumbens injections of 10.0 µg phenylephrine given 24 hours after intra-accumbens administration of 10.0 µg dexamphetamine (left) or 10.0 µg cocaine (right) in otherwise naive animals (*n* = 9/test-group). The upper panels show the response to priming injections and the lower panels the response to phenylephrine given 24 hours later

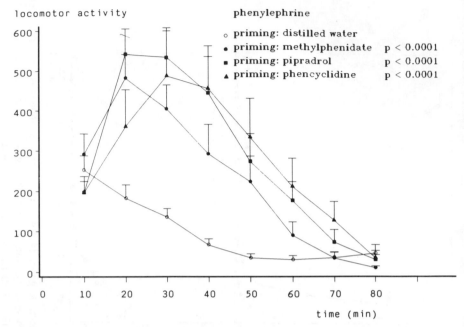

Figure 12. Effect of intra-accumbens injections of 10.0 μg phenylephrine given 24 hours after intra-accumbens administration of distilled water, 10.0 μg methylphenidate, 10.0 μg pipradrol, and 10.0 μg phencyclidine in otherwise naive animals (*n* = 9/test-group)

the mesolimbic α-receptors may also play an important role in such environmentally conditioned activity. To investigate this possibility, the following experiment was performed. Two groups of nine rats were handled and habituated as described above. The animals of the first group received a systemic priming injection of dexamphetamine (1 mg/kg, given subcutaneously) and were immediately returned to their home cages, whereas the animals of the second group received the same treatment, but were put in the experimental locomotor cages, to which they were already habituated. On the test-day, both groups received intra-accumbens injections of phenylephrine (10.0 μg/0.5 μl per side) and were tested in the experimental locomotor cages. As shown in Figure 13, dexamphetamine only sensitized the mesolimbic α-receptors in the ventral striatum of animals which received the priming injection of dexamphetamine in their actual testing environment. Thus, the conditioning environment is able to control the expression of dexamphetamine-induced sensitization to α-adrenergic agonists injected into the ventral striatum. The above-mentioned notion that dexamphetamine may open the amygdaloid gate and, accordingly, allow the organism to

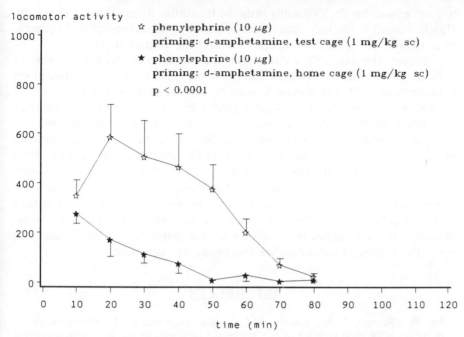

Figure 13. Environmental conditioning of the sensitization induced by systemic administration of 1.0 mg/kg dexamphetamine to subsequent intra-accumbens injections of 10.0 μg phenylephrine, given 24 hours later (*n* = 9/test-group)

associate previously neutral stimuli with primary reinforcers provides an adequate explanation for this phenomenon. The finding that *intra-accumbens* injections of dexamphetamine do not lead to environmental conditioning may simply imply that the strength of the internal stimuli elicited by intra-accumbens injections of dexamphetamine overshadows the influence of the external stimuli; this apparently does not occur after the systemic administration of a relatively low dose of dexamphetamine. Further research is required to validate the latter hypothesis.

OVERALL CONCLUSION: EXPERIMENTAL DATA

These data show that intra-accumbens injections of dexamphetamine alter the neurochemical state within the ventral striatum in such a way that behavioural responses can be elicited by activation of α-adrenergic receptors within the ventral striatum; this phenomenon does not occur in well-habituated and well-handled animals which are not challenged by environmental or pharmacological stimuli. This effect is ascribed to the ability of dexamphetamine to accelerate ultimately the transition from the hippocampal–amygdaloid seesaw II to seesaw I; this transition is a mechanism to compensate for the originally induced transition from seesaw I to seesaw II, which itself is the consequence of the dexamphetamine-induced increase in activity at the level of α-receptors within the ventral striatum.

Together, the available data suggest that α-receptors within the ventral striatum are critically involved in the mechanisms by which transitions between seesaw II and seesaw I come to control behavioural responses to environmental and pharmacological challenges. In other words, our data not only support Antelman's concept of the critical role of NA in stressor-induced sensitization to subsequent stressors, be they environmental or pharmacological (Antelman et al., 1980, 1989; Antelman and Chiodo, 1983; Antelman, 1988), but also extend it by demonstrating that mesolimbic α-receptors in particular are implicated in this process. Like Antelman, we believe that deficits in the mechanisms under discussion may play a critical role in a great variety of human disorders varying from depression, panic disorders and schizophrenia to addiction and amphetamine psychosis. It is up to the reader to conceptualize the nature of such deficits.

REFERENCES

Allin, R., Russell, V.A., Lamm, M.C.L. and Taljaard, J.J.F. (1988) Regional distribution of monoamines in the nucleus accumbens of the rat. *Neurochemical Research* **13**, 937–942.

Antelman, S.M. (1988) Time-dependent sensitization as the cornerstone for a new approach to pharmacotherapy: drugs as foreign/stressful stimuli. *Drug Review* **14**, 1–30.

Antelman, S.M. and Caggiula, A.R. (1977) Norepinephrine-dopamine interactions and behavior. A new hypothesis of stress-related interactions between brain norepinephrine and dopamine is proposed. *Science* **19**, 646–653.

Antelman, S.M. and Chiodo, L.A. (1983) Amphetamine as a stressor. In: Creese, I. (ed.) *Stimulants: Neurochemical, Behavioral and Clinical Perspectives* New York: Raven Press, pp. 269–299.

Antelman, S.M., Eichler, A.J., Black, C.A. and Kocan, D. (1980) Interchangeability of stress and amphetamine in sensitization. *Science* **207**, 329–331.

Antelman, S.M., Knopf, S., Kocan, D. and Edwards, D.J. (1989) Persistent sensitization of clonidine-induced hypokinesia following one exposure to a stressor: possible relevance to panic disorder and its treatment. *Psychopharmacology* **98**, 97–101.

Arnt, J. (1981) Hyperactivity following injection of a glutamate agonist and 6, 7-ADTN into rat nucleus accumbens and its inhibition by THIP. *Life Sciences* **28**, 1597–1603.

Beninger, R.J. (1983) The role of dopamine in locomotor activity and learning. *Brain Research Reviews* **6**, 173–196.

Braestrup, C. (1977) Changes in drug-induced stereotyped behavior after 6-OHDA lesions in noradrenaline neurons. *Psychopharmacology* **51**, 199–204.

Cador, M., Robbins, T.W. and Everitt, B.J. (1989) Involvement of the amygdala in stimulus-reward associations: interaction with the ventral striatum. *Neuroscience* **30**, 77–86.

Carboni, E., Imperato, A., Perezzani, L. and Di Chiara, G. (1989) Amphetamine, cocaine, phencyclidine and nomifensine increase extracellular dopamine concentrations preferentially in the nucleus accumbens of freely moving rats. *Neuroscience* **28**, 653–661.

Cedarbaum, J.M. and Aghajanian, G.K. (1978) Afferent projections to the rat locus coeruleus as determined by a retrograde tracing technique. *Journal of Comparative Neurology* **178**, 1–16.

Christie, M.J., Summers, R.J., Stephenson, J.A., Cook, C.J. and Beart, P.M. (1987) Excitatory amino acid projections to the nucleus accumbens septi in the rat: a retrograde transport study utilizing D[^{3}H]GABA. *Neuroscience* **22**, 425–439.

Clarke, P.B.S., Jakubovic, A. and Fibiger, H.C. (1988) Anatomical analysis of the involvement of mesolimbocortical dopamine in the locomotor stimulant actions of d-amphetamine and apomorphine. *Psychopharmacology* **96**, 511–520.

Cools, A.R. (1977) Two functionally and pharmacologically distinct dopamine receptors in the rat brain. In: Costa, E. and Gessa, G.L. (eds) *Advances in Biochemical Psychopharmacology*. New York: Raven Press, pp. 215–225.

Cools, A.R. (1980) Rapid development of hypersensitivity and hyposensitivity to apomorphine and haloperidol: role of norepinephrine receptor mechanisms in CNS. In: Cattabeni, F. (ed.) *Long-Term Effects of Neuroleptics*. New York: Raven Press, pp. 215–222.

Cools, A.R. (1986) Mesolimbic dopamine and its control of locomotor activity in rats: differences in pharmacology and light/dark periodicity between the olfactory tubercle and the nucleus accumbens. *Psychopharmacology* **88**, 451–459.

Cools, A.R. (1988) Transformation of emotion into motion: role of mesolimbic noradrenaline and neostriatal dopamine. In: Hellhammer, D., Florin, I. and Weiner, H. (eds) *Neurobiological Approaches to Human Disease*. Toronto: Hans Huber Publishers, pp. 15–28.

Cools, A.R. and Oosterloo, S.K. (1983) (3, 4-Dihydroxyphenylimino)-2-imidazoline (DPI) and its action at noradrenergic and dopaminergic receptors in the nucleus accumbens of rats: mesolimbic catecholamine receptors and hyperactivity. *Journal of Neural Transmission* **18**, 181–188.

Cools, A.R. and Van Rossum, J.A.M. (1980) Multiple receptors for brain dopamine in behavior regulation: concept of dopamine-E and dopamine-I receptors. *Life Sciences* **27**, 1237–1253.

Cools, A.R., Dongen, P.A.M. van and Well, P. van (1979) Mesolimbic norepinephrine and changes in behavioral responsiveness to apomorphine in rats. In: Usdin, E., Kopin, I.J. and Banchas, J. (eds) *Catecholamines: Basic and Clinical Frontiers*. New York: Pergamon Press, pp. 592–594.

Cools, A.R., Ellenbroek, B., Bos, R. van den and Gelissen, M. (1987) Mesolimbic noradrenaline: specificity, stability and dose-dependency of individual-specific responses to mesolimbic injections of α-noradrenergic agonists. *Behavioral Brain Research* **25**, 49–61.

Cools, A.R., Spooren, W., Cuypers, E., Bezemer, R. and Jaspers, R. (1988a) Heterogeneous role of neostriatal and mesostriatal pathology in disorders of movement: a review and new facts. In: Crossman, A.R. and Sambrook, M.A. (eds) *Neural Mechanisms in Disorders of Movement*. London: John Libbey and Company Ltd, pp. 111–119.

Cools, A.R., Hoeboer W. and de Vries, T. (1988b) Role of D1 and D2 dopaminergic receptors in dopamine-mediated locomotion elicited from the nucleus accumbens and the tuberculum olfactorium. *Psychopharmacology* **96**, 33.

Cools, A.R., Brachten, R., Heeren, D., Willemen, A. and Ellenbroek, B. (1990) Search after neurobiological profile of individual-specific features of Wistar rats. *Brain Research Bulletin* **24**, 49–69.

Costall, B. and Naylor, R.J. (1976) Apomorphine as an antagonist of the dopamine response from the nucleus accumbens. *Journal of Pharmacy and Pharmacology* **28**, 592–595.

Costall, B., Marsden, C.F.D., Naylor, R.J. and Pycock, C.J. (1977) Stereotyped behaviour patterns and hyperactivity induced by amphetamine and apomorphine after discrete 6-hydroxydopamine lesions of extrapyramidal and mesolimbic nuclei. *Brain Research* **123**, 89–111.

Costall, B., Hui, S.-C. G. and Naylor, R.J. (1979) The importance of serotonergic mechanisms for the induction of hyperactivity by amphetamine and its antagonism by intra-accumbens (3,4-dihydroxyphenylamino)-2-imidazoline (DPI). *Neuropharmacology* **18**, 605–609.

DeFrance, J.F., Sikes, R.W. and Chronister, R.B. (1985) Dopamine action in the nucleus accumbens. *Journal of Neurophysiology* **54**, 1568–1577.

Dickinson, S.L., Gadie, B. and Tulloch, I.F. (1988) $\alpha 1$- and $\alpha 2$-adrenoceptor antagonists differentially influence locomotor and stereotyped behaviour induced by d-amphetamine and apomorphine in the rat. *Psychopharmacology* **96**, 521–527.

Dreher, J.K. and Jackson, D.M. (1989) Role of D1 and D2 dopamine receptors in mediating locomotor activity elicited from the nucleus accumbens of rats. *Brain Research* **487**, 267–277.

Ellenbroek, B.A., Hoven, van den, J. and Cools, A.R. (1988). The nucleus accumbens and forelimb muscular rigidity in rats. *Experimental Brain Research* **72**, 299–304.

Everitt, B.J., Cador, M. and Robbins, T.W. (1989) Interactions between the amygdala and ventral striatum in stimulus-reward associations: studies using a second-order schedule of sexual reinforcement. *Neuroscience* **30**, 63–75.

Fletcher, G.H. and Starr, M.S. (1987) Behavioural evidence for the functionality of D-2 but not D-1 dopamine receptors at multiple brain sites in the 6-hydroxydopamine-lesioned rat. *European Journal of Pharmacology* **138**, 407–411.

Gold, L.H., Swerdlow, N.R. and Koob, G.F. (1988) The role of mesolimbic dopamine in conditioned locomotion produced by amphetamine. *Behavioral Neuroscience* **102**, 544–552.

Greenberg, D.A., U'Prichard, D.C., Sheehan, P. and Snyder, S.H. (1978) α-Noradrenergic receptors in the brain: differential effects of sodium on binding of [^{3}H]agonists and [^{3}H]antagonists. *Brain Research* **140**, 378–384.

Groenewegen, H.J., Vermeulen-van der Zee, E., te Kortschot, A. and Witter, M.P. (1987) Organization of the projections from the subiculum to the ventral striatum in the rat. A study using anterograde transport of Phaseolus vulgaris leucoagglutinin. *Neuroscience* **23**, 103–120.

Hamilton, M.H., de Belleroche, J.S., Gardiner, I.M. and Herberg, L.J. (1986) Stimulatory effect of N-Methyl aspartate on locomotor activity and transmitter release from rat nucleus accumbens. *Pharmacology Biochemistry and Behavior* **25**, 943–948.

Hannigan, J.H., Springer, J.E. and Issacson, R.L. (1984) Differentiation of basal ganglia dopaminergic involvement in behavior after hippocampectomy. *Brain Research* **291**, 83–91.

Hata, F., Uchida, S., Takeyasu, K., Ishida, H. and Yoshida, H. (1980) Changes in α-adrenergic receptors in rat brain in vitro by preincubation with α-adrenergic ligands. *Japanese Journal of Pharmacology* **30**, 570–574.

Hernandez, L., Lee, F. and Hoebel, B.G. (1987) Simultaneous microdialysis and amphetamine infusion in the nucleus accumbens and striatum of freely moving rats: increase in extracellular dopamine and serotonin. *Brain Research Bulletin* **19**, 623–628.

Kolta, M.G., Shreve, P. and Uretsky, N.J. (1989) Effect of pretreatment with amphetamine on the interaction between amphetamine and dopamine in the nucleus accumbens. *Neuropharmocology* **28**, 9–14.

Kuczenski, R. and Segal, D. (1989) Concomitant characterization of behavioral and striatal neurotransmitter response to amphetamine using in vivo microdialysis. *Journal of Neuroscience* **9**, 2051–2065.

Lindvall, O. and Bjorklund, A. (1978) Organization of catecholamine neurons in the rat central nervous system. In: Versen, L.L., Versen, J.D. and Snyder, S.H. (eds) *Handbook of Psychopharmacology*. New York: Plenum Press, pp. 139–231.

Louilot, A., le Moal, M. and Simon, H. (1986) Differential reactivity of dopaminergic neurons in the nucleus accumbens in response to different behavioral situations. An in vivo voltametric study in free moving rats. *Brain Research* **397**, 395–400.

Mogenson, G.J. and Nielsen, M. (1984) A study of the contribution of hippocampal-accumbens-subpallidal projections to locomotor activity. *Behavioral and Neural Biology* **42**, 38–51.

Mogenson, G.J. and Yim, C.Y. (1980) Electrophysiological and neuropharmacological behavioral studies of the nucleus accumbens: implications for its role as a limbic-motor interface. In: Chronister, R.B. and DeFrance, J.F. (eds) *The Neurobiology of the Nucleus Accumbens*. Brunswick, Maine: Haer Institute for Electrophysiological Research, pp. 210–229.

Mogilnicka, E. and Braestrup, C. (1976) Noradrenergic influence on the stereotyped behaviour induced by amphetamine, phenylethylamine and apomorphine. *Journal of Pharmacy and Pharmacology* **28**, 253–255.

Nurse, B., Russell, V.A. and Taljaard, J.J.F. (1985) Effect of chronic desipramine treatment on adrenoceptor modulation of [^{3}H]dopamine release from rat nucleus accumbens slices. *Brain Research* **334**, 235–242.

Oades, R.D. (1985) The role of noradrenaline in tuning and dopamine in switching between signals in the CNS. *Neuroscience and Behavioral Reviews* **9**, 261–282.

Oades, R.D. and Halliday, G.M. (1987) Ventral tegmental (A10) system: neurobiology. I. Anatomy and connectivity. *Brain Research Reviews* **12**, 117–165.

O'Donohue, T.L., Crowley, W.R. and Jacobowitz, M. (1979) Biochemical mapping of the noradrenergic ventral bundle projection sites: evidence for a noradrenergic-dopaminergic interaction. *Brain Research* **172**, 87–100.

Palmer, G.C. and Chronister, R.B. (1980) The biochemical pharmacology of the nucleus accumbens. In: Chronister, R.B. and DeFrance, J.F. (eds) *The Neurobiology of the Nucleus Accumbens*. Brunswick, Maine: Haer Institute for Electrophysiological Research, pp. 273–315.

Peris, J. and Zahniser, N.R. (1989) Persistent augmented dopamine release after acute cocaine requires dopamine receptor activation. *Pharmacology Biochemistry and Behavior* **32**, 71–76.

Phillipson, O.T. and Griffiths, A.C. (1985) The topographic order of inputs to nucleus accumbens in the rat. *Neuroscience* **16**, 275–296.

Pijnenburg, A.J.J. (1976) *The Nucleus Accumbens; Psychopharmacological Investigations on the Mesolimbic Dopamine System*. Thesis, Nijmegen, Stichting Studentenpers.

Pisa, M., Martin-Iverson, M.T. and Fibiger, H.C. (1988) On the role of the dorsal noradrenergic bundle in learning and habituation to novelty. *Pharmacology Biochemistry and Behavior* **30**, 835–845.

Plaznik, A., Danysz, W. and Kostowski, W. (1985) A stimulatory effect of intraaccumbens injections of noradrenaline on the behavior of rats in the forced swim test. *Psychopharmacology* **87**, 119–123.

Pycock, C. (1977) Noradrenergic involvement in dopamine-dependent stereotyped and cataleptic responses in the rat. *Naunyn-Schmiedeberg's Archiv für Experimentelle Pathologie und Pharmacologie* **298**, 15–22.

Reinstein, D.K., Hannigan, J.H. and Isaacson, R.L. (1982) Time course of certain behavioral changes after hippocampal damage and their alteration by dopaminergic intervention into nucleus accumbens. *Pharmacology Biochemistry and Behavior* **17**, 193–202

Reisine, T. (1981) Adaptive changes in catecholamine receptors in the central nervous system. *Neuroscience* **6**, 1471–1502.

Robinson, T.E. and Becker, J.B. (1986) Enduring changes in brain and behavior produced by chronic amphetamine administration: a review and evaluation of animal models of amphetamine psychosis. *Brain Research Reviews* **11**, 167–198.

Robinson, T.E., Jurson, P.A., Bennett, J.A. and Bentgen, K.M. (1988) Persistent sensitization of dopamine neurotransmission in ventral striatum (nucleus accumbens) produced by prior experience with (+)-amphetamine: a microdialysis study in freely moving rats. *Brain Research* **462**, 211–222.

Robinson, T.G. and Beart, P.M. (1988) Excitant amino acid projections from rat amygdala and thalamus to nucleus accumbens. *Brain Research Bulletin* **20**, 467–471.

Rolinski, Z. and Scheel-Krüger, J. (1973) The effect of dopamine and noradrenaline antagonists on amphetamine induced locomotor activity in mice and rats. *Acta Pharmacologica et Toxicologica* **33**, 385–399.

Sawaya, M.C.B., Dolphin, A., Jenner, P., Marsden, C.D. and Meldrum, B.S. (1977) Noradrenaline-sensitive adenylate cyclase in slices of mouse limbic forebrain: characterization and effect of dopaminergic agonists. *Biochemical Pharmacology* **26**, 1877–1884.

Segal, D.S., Geyer, M.A. and Weiner, B.E. (1975) Strain differences during intraventricular infusion of norepinephrine: possible role of receptor sensitivity. *Science* **189**, 301–303.

Simon, H. and LeMoal, M. (1984) Mesencephalic dopaminergic neurons: functional role. In: Usdin, E., Carlsson, A., Dahlström, A. and Engel, J. (eds) *Catecholamines: Neuropharmacology and Central Nervous System*. New York: Alan R. Liss, pp. 293–307.

Speciale, S.G., Crowley, W.R., O'Donohue, T.L. and Jacobowitz, D.M. (1978) Forebrain catecholamine projections of the A5 cell group. *Brain Research* **154**, 128–133.

Springer, J.E. and Isaacson, R.L. (1982) Catecholamine alterations in basal ganglia after hippocampal lesions. *Brain Research* **252**, 185–188.

Starke, K. (1979) Presynaptic regulation of release in the central nervous system. In: Paton, D.M. (ed.) *The Release of Catecholamines from Adrenergic Neurons*. New York: Pergamon Press, pp. 143–183.

Steinbusch, H.W.H. (1981) Distribution of serotonin immunoreactivity in the central nervous system of the rat. *Neuroscience* **6**, 557–618.

Sutanto, W., de Kloet, E.R., de Bree, F. and Cools, A.R. (1989) Differential corticosteroid binding characteristics to the mineralocorticoid (type I) and glucocorticoid (type II) receptors in the brain of pharmacogenetically-selected apomorphine-susceptible and apomorphine-unsusceptible Wistar rats. *Neuroscience Research Communications* **5**, 19–27.

Svensson, L. and Ahlenius, S. (1983) Suppression of exploratory locomotor activity by the local application of dopamine or 1-noradrenaline to the nucleus accumbens of the rat. *Pharmacology Biochemistry and Behavior* **19**, 693–699.

Taghzouti, K., Simon, H., Louilot, A., Herman, J.P. and LeMoal, M. (1985) Behavioral study after local injection of 6-hydroxydopamine into the nucleus accumbens in the rat. *Brain Research* **344**, 9–20.

Taylor, K.M. and Snyder, S.H. (1971) Differential effects of D- and L-amphetamine on behavior and on catecholamine disposition in dopamine and norepinephrine containing neurons of rat brain. *Brain Research* **28**, 295–309.

Unemoto, H., Sasa, M. and Takaori, S. (1985a) Inhibition from locus coeruleus of nucleus accumbens neurons activated by hippocampal stimulation. *Brain Research* **338**, 376–379.

Unemoto, H., Sasa, M. and Takaori, S. (1985b) A noradrenaline-induced inhibition from locus coeruleus of nucleus accumbens neuron receiving input from hippocampus. *Japanese Journal of Pharmacology* **39**, 233–239.

U'Prichard, D.C., Greenberg, D.A. and Snijder, S.H. (1977) Binding characteristics of a radiolabelled agonist and antagonist at central nervous system α-noradrenergic receptors. *Molecular Pharmacology* **13**, 454–473.

R. van den Bos, Cools, A.R. and Ögren, S.O. (1988) Differential effects of the selective D2-antagonist raclopride in the nucleus accumbens of the rat on spontaneous and d-amphetamine-induced activity. *Psychopharmacology* **95**, 447–451.

Walaas, I. and Fonnum, F. (1979) The effects of surgical and chemical lesions on neurotransmitter candidates in the nucleus accumbens of the rat. *Neuroscience* **4**, 209–216.

Waterhouse, B.D., Sessler, F.M., Cheng, J.T., Woodward, D.J., Azizi, S.A. and Moises, H.C. (1988) New evidence for a gating action of norepinephrine in central neuronal circuits of mammalian brain. *Brain Research Bulletin* **21**, 425–432.

Weinstock, M. and Speiser, Z. (1974) Modification by propranolol and related compounds of motor activity and stereotype behaviour induced in the rat by amphetamine. *European Journal of Pharmacology* **25**, 29–35.

Weiss, B. (1988) Modulation of adrenergic receptors during aging. *Neurobiology of Aging* **9**, 61–62.

Yang, C.R. and Mogenson, G.J. (1986) Dopamine enhances terminal excitability of hippocampal-accumbens neurons via D2 receptor: role of dopamine in presynaptic inhibition. *Journal of Neuroscience* **6**, 2470–2478.

Yang, C.R. and Mogenson, G.J. (1987) Hippocampal signal transmission to the pedunculopontine nucleus and its regulation by dopamine D2 receptors in the nucleus accumbens: an electrophysiological and behavioural study. *Neuroscience* **23**, 1041–1055.

Yim, C.Y. and Mogenson, G.J. (1986) Mesolimbic dopamine projection modulates amygdala-evoked EPSP in nucleus accumbens neurons: an in vivo study. *Brain Research* **369**, 347–352.

Yim, C.Y. and Mogenson G.J. (1988) Neuromodulatory action of dopamine in the nucleus accumbens: an in vivo intracellular study. *Neuroscience* **26**, 403–415.

Zebrowska-Lupina, I., Kleinrok, Z., Kozyrska, C. and Wielosz, M. (1978) The effect of α-adrenergic receptor stimulant drugs on amphetamine or apomorphine-induced stereotypy in rats. *Polish Journal of Pharmacology* **30**, 459–467.

7

Relationships between Mesocortical and Mesolimbic Dopamine Neurons: Functional Correlates of D1 Receptor Heteroregulation

JEAN-POL TASSIN, DENIS HERVÉ, PAUL VEZINA,
FABRICE TROVERO, GÉRARD BLANC AND JACQUES
GLOWINSKI

Chaire de Neuropharmacologie, INSERM U. 114, College de France, Paris,
75005, France

INTRODUCTION

In the rat, the ventral tegmental area (VTA) and the substantia nigra (SN), two mesencephalic structures, contain the cell bodies of most of the ascending dopamine (DA) neurons (Björklund and Lindvall, 1984). In this VTA–SN complex, only 3 per cent of these DA neurons send axonal arborizations to prefrontal, rhinal and cingular cortices. Although these neurons clearly represent a minority, they exhibit many characteristics suggesting that they play a major role in the regulation of affective responses. First, they project to restricted cortical areas connected with the dorsomedial nucleus of the thalamus, a connection which usually defines the cortical regions controlling cognitive and emotional processes (Akert, 1964; Divac et al., 1978). Second, stressful situations specifically increase the release of DA in these cortical areas and this effect can be prevented by prior treatment with benzodiazepines (Lavielle et al., 1979). Moreover, in the rat, an environmental change such

The Mesolimbic Dopamine System: From Motivation to Action.
Edited by P. Willner and J. Scheel-Krüger

© 1991 John Wiley & Sons Ltd

as a few weeks' isolation is sufficient to reduce the activity of mesocortical DA neurons and to render them hypersensitive to stressful stimuli (Blanc et al., 1980). Finally, the destruction of these cortical DA projections seems to be related to the appearance of a syndrome characterized by locomotor hyperactivity and the loss of the behavioral inhibitory functions responsible for the performance of coordinated tasks (Le Moal et al., 1969; Tassin et al., 1978a).

Mesocortical DA neurons should not, however, be considered as an isolated entity. Indeed, experiments have provided evidence that the different ascending DA neurons innervating cortical and subcortical structures are interrelated. Initially, Pycock and his colleagues reported that the destruction of prefrontocortical DA nerve endings induces an increase in DA utilization in the nucleus accumbens (Pycock et al., 1980). Although these findings have not always been replicated by other laboratories, the relationships between DA neurons they suggested have now been demonstrated with different experimental models. For example, interruption of DA transmission in the amygdala, achieved by locally injecting either a DA antagonist (Louilot et al., 1985) or the neurotoxin 6-hydroxydopamine (6-OHDA), induces an increased utilization of DA in the nucleus accumbens as well as a decrease in the DOPAC:DA ratio in the prefrontal cortex (Simon et al., 1988). Similarly, indirect support for these interrelations has been obtained in experiments which measured DA utilization in cortical and subcortical structures following lesions of nuclei (median and dorsal raphe, habenula, locus coeruleus) sending projections to the VTA–SN complex (Hervé et al., 1979, 1981, 1982; Lisoprawski et al., 1980). Generally, changes in DA utilization produced in the nucleus accumbens always differed from those produced in the prefrontal cortex and, in some cases, were completely opposite in direction. Moreover, prolonged isolation in the rat which, as mentioned above, induces a reduction in DA utilization in the prefrontal cortex, is accompanied by an increase in the DOPAC:DA ratio in the nucleus accumbens and the striatum (Blanc et al., 1980). Finally Louilot et al. (1989), using voltammetric detection techniques, have recently shown that the blockade by a DA antagonist of DA transmission in the prefrontal cortex increases DA release in the nucleus accumbens.

The mechanisms responsible for these interactions between the cortical and subcortical DA systems are not yet completely understood. It is very likely, however, that information is conveyed between DA neurons by non-DA cells which bear the DA receptors, or which are under the control of interneurons bearing these receptors, and connect the different DA projection areas. The aim of this paper is to present data suggesting that changes in

DA receptors following lesions of DA and/or non-DA cells can provide information on the functional relationships which exist between ascending DA neurons.

Binding studies on membranes (Seeman, 1980; Billard et al., 1984) and autoradiographic analyses of slices exposed to selective ligands (Palacios et al., 1981; Savasta et al., 1986; Bouthenet et al., 1987) have allowed DA receptors to be divided into at least two types: those positively coupled to adenylate cyclase which lead to an enhanced activity of the enzyme when they are exposed to agonists (D1 receptors) and those not associated with this enzyme or which could inhibit its activity when they are stimulated (D2 receptors) (Kebabian et al., 1972; Stoof and Kebabian, 1981; Onali et al., 1985; Memo et al., 1986).

In this paper, we focus on D1 receptors. Although for many years the function of the D1 receptor was questioned by several workers, this no longer seems to be the case. The discovery of the potent selective D1 antagonist SCH 23390 (Ioro et al., 1983) has allowed the demonstration that some behavioural responses, induced either by DA or by some of its agonists, are mediated through D1 receptors (Christensen et al., 1984). Moreover, some behaviours which were attributed to stimulation of D2 receptors have now been shown to necessitate the previous stimulation of D1 receptors (Walters et al., 1987). Finally, the elegant investigations of Greengard and his colleagues have revealed the existence of a specific protein, DARPP 32, that is distributed in target areas of DA ascending neurons (Walaas et al., 1983). Through protein kinase A, DARPP 32 can be phosphorylated as a result of the interaction of DA with D1 receptors and the subsequent activation of adenylate cyclase and production of cyclic AMP. Once phosphorylated, DARPP 32 acts as a potent inhibitor of protein phosphatase 1, which has a broad spectrum of action, such as glycogen metabolism or protein synthesis (Hemmings et al., 1984, 1987; Ingebritsen and Cohen, 1983). Stimulation of D1 receptors may therefore have important metabolic consequences for the neuronal cells which possess them.

Although both types of receptors exist in most areas innervated by DA neurons, some structures, such as the prefrontal cortex or the pars reticulata of the SN, exhibit much higher densities of D1 than D2 receptors (Tassin et al., 1978b; Marchais et al., 1980; Boyson et al., 1986; Savasta et al., 1986). While a good parallel has been found between the localization of DA nerve terminals and D1 receptors in several structures, especially in the anterior parts of the cerebral cortex, it should be noted that the ratio between the two is not always the same from one structure to the other. Indeed, it has been shown that the density of D1 receptors (as indexed by

DA-sensitive adenylate cyclase activity) relative to the level of DA in the structure, is tenfold higher in the prefrontal and cingular cortices than in the striatum or the nucleus accumbens (Tassin et al., 1982a). The functional significance of this relatively high density of D1 receptors is presently unknown, but it has led us to analyse the properties of these cortical receptors further and to compare them with those found in subcortical structures.

In the first group of experiments, we performed 6-OHDA lesions of the VTA to study the development of denervation supersensitivity of cortical and subcortical DA-sensitive adenylate cyclase activity following the destruction of the ascending DA neurons. Results indicated that, despite an almost complete disappearance of DA in the prefrontal cortex and the nucleus accumbens 6 weeks after the lesion, there was no increase in DA-sensitive adenylate cyclase activity measured in homogenates of tissue punched out from these structures. Surprisingly, when DA neurons were destroyed by an electrolytic lesion of the VTA, an increase in DA-sensitive adenylate cyclase in the prefrontal cortex (48 per cent) and no change in the nucleus accumbens were obtained. We concluded that the presence or absence of non-DA fibres could affect the development of denervation supersensitivity of the adenylate cyclase activity linked to D1 receptors (Tassin et al., 1982b). In other words, neurotransmitters released from non-DA (heterologous) nerve terminals could modify the sensitivity of D1 receptors in the prefrontal cortex.

Further experiments indicated that subcortical D1 receptors were also submitted to these heteroregulation processes. They revealed that cortico-subcortical neurons interconnecting the different DA projecting areas were of major importance. We will first describe these experiments which demonstrate the role of these cortico-subcortical pathways in the regulation of D1 receptors in the nucleus accumbens and the stratium. Furthermore, it will be shown that modulations in the sensitivity of subcortical D1 receptors obtained by specific lesions of DA or non-DA neurons can induce modifications in the behavioural response to pharmacological treatments. In the second part of this paper, data indicating that cortical D1 receptors are also subject to heteroregulation by noradrenergic (NA) neurons will be reviewed (Tassin et al., 1986). Moreover, since the specific presence of neurotensin (NT) in mesocortical DA neurons has been demonstrated (Studler et al., 1988), we will present recent data suggesting that NT binding sites, co-localized with D1 receptors in prefrontal and rhinal cortices, are also submitted to heteroregulation by NA neurons. Finally, behavioural data will be presented indicating the possible influence of the heteroregulation of cortical D1 receptors via stimulation of α-1-adrenergic receptors on the control of spontaneous alternation and locomotor activity.

HETEROREGULATION OF D1 RECEPTORS IN THE NUCLEUS ACCUMBENS: INFLUENCE OF NON-DA PREFRONTOCORTICAL EFFERENT FIBRES

As mentioned previously, neither chemical (6-OHDA) nor electrolytic lesions of the VTA affected the sensitivity of D1 receptors in the nucleus accumbens, although both types of lesions reduce the levels of DA in this subcortical structure by 95 per cent. In fact, cells of the nucleus accumbens receive two types of information originating from DA neurons in the VTA. One type is direct and mediated by the mesoaccumbens DA fibres. The other is indirect and is mediated by the mesocortical DA neurons which in turn control the corticonucleus accumbens excitatory pathway (Figure 1). The absence of D1 denervation supersensitivity in the nucleus accumbens could therefore be due to the disinhibition of this cortico-nucleus accumbens pathway which may occur following the destruction of the mesocortical DA system. Bilateral ablations of the prefrontal cortex were therefore performed to prevent the effects of this disinhibition (Reibaud et al., 1984). These lesions induced a 55 per cent decrease in the activity of the high affinity uptake of [³H]glutamic acid in synaptosomes from the nucleus accumbens, confirming anatomical and biochemical observations indicating that numerous

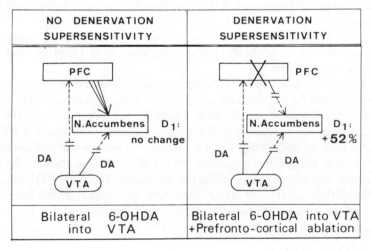

Figure 1. Effects of the bilateral 6-OHDA lesion of the VTA (left) and of the simultaneous bilateral 6-OHDA lesion of the VTA plus the bilateral ablation of the prefrontal cortex (right) on D1 receptor sensitivity in the nucleus accumbens. Animals were sacrificed 6 weeks after the lesions. DA-sensitive adenylate cyclase activity (D1 receptors) was estimated from homogenates of microdiscs of tissue punched out in the nucleus accumbens (N. accumbens). Changes in DA-sensitive adenylate cyclase activity are expressed as percentage of control values. PFC, prefrontal cortex

subcortical structures are innervated by glutamatergic neurons originating from the prefrontal cortex (Beckstead, 1979; Fonnum et al., 1981).

When the prefrontocortical ablation was performed simultaneously with the bilateral injection of 6-OHDA into the VTA, a marked hypersensitivity of the DA-sensitive adenylate cyclase activity was observed in the nucleus accumbens (+52 per cent). This modification corresponded to a change in maximal activity since experiments were performed at saturating concentrations of DA (10^{-4} M), and dose-response curves indicated only a twofold increase in the apparent affinity of the receptor adenylate cyclase complex for DA. The ablation of the prefrontal cortex alone induced a small increase (14 per cent, $P<0.01$) in DA-sensitive adenylate cyclase activity in the nucleus accumbens (Reibaud et al., 1984). Complementary experiments further indicated that the expression of the D1-linked adenylate cyclase denervation supersensitivity in the nucleus accumbens was dependent on the activity of cortico-nucleus accumbens neurons (Tassin et al, 1982b). Indeed, a 39 per cent increase in DA-sensitive adenylate cyclase activity occurred in the nucleus accumbens when the animals were pretreated with desipramine 30 minutes before the bilateral injection of 6-OHDA into the VTA, a procedure which allowed for a partial protection of the mesocortical DA neurons (Hervé et al., 1986a), and possibly prevented the disinhibition of the cortico-nucleus accumbens glutamatergic pathway. However, since the descending prefrontocortical neurons innervate several subcortical structures also interconnected with the nucleus accumbens, it cannot be completely excluded that neurons other than those projecting to the nucleus accumbens contribute to the observed effect (Krettek and Price, 1978; Kelley et al., 1982).

The heteroregulation of D1 receptors demonstrated here reveals the existence of specific interactions between identified neuronal systems that may have physiological significance. Indeed, the target cells of the VTA DA neurons in the nucleus accumbens also integrate information from the prefrontal cortex, and changes in the activity of cortico-nucleus accumbens neurons can modulate the sensitivity of D1 receptors on these cells. It can be assumed, therefore, that in different structures containing D1 receptors, heteroregulation specific to these receptors can occur depending on the nature and the origin of fibres afferent to the structure, and that behavioural expressions of such heteroregulation would be expected in certain conditions.

HETEROREGULATION OF D1 RECEPTORS IN THE STRIATUM: INFLUENCE OF NON-DA IPSILATERAL AND CONTRALATERAL AFFERENT FIBRES

The striatum is innervated not only by nigrostriatal DA neurons but also by VTA DA cells that predominantly innervate the anteromedial part of the striatum (Tassin et al., 1976; Fallon and Moore, 1978). A good correlation exists between the distribution of DA nerve terminals and D1 receptors which are more abundant in the anterior part of the striatum (Bockaert et al., 1976). It is also well established that the striatum is innervated by cells from all cortical areas (Heimer et al., 1985).

Destruction of the striatal DA innervation was performed by an injection of 6-OHDA into the Fields of Forel, a site through which all ascending DA fibres pass, including those of the ipsilateral cortex. This lesion induced the expected denervation supersensitivity of D1-linked adenylate cyclase in the anteromedial part of the striatum 6–12 weeks later (+ 45 per cent; Figure 2), but no change in the laterodorsal part of the striatum (Hervé et al., 1989). In this context, Savasta et al. (1988) have reported that the denervation-induced supersensitivity of D2 receptors (visualized by autoradiographic studies) is more pronounced in the laterodorsal part than in the anteromedial part of the striatum.

This suggests that DA receptors found in different striatal areas could be subject to different kinds of heteroregulation depending on the origin of the afferent fibres present. Interestingly, wheat germ agglutinin horseradish peroxidase (WGA-HRP, Sigma) (Mesulam, 1978) experiments, performed in collaboration with Dr Thierry, have shown that the anteromedial striatum

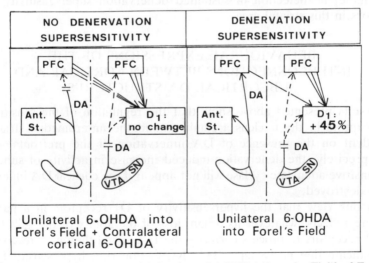

Figure 2. Effects of the unilateral injection of 6-OHDA into the Field of Forel and of the simultaneous unilateral injection of 6-OHDA into the Field of Forel plus a contralateral 6-OHDA injection into the prefrontal cortex on the sensitivity of D1 receptors in the anterior ipsilateral striatum. Details are as described in the legend to Figure 1 with the exception that microdiscs of tissue were punched out from the anterior part of the ipsilateral striatum. Ant. St., Anterior striatum; PFC, prefrontal cortex; SN, substantia nigra

receives bilateral projections from cells located in the prefrontal DA cortical field, while the laterodorsal striatum receives projections from cells which lie essentially in the ipsilateral dorsolateral cortex, ouside the DA cortical field (Hervé et al., 1989). Denervation-induced supersensitivity of D1 receptors in the anteromedial striatum following a unilateral 6-OHDA lesion in the Fields of Forel could therefore be related to the preserved DA innervation in the contralateral prefrontal cortex and thus to the unaffected activity of these contralateral prefrontal cells which innervate both striata. In agreement with this hypothesis, the denervation-induced supersensitivity of D1 receptors in the anteromedial striatum was no longer observed when a 6-OHDA lesion of the contralateral prefrontal cortex was added to the lesion made in the Fields of Forel (Figure 2).

This result can be compared to those obtained in the nucleus accumbens following bilateral 6-OHDA lesions of the VTA that also bilaterally destroy the DA nerve terminals in the prefrontal cortex (Figure 1, left; Reibaud et al., 1984). Together these data suggest that in both cases, it is a change in the regulation of prefrontal cells induced by DA denervation which is responsible for the lack of development of denervation supersensitivity of subcortical D1 receptors. It remains to be determined, however, whether lesions of cortical cells projecting to the laterodorsal part of the striatum will enable the detection of sustained denervation supersensitivity of D1 receptors in this striatal area.

BEHAVIOURAL EXPRESSIONS OF THE INTERCONNECTIONS BETWEEN CORTICAL AND SUBCORTICAL DA STRUCTURES

The results presented above show that the regulation of the sensitivity of D1 receptors in the nucleus accumbens and the anteromedial striatum is dependent on the presence of DA innervation of the prefrontal cortex. More precisely, the denervation-induced increase in activity of subcortical DA-sensitive adenylate cyclase will not appear if the cortical DA innervation is also destroyed.

It is our view that the hypersensitivity of D1 receptors in a particular structure reflects, whatever its origin, loss of the ability of the cells bearing the D1 receptors to process correctly the DA signal they may receive. Our data indicate that postsynaptic DA dysfunction (i.e. hypersensitivity) in a subcortical structure can be compensated for by DA denervation of the prefrontal cortex. Accordingly, this suggests that the cortical and subcortical DA projections may play opposite roles in the modulation of the outputs arising from accumbens and anterior striatal neurons.

To verify this hypothesis, behavioural experiments were recently performed on models assumed to indicate DA function in either the nucleus accumbens or the striatum, i.e. locomotor activity and turning behaviour induced by DA agonists.

Respective Roles in Locomotor Activity of DA Stimulation of Prefrontal Cortex and Nucleus Accumbens

It is generally agreed that the locomotor activating effects induced by the injection of amphetamine into the nucleus accumbens are related to the increased release of DA in this nucleus (Kelly et al., 1975). Rats were implanted with chronic bilateral injection cannulae aimed at both the prefrontal cortex and the nucleus accumbens. When amphetamine (1.5 µg/0.5 µl/side) was injected into the nucleus accumbens, a mean increase in locomotor activity of 314 per cent compared to control saline injections was obtained. No significant effect was obtained when amphetamine (2.5 µg/0.5 µl/side) was injected into the prefrontal cortex only. However, when amphetamine was injected into both sites, prefrontal cortex amphetamine reduced the hyperactivity produced by nucleus accumbens amphetamine alone injections by a mean of 42 per cent (Tassin et al., 1988a). More recent experiments indicate that this cortical effect is mediated via D1 receptors. Indeed, the injection of SCH 23390 (a D1 antagonist) (0.25 µg/0.5 µl/side) into the prefrontal cortex increases the locomotor activity induced by the injection of amphetamine into the nucleus accumbens by 110 per cent, while the injection of sulpiride (a D2 antagonist) (1 µg/0.5 µl/side) is without significant effect. Both of these antagonists, at the doses tested, blocked the locomotor activating effects of amphetamine when co-injected with amphetamine into the nucleus accumbens (Vezina et al., 1990). These results suggest that prefrontocortical DA plays an inhibitory role in locomotor behaviour; i.e. that it exerts an effect on this behaviour opposite to that produced by the stimulation of DA receptors in the nucleus accumbens.

Bilateral Cortical DA Denervation Decreases the Turning Behaviour Induced by Apomorphine in Animals with Unilateral Striatal DA Lesions

It is well known that the unilateral 6-OHDA denervation of the striatum induces, 4 weeks after the lesion, a turning behaviour when animals are treated with DA agonists (Ungerstedt and Arbuthnott, 1970). This effect has been related to the development of hypersensitivity of DA receptors in the lesioned striatum, the treatment with DA agonists revealing the functional disequilibrium induced by the lesion (Ungerstedt, 1971).

As described above, the denervation supersensitivity of D1 receptors in the anteromedial striatum produced by a unilateral lesion of the Fields of

Forel could be blocked by simultaneously performing a DA lesion of the contralateral cortex. In collaboration with Dr Piazza, lesioned animals were injected intraperitoneally with apomorphine (50 μg/kg) or SKF 38393 (1 mg/kg). Animals were lesioned either unilaterally in the Fields of Forel (a treatment which destroys DA fibres both in the striatum and the ipsilateral prefrontal cortex) or both in the Fields of Forel and the contralateral prefrontal cortex. The superimposed DA denervation of the prefrontal cortex did indeed decrease the turning behaviour induced by apomorphine (-42 per cent: 147 ± 17 turns/hour versus 88 ± 19 turns/hour) or SKF 38393 (-56 per cent: 446 ± 78 turns/hour versus 197 ± 58 turns/hour) in unilateral Fields of Forel-lesioned animals (Piazza et al., 1990). This cannot be due to modifications of the sensitivity of cortical D1 receptors since, as shown in the following section, simultaneous destruction of DA and NA ascending fibres blocks the development of cortical D1 receptor denervation hypersensitivity. The respective role in the effect of striatal D1 and D2 receptors observed remains to be determined, however. It would seem, none the less, that D1 receptors are at least implicated since the expression of the inhibition produced by lesion of the prefrontal cortex is slightly greater with SKF 38393, a D1 agonist, than with apomorphine, a mixed D1/D2 agonist.

In both of these examples, modifying DA transmission in the prefrontal cortex antagonizes the effects obtained by modifying DA transmission in a subcortical structure. There is an important difference between the two situations, however. In the first case, it is the *stimulation* of cortical DA transmission which inhibits the behaviour induced by *increased* DA stimulation in the subcortical structure. This result is in agreement with previous studies indicating that the mesocortical DA system plays an inhibitory role in locomotor activity (Tassin et al., 1978a). In the second case, it is the *destruction* of the cortical DA innervation which diminishes or compensates for the effects induced by *destruction* of subcortical DA innervation. Indeed, it is a cortical denervation which compensates for the effects produced by a striatal denervation. Thus, as in the first case, cortical and striatal DA innervations would seem to act in an opposite manner.

The above studies of D1 receptor heteroregulation in the nucleus accumbens and in the striatum have led us to characterize some of the privileged relations between these subcortical structures and the prefrontal cortex. We will now show that such heteroregulation also exists for cortical D1 receptors and that, as has been demonstrated for subcortical areas, these cortical heteroregulations can be associated with some behavioural modulations. Furthermore, it cannot be excluded that modifications of the sensitivity of cortical D1 receptors might influence the behavioural expression of the DA cortico-subcortical relationships.

INFLUENCE OF THE CORTICAL NORADRENERGIC INNERVATION ON THE REGULATION OF D1 RECEPTORS AND NT BINDING SITES IN THE PREFRONTAL CORTEX: RELATIONSHIPS WITH LOCOMOTOR ACTIVITY

Among the ascending DA systems, the mesocortical neurons seem to be the only ones to synthesize NT, a 13 amino-acid neuropeptide, extensively (Studler et al., 1988). The autoradiographic analysis of cortical slices in the presence of ^{3}[H]SCH 23390 and unlabelled spiroperidol (to eliminate 5-HT$_2$ binding) has shown, as has been found with DA-sensitive adenylate cyclase activity, a very good correlation between the localization of D1 receptors and DA nerve terminals (Tassin et al., 1982a; Savasta et al., 1986; Trovero et al., 1988). In collaboration with Drs Kitabgi and Rostène, cortical slices were also incubated with [^{125}I]NT (Hervé et al., 1986b). This revealed that cortical NT binding sites were concentrated in areas strikingly similar to those of D1 receptors, such as prefrontal and rhinal cortices (Figure 3).

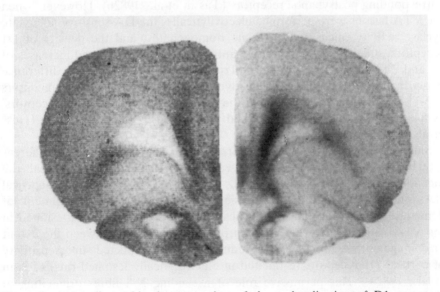

Figure 3. Autoradiographic demonstration of the co-localization of D1 receptors and NT binding sites in the anterior cerebral cortex of the rat. The left hemicortex was incubated with tritiated SCH 23390 in the presence of unlabelled spiroperidol to avoid any binding to 5-HT$_2$ receptors. The right hemicortex was incubated with ^{125}[I]NT. Prefrontal and rhinal cortices are clearly labelled in their deep layers as are the dorsal zones of the olfactory tubercles. Background differences between the left and right hemicortices are due to the different specific activities of the two ligands used (70 and 2000 ci/mmole for SCH 23390 and iodinated NT, respectively). The photomontage and the photograph were obtained with an IMSTAR image analyser (Paris). From Tassin et al., 1988b

Lesion studies were therefore performed to determine whether these receptors were presynaptic or postsynaptic and whether they were, like subcortical D1 receptors, subject to heteroregulation processes.

Cortical D1 Receptors

As mentioned above, 6-OHDA injections into the VTA did not produce any changes in the activity of the prefrontocortical D1-linked adenylate cyclase even though cortical DA levels were reduced by more than 98 per cent. These results showed that cortical D1 receptors were postsynaptic to DA nerve terminals and indicated that, in the central nervous system, even the total destruction of a homogeneous population of afferent presynaptic fibres does not necessarily produce denervation hypersensitivity of the corresponding postsynaptic receptors (Tassin et al., 1982b). However, when the VTA lesions were performed electrolytically, the DA-sensitive adenylate cyclase activity, measured on tissue homogenates, and the density of D1 receptors, obtained by quantitative autoradiography, presented increases of 48 and 24 per cent, respectively (Trovero et al., 1990a). This difference between the increases in DA-sensitive adenylate cyclase and D1 receptors is probably due to the presence in the prefrontal cortex of 'spare receptors' as has been proposed by Creese and his colleagues for the striatum (Hess et al., 1987).

Since electrolytic VTA lesions spare the cortical NA innervation whereas 6-OHDA VTA lesions destroy ascending NA fibres that pass near the location of the DA cells (Tassin et al., 1982b), the destruction of the cortical NA innervation could be responsible for the lack of development of denervation supersensitivity of cortical D1 receptors in animals lesioned in the VTA with 6-OHDA. A good correlation was found between the extent of damage to NA fibres and the reduction of the expected supersensitivity of cortical D1 receptors (estimated in electrolytically lesioned rats) (Tassin et al., 1982a). This permissive role of ascending NA fibres originating in the locus coeruleus in the appearance of denervation supersensitivity of cortical D1 receptors was also supported by experiments conducted on rats with simultaneous bilateral electrolytic lesions of the VTA and bilateral 6-OHDA lesions of the dorsal NA bundle (made near the pedunculus cerebellaris superior). Indeed, no significant change in DA-sensitive adenylate cyclase activity was found in the prefrontal cortex of rats with the two types of lesions. Lesions of NA neurons alone were without effect on enzyme activity (Tassin et al., 1986) (Figure 4).

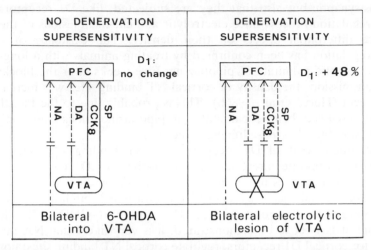

Figure 4. Effects of bilateral 6-OHDA or electrolytic lesions of the VTA on D1 receptor sensitivity in the prefrontal cortex. Details are as described in the legend of Figure 1 with the exception that microdiscs of tissue were punched out from the prefrontal cortex. It should be added that, as mentioned in the text, the mesocortical DA neurons co-synthesize NT (Studler et al., 1988), and that the substance P fibres projecting to the medial prefrontal cortex originate from the nucleus laterodorsalis tegmenti (Sakanaka et al., 1983). CCK_8, Cholecystokinin; PFC, prefrontal cortex; SP, substance P

Cortical NT Binding Sites

In 1981, Palacios and Kuhar showed that most of the NT binding sites localized by autoradiography with ^{3}[H]NT in the mesencephalon were located on DA cells (Palacios and Kuhar, 1981). Moreover, following a 6-OHDA injection into the VTA–SN complex, they obtained an important decrease of the density of NT binding sites in the striatum. These data suggested that DA cell bodies and axons bore high densities of NT binding sites and could explain why the topographical distribution of the mesocortical DA nerve terminals was so strikingly similar to that of cortical NT binding sites (Tassin et al., 1988b). Other findings, however, suggested that these cortical NT binding sites were postsynaptic to the mixed NT/DA mesocortical neurons since an electrolytic lesion of the VTA did not modify the autoradiographic density of ^{125}[I]NT in the prefrontal and rhinal cortices (Trovero et al., 1990a). Moreover, when, in collaboration with Drs Kitabgi and Rostène, the ascending DA neurons were destroyed by a 6-OHDA lesion in the VTA, an increased density of these cortical NT binding sites (35 per cent) was obtained (Hervé et al., 1986b).

These results indicate not only that most of the cortical NT binding sites are postsynaptic but also that they are subjected, like D1 receptors, to a heteroregulation process since electrolytic and chemical lesions of the VTA produce differential effects on their density. The existence of such a heteroregulation has been confirmed by treating animals with a long-acting neuroleptic, the palmitate of pipotiazine. Five weeks after the blockade of DA transmission, the density of cortical NT binding sites was increased by 54 per cent (Hervé et al., 1986b). This is probably due to the fact that, as will be discussed below, palmitate of pipotiazine blocks not only DA transmission but also α-1-adrenergic receptors.

Interestingly, cortical D1 receptors and NT binding sites seem to be regulated in opposite directions: hypersensitivity of D1 cortical receptors develops when there is no change in cortical NT binding sites (electrolytic VTA lesion), and increased density of cortical NT binding sites appears when there is no change in cortical D1 receptors (6-OHDA/VTA lesion). Although it has yet to be demonstrated, it is very likely that NA fibres, as shown for cortical D1 receptors, regulate cortical NT binding sites; however, in this case, it is the absence of NA innervation that would be necessary for the denervation supersensitivity of cortical NT binding sites to develop.

INFLUENCE OF ASCENDING NA FIBRES AND α-1-ADRENERGIC RECEPTORS ON THE LOCOMOTOR HYPERACTIVITY INDUCED BY ELECTROLYTIC VTA LESIONS

Bilateral electrolytic lesions of the VTA in the rat induce deficits such as locomotor hyperactivity and the disappearance of spontaneous alternation ('VTA syndrome') (Le Moal et al., 1969). Correlational studies have indicated that the amplitude of the locomotor hyperactivity is proportional to the extent of destruction of the DA fibres innervating the prefrontal cortex and, more interestingly, to the development of a D1 receptor supersensitivity in this area (Tassin et al., 1978a, 1982a). Since destruction of the ascending NA pathways down-regulates cortical D1 receptor denervation supersensitivity induced by the electrolytic lesion of the VTA, it was tempting to investigate whether chemical (6-OHDA) lesions of the cortical NA innervation could affect the locomotor hyperactivity induced by the electrolytic lesion of the VTA.

In experiments conducted in collaboration with Drs Taghzouti, Simon and Le Moal, animals were either lesioned by bilateral electrocoagulations of the VTA, by bilateral injections of 6-OHDA made laterally into the pedunculus cerebellaris superior (PCS, site of ascending NA fibres), or simultaneously by both types of lesions. These experiments revealed that the NA neurons play a permissive role in the expression of the behavioural deficits induced by the electrocoagulation of the VTA. Indeed, while animals lesioned only in the VTA exhibited, as expected, increased nocturnal locomotor activity (56 per cent) and reduced spontaneous alternation behaviour (59 per cent instead of 76 per cent for the sham-operated animals), no significant changes in locomotor activity or in spontaneous alternations were seen in rats with simultaneous bilateral electrolytic lesion of the VTA and bilateral 6-OHDA lesion of the dorsal NA bundle when compared to sham-operated rats. Chemical lesions of the NA fibres alone had no effect, either on locomotor activity or on spontaneous alternation (Taghzouti et al., 1988).

Therefore, the simultaneous destruction of NA neurons and of VTA DA neurons markedly reduced the deficits observed in rats with electrolytic VTA lesions. This functional recovery indicates that deficits induced by a given lesion can be abolished by another type of lesion, and provides new insights into the antagonistic properties of ascending NA and DA neurons. It is proposed that a functional hierarchy exists between these systems since no significant modification of locomotor activity or spontaneous alternation was observed in rats with NA lesions alone. These results may explain why many deficits of the VTA syndrome are more pronounced in rats with electrolytic lesions than in animals with 6-OHDA lesions (Le Moal et al., 1969; Galey et al., 1977; Tassin et al., 1978a).

Since the modulation of D1 receptors and NT binding sites by ascending NA neurons seems to occur in the prefrontal cortex, this structure could be an important site of interaction between NA fibres and the target cells of the mixed mesocortical NT/DA neurons, and could be involved in the expression of the behavioural deficits examined. It cannot be excluded, however, that this type of interaction also occurs in other structures innervated by the VTA DA cells such as the different subcortical structures (see Cools et al., Chapter 6, this volume). Nevertheless, we have recently tried to determine which type of NA receptor (α or β) is implicated in this interaction, assuming that it occurred in the prefrontal cortex. Biochemical experiments, which will be described more precisely elsewhere (Trovero et al., 1990b) indicated that EEDQ, a ligand which binds irreversibly to α-adrenergic, but not to β-adrenergic receptors (Meller et al., 1985), could modify the sensitivity of cortical D1 receptors. Moreover, the fact that pretreating the animals with prazosin, an α-1-adrenergic antagonist, could block the effect of N-ethoxycarbonyl-2-ethoxy-1,2-dihydroquinoline (EEDQ) further suggested that these latter receptors were responsible for the heteroregulation of cortical D1 receptors.

This hypothesis has recently been confirmed in behavioural experiments in which animals rendered hyperactive by electrolytic lesions of the VTA were treated with low doses (0.5 mg/kg i.p.) of prasozin 1 hour before recording of nocturnal locomotor activity. This treatment, which had no effect on sham-operated animals, completely reversed the locomotor hyperactivity seen in lesioned animals up to 48 hours after injection. This interaction seems specific to α-1-adrenergic receptors occupied by prasozin since the same experiment performed with WB 4101, another α-1-adrenergic antagonist which binds to α-1A- and α-1B-adrenergic receptors (Morrow and Creese, 1986; Minneman, 1989), did not modify the locomotor hyperactivity of lesioned animals. Indeed, autoradiographic experiments using tritiated prasozin and WB 4101 as ligands have demonstrated different patterns in the cortical binding sites of these two ligands (Trovero et al., 1990c).

CONCLUSION

To study the interrelations between the ascending DA systems, we have focused our attention on the regulation of one type of DA receptor, the D1 receptor, which is positively coupled to adenylate cyclase. The initial experiments revealed that the sensitivity of D1 receptors was not only regulated by afferent DA fibres but also by neurotransmitters released by non-DA nerve terminals. Cortical as well as subcortical D1 receptors seem to be subject to this heteroregulation process. Analyses of the nature and the origin of the non-DA fibres implicated in the heteroregulation of D1 receptors indicated that these neurons were part of well-defined anatomical circuits and suggested that this heteroregulation had functional significance. For example, an intact cortical DA innervation appeared to be of major importance to obtain a denervation hypersensitivity of the D1 receptors in the nucleus accumbens as well as in the striatum. This indicated that the DA stimulation of cortical or subcortical structures might have opposite effects on functions regulated by these structures. Behavioural experiments have indeed confirmed the antagonistic functional roles of cortical and subcortical DA innervations.

In the prefrontal cortex, sensitivity of D1 receptors appears to be regulated by ascending NA fibres; in other words, the presence of an intact NA cortical innervation is necessary to obtain a denervation hypersensitivity of cortical D1 receptors. Interestingly, NT binding sites, which are co-localized with D1 receptors in the anterior cortex, are submitted to a heteroregulation opposite to that observed for cortical D1 receptors. That is, the absence of ascending NA fibres seems necessary to obtain a denervation hypersensitivity of the NT binding sites following the destruction of the mixed mesocortical NT/DA pathway. The physiological role of these NA ascending fibres, and more particularly of the α-1-adrenergic receptors, has been confirmed in behavioural experiments which indicated that the deficits induced by the destruction of the mixed NT/DA mesocortical pathway could be compensated either by the superimposed destruction of the ascending NA fibres or by the pharmacological blockade of the α-1-adrenergic receptors.

It should be noted that the presence of a hypersensitivity of DA receptors in subcortical structures has been related to human nervous diseases such as tardive dyskinesia (Muller and Seeman, 1978; Rupniak et al., 1983). Indeed, long-term treatments with DA antagonists produce supersensitivity of subcortical DA receptors (Burt et al., 1977; Muller and Seeman, 1978; Christensen et al., 1984; Creese and Chen, 1985). Interestingly, the same treatments do not modify D1 or D2 receptors in the prefrontal cortex (Memo et al., 1987). According to our demonstration of the role of the cortical NA innervation in the development of cortical D1 receptor hypersensitivity, it can be proposed that some neuroleptics, because of their influence on NA transmission, and particularly on α-1-adrenergic receptors, do not induce cortical D1 receptor hypersensitivity. Moreover, the modification of cortical NT binding sites by these neuroleptic treatments might also be important. It may be that tardive dyskinesia is the behavioural expression of the disequilibrium between mesocortical and mesolimbic DA transmission induced by neuroleptics. If this hypothesis is correct, it would be expected that either NA or NT agonists might improve the condition of patients afflicted by this disease.

REFERENCES

Akert, K. (1964) Comparative anatomy of the frontal cortex and thalamocortical connections. In: Warren, J.M. and Akert, K. (eds) *The Frontal and Agranular Cortex and Behaviour*. New York: McGraw-Hill, pp. 372–396.

Beckstead, R.M. (1979) An autoradiographic examination of cortico-cortical and subcortical projections of the medio-dorsal (prefrontal) cortex in the rat. *Journal of Comparative Neurology* **18**, 43–62.

Billard, W., Rupert, V., Crosby, G., Ioro, L.C. and Barnett, A. (1984) Characterization of the binding of (3H)SCH 23390, a selective D1 antagonist receptor ligand, in rat striatum. *Life Sciences* **35**, 1885–1893.

Björklund, A. and Lindvall, O. (1984) Dopamine containing systems in the CNS. In: Björklund, A. and Hökfelt, T. (eds) *Handbook of Chemical Neuroanatomy*. Amsterdam: Elsevier, pp. 55–122.

Blanc, G., Hervé, D., Simon, H., Lisoprawski, A., Glowinski, J., and Tassin, J.-P. (1980) Response to stress of mesocortico-prefrontal DA neurons in rats after long-term isolation. *Nature* **284**, 265–267.

Bockaert, J., Prémont, J., Glowinski, J., Thierry, A.M. and Tassin, J.-P. (1976) Topographical distribution of dopaminergic innervation and of dopaminergic receptors in the rat striatum. II. Distribution and characteristics of dopamine adenylate cyclase. Interaction of D-LSD with dopaminergic receptors. *Brain Research* **107**, 303–315.

Bouthenet, M.L., Martres, M.P., Sales, N. and Schwartz, J.C. (1987) A detailed mapping of D2 receptors in rat central nervous system by autoradiography with (125I)iodosulpiride. *Neuroscience* **20**, 117–155.

Boyson, S.J., McGonicle, P. and Molinoff, P.B. (1986) Quantitative autoradiographic localization of the D1 and D2 subtypes of dopamine receptors in rat brain. *Journal of Neuroscience* **6**, 3177–3188.

Burt, D.R., Creese, I. and Snyder, S.H. (1977) Antischizophrenic drugs: chronic treatment elevates dopamine receptor binding in brain. *Science* **196**, 326–328.

Christensen, A.V., Arnt, J., Hyttel, J., Larsen, J.J. and Svensen, O. (1984) Pharmacological effects of a specific dopamine D1 antagonist SCH 23390 in comparison with neuroleptics. *Life Sciences* **34**, 1529–1540.

Creese, I. and Chen, A. (1985) Selective D1 receptor increase following chronic treatment with SCH 23390. *European Journal of Pharmacology* **109**, 127–128.

Divac, I., Björklund, A., Lindvall, O. and Passingham, R.E. (1978) Converging projections from the medio-dorsal nucleus and mesencephalic dopaminergic neurons to the neocortex in three species. *Journal of Comparative Neurology* **180**, 59–72.

Fallon, J.H. and Moore, R.Y. (1978) Catecholaminergic innervation of the basal forebrain. IV. Topography of the dopaminergic projection of the basal forebrain and neostriatum. *Journal of Comparative Neurology* **180**, 545–580.

Fonnum, F., Storm-Mathisen, J. and Divac, I. (1981) Biochemical evidence for glutamate as neurotransmitter in cortico-striatal and cortico-thalamic fibres in rat brain. *Neuroscience* **6**, 863–873.

Galey, D., Simon, H. and Le Moal, M. (1977) Behavioural effects of lesions of the A10 area DA of the rat. *Brain Research* **124**, 83–97.

Heimer, L., Alheid, G.F. and Zaborsky, L. (1985) Basal ganglia. In: Paxinos, G. (ed.) *The Rat Nervous System*. New York: Academic Press, pp. 37–85.

Hemmings, H.C., Greengard, P. and Lim Tung, H.Y. (1984) DARPP-32, a dopamine-regulated neuronal phosphoprotein, is a potent inhibitor of protein phosphatase-1. *Nature* **310**, 503–505.

Hemmings, Jr, H.C., Walaas, S.I., Ouimet, C.C. and Greengard, P. (1987) Dopaminergic regulation of protein phosphorylation in the striatum: DARPP-32. *Trends in Neurosciences* **10**, 377–383.

Hervé, D., Simon, H., Blanc, G., Lisoprawski, A., Le Moal, M., Glowinski, J. and Tassin, J.-P. (1979) Increased utilization of dopamine in the nucleus accumbens but not in the cerebral cortex after dorsal raphé lesion in the rat. *Neuroscience Letters* **15**, 877–888.

Hervé, D., Simon, H., Blanc, G., Glowinski, J. and Tassin, J.-P. (1981) Opposite changes in dopamine utilization in the nucleus accumbens and the frontal cortex after electrolytic lesion of the median raphé in the rat. *Brain Research* **216**, 422–428.

Hervé, D., Blanc, G., Glowinski, J. and Tassin, J.-P. (1982) Reduction of dopamine utilization in the prefrontal cortex but not in the nucleus accumbens after selective destruction of noradrenergic fibers innervating the ventral tegmental area in the rat. *Brain Research* **237**, 510–516.

Hervé, D., Studler, J.M., Blanc, G., Glowinski, J. and Tassin, J.-P. (1986a) Partial protection by Desmethylimipramine of the mesocortical DA neurons from the neurotoxic effect of 6-OHDA injected in ventral mesencephalic tegmentum. The role of noradrenergic innervation. *Brain Research* **383**, 47–53.

Hervé, D., Tassin, J.-P., Studler, J.M., Dana, C., Kitabgi, P., Vincent, J.P., Glowinski, J. and Rostène, W. (1986b) Dopaminergic control of 125I-labeled neurotensin binding site density in corticolimbic structures of the rat brain. *Proceedings of the National Academy of Sciences (USA)* **83**, 6203–6207.

Hervé, D., Trovero, F., Blanc, G., Thierry, A.M., Glowinski, J. and Tassin, J.-P. (1989) Non-dopaminergic prefronto-cortical efferent fibers modulate D1 receptor denervation supersensitivity in specific regions of the rat striatum. *Journal of Neuroscience* **9**, 3699–3708.

Hess, E.J., Battaglia, G., Norman, A. and Creese, I. (1987) Differential modification of striatal D1 dopamine receptor and effector moieties by N-ethoxycarbonyl-2-ethoxy-1,2-dihydroxyquinoline in vivo and in vitro. *Molecular Pharmacology* **31**, 50–57.

Ingebritsen, T.S. and Cohen, P. (1983) Protein phosphatases: properties and role in cellular regulation. *Science* **221**, 331–338.

Ioro, L.C., Barnett, A., Leitz, F.H., Houser, V.P. and Korduba, C.A. (1983) SCH 23390, a potential benzazepine antipsychotic with unique interactions on dopaminergic systems. *Journal of Pharmacological and Experimental Therapeutics* **226**, 462–468.

Kebabian, J.W., Petzold, G.L. and Greengard, P. (1972) Dopamine-sensitive adenylate cyclase in caudate nucleus of rat brain and its similarity to the 'dopamine' receptor. *Proceedings of the National Academy of Sciences (USA)* **69**, 2145–2149.

Kelley, A.E., Domesick, V.B. and Nauta, W.J.H. (1982) The amygdalostriatal projection in the rat: an anatomical study by anterograde and retrograde tracing methods. *Neuroscience* **7**, 615–630.

Kelly, P.H., Seviour, P.W. and Iversen, S.D. (1975) Amphetamine and apomorphine responses in the rat following 6-OHDA lesions of the nucleus accumbens septi and corpus striatum. *Brain Research* **94**, 507–522.

Krettek, J.E. and Price, J.L. (1978) Amygdaloid projections to subcortical structures within the basal forebrain and brainstem in the rat and cat. *Journal of Comparative Neurology* **178**, 225–280.

Lavielle, S., Tassin, J.-P., Thierry, A.M., Blanc, G., Hervé, D., Bathélémy, C. and Glowinski, J. (1979) Blockade by benzodiazepines of the selective high increase in DA turnover induced by stress in mesocortical DA neurons in the rat. *Brain Research* **168**, 585–594.

Le Moal, M., Cardo, B. and Stinus, L. (1969) Influence of ventral mesencephalic lesions on various spontaneous and conditional behaviours in the rat. *Physiology and Behaviour* **4**, 567–574.

Lisoprawski, A., Hervé, D., Blanc, G., Glowinski, J. and Tassin, J.-P. (1980) Selective activation of the mesocortico-frontal dopaminergic neurons induced by lesion of the habenula in the rat. *Brain Research* **183**, 229–234.

Louilot, A., Simon, H., Taghzouti, K. and Le Moal, M. (1985) Modulation of dopaminergic activity in the nucleus accumbens following facilitation or blockade of the dopaminergic transmission in the amygdala: a study by in vivo differential pulse voltammetry. *Brain Research* **346**, 141–145.

Louilot, A., Le Moal, M. and Simon, H. (1989) Opposite influences of dopaminergic pathways to the prefrontal cortex or the septum on the dopaminergic transmission in the nucleus accumbens. An in vivo voltammetric study. *Neuroscience* **29**, 45–56.

Marchais, D., Tassin, J.-P. and Bockaert, J. (1980) Dopaminergic component of (3H)Spiroperidol binding in the rat anterior cortex. *Brain Research* **183**, 235–240.

Meller, E., Bohmaker, K., Goldstein, M. and Friedhoff, A.J. (1985) Inactivation of D1 and D2 dopamine receptors by N-ethoxy-2-ethoxy-1,2-dihydroquinoline in vivo: selective protection by neuroleptics. *Journal of Experimental Therapeutics* **233**, 656–662.

Memo, M., Missale, C., Valerio, A., Carruba, M.O. and Spano, P.F. (1986) Dopaminergic inhibition release and calcium influx induced by neurotensin in anterior pituitary is independent of cyclic AMP system. *Journal of Neurochemistry* **47**, 1689–1695.

Memo, M., Pizzi, M., Nisoli, E., Missale, C., Carruba, M.O. and Spano, P. (1987) Repeated administration of (-)sulpiride and SCH 23390 differentially up-regulate

D1 and D2 dopamine receptor function in rat mesostriatal areas but not in cortico-limbic brain regions. *European Journal of Pharmacology* **138**, 45–51.

Mesulam, M.M. (1978) Tetramethyl benzidine for horseradish peroxidase neurohisto-chemistry: A non-carcinogenic blue reaction product with superior properties for visualizing neural afferents and efferents. *Journal of Histochemistry and Cytochemistry* **26**, 106–117.

Minneman, K.P. (1989) α-1-adrenergic receptor subtypes, Inositol phosphates, and sources of cell Ca^{++}. *Pharmacological Reviews* **40**, 87–119.

Morrow, A.L. and Creese, I. (1986) Characterization of α-1-adrenergic receptor subtypes in rat brain: a reevaluation of 3H-WB-4101 and 3H-Prasozin binding. *Molecular Pharmacology* **29**, 321–330.

Muller, P. and Seeman, P. (1978) Dopaminergic supersensitivity after neuroleptics. *Psychopharmacology* **60**, 1–11.

Onali, P.L., Olianas, M.C. and Gessa, G.L. (1985) Characterization of dopamine receptors mediating inhibition of adenylate cyclase activity in rat striatum. *Molecular Pharmacology* **28**, 138–145.

Palacios, J.M. and Kuhar, M.J. (1981) Neurotensin receptors are located on dopamine-containing neurons in rat midbrain. *Nature* **294**, 587–589.

Palacios, J.M., Niehoff, D.L. and Kuhar, M.J. (1981) 3H-Spiperone binding sites in brain: autoradiographic localization of multiple receptors. *Brain Research* **213**, 277–289.

Piazza, P.V., Hervé, D., Glowinski, J. and Tassin, J.-P. (1990) Turning behaviour induced by unilateral 6-OHDA destruction of DA nigro-striatal pathway is decreased by lesion of the DA innervation of the contralateral prefrontal cortex. In preparation.

Pycock, C.J., Kerwin, R.W. and Carter, C.J. (1980) Effect of 6-hydroxydopamine lesions of the medial prefrontal cortex on neurotransmitter systems in subcortical sites in the rat. *Journal of Neurochemistry* **34**, 91–99.

Reibaud, M., Blanc, G., Studler, J.M., Glowinski, J. and Tassin, J.-P. (1984) Non-dopaminergic prefronto-cortical efferents modulate D1 receptors in the nucleus accumbens. *Brain Research* **305**, 43–50.

Rupniak, N.M.J., Jenner, P. and Marsden, C.D. (1983) The effect of chronic neuroleptic administration on cerebral dopamine receptor function. *Life Sciences* **32**, 2289–2311.

Sakanaka, M., Shiosaka, S., Takatsuki, K. and Tohyama, M. (1983) Evidence for the existence of substance P-containing pathway from the nucleus laterodorsalis tegmenti (castaldi) to the medial frontal cortex of the rat. *Brain Research* **259**, 123–126.

Savasta, M., Dubois, A. and Scatton, B. (1986) Autoradiographic localization of D1 dopamine receptors in the rat brain with (3H)SCH 23390. *Brain Research* **375**, 291–301.

Savasta, M., Dubois, A., Benavides, J. and Scatton, B. (1988) Different plasticity changes in D1 and D2 receptors in rat striatal subregions following impairment of dopaminergic transmission. *Neuroscience Letters* **85**, 119–124.

Seeman, P. (1980) Brain dopamine receptors. *Pharmacological Reviews* **32**, 229–313.

Simon, H., Taghzouti, K., Gozlan, H., Studler, J.M., Louilot, A., Hervé, D., Glowinski, J., Tassin, J.-P. and Le Moal, M. (1988) Lesion of dopaminergic terminals in the amygdala produces enhanced locomotor response to D-amphetamine and opposite changes in dopaminergic activity in prefrontal cortex and nucleus accumbens. *Brain Research* **447**, 335–340.

Stoof, J.C. and Kebabian, J.W. (1981) Opposing role for D1 and D2 dopamine receptors in efflux of cyclic AMP from rat neostriatum. *Nature* **294**, 366–368.

Studler, J.M., Kitabgi, P., Tramu, G., Hervé, D., Glowinski, J. and Tassin, J.-P. (1988) Extensive co-localization of neurotensin with dopamine in rat meso-cortico-frontal dopaminergic neurons. *Neuropeptides* **11**, 95–100.

Taghzouti, K., Simon, H., Hervé, D., Blanc, G., Studler, J.M., Glowinski, J., Le Moal, M. and Tassin, J.-P. (1988) Behavioural deficits induced by an electrolytic lesion of the rat ventral mesencephalic tegmentum are corrected by a superimposed lesion of the dorsal noradrenergic system. *Brain Research* **440**, 172–176.

Tassin, J.-P., Cheramy, A., Blanc, G., Thierry, A.M. and Glowinski, J. (1976) Topographical distribution of dopaminergic innervation and of dopaminergic receptors in the rat striatum. I. Microestimations of (3H)dopamine uptake and dopamine content in microdiscs. *Brain Research* **107**, 291–301.

Tassin, J.-P., Stinus, L., Simon, H., Blanc, G., Thierry, A.M., Le Moal, M., Cardo, B. and Glowinski, J. (1978a) Relationship between the locomotor hyperactivity induced by A_{10} lesions and the destruction of fronto-cortical DA innervation in the rat. *Brain Research* **141**, 267–281.

Tassin, J.-P., Bockaert, J., Blanc, G., Stinus, L., Thierry, A.M., Lavielle, S., Premont, J. and Glowinski, J. (1978b) Topographical distribution of dopaminergic innervation and dopaminergic receptors of the anterior cerebral cortex of the rat. *Brain Research* **154**, 241–251.

Tassin, J.-P., Simon, H., Glowinski, J. and Bockaert, J. (1982a) Modulations of the sensitivity of dopaminergic receptors in the prefrontal cortex and the nucleus accumbens: relationship with locomotor activity. In: Collu, R., Ducharme J.R., Barbeau, A. and Tobis, G. (eds) *Brain Peptides and Hormones* New York: Raven Press, pp. 17–30.

Tassin, J.-P., Simon, H., Hervé, D., Blanc, G., Le Moal, M., Glowinski, J. and Bockaert, J. (1982b) Non-dopaminergic fibres may regulate dopamine-sensitive adenylate cyclase in the prefrontal cortex and nucleus accumbens. *Nature* **295**, 696–698.

Tassin, J.-P., Studler, J.M., Hervé, D., Blanc, G. and Glowinski, J. (1986) Contribution of noradrenergic neurons to the regulation of dopaminergic (D1) receptor denervation supersensitivity in rat prefrontal cortex. *Journal of Neurochemistry* **46**, 243–248.

Tassin, J.-P., Vezina, P., Blanc, G. and Glowinski, J. (1988a) Amphetamine injected into the medial prefrontal cortex attenuates the locomotor activating effects of amphetamine in the nucleus accumbens. *Society for Neuroscience Abstracts* **14**, 662.

Tassin, J.-P., Kitabgi, P., Tramu, G., Studler, J.M., Hervé, D., Trovero, F. and Glowinski, J. (1988b) Rat mesocortical dopaminergic neurons are mixed Neurotensin/Dopamine neurons: immunohistochemical and biochemical evidence. *Annals of the New York Academy of Sciences* **537**, 531–533.

Trovero, F., Hervé, D., Blanc, G., Glowinski, J. and Tassin, J.-P. (1988) Quantitative autoradiography as a tool to study distribution and regulation of central neurotransmitter receptors; further evidence for dopaminergic receptor heteroregulation. Munich: XVIth CNIP Congress, abstract.

Trovero, F., Hervé, D., Blanc, G., Glowinski, J. and Tassin, J.-P. (1990a) Opposite regulation of postsynaptic D1 receptors and Neurotensinergic binding sites of the mixed DA/NT meso-cortical pathway. Submitted.

Trovero, F., Hervé, D., Blanc, G., Glowinski, J. and Tassin, J.-P. (1990b) Partial irreversible blockade of cortical D1 receptors by EEDQ induces an increase of DA-sensitive adenylate cyclase activity: role of α-1-adrenergic receptors. Submitted.

Trovero, F., Blanc, G., Hervé, D., Glowinski, J. and Tassin, J.-P. (1990c) Prazosin, an antagonist of α-1-adrenergic receptors, blocks specifically the locomotor activity induced by an electrolytic lesion of ventral tegmental area. Submitted.

Ungerstedt, U. (1971) Postsynaptic supersensitivity after 6-hydroxydopamine induced degeneration of the nigro-striatal dopamine system. *Acta Physiologica Scandinavica* **367**, 1–48 (suppl).

Ungerstedt, U. and Arbuthnott, G. (1970) Quantitative recording of rotational behaviour in rats after 6-hydroxydopamine of the nigro-striatal dopamine system. *Brain Research* **24**, 485–493.

Vezina, P., Blanc, G., Glowinski, J. and Tassin, J.-P. (1990) Evidence for prefrontal cortex inhibition of locomotor behaviour. A role for the D1 dopamine receptor. Submitted.

Walaas, S.I., Aswad, D.W. and Greengard, P. (1983) A dopamine-and cyclic AMP-regulated phosphoprotein enriched in dopamine-innervated brain regions. *Nature* **301**, 69–71.

Walters, J.R., Bergström, D.A., Carlson, J.H., Chase, T.N. and Braun, A.R. (1987) D1 dopamine receptor activation required for postsynaptic expression of D2 agonist effects. *Science* **236**, 719–722.

Part 2

BEHAVIOURAL PHARMACOLOGY OF MESOLIMBIC DOPAMINE

8

Dopamine and Motivated Behavior: Insights Provided by *In Vivo* Analyses

A.G. PHILLIPS[1], J.G. PFAUS[1] AND C.D. BLAHA[1,2]

[1]Department of Psychology and [2]Division of Neurological Sciences, Department of Psychiatry, University of British Columbia, Vancouver, BC, Canada V6T 1Y7

INTRODUCTION

On a superficial level, there is a clear relationship between dopaminergic activity in the brain and the behavior of mammals. The challenge to specialists in this field is to specify the precise aspects of behavior that are related to dynamic changes in dopamine (DA) release. One of the main objectives of this paper is to review the evidence in support of the link between DA, preparatory behavior and incentive motivation, particularly in light of recent behavioral experiments employing techniques for the *in vivo* analyses of DA release.

The classical studies of Ungerstedt (1971) using the selective neurotoxin 6-hydroxydopamine (6-OHDA) to destroy the mesotelencephalic DA pathways, identified a number of behavioral deficits ranging from a transient period of akinesia to more chronic disruptions of ingestive behaviors. Particular attention was paid to the aphagic and adipsic syndromes previously associated with selective damage to the lateral hypothalamic drive systems that were thought to control different aspects of basic motivation (Stellar, 1954). A number of related studies with 6-OHDA provided good evidence for dopaminergic substrates of self-stimulation behavior in certain regions of the brain (Fibiger and Phillips, 1987). A natural extension of these findings was the suggestion that dopaminergic systems may play an essential role in motivation and reward (Stellar and Stellar, 1985). However, a simple

The Mesolimbic Dopamine System: From Motivation to Action.
Edited by P. Willner and J. Scheel-Krüger

© 1991 John Wiley & Sons Ltd

link between dopaminergic activity, drive states and reward mechanisms may not be justified in light of contemporary theories of motivation and recent empirical studies employing new methodology for *in vivo* analysis of DA in the behaving animal.

For the purpose of the present discussion, motivation is defined as a theoretical construct that encompasses the processes underlying the initiation and termination of purposive or goal-directed behaviors. As indicated above, one prominent school of thought has emphasized the role of drive states, arising from homeostatic imbalances in physiological regulatory systems, as causal factors in motivation (Hull, 1943). Accordingly, motivated behaviors such as feeding or drinking were thought to be pursued for the sole purpose of redressing an underlying physiological disturbance. Drive theory has been challenged on many occasions by the concept of incentive motivation (Bindra, 1968; Bolles, 1972; Toates, 1981; Weingarten, 1985). In contrast to the 'push' of drive states, incentive motivation emphasizes the 'pull' of expectancy or anticipation triggered by salient external incentive stimuli. Expectancies develop as a consequence of repeated association between salient environmental stimuli and biologically significant stimuli (i.e. rewards). After becoming reliable predictors of rewarding stimuli, incentives acquire the capacity to initiate and sustain a wide variety of behaviors long before the consumption of a natural reward.

Students of animal behavior have paid particular attention to the distinction between preparatory and consummatory behaviors (Konorski, 1967; Woodworth, 1918). Preparatory behaviors, including foraging and hoarding, are responses that lead to and facilitate a separate class of consummatory behaviors that occur after the animal has made contact with a reward such as food. Consummatory acts, such as chewing and swallowing, can be readily identified and described. They have rigidly defined topographies and clearly defined objectives. In contrast, preparatory responses such as foraging behaviors are more flexible. They have less immediate objectives and have more variable topographies. Several different preparatory patterns may lead to identical consummatory reactions.

DA AND PREPARATORY FEEDING BEHAVIOR

Numerous studies suggest that dopaminergic activity may play a more important role in preparatory than in consummatory feeding behaviors. Hoarding behavior is disrupted by the DA receptor antagonist pimozide (Blundell et al., 1977), and is virtually abolished by lesions of the mesolimbic DA system at the level of the ventral tegmental area (VTA) which do not significantly alter food or water intake in these animals (Le Moal et al., 1977; Koob et al., 1978; Kelley and Stinus, 1985). Autoshaped behavior, identified as a form of preparatory responding by Woodruff and Williams

(1976), is attenuated by moderate doses of pimozide or haloperidol (Phillips et al., 1981). Similarly, instrumental responding for food reward is attenuated by central DA lesions in animals that are not aphagic (Fibiger et al., 1974; Heffner and Seiden, 1983), and by low or moderate doses of pimozide (Wise et al., 1978; Tombaugh et al., 1979; Wise and Schwartz, 1981).

Preparatory behaviors can also be studied through the use of classical conditioning procedures to ensure their clear separation from consummatory behaviors. Recent experiments in our laboratory have observed preparatory responses to conditional stimuli that have previously signalled the delivery of food (Blackburn et al., 1987, 1989 a, b). The procedure was derived from a conditioned feeding paradigm developed by Weingarten (1984). Rats responded to the conditional stimulus (CS+) by orientating to the cue light and exploring the niche into which food was about to be delivered. Pimozide (0.4–0.6 mg/kg) increased the latency to enter the niche and decreased the number of entries occurring prior to food delivery. In contrast, once food was delivered, the animals entered the niche with a short latency and consumed the meal in a normal manner. Thus, unlike preparatory responses, consummatory feeding responses were not disrupted by pimozide. These results were consistent with previous reports that the DA receptor antagonist chlorpromazine disrupts responding in the presence of conditional stimuli signalling food delivery by monkeys (Migler, 1975) and rats (Clody and Carlton, 1980).

Further support for the involvement of DA neurons in preparatory feeding behavior comes from a study by Simansky et al. (1985), who reported that DA utilization was increased when rats were exposed to stimuli signalling a subsequent meal. Increased DA utilization, as reflected by the ratio of the DA metabolite 3,4-dihydroxyphenylacetic acid (DOPAC) to DA (DOPAC:DA ratio), was observed in the hypothalamus but not in the striatum, nucleus accumbens, amygdala or olfactory tubercle. The failure to observe increased dopaminergic activity in the telencephalon is somewhat surprising in view of the proposed involvement of mesostriatal DA neurons in sensorimotor responses (Marshall et al., 1974; Ungerstedt, 1974; White, 1986) and the suggestion of a role for mesolimbic DA neurons in preparatory feeding responses such as hoarding (Blundell et al., 1977; Le Moal et al., 1977; Kelley and Stinus, 1985), foraging (Panksepp, 1982), and reaction to cues predictive of food (Blackburn et al., 1987; 1989a, b).

In a related study, neurochemical changes in dopaminergic activity in the nucleus accumbens and striatum were measured *ex vivo* following preparatory or consummatory feeding behaviors (Blackburn et al., 1989a). In one experiment, rats were conditioned to associate food delivery with the presentation of a conditional stimulus (CS+). When sacrificed after exposure to the CS+ alone on a test trial, the DOPAC:DA ratio was increased significantly in the nucleus accumbens (Figure 1A). A similar trend in the ratio of homovanillic acid (HVA) to DA (HVA:DA ratio) was also observed. Similar increases were observed in the striatum, but these were not statistically significant. In contrast, no increases were observed in the DOPAC:DA ratio or the HVA:DA ratio in either brain region when rats were permitted to consume an unsignalled meal for 7 minutes (Figure 1B). These findings suggest that activation of DA terminals in the nucleus accumbens occurs during the anticipation of a meal, at which time the rat is engaged in preparatory feeding behaviors; and that similar changes do not accompany short bouts of consummatory feeding behavior. As such, these results complement the previously described observation that DA receptor antagonists selectively disrupt appetitive behaviors elicited by food-related stimuli at doses that do not decrease food intake (Blackburn et al., 1987, 1989b). Together, these results support the hypothesis that DA systems are more importantly involved in preparatory than in consummatory feeding behaviors.

In an effort to gain a more direct assessment of the relationship between feeding behavior and neurochemical activity in various terminal regions of the mesotelencephalic DA systems, we have adopted the methodology of *in vivo* electrochemistry. This procedure involves the chronic implantation of stearate-modified graphite paste working electrodes developed by Blaha and Lane (1983), and has been used successfully to monitor changes in DA release following self-stimulation of the VTA (Phillips et al., 1989). As part of a continuing program to validate the use of stearate-modified electrodes in conjunction with chronoamperometry, and for assessing behavioral correlates of dynamic changes in extracellular DA levels, we have examined the effects of d-amphetamine and γ-butyrolactone (GBL), alone or in combination, on chronoamperometric signals obtained from these chronic electrodes. As predicted from *in vivo* microdialysis studies (Imperato and Di Chiara, 1984, 1985), d-amphetamine (2 mg/kg s.c.) increased the chronoamperometric signal, while GBL (200 mg/kg i.p.) had a pronounced inhibitory effect. Importantly, administration of d-amphetamine reversed the inhibitory effects of GBL. Parallel experiments are under way to confirm that oxidation of ascorbic acid or DOPAC does not contribute to this electrochemical signal. All of the data obtained to date are consistent with the claim that the stearate-modified graphite paste electrode is suitable for monitoring the extracellular overflow of DA *in vivo*. Nevertheless, it is imperative that the long-term viability of these electrodes is examined rigorously, to ensure that the procedure described here can be used reliably to study neurochemical correlates of behavior.

Preliminary experiments have monitored DA levels by chronoampero-metric techniques in both the nucleus accumbens and anterior striatum of the rats trained previously on the conditioned feeding schedule described above. A chronoamperometric measurement of DA oxidation current was taken every 30 seconds throughout several 24-hour periods, in which a

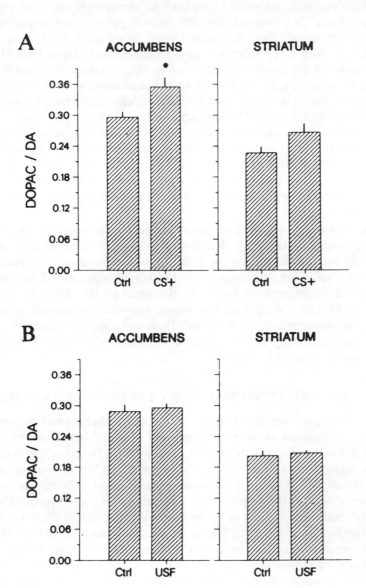

Figure 1. Ratio of DOPAC to DA in the nucleus accumbens and striatum. **A.** following 4-minute exposure to the CS+ (bars represent mean of seven rats). Difference from control value *P* <0.025. **B.** Seven minutes after the onset of unsignalled food (USF) (bars represent mean of eight rats). Adapted from Blackburn et al. (1989a)

tone–light combination served as a CS+ to signal eight meals of liquid diet per day. Each CS+ was initiated 270 seconds prior to delivery of the meal and was terminated 60 seconds after delivery of the meal. Eight presentations of a buzzer, with no programmed consequences, served as a CS−. The data were analysed by monitoring changes in the chronoamperometric signals during presentation of: (1) the CS+; (2) consumption of the meal; or (3) during and after presentation of the CS−. Representative examples of the data obtained in a single 24 hour experiment are shown in Figure 2. During this session, a clear elevation in the DA oxidation current was observed in 5 of 5 CS+ trials that had a stable pre-CS baseline. In the nucleus accumbens, the magnitude of the changes recorded during the CS+ trials averaged 6.6 nA. Smaller changes were observed in the striatum ($\overline{X}=3.0$ nA), and these changes confirm the trends observed previously with *ex vivo* measurements (Blackburn et al., 1989a).

A distinct advantage of chronoamperometry is the relatively fast sampling rate it provides. In the study described above, clear increases were observed within 20 seconds of the onset of the CS+, reaching an asymptote at the time the liquid diet was dispensed. Further changes could be monitored during and following each meal. At the onset of the meal, an immediate drop in the chronoamperometric signal was often observed in both the nucleus accumbens and the striatum. These data suggest that an increase in dopaminergic activity may be elicited by stimuli that reliably predict that the presence of food is imminent.

DA AND CONSUMMATORY FEEDING BEHAVIOR

The experiments described above all indicate that, while dopaminergic activity is involved in certain aspects of feeding behavior, there is no evidence for the direct activation of these systems by the act of feeding *per se*. As such, these results appear to contradict earlier reports of increased DA utilization following the consumption of food (Chance et al., 1985; Heffner et al., 1980). However, the time course of these reported increases indicates that they may not be immediate consequences of the act of feeding. For example, although both Biggio et al. (1977) and Heffner et al. (1984) found increases in DA utilization 1 hour after feeding began, further substantial increases were observed at subsequent sampling times, even though little ingestion occurred after the first hour. Blackburn et al. (1986) found evidence of increased DA utilization 1 hour after access to food pellets or to a liquid diet, but did not observe increases when rats consumed similar quantities of a palatable but non-nutritive saccharin solution. Together, these results suggest that increases in DA utilization observed in the brains of rats 1 hour after the onset of a feeding session may be due to postingestive events.

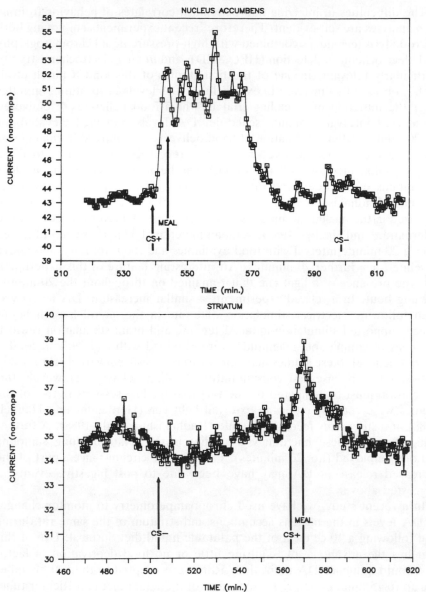

Figure 2. Changes in DA oxidation current in the nucleus accumbens (upper panel) and striatum (lower panel) following presentation of a CS+ signalling a meal 270 seconds after onset, or a CS− with no signal value. Data represent the chronoamperometric record (20-second sampling rate) from a stearate-modified carbon paste electrode implanted chronically in a male rat. Note, baseline current values prior to CS presentation represent the sum of both background current and DA oxidation current

The difficulties in inferring neurochemical correlates of behavior from *ex vivo* analyses are self-evident. Therefore, recent experiments employing both microdialysis techniques combined with high-pressure liquid chromatography and electrochemical detection (HPLC-ED), and *in vivo* electrochemistry are particularly relevant. In one of the first studies of this kind, Church et al. (1987) observed an increase in extracellular DA levels in striatum 5 minutes after the initiation of a feeding trial in which food pellets were delivered on a fixed interval 1 minute schedule. DA levels remained elevated for 15–20 minutes after termination of food delivery. A comparable change was not observed in food-deprived rats given free access. In contrast to these latter results, increased release of DA has been observed in the nucleus accumbens of food-deprived rats given access to food pellets for 4 hours per day (Radhakishun et al., 1988). Increased DA release has also been reported in the nucleus accumbens when rats pressed a lever for food reward (Hernandez and Hoebel, 1988). A mean increase of 37 per cent was obtained over a 20-minute interval with food available, and the level remained above baseline for a further 20 minutes. An interesting feature of this experiment was the presence of a light cue that remained on throughout the 20-minute feeding bout. In a related experiment, a similar increase in DA levels was seen following electrical stimulation of a site in the lateral hypothalamus which supported stimulation-induced feeding and brain stimulation reward. Changes of comparable magnitude were obtained with and without food.

On one level, these studies may appear to be consistent with a relationship between DA release and consummatory feeding behavior. However, this conclusion must be tempered by the fact that feeding sessions in two of the studies were cued by either an external light cue (Hernandez and Hoebel, 1988) or a strict daily feeding schedule (Radhakishun et al., 1988). A further difficulty with these microdialysis studies is the relatively long sampling periods employed (i.e. 20 minutes). Under these circumstances, part of the increased release of DA may have been due to post ingestive events as suggested above.

In a recent study, we have used chronoamperometry to monitor changes in DA levels in the nucleus accumbens and striatum of the same rat during and following a 10 cc meal of the palatable liquid diet Sustacal. Use of this diet has the advantage of requiring little or no food deprivation, a factor that could influence DA utilization. Rats were adapted to the test chamber for up to 15 minutes before presentation of the liquid diet in a Richter tube. Chronoamperometric recordings were taken every 20 seconds during the baseline period and for a further 20 minutes after presentation of the meal. Tests were conducted daily with four animals for 7 days. The meal was initiated within 60 seconds of exposure to the spout and continued for 3–7 minutes (X=4 minutes 56 seconds). On the first day, little or no change in DA oxidation current was observed. However, as shown in Figure 3, a

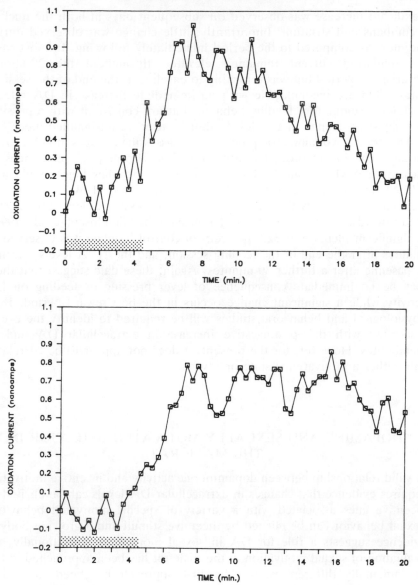

Figure 3. Changes in dopamine oxidation current from baseline in the nucleus accumbens (upper panel) and striatum (lower panel) during (stippled area) and following consumption of 10 cc of a palatable liquid diet. Each data point represents the average of six consecutive daily chronoamperometric measurements at a 20-second sampling rate. These data from an individual subject are representative of four rats that were given a meal of liquid diet in addition to *ad libitum* food for 7 days

significant increase was observed on subsequent days in both the nucleus accumbens and striatum. Importantly, little change was observed during the meal as compared to the period immediately following. In most cases the oxidation current remained elevated throughout the 20-minute observation period but was returning to baseline at the end of the session. These data are incompatible with an immediate increase in DA release during consummatory feeding behavior but are consistent with a possible postingestive change in DA levels shortly after an unsignalled meal.

An alternate voltammetric procedure for assessing changes in DA activity during behavior involves the use of carbon/silicone-paste electrodes to measure methylated catecholamine metabolites, including homovanillic acid (HVA), in the caudate nucleus (O'Neill et al., 1983). This technique was used recently to study the effect of a 30-minute session of lever pressing for food reward on a variable interval 10-second schedule (Joseph et al., 1990). A significant increase of 32.8 per cent of control baseline was observed 30 minutes after the end of the feeding session, and the HVA levels returned to baseline after a further 30 minutes. Again, these data suggest that there may be no immediate consequence of lever pressing or feeding on DA activity while a significant change occurs in the post-reward period. Both physiological and behavioral studies will be required to identify the events associated with this postingestive increase in extracellular DA and its metabolites. However, for the present, it does not appear to be correlated with either a motivational state or reward.

DOPAMINE AND SEXUALLY MOTIVATED BEHAVIOR IN THE MALE RAT

A valid relationship between dopaminergic activity and incentive motivation requires evidence that changes in extracellular DA levels can be elicited by incentive cues associated with a variety of specific motivated behaviors. Sexual behavior can be elicited by incentive stimuli and a growing body of evidence suggests a role for DA in sexual motivation. Traditionally, the evaluation of sexual motivation in the male rat has been approached in two fundamentally different ways. The first approach has been to analyse measures of behavior performed by the male in interaction with the female rat. Special status has been accorded to mount and intromission latencies because they reflect the first copulatory contact made by the male. However, it should be recognized that both may consist of motivational and performance components (Cherney and Bermant, 1970; Sachs and Barfield, 1976). The number of intromissions preceding ejaculation, the interintromission interval, and the ejaculation latency have also been viewed as measures of sexual motivation that reflect either the rate of copulation or the amount of genital stimulation required for ejaculation. The second approach involves the analysis of behaviors performed by the male either to gain access to, or in anticipation of, a sexually receptive female rat. Such behaviors have included performance in obstruction boxes (Warner, 1927), straight alley running (Sheffield et al., 1951), maze learning (Whalen, 1961), crossing of electrified grids (Moss, 1924), and bar-pressing behavior (Schwartz, 1956; Jowaisas et al., 1971; Sachs et al., 1974; Everitt et al., 1987). Although the interpretation of data derived from this second approach is straightforward and theoretically elegant, some of the situations are relatively artificial and the establishment of baseline rates of performance is often extremely time-consuming. Unfortunately, the analysis of anticipatory sexual behaviors is not commonly employed in assessments of sexual motivation.

Based on measures of the direct interaction between the sexes, Beach (1956) proposed a two-factor theory of sexual motivation that essentially re-stated the distinction noted above between preparatory and consummatory aspects of behavior. He suggested that the initiation and consummation of copulatory behavior were under the control of two independent motivational processes. The first process, called the 'sexual arousal mechanism' was thought to orientate the male toward the female and initiate mounts. The second process, called the 'intromission and ejaculation mechanism' was thought to drive the stereotyped pattern of penile intromissions that culminates in ejaculation. More recently, Sachs (1978) published the results of a factor analysis of ten measures of sexual behavior performed by the male in interaction with the female. From the results of this analysis, Sachs proposed the existence of at least four independent processes underlying the performance of sexual behavior by the male rat. These processes were characterized by factors called the initiation factor, the copulatory rate factor, the hit rate (the percentage of mounts resulting in intromission), and the intromission count. Although Sachs' approach retained a distinction between preparatory and consummatory aspects of copulatory behavior, it separated the consummatory aspect into three independent, but obviously interactive, processes (copulatory rate factor, hit rate and intromission count).

Separating sexual behavior into anticipatory/preparatory and consumma-tory components may be a valuable heuristic for identifying the neural mechanisms that control particular aspects of sexual behavior. Several studies have noted that the active pursuit of a sexually receptive female does not necessarily result in copulation. For example, castrated male rats will maintain a high rate of precopulatory investigation of the female's anogenital area long after their display of copulatory behavior has ceased (Madlafousek et al., 1976). Treatment with opioid drugs (Meyerson, 1981) or lesions of the medial preoptic area (Heimer and Larsson, 1966) eliminate male copulatory behavior but leave precopulatory investigation and pursuit of the female intact. Perhaps the most convincing demonstration of a preparatory and consummatory distinction in sexual behavior was made by Everitt and Stacey (1987), in which lesions of the medial preoptic area eliminated copulatory behavior but had no effect on rates of bar pressing to gain access to a sexually receptive female. If mount or intromission latencies had been the only measures of preparatory sexual behavior in those studies, it could have been suggested that the treatments eliminated copulatory behavior by disrupting a sexual arousal mechanism or an initiation factor. It may be that precopulatory behaviors are driven by the same mechanism that initiates mounting, but are simply less sensitive to the particular surgical or chemical treatments described above. However, it is also possible that behaviors performed by the male to gain access to a sexually receptive female may be dissociated from the initiation of copulatory behavior, much like foraging can be dissociated from the initiation of feeding.

Numerous reviews of the neuropharmacology of DA and the sexual behavior of male rats conclude that elevated DA activity serves to increase sexual arousal in the presence of appropriate incentive stimuli (Crowley and Zemlan, 1981; Bitran and Hull, 1987; Sachs and Meisel, 1988). This evidence is generally taken from studies using both systemic and central administration of DA agonists or antagonists. In rats, the systemic administration of DA agonists, such as L-DOPA or apomorphine, can reduce the latency to initiate copulatory behavior, reduce the number of intromissions required for ejaculation, reduce the ejaculation latency and postejaculatory interval (PEI), and stimulate copulatory activity in sexually inactive rats. Central infusions of apomorphine to the medial preoptic area (MPOA), a region critical for the expression of copulatory behavior and a terminal region of the incertohypothalamic DA system, increased the number of ejaculations and decreased the interintromission interval, the ejaculation latency and the PEI (Hull et al., 1986). Although apomorphine infused into the nucleus accumbens decreased the intromission latencies in that study, that effect was of borderline statistical significance only. Apomorphine had no effect on copulatory behavior following infusions to either the striatum or lateral septum. In contrast, infusions of d-amphetamine into the nucleus accumbens significantly decreased the mount and intromission latencies of sexually active male rats (Everitt et al., 1989).

Conversely, the systemic administration of a variety of DA antagonists disrupts these aspects of copulatory behavior in male rats. Low-to-moderate doses of the typical neuroleptics haloperidol or pimozide increase mount and intromission latencies, decrease the proportion of intromissions, and in some cases decrease the ejaculation latency and increase the PEI (Ahlenius and Larsson, 1984; McIntosh and Barfield, 1984; Pfaus and Phillips, 1989). Higher doses of these drugs typically abolish copulatory behavior. These effects are believed to reflect the blockade of central DA receptors because domperidone, a DA antagonist that does not readily cross the blood–brain barrier, does not affect the copulatory behavior of intact, sexually active male rats (Falaschi et al., 1981). Central infusions of *cis*-flupenthixol to the MPOA have been reported to reduce the proportion of male rats that initiate copulation (Pehek et al., 1988a). In rats that did initiate copulation, *cis*-flupenthixol reduced the total number of ejaculations, and increased both the interintromission interval and the ejaculation latency without affecting other aspects of copulatory behavior or general motor activity.

Another method for assessing the role of brain DA systems in male sexual behavior involves electrolytic or neurotoxic lesions of DA cell bodies, projection fibers, or terminal regions, or a general depletion of DA by intraventricular infusions of 6-OHDA along with systemic administration of pargyline. Caggiula et al. (1976) employed the latter procedure, and despite the fact that the combination of 6-OHDA and pargyline produced a 74 per cent depletion of caudate DA, and 81 per cent and 54 per cent depletions of cortical and hypothalamic noradrenaline (NA) respectively, they observed only a transient reduction in the total number of ejaculations relative to control rats given sham treatment. However, subsequent administration of the tyrosine hydroxylase inhibitor α-methylparatyrosine at a dose that did not affect the copulatory behavior of non-lesioned rats, increased the intromission latencies and dramatically reduced the proportion of rats that achieved ejaculation.

Both unilateral and bilateral electrolytic lesions of the A9 cell bodies in the substantia nigra have been reported to increase mount and intromission latencies, decrease the number of intromissions and ejaculations, and increase the PEI in sexually active rats (McIntosh and Barfield, 1984; Brackett et al., 1986). Although these effects are similar to those produced by systemic administration of DA antagonists, unilateral infusions of 6-OHDA to A9 produced only a small, but significant, increase in the PEI.

Bilateral electrolytic lesions of the A10 cell bodies in the VTA have also been reported to increase mount latencies and PEIs in sexually active rats (Brackett et al., 1986). Lesions of the corticomedial amygdala, a terminal region of the A10 DA projections, increased the number of intromissions and the ejaculation latency, and decreased the total number of ejaculations to sexual exhaustion (Giantonio et al., 1970; Harris and Sachs, 1975). However, some of these effects were reproducible only if the stimulus females were primed with estrogen alone, a treatment that reduces the display of proceptive behaviors (Perkins et al., 1980). Everitt et al. (1989) observed that bilateral N-methyl-D-aspartate lesions of basolateral amygdala had no effect on copulatory behavior in male rats; however, these lesions reduced the rate of operant responding for a secondary sexual reward. Interestingly, infusions of amphetamine to the nucleus accumbens of rats with basolateral amygdala lesions restored rates of operant responding for the secondary sexual reward (see Cador et al., Chapter 9, this volume). Together, these results indicate that diencephalic, mesostriatal and mesolimbic DA projections play a complicated role in the control of both arousal and performance aspects of male copulatory behavior.

Although inferences about the role of DA in motivational aspects of male copulatory behavior can be made from these studies, some of the effects on copulatory behavior are paradoxical. For example, the increased mount or intromission latencies typically observed following lesions of DA cell bodies or treatment with DA antagonists can be interpreted as a disruption of sexual motivation whereas the decreased number of intromissions before ejaculation can be interpreted as a facilitation (Sachs and Barfield, 1976). However, there is evidence that DA antagonists such as haloperidol decrease the number of penile erections displayed by intact male rats (Pehek et al., 1988b), an effect that could explain both the increased intromission latency and decreased number of intromissions. Although mount latencies may be a more appropriate measure of the motivation to initiate copulatory activity, they can be confounded by several factors, including the female's level of sexual receptivity. Moreover, had mount or intromission latencies been the only measure of sexual motivation in the recent studies by Everitt and associates, there would have been no reason to suspect that lesions of the basolateral amygdala had any effect on aspects of sexual motivation. Thus, it is difficult to determine the role of DA in the sexual motivation of male rats by examining measures of consummatory copulatory behavior alone.

A new form of anticipatory sexual motivation was recently characterized in male rats by Mendelson and Pfaus (1989), in the bilevel chambers designed by Mendelson and Gorzalka (1987). This behavior appeared as high rates of changing between the two levels of the chamber during the 5-minute adaptation periods prior to the introduction of a sexually receptive female for a test of copulation. The increased rates of level changing did not develop in sexually active males given access to either sexually non-receptive females or other males following the 5-minute adaptation periods. Unlike training rats to run mazes or bar-press for sexually receptive females, baseline rates of level changing were acquired rapidly and spontaneously in the bilevel chambers. Recent experiments (Pfaus and Phillips, in preparation) using level changing as a measure of anticipatory sexual motivation revealed a striking effect of DA antagonists. Systemic administration of haloperidol, pimozide, clozapine, SCH 23390 and sulpiride all decreased rates of level changing at doses that had no effect on copulatory behavior. Higher doses of these drugs affected copulatory behavior and decreased rates of level changing further. Central infusions of haloperidol to either the nucleus accumbens or MPOA also decreased rates of level changing, whereas infusions to the striatum did not. Interestingly, infusions to the MPOA also increased mount and intromission latencies and decreased the number of ejaculations, whereas infusions to the nucleus accumbens had no effect on copulatory behavior, and infusions to the striatum increased, rather than decreased, the number of ejaculations. As with feeding, these results suggested that central DA systems play a preferential role in anticipatory or preparatory aspects of sexual motivation, and indicated that at least two DA terminal regions, the nucleus accumbens and MPOA, are involved.

Recent advances in the electrochemical detection of transmitter substances and their metabolites with HPLC have given investigators a new tool for assessing transmitter activity in various brain regions following controlled periods of behavior. Several studies have recently examined regional DA activity following periods of copulatory behavior in intact, sexually active rats. Ahlenius et al. (1987) examined the accumulation of DOPA in the striatum, septum, nucleus accumbens and anterior hypothalamus following either 10 minutes of relatively unspecified sexual activity (at least one ejaculation) with a receptive female, 25 minutes of treadmill locomotion, or 10 minutes in the home cage. Sexual activity increased DOPA accumulation in the striatum and nucleus accumbens, but not in the septum or anterior hypothalamus, in comparison with control rats left in the home cage. Treadmill locomotion increased DOPA accumulation in the striatum, but not in the other three regions, suggesting that catecholamine synthesis (as determined by DOPA accumulation) increases in the nucleus accumbens as a specific function of sexual activity, and in the striatum as a non-specific function of either sexual activity or treadmill locomotion. Although suggestive, these results do not specify exactly what aspects of copulatory activity contributed to the increased DOPA accumulation in either the nucleus accumbens or striatum.

Levels of DA and DOPAC in the parietal cortex, preoptic region, mediobasal hypothalamus and lumbosacral spinal cord have been examined in rats that achieved either one ejaculation, or intromissions but no ejaculation, compared to sexually inactive rats that did not initiate copulatory behavior with receptive females (Mas et al., 1987). In that study, both DA and DOPAC levels were significantly elevated in the preoptic region after ejaculation. Although both DA and DOPAC levels were elevated in the preoptic region after intromission alone, only the DOPAC elevation reached statistical significance. DA levels in the lumbosacral cord were also elevated significantly after intromission alone, but not after ejaculation, suggesting that DA mechanisms in this region of the cord may contribute to the descending inhibition of ejaculatory reflexes during intromission. Unfortunately, DOPAC levels in the cord were undetectable, thus DA utilization could not be evaluated. Changes in DA or DOPAC levels did not occur in either the parietal cortex or mediobasal hypothalamus. These results suggest that DA release and utilization in the preoptic region is increased following an ejaculation. Intromission alone increases DA utilization but not necessarily DA release in the preoptic region.

Finally, a study by Hoffman et al. (1987) examined DA and DOPAC levels in the MPOA, arcuate nucleus/median eminence, or medial forebrain bundle of intact, sexually active rats that had either copulated to sexual exhaustion or were run in a motor-driven wheel, compared to intact, sexually inactive control rats. Each rat in the wheel-running condition was yoked to a rat in the sexual exhaustion condition such that the wheel started rotating when mounts were initiated and stopped rotating after ejaculation. DA levels in the MPOA, but not in the arcuate nucleus or medial forebrain bundle, were elevated significantly in both sexually exhausted and active rats. Although no differences in DOPAC concentration were detected among groups in the three brain regions, there was a significant negative correlation between the number of ejaculations and DOPAC concentration in the medial forebrain bundle. This suggests that DA utilization in this region was inversely related to the number of ejaculations. The increased DA concentration in the MPOA, together with the lack of change in DOPAC concentration, suggests that DA utilization and/or release was attenuated in the MPOA following lengthy bouts of locomotor activity, the manipulation common to both the sexual exhaustion and forced activity groups. Taken together, these results indicate that DA synthesis, release and/or utilization may increase during copulation in several DA terminal regions, notably the nucleus accumbens, neostriatum and MPOA. However, in the two studies that controlled for locomotor activity, the effects observed in the neostriatum and MPOA were not specific to copulatory behavior.

We have recently conducted a study in collaboration with G. Damsma, G. Nomikos and H.C. Fibiger (Pfaus et al., 1990) using *in vivo* microdialysis to examine DA release in the nucleus accumbens and striatum during the copulatory behavior of male rats. The behavioral tests consisted of three distinct phases: (*1*) separation of the partners for 10 minutes behind a wire mesh screen; (*2*) a 30-minute bout of copulatory behavior following removal of the screen partition; and (*3*) an 80-minute postcopulatory period in which the male was observed in the absence of the female. Biochemical analyses of DA in the dialysates at 10-minute intervals revealed three distinct patterns of change in DA levels in the nucleus accumbens. In phase 1 of the test, exposure to the female without physical contact was accompanied by a significant rise in the DA level. A further increase was observed during active copulation and DA levels decreased throughout phase 3, but still remained above baseline levels. In contrast, a much smaller increase was observed in the striatum in phase 1 and DA levels increased gradually during active copulation and returned to baseline levels during phase 3 of the test. These results confirmed that DA release in the nucleus accumbens and striatum increases during the anticipatory and consummatory phases of sexual behavior in the male rat. The different patterns of release suggested that these mesocorticolimbic and striatal DA systems may contribute differentially to the regulation of copulatory behavior. This suggestion was consistent with effects following local infusions of haloperidol into these areas. However, a further description of the specific aspects of copulatory behavior associated with increased DA release in these brain regions will require an analytical procedure with finer temporal resolution.

With this objective in mind, we have undertaken a study in which DA levels in both the nucleus accumbens and striatum were measured with chronoamperometry during various phases of sexual behavior in the male rat. All males were experienced copulators prior to implantation of the chronic electrode assemblies, and subsequent tests while connected to an electrical cable and commutator confirmed that neither the surgery nor the cable interfered with their copulatory behavior. The procedure for testing sexual behavior was similar to that used in the microdialysis experiments, except that the female was placed behind the screen for only 5 minutes.

As may be seen in Figure 4, a dramatic and immediate increase in the chronoamperometric signal was observed upon placing the female behind the screen. This elevated signal was maintained through the first intromission up to the first ejaculation. The first ejaculation was followed by a decline in the signal. Towards the end of the first PEI, the signal rose again and a second copulatory sequence was initiated by an intromission. This pattern was repeated throughout the 30-minute session.

The changes observed in the striatum were markedly different (Figure 4). A slight increase in the current was seen when the female was placed behind the screen and there was no large change during the first copulatory sequence. The first ejaculation was followed by an increase in the signal which tended to increase slowly and moderately throughout the test. The differences between the striatum and nucleus accumbens are summarized in Figure 5, which shows the average magnitude of change in current to the presence of the female and during the first intromission, the ejaculation and the PEI of each copulatory sequence. The DA signal changed dynamically in the nucleus accumbens, while exhibiting a steady rise in the striatum across the entire test session. These results are quite consistent with the results of the microdialysis experiments described above.

Control experiments with either a male, a non-receptive female, or a slide containing estrous vaginal secretions revealed a significant but small increase in the DA signal in the nucleus accumbens (Figure 6), indicating that the magnitude of the previous observation was not due simply to the presence of another animal behind the screen. None of the control stimuli evoked a significant rise in the signal in the striatum. Thus it would appear that the presence of an estrous female is a particularly salient stimulus for evoking an increase in DA release in the nucleus accumbens. This is consistent with

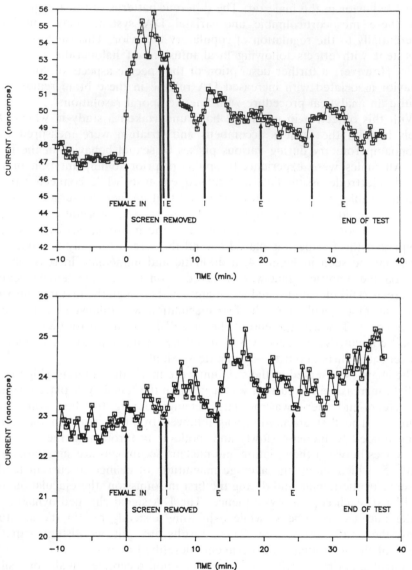

Figure 4. Changes in DA oxidation current in the nucleus accumbens (upper panel) and striatum (lower panel) during various phases of sexual behavior by a male rat. Chronoamperometric records were obtained from a stearate-modified carbon paste electrode with a 20-second sampling rate. Baseline current values in the 10-minute period prior to the behavioral test represent the sum of both background current and DA oxidation current. The behavioral test started by placing an estrus female rat into the observation chamber behind a wire screen for 5 minutes, I, Intromission; E, ejaculation

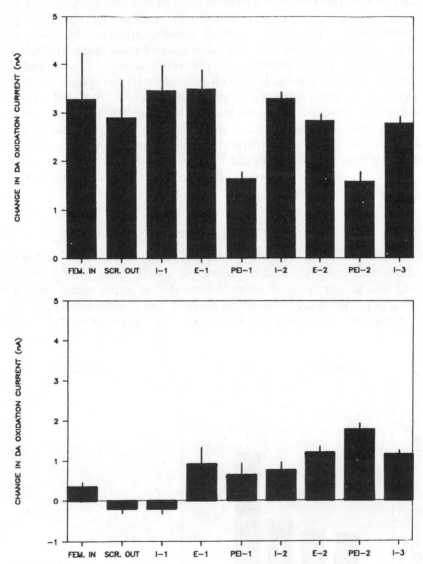

Figure 5. Mean changes in DA oxidation current in nucleus accumbens ($n=5$, upper panel) and striatum ($n=5$, lower panel), coinciding with specific phases of a 5-minute precopulatory period and a 30-minute bout of sexual activity in male rats. FEM. IN, Female in chamber behind screen; SCR. OUT, screen out to permit contact between male and female; I-1, first intromission of copulatory sequence one; E-1, first ejaculation; PEI-1, midpoint of first postejaculation interval; I-2, first intromission of copulatory sequence two; E-2, second ejaculation; PEI-2, midpoint of second postejaculation interval; I-3, first intromission of copulatory sequence three

an activation of this system by incentive cues, in this case the proprioceptive cues and odour of a receptive female. This pattern of results is quite compatible with Toates' (1986) model of sexual motivation which recognizes a complex interaction between external incentive stimuli and hormonal state in determining sexual arousal and the sensitization of an ejaculation mechanism. The increase in DA levels elicited by the receptive female may be an essential neural substrate for processes of sexual arousal. Toates also postulates that ejaculation in turn leads to the desensitization of the sexual arousal mechanism. The clear and dramatic drop in the DA signal in the nucleus accumbens following ejaculation is entirely consistent with this model. Together these data suggest that dopaminergic activity in the limbic system may be critically involved in the dynamic control of sexual behavior in the mammalian brain.

CONCLUSIONS

Neurochemical analyses of extracellular DA, using both *ex vivo* and *in vivo* procedures indicate increased dopaminergic activity prior to and following feeding and sexual behavior in male rats. Recent experiments employing procedures for the segregation of preparatory and consummatory phases of these behaviors, in conjunction with *in vivo* measurement of DA release,

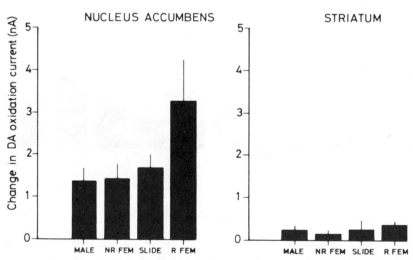

Figure 6. Changes in DA oxidation current from baseline in the nucleus accumbens (left panel) or striatum (right panel) observed during a 10-minute test in which either a male rat (MALE), a non-estrous female (NR FEM), a glass slide (SLIDE) containing the odour of an estrous female, or an estrous female (R FEM) was placed behind a wire mesh screen in the same chamber with the experimental male rat

provide compelling evidence for elevated transmitter release during preparatory behaviors. This pattern of results is compatible with a link between increased dopaminergic activity and behavioral arousal associated with incentive motivation. In the context of the title of this volume, this would form the motivational state that leads to action.

Although still highly speculative, the hints of a decrease in dopaminergic activity following consumption of a signalled meal in hungry animals or ejaculation in sexually aroused males, has important implications for the dopaminergic hypothesis of reward (Wise et al., 1978; see also Beninger, Chapter 11, this volume). Rather than increased dopaminergic activity being a neurochemical correlate of reward, the opposite relationship may hold. Anticipation of reward may enhance dopaminergic activity, producing a concomitant increase in arousal, which is rapidly reduced by the rewarding effects of feeding or ejaculation. In this manner, dopaminergic activity (mainly in the mesolimbic region) could be characterized as playing a major role in incentive motivation, while a phasic reduction in release may signal satisfaction. Hopefully, further experiments with other classes of motivated behavior, in conjunction with *in vivo* electrochemical and microdialysis measures of extracellular levels of DA and other monoamines, will clarify these issues in the near future.

ACKNOWLEDGEMENTS

The voltammetry experiments described in this paper were supported by Program Grant-23, from the Medical Research Council of Canada. The helpful comments of H.C. Fibiger are acknowledged gratefully. We thank E. McCririck for excellent assistance in typing the manuscript.

REFERENCES

Ahlenius, S. and Larsson, K. (1984) Lisuride, LY-141865, and 8-OH-DPAT facilitate male rat sexual behaviour via a non-dopaminergic mechanism. *Psychopharmacology* **83**, 137–140.
Ahlenius, S., Carlsson, A., Hillegaart, V., Hjorth, S. and Larsson, K. (1987) Region-selective activation of brain monoamine synthesis by sexual activity in the male rat. *European Journal of Pharmacology* **114**, 77–82.
Beach, F.A. (1956) Characteristics of masculine 'sex drive'. *Nebraska Symposium on Motivation* **4**, 1–32.
Biggio, G., Porceddu, M.L., Fratta, W. and Gessa, G.L. (1977) Changes in dopamine metabolism associated with fasting and satiation. In: Costa, E. and Gessa, G.L. (eds) *Advances in Biochemical Psychopharmacology*. New York: Raven, pp. 377–380.
Bindra, D. (1968) Neuropsychological interpretation of the effects of drive and incentive motivation on general activity and instrumental behavior. *Psychological Review* **75**, 1–22.

Bitran, D. and Hull, E.M. (1987) Pharmacological analysis of male rat sexual behavior. *Neuroscience and Biobehavioral Reviews* **11**, 365–389.

Blackburn, J.R., Phillips, A.G., Jakubovic, A. and Fibiger, H.C. (1986) Increased dopamine metabolism in the nucleus accumbens and striatum following consumption of a nutritive meal but not a palatable non-nutritive saccharin solution. *Pharmacology Biochemistry and Behavior* **25**, 1095–1100.

Blackburn, J.R., Phillips, A.G. and Fibiger, H.C. (1987) Dopamine and preparatory behavior: I. Effects of pimozide. *Behavioral Neuroscience* **101**, 352–360.

Blackburn, J.R., Phillips, A.G., Jakubovic, A. and Fibiger, H.C. (1989a) Dopamine and preparatory behavior: II. A neurochemical analysis. *Behavioral Neuroscience* **103**, 15–23.

Blackburn, J.R., Phillips, A.G. and Fibiger, H.C. (1989b) Dopamine and preparatory behavior: III. Effects of metoclopromide and thioridazine. *Behavioral Neuroscience* **103**, 903–906.

Blaha, C.D. and Lane, R.F. (1983) Chemically modified electrode for *in vivo* monitoring of brain catecholamines. *Brain Research Bulletin* **10**, 861–864.

Blundell, J.E., Strupp, B.J. and Latham, C.J. (1977) Pharmacological manipulation of hoarding: further analysis of amphetamine isomers and pimozide. *Physiological Psychology* **5**, 462–468.

Bolles, R.C. (1972) Reinforcement, expectancy and learning. *Psychological Reviews* **79**, 394–409.

Brackett, N.L., Iuvone, P.M. and Edwards, D.A. (1986) Midbrain lesions, dopamine, and male sexual behavior. *Behavioral Brain Research* **20**, 231–240.

Caggiula, A.R., Shaw, D.H., Antelman, S.M. and Edwards, D.A. (1976) Interactive effects of brain catecholamines and variations in sexual and nonsexual arousal on copulatory behavior of male rats. *Brain Research* **111**, 321–336.

Chance, W.T., Foley-Nelson, T., Nelson, J.L., Kim, M.W. and Fischer, J.E. (1985) Changes in neurotransmitter levels associated with feeding and satiety. *Society for Neuroscience Abstracts* **11**, 61.

Cherney, E.F. and Bermant, G. (1970) The role of stimulus female novelty in the rearousal of copulation in male laboratory rats (*Rattus norvegicus*). *Animal Behaviour* **18**, 567–574.

Church, W.H., Justice, Jr., J.B. and Neill, D.B. (1987) Detecting behaviorally relevant changes in extracellular dopamine with microdialysis. *Brain Research* **412**, 397–399.

Clody, D.E. and Carlton, P.E. (1980) Stimulus efficacy, chlorpromazine, and schizophrenia. *Psychopharmacology* **34**, 1127–1131.

Crowley, W.R. and Zemlan, F.P. (1981) The neurochemical control of mating behavior. In: Adler, N.T. (ed.) *Neuroendocrinology of Reproduction*. New York: Plenum, pp. 451–482.

Everitt, B.J. and Stacey, P. (1987) Studies of instrumental behavior with sexual reinforcement in male rats (*Rattus norvegicus*). II: Effects of preoptic area lesions, castration, and testosterone. *Journal of Comparative Psychology* **101**, 407–419.

Everitt, B.J., Fray, P., Kostarczyk, E., Taylor, S. and Stacey, P. (1987) Studies of instrumental behavior with sexual reinforcement in male rats (*Rattus norvegicus*): I. Control by brief visual stimuli paired with a receptive female. *Journal of Comparative Psychology* **101**, 395–406.

Everitt, B.J., Cador, M. and Robbins, T.W. (1989) Interactions between an amygdala and ventral striatum in stimulus-reward associations: studies using a second-order schedule of sexual reinforcement. *Neuroscience* **20**, 63–75.

Falaschi, P., Rocco, A., De Georgio, G., Frajese, G., Fratta, W. and Gessa, G.L.

(1981) Brain dopamine and premature ejaculation: results of treatment with dopamine antagonists. In: Gessa, G.L. and Corsini, G.U. (eds) *Apomorphine and other dopaminomimetics. Vol. 1: Basic Pharmacology.* New York: Raven, pp. 117–121.

Fibiger, H.C. and Phillips, A.G. (1987) Role of catecholamine neurotransmitters in brain reward systems: implications for the neurobiology of affect. In: Engel, J. and Oreland, L. (eds) *Brain Reward Systems and Abuse.* New York: Raven, pp. 61–74.

Fibiger, H.C., Phillips, A.G. and Zis, A.P. (1974) Deficits in instrumental responding after 6-hydroxydopamine lesions of the nigro-neostriatal dopaminergic projection. *Pharmacology Biochemistry and Behavior* **2**, 87–96.

Giantonio, G.W., Lund, N.L. and Gerall, A.A. (1970) Effect of diencephalic and rhinencephalic lesions on the male rat's sexual behavior. *Journal of Comparative and Physiological Psychology* **73**, 38–46.

Harris, V.S. and Sachs, B.D. (1975) Copulatory behavior in male rats following amygdaloid lesions. *Brain Research* **86**, 514–518.

Heffner, T.G. and Seiden, L.S. (1983) Impaired acquisition of an operant response in young rats depleted of brain dopamine in neonatal life. *Psychopharmacology* **79**, 115–119.

Heffner, T.G., Hartman, J.A. and Seiden, L.S. (1980) Feeding increases dopamine metabolism in the rat brain. *Science* **208**, 1168–1170.

Heffner, T.G., Vosmer, G. and Seiden, L.S. (1984) Time-dependent changes in hypothalamic dopamine metabolism during feeding in the rat. *Pharmacology Biochemistry and Behavior* **20**, 947–949.

Heimer, L. and Larsson, K. (1966) Impairment of mating behavior in male rats following lesions in the preoptic-anterior-hypothalamic continuum. *Brain Research* **3**, 238–263.

Hernandez, L. and Hoebel, B.G. (1988) Feeding and hypothalamic stimulation increase dopamine turnover in the accumbens. *Physiology and Behavior* **44**, 599–606.

Hoffman, N.W., Gerall, A.A. and Kalivas, P.W. (1987) Sexual refractoriness and locomotion effects on brain monoamines in the male rat. *Physiology and Behavior* **41**, 563–569.

Hull, C.L. (1943) *Principles of Behavior.* New York: Appleton-Century-Crofts.

Hull, E.M., Bitran, D., Pehek, E.A., Warner, R.K., Band, L.C. and Holmes, G.M. (1986) Dopamine control of male sex behavior in rats: effects on an intracerebrally-infused agonist. *Brain Research* **370**, 73–81.

Imperato, A. and Di Chiara, G. (1984) Trans-striatal dialysis coupled to reverse-phase high performance liquid chromatography with electrochemical detection: a new method for the study of the *in vivo* release of endogenous dopamine and metabolites. *Journal of Neuroscience* **4**, 966–984.

Imperato, A. and Di Chiara, G. (1985) Dopamine release and metabolism in awake rats after systemic neuroleptics as studied by trans-striatal dialysis. *Journal of Neuroscience* **5**, 297–306.

Joseph, M.H., Hodges, H. and Gray, J.A. (1990) Lever pressing for food reward and *in vivo* voltammetry: evidence for increases in extracellular homovanillic acid, the dopamine metabolite and uric acid in the rat caudate nucleus. *Neuroscience* (in press).

Jowaisas, D., Taylor, J., Dewsbury, D.A. and Malagodi, E.F. (1971) Copulatory behavior of male rats under an imposed operant requirement. *Psychonomic Science* **25**, 287–290.

222   *Phillips et al.*

Kelley, A.E. and Stinus, L. (1985) Disappearance of hoarding behavior after 6-hydroxydopamine lesions of the mesolimbic dopamine neurons and its reinstatement with L-dopa. *Behavioral Neuroscience* **99**, 531–545.

Konorski, J. (1967) *Integrative Activity of the Brain*. Chicago: University of Chicago Press.

Koob, G.F., Riley, S.J., Smith, S.C. and Robbins, T.W. (1978) Effects of 6-hydroxydopamine lesions of the nucleus accumbens septi and olfactory tubercle on feeding, locomotor activity, and amphetamine anorexia in the rat. *Journal of Comparative and Physiological Psychology* **92**, 917–927.

Le Moal, M., Stinus, L., Simon, H., Tassin, J.-P., Thierry, A.M., Blanc, G., Glowinski, J. and Cardo, B. (1977) Behavioral effects of a lesion in the ventral mesencephalic tegmentum: evidence for involvement of A10 dopaminergic neurons. In: Costa, E. and Gessa, G.L. (eds) *Advances in Biochemical Psychopharmacology*. New York: Raven, pp. 237–245.

Madlafousek, J., Hlinak, Z. and Beran, J. (1976) Decline of sexual behavior in castrated male rats: effects of female precopulatory behavior. *Hormones and Behavior* **7**, 245–252.

Marshall, J.F., Richardson, J.S. and Teitelbaum, P. (1974) Nigrostriatal bundle damage and the lateral hypothalamic syndrome. *Journal of Comparative and Physiological Psychology* **87**, 808–830.

Mas, M., del Castillo, A.R., Guerra, M., Davidson, J.M. and Battaner, E. (1987) Neurochemical correlates of male sexual behavior. *Physiology and Behavior* **41**, 341–345.

McIntosh, T.K. and Barfield, R.J. (1984) Brain monoaminergic control of male reproductive behavior: II: Dopamine and the post-ejaculatory refractory period. *Behavioral Brain Research* **12**, 267–273.

Mendelson, S.M. and Gorzalka, B.B. (1987) An improved chamber for the observation and analysis of the sexual behavior of the female rat. *Physiology and Behavior* **39**, 67–71.

Mendelson, S.M. and Pfaus, J.G. (1989) Level searching: a new assay of sexual motivation in the male rat. *Physiology and Behavior* **45**, 337–341.

Meyerson, B.J. (1981) Comparison of the effects of endorphin and morphine on exploratory and socio-sexual behavior in the male rat. *European Journal of Pharmacology* **69**, 453–463.

Migler, B. (1975) Conditioned approach: an analogue of conditioned avoidance: effects of chlorpromazine and diazepam. *Pharmacology Biochemistry and Behavior* **3**, 961–965.

Moss, F.A. (1924) A study of animal drives. *Experimental Psychology* **7**, 165–185.

O'Neill, R.D., Fillenz, M., Albery, W.J. and Goddard, N.J. (1983) The monitoring of ascorbate and monoamine transmitter metabolites in the striatum of unanaesthetized rats using microprocessor-based voltammetry. *Neuroscience* **9**, 87–93.

Panksepp, J. (1982) Toward a general psychobiological theory of emotions. *Behavioral and Brain Sciences* **5**, 407–467.

Pehek, E.A., Thompson, J.T., Eaton, R.C., Bazzett, T.J. and Hull, E.M. (1988a) Apomorphine and haloperidol, but not domperidone affect penile reflexes in rats. *Pharmacology, Biochemistry and Behavior* **31**, 201–208.

Pehek, E.A., Thompson, J.T., Eaton, R.C., Bazzett, T.J. and Hull, E.M. (1988b) Microinjection of cis-flupenthixol, a dopamine antagonist, into the medial preoptic area impairs sexual behavior of male rats. *Brain Research* **443**, 70–76.

Perkins, M.S., Perkins, M.N. and Hitt, J.C. (1980) Effects of stimulus female on sexual behavior of male rats given olfactory tubercle and corticomedial amygdaloid lesions. *Physiology and Behavior* **25**, 495–500.

Pfaus, J.G. and Phillips, A.G. (1989) Differential effects of dopamine receptor antagonists on the sexual behavior of male rats. *Psychopharmacology* **98**, 363–368.

Pfaus, J.G., Damsma, G., Nomikos, G.G., Wenkstern, D., Blaha, C.D., Phillips, A.G. and Fibiger, H.C. (1990) Sexual behavior enhances central dopamine transmission in the male rate. *Brain Research* (in press).

Phillips, A.G., McDonald, A.C. and Wilkie, D.M. (1981) Disruption of autoshaped responding to a signal of brain-stimulation reward by neuroleptic drugs. *Pharmacology Biochemistry and Behavior* **14**, 543–548.

Phillips, A.G., Blaha, C.D. and Fibiger, H.C. (1989) Neurochemical correlates of brain-stimulation reward measured by ex vivo and in vivo analyses. *Neuroscience and Biobehavioral Reviews* **13**, 99–104.

Radhakishun, F.S., van Ree, J.M. and Westerink, B.H.C. (1988) Scheduled eating increases dopamine release in the nucleus accumbens of food deprived rats as assessed with on-line brain dialysis. *Neuroscience Letters* **85**, 351–356.

Sachs, B.D. (1978) Conceptual and neural mechanisms of masculine copulatory behavior. In: McGill, T.E., Dewsbury, D.A. and Sachs, B.D. (eds) *Sex and Behavior: Status and Prospectus*, New York: Plenum Press, pp. 267–295.

Sachs, B.C. and Barfield, R.J. (1976) Functional analysis of masculine copulatory behavior in the rat. *Advances in the Study of Behaviour* **7**, 91–145.

Sachs, B.D. and Meisel, R.L. (1988) The physiology of male sexual behavior. In: Knobil, E. and Neill, J. (eds) *The Physiology of Reproduction*. New York: Raven, pp. 1393–1485.

Sachs, B.D., Macaione, R. and Fagy, L. (1974) Pacing of copulatory behavior in the male rat: effects of receptive females and intermittent shocks. *Journal of Comparative and Physiological Psychology* **87**, 326–331.

Schwartz, M. (1956) Instrumental and consummatory measures of sexual capacity in the male rat. *Journal of Comparative and Physiological Psychology* **49**, 328–333.

Sheffield, F.D., Wulff, J.J. and Backer, R. (1951) Reward value of copulation without sex drive reduction. *Journal of Comparative and Physiological Psychology* **44**, 3–8.

Simansky, K.J., Bourbonais, K.A. and Smith, G.P. (1985) Food-related stimuli increase the ratio of 3,4-dihydroxyphenylacetic acid to dopamine in the hypothalamus. *Pharmacology Biochemistry and Behavior* **23**, 253–258.

Stellar, E. (1954) The physiology of motivation. *Psychological Review* **61**, 5–22.

Stellar, J.R. and Stellar, E. (1985) *The Neurobiology of Motivation and Reward*. New York: Springer-Verlag.

Toates, F.M. (1981) The control of ingestive behaviour by internal and external stimuli—A theoretical review. *Appetite* **2**, 35–50.

Toates, F.M. (1986) *Motivational Systems*. Cambridge: Cambridge University Press.

Tombaugh, T.N., Tombaugh, J. and Anisman, H. (1979) Effects of dopamine receptor blockade on alimentary behaviors: home cage food consumption, operant acquisition, and performance. *Psychopharmacology* **66**, 219–225.

Ungerstedt, U. (1971) Adipsia and aphagia after 6-hydroxydopamine induced degeneration of the nigro-striatal dopamine system. *Acta Physiologica Scandinavica Supplementum* **367**, 95–122.

Ungerstedt, U. (1974) Brain dopamine neurons and behavior. In: Schmitt, F.O. and Worden, F.G. (eds) *The Neurosciences, Third Study Program*. Cambridge MA: MIT Press, pp. 695–703.

Warner, W.H. (1927) A study of sex drive in the white rat by means of an obstruction method. *Comparative Psychology Monographs* **4**, 1–67.

Weingarten, H.P. (1984) Meal initiation controlled by learned cues: basic behavioral properties. *Appetite* **5**, 147–158.

Weingarten, H.P. (1985) Stimulus control of eating: implications for a two-factor theory of hunger. *Appetite* **6**, 387–401.

Whalen, R.E. (1961) Effects of mounting without intromission and intromission without ejaculation on sexual behavior and maze learning. *Journal of Comparative Physiological Psychology* **54**, 409–415.

White, N.M. (1986) Control of sensorimotor function by dopaminergic nigrostriatal neurons: influence on eating and drinking. *Neuroscience and Biobehavioral Reviews* **10**, 15–36.

Wise, R.A. and Schwartz, H.V. (1981) Pimozide attenuates acquisition of lever pressing for food in rats. *Pharmacology Biochemistry and Behavior* **15**, 655–656.

Wise, R.A., Spindler, J., de Wit, H. and Gerber, G.J. (1978) Neuroleptic-induced 'Anhedonia' in rats: pimozide blocks reward quality of food. *Science* **201**, 262–264.

Woodruff, G. and Williams, D.R. (1976) The associative relation underlying autoshaping in the pigeon. *Journal of the Experimental Analysis of Behavior* **16**, 1–13.

Woodworth, R.S. (1918) *Dynamic Psychology*. New York: Columbia University Press.

9

Limbic–Striatal Interactions in Reward-Related Processes: Modulation by the Dopaminergic System

M. CADOR[1], T.W. ROBBINS[2], B.J. EVERITT[3],
H. SIMON[1], M. LE MOAL[1] AND L. STINUS[1]

[1]Psychobiologie des Comportements Adaptatifs, INSERM U. 259,
Université de Bordeaux II, Domaine de Carreire, rue Camille Saint-Saëns,
33077 Bordeaux Cedex, France; [2]Department of Experimental Psychology;
and [3]Department of Anatomy, University of Cambridge, Downing Street,
Cambridge CB2 3EB, UK

INTRODUCTION

Animals are in constant dynamic interaction with their internal as well as external environment. Any modification of either of these environments leads to the emergence of behavior which restores homeostasis and is expressed through specific acts or actions. As stated by Bolles (1975): 'Actions or acts are the way by which the organism demonstrates interest in the environment, searches out the goal for its current needs and initiates specific motor acts once the goal has been found'. Acts or action can vary in strength, speed or direction; they depend on sensory integration and level of motivation which give the activation and choice of direction to control behavior. The level of motivation can be influenced by internal events. For example, deprivation induces an internal drive state which leads animals to seek for specific goal-objects. However, it is clear that not all behaviors are only the consequence of homeostatic imbalance. Indeed, motivated behaviors can also be initiated by external stimuli; for instance, objects which have gained motivational significance by being associated with a primary reward

The Mesolimbic Dopamine System: From Motivation to Action.
Edited by P. Willner and J. Scheel-Krüger

© 1991 John Wiley & Sons Ltd

or a primary goal-object (Bolles, 1975) may create what has been called an incentive–motivational state (Bindra, 1969).

The computation of information leading to this 'central motive state' as defined by Bindra occurs principally in a set of structures which can be neuroanatomically and functionally differentiated from the brain circuits which compute sensorial inputs and outputs. These two neural circuits, besides being different in the nature of the information they transfer, can also be differentiated as to the specific way they compute this information. Somatosensorial inputs and outputs are more generally computed in a serial way, layer by layer, cortex by cortex, according to the sensory modality of the inputs, whereas the second circuit is composed of structures which are all interconnected and function in an interdependent manner. The second circuit is composed of classically recognized limbic structures such as the amygdala, the septum, the hippocampus, and the mediofrontal cortex, and motor-related structures such as the ventral striatum, which compute respectively the affective, emotional, motivational aspects of behavior, and the initiation of action. These structures must function harmoniously to allow the coordination of behavioral outputs. It has been proposed that this coordinated and interdependent functioning is orchestrated by widely diverging systems, such as the dopamine (DA) system, which innervate each of these structures, and ensure both the optimal functioning of the structure innervated and the facilitation of the transfer of information from one structure to another (Simon and Le Moal, 1984; Louilot et al., 1987; 1989). In Figure 1 the projections of the DA system, the cell bodies of which are located in the mesencephalic reticular formation at the level of the ventromedial mesencephalon, within the ventral tegmental area (VTA) (Dahlström and Fuxe, 1964) are schematically represented. These DA neurons innervate different structures such as the nucleus accumbens, olfactory tubercle, anteromedial part of the striatum, septum, amygdala, hippocampus and different cortical regions (Lindvall and Björklund, 1974; Lindvall et al., 1974; Fuxe et al., 1974; Lindvall, 1975; Simon et al., 1976; Fallon and Moore, 1978a, b; Emson and Koob, 1978; Fallon et al., 1978; Lindvall and Steveni, 1978; Simon et al., 1979; Swanson, 1982; Berger et al., 1985; Descarries et al., 1987; see Björklund and Lindvall, 1984 for a review).

This coordinating role of the mesolimbic DA system appears to be particularly crucial at the level of the ventral striatum, since this has been demonstrated to be a key structure in the translation of motivated states into acts. Indeed, on the basis of anatomical and electrophysiological data, Mogenson and colleagues (1982) proposed that the ventral striatum may represent a functional interface between the limbic system and the motor system. Several data support this hypothesis. Anatomical studies using retrograde and anterograde tracers revealed that the nucleus accumbens

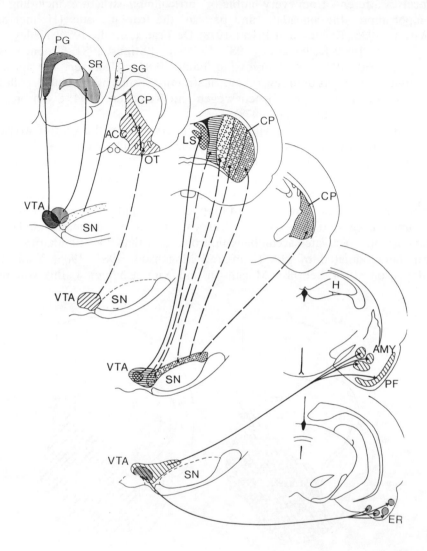

Figure 1. Schematic representation of the different dopaminergic structures innervated by DA cells located in the ventral mesencephalon. Since there is a continuum between the DA cells of the VTA and the SN, both mesolimbic and mesostriatal systems are represented. ACC, nc. accumbens; AMY, amygdala; CP, nc. caudatus-putamen; ER, entorhinal cortex; H, hippocampus; LS, lateral septal nucleus; OT, olfactory tubercle; PF, piriform cortex; PG, pregenual cortex; SG, supragenual cortex; SN, substantia nigra; SR, suprarhinal cortex; VTA, ventral tegmental area (A10). (Modified with permission from Björklund and Lindvall, 1984)

receives afferents from every limbic or corticolimbic structure, including the hippocampus, the amygdala, and parts of the frontal cortex (Heimer and Wilson, 1975; Krettek and Price, 1978; De France et al., 1980; Kelley and Domesick, 1982; Kelley et al., 1982; Kelley and Stinus, 1984; Groenewegen et al., 1980, 1987; McGeorge and Faull, 1989). However, the nucleus accumbens projects onto several motor structures, such as the globus pallidus and the substantia nigra (Groenewegen and Russchen, 1964; Swanson and Cowan, 1975; Nauta et al., 1978).

A functional interaction with the DA innervation of the ventral striatum is supported by the striking overlap schematically represented in Figure 2 between the limbic afferents from the amygdala, the hippocampus and the DA terminals arising in the VTA. The functional nature of these interactions has been addressed mainly by means of electrophysiological studies concerned with the influence of amygdala and hippocampal inputs on activity of nucleus accumbens cells. It appears that electrical stimulation of the amygdala and hippocampus activates accumbens neurons, and that this stimulatory effect can be modulated by DA (Yim and Mogenson, 1982, 1986; Yang and Mogenson, 1984; see also Mogenson and Yim, Chapter 4, this volume).

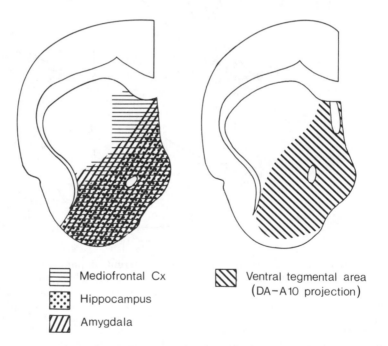

Mediofrontal Cx

Hippocampus

Amygdala

Ventral tegmental area
(DA–A10 projection)

Figure 2. Schematic drawing of the convergence of inputs at the level of the ventral striatum from three considered limbic areas: the mediofrontal cortex, the hippocampus and the amygdala. (Modified from Kelley and Stinus, 1984)

However, these studies are indirect and did not address specifically the implications of limbic–striatal interactions and their modulation by the DA system in adaptive behaviors.

In the present chapter, we present some data which have been proposed to enlighten the two major roles of the DA system: first, the permissive role of the DA system at the level of the structures innervated; and second, the facilitatory or gain-amplifying action that DA appears to play in the transfer of information from one integrative structure to another.

BEHAVIORAL APPROACH TO THE PHYSIOLOGY OF THE MESOCORTICOLIMBIC DA SYSTEM: A PERMISSIVE ROLE

The role of the mesolimbic DA system has been extensively studied in our laboratory. For years, Le Moal, Simon and Stinus studied systematically the effect of selective lesions of the DA cell bodies and terminals on adaptive behavior. One of the best examples of the non-specific function of the DA system is a study by Kelley and Stinus (1985) on hoarding behavior. Hoarding is quite a complex behavior, frequently observed in rodents, which induces animals in the presence of a large amount of food to collect and hoard this food in a particular place, such as the home cage, instead of eating the food at once. As shown in Table 1, specific lesions of the DA cell bodies in the VTA completely disrupt this behavior. Lesioned animals failed to hoard any pellets, but rather ate the pellet in a completely disorganized manner in the open field. Replacement treatment with L-DOPA (an indirect dopaminergic agonist) (given orally) completely restored this behavior in such a way that lesioned animals behaved like controls and hoarded the whole amount of pellets (see Table 1).

Thus, the simple reinstatement of a certain level of DA transmission is

Table 1. Effect of 6-OHDA lesion of DA cell bodies in the VTA on hoarding behavior and recovery of the deficit following peripheral administration of L-DOPA. Sixty pellets were disposed in an open field, and food-deprived animals were allowed to hoard for 90 minutes. The two groups of animals were not different regarding the amount of food intake during a 24-hour period. (Modified with permission from Kelley and Stinus, 1985)

Group	Pellets hoarded	Food intake over 24-hour period (g)
Sham	52.0 ± 6.0	23.9 ± 0.7
VTA lesion	3.0 ± 2*	26.2 ± 2.0
VTA lesion + L-DOPA	59.0 ± 2.0	—

*$P < 0.001$ compared to control group.

sufficient to permit quite complex behavior to occur, and suggests that DA does not transmit specific messages but has only a permissive action on the integrative message computed by the structure innervated. Such recovery of the deficit induced by DA lesion has been obtained by several types of treatment which have in common the ability to increase the availability of DA at the synapse. For instance, stimulation of DA grafts in the nucleus accumbens by d-amphetamine, after destruction of the DA terminals at this level, has been shown to reinstate normal hoarding behavior (Herman et al., 1986). Increasing arousal, which is accompanied by increased DA transmission, may also provide a way to recover some of the deficits induced by DA lesions. Thus, selective depletion of septal DA impaired performance in both the Y and the radial mazes. However, the deficit disappeared when the lesioned animals were deprived of food (Taghzouti et al., 1986). Studies conducted by H. Simon and his colleagues are in favor of this non-specific role of the DA system. They studied the effect of 6-hydroxydopamine (6-OHDA) lesions of the DA terminals in the different areas innervated, and found that DA lesions induce deficits of the same nature as those induced by imbalance of the activity of the structure itself. They found, for example, that 6-OHDA lesions of the prefrontal cortex in the rat induce the same deficit in delayed alternation (Simon et al., 1980; Simon, 1981) as has been reported after 6-OHDA lesion or damage to the whole structure itself in monkeys (Brozoski et al., 1979). 6-OHDA lesions of septal DA terminals increased the frustrative energizing effect on behavior induced by omission of an expected reward (Taghzouti et al., 1985a). These results correlate well with the increased responding and emotional behavior observed after electrolytic lesion of the septum (Isaacson, 1982).

Finally, at the level of the nucleus accumbens several types of deficit have been observed after DA lesions, some of which can be classified as limbic because they have been typically seen after lesions of limbic structures, whereas others are classified as motor deficits. A limbic deficit has been shown in the spatial discrimination and reversal test (Taghzouti et al., 1985b). During this test, food-deprived animals had to learn to eat always in the same arm of a T-maze. The criterion for the spatial discrimination was a correct response on 5 consecutive days. Immediately after acquisition, the food was transferred to the opposite arm of the T-maze, and training was continued to the same learning criterion. This procedure was repeated for 5 days. The results showed that the experimental animals were impaired during the first 3 days of spatial discrimination but not during the last 2 days (Figure 3, left). During the reversal situation, control animals were very quick to change from one arm to the other. On the contrary, animals with lesions in the nucleus accumbens had difficulty in choosing the arm opposite to the one previously rewarded and persevered in the previously baited arm (Figure 3, right). This apparent difficulty in switching their behavior has been reported after lesions of other limbic structures such as the septohippocampal system.

A motor-related deficit after 6-OHDA lesion of the nucleus accumbens has also been reported (Taghzouti et al., 1985c). Performance of sham or 6-OHDA nucleus accumbens-lesioned animals was studied in a series of behavioral tasks such as an open field, a four-hole box, and a two-compartment exploration test. In each of these tasks, the latency to initiate a behavioral response, i.e. a locomotor response in the open field, a visit to a hole in the hole box, or a visit to the second chamber in the two-compartment box test was measured. The lesioned animals in all four tasks showed an increased latency to initiate these behavioral responses (Table 2).

Thus, from these experiments it appears that both limbic and motor deficits can be clearly seen after lesion of the DA terminals in the nucleus accumbens. The anatomical position of the nucleus accumbens described previously may explain the behavioral deficits observed after 6-OHDA lesions. The limbic deficit could then be explained by an interruption of the transfer of limbic information, whereas the motor deficit could be explained by an absence of modulation of the accumbens neural outputs towards the motor structures.

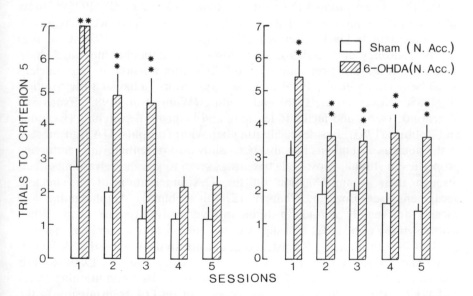

Figure 3. Effect of 6-OHDA lesion at the level of the nucleus accumbens in a spatial discrimination test (left) and its reversal (right) in a T-maze. Means number of trials + SEM to achieve criterion of five correct responses during the 5 days of test. **$P < 0.01$, Student t-test. (Modified from Taghzouti et al., 1986)

Table 2. Effects of 6-OHDA lesion of DA terminals in the nucleus accumbens on latency (s) to induce behavioral response in a hole box (latency of the first visit to a hole), in an open field (latency for the first move), and a two-compartment field (latency of the first visit to the second compartment)

Group	Behavioral situations		
	Open field (s)	4-hole box (s)	Two-compartment field (s)
Sham	7 ± 2	7 ± 2	20 ± 3
6-OHDA	32 ± 3*	28 ± 3*	100 ± 10*

*$P < 0.05$ compared to control group.

These results agree with the concept of the nucleus accumbens as an interface between limbic and motor systems, which, through its DA innervation, gates the effect of motivational influences on response outputs. If lesioning the DA system at this level induces limbic and motor deficits, increasing DA function in this area may energize or amplify limbic and motor influences on behavior. Indeed, it is clear that DA agonists, such as amphetamine, exert their psychomotor stimulant effects through their action on the DA innervation of the ventral striatum (Kelly et al., 1975). Direct intra-accumbens injections of d-amphetamine or DA produce increases in locomotor activity (Jackson et al., 1975; Pijnenburg et al., 1976; Costall et al., 1984; Kelley et al., 1988). Low doses of d-amphetamine which have been shown to act predominantly on DA transmission in the nucleus accumbens (Kelly et al., 1975) increase exploratory behavior (Taghzouti et al., 1985c; Kelley et al., 1986) and feeding (Winn et al., 1982; Evans and Vaccarino, 1986), and facilitate learning and behavioral switching (Evenden and Robbins, 1983). Besides facilitating behavioral outputs, DA transmission in the nucleus accumbens has also been shown to potentiate the reinforcing properties of stimuli. Most addictive drugs seem to possess rewarding effects through their common action on the DA innervation of the nucleus accumbens (see Bozarth, Chapter 12, this volume). Amphetamine and cocaine are readily self-administered intravenously (Roberts et al., 1980; Roberts and Koob, 1982) and directly into the nucleus accumbens (Hoebel et al., 1983); both self-administrations disappeared after 6-OHDA lesions of the nucleus accumbens (Lyness et al., 1979; Roberts et al., 1980; Roberts and Koob, 1982). D-amphetamine also supports place conditioning (Carr and White, 1983), which is likewise dependent on DA transmission in the nucleus accumbens (Spyraki et al., 1982). Furthermore, a role for DA in incentive motivation has also been demonstrated since it has been shown that d-amphetamine increases the control over behavior exerted by conditioned reinforcers (previously neutral stimuli which come to control behavior by prior association with primary reinforcers such as food or water) (Hill, 1970; Robbins, 1975, 1978; Robbins and Koob, 1978; Beninger et al., 1981; Robbins et al., 1983). More recently, the specific implication of DA transmission in the ventral striatum in incentive motivation has been demonstrated by Taylor and Robbins (1984), so raising the problem of limbic influences on DA-dependent processes in the ventral striatum.

DOPAMINE FACILITATORY ROLE OF LIMBIC–STRIATAL INTERACTIONS IN CONDITIONED REINFORCEMENT PARADIGMS

A stringent criterion for designating a stimulus as a conditioned reinforcer is the capacity to reinforce the acquisition of a new response in the absence of the primary reward. In the study of Taylor and Robbins (1984) thirsty animals were first trained to drink from a dipper. Then, during a conditioning phase (14 days with one session per day), these animals were trained to associate a dipper noise compound stimulus (conditioned stimulus or CS) with the delivery of water (unconditioned stimulus or US) by means of sessions of 30 presentations of the CS followed by the US, at random time intervals. During a testing phase in which water was no longer presented, the capacity of the CS to be a reinforcer by itself was tested by measuring the acquisition of a new instrumental response controlled by the CS alone. Two levers were introduced in the cage. Pressing one of these levers (the CR, conditioned response, lever) elicited the delivery of the CS (the light dipper noise compound stimulus); pressing the other lever (the NCR, non-conditioned response, lever) did not elicit anything.

Control animals responded significantly more on the CR lever than on the NCR lever. However, intra-accumbens d-amphetamine selectively enhanced responding on the lever providing the compound stimulus (CR lever), whereas no increased responding was observed on a control lever (NCR lever) (see Figure 4, left).

This effect has been shown to be behaviorally and neurochemically specific, since stimulation of CR lever responding failed to occur if the CS had been only randomly correlated with water (and was therefore unpredictive of it) (Taylor and Robbins, 1984), and intra-caudate injections, compared to intra-accumbens injections, produced more variable responses (Taylor and Robbins, 1986). Furthermore, this effect of d-amphetamine is biochemically specific and depends upon the integrity of the DA innervation of the ventral striatum since 6-OHDA lesion at this level completely abolishes the potentiating effect of d-amphetamine (Taylor and Robbins, 1984) but a lesion of the noradrenergic system had no effect (Cador et al., unpublished results). These results suggest, in accordance with previous suggestions, that

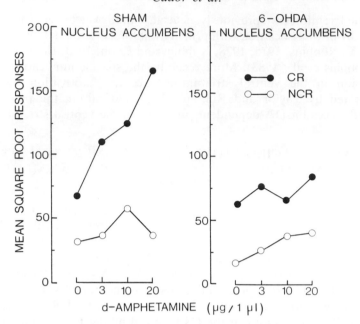

Figure 4. Dose-related responding on a lever providing a conditioned reinforcer (CR) and on a control lever (NCR), following d-amphetamine (3, 10, 20 µg/µl) or saline infusion into the nucleus accumbens, in sham- or 6-OHDA-lesioned animals at the level of the nucleus accumbens. (Modified from Taylor and Robbins, 1984)

increasing DA transmission at the level of the ventral striatum facilitates and amplifies behavior observed in normal conditions. However, although the facilitatory effect of d-amphetamine on CR was prevented by ventral striatal DA depletion, it is important to note that the behavioral control exerted by CR in the absence of the drug (after saline infusion) is intact (Figure 4, right). This suggests that ventral striatal DA may mediate the amphetamine-induced potentiation of behavior dictated by environmental contingencies, while implicating other, possibly limbic, mechanisms in the process by which stimuli act as conditioned reinforcers under normal circumstances.

Several lines of evidence suggest a particular role of the amygdaloid input in mediating associative influences, such as those involved in conditioned reinforcement, which could control the outputs of the ventral striatum. Firstly, the amygdala has long been associated with associative aspects of emotions, such as the formation of stimulus–reward associations (Weiskrantz, 1956; Jones and Mishkin, 1972; Mishkin, 1978; Spiegler and Mishkin, 1981; Cormier, 1981), and more specifically in conditioned reinforcement (Gaffan and Harrison, 1987). Second, as already noted, there is a complete overlap between afferents from the basolateral nucleus of the amygdala and the DA afferents from the ventral tegmentum (Krettek and Price, 1978; Kelley et al., 1982; Phillipson and Griffiths, 1985; Groenewegen et al., 1987), and some functional aspects of this interaction have been evidenced (Mogenson et al., 1982).

We have examined how the effects on behavior exerted by conditioned reinforcers or secondary reinforcers may be mediated through the amygdala via DA-dependent functions in the ventral striatum (Cador et al., 1989; Everitt et al., 1989a). We used two different types of experiment in parallel to study the behavioral consequences of amygdala–ventral striatum interactions; both experiments strongly implicate stimulus–reward associations. In a first study, we used the same protocol as that used by Taylor and Robbins (1984), in which we measured the acquisition of a new instrumental response to obtain a conditioned reinforcer, a stimulus which was previously paired with primary reward. In a second experiment, a second-order schedule of sexual reinforcement was used. Male rats were trained to respond under a fixed-interval schedule to obtain a receptive female. Responding during the interval was maintained by making contingent on each 10 consecutive lever presses the presentation of a CS, which was paired with the presentation of the female at the end of the session. The difference between the two protocols is that the strength of the CS–US association is tested in two different situations. The first experiment used an extinction situation, i.e. the US (the primary reward) is not presented any more and the strength of the association decreases with the repetition of the test session. In the second situation the primary reward is always presented at the end of the session and responding elicited by this type of schedule can be maintained for months and remain stable.

In the two experiments, the rats were trained first under the different schedules. Surgical manipulations were then performed. All animals received cannula implantation aimed at the nucleus accumbens to receive later intra-accumbens infusions of d-amphetamine. At the time of surgery, experimental groups also received excitotoxic lesion of the basolateral part of the amygdala using N-methyl-D-aspartate (NMDA), whereas control groups received injections of vehicle (for detailed procedure and description of the extent of the lesions, see Cador et al., 1989).

Effects of Lesion of the Amygdala on the Acquisition of Responding with Conditioned Reinforcement and its Potentiation by d-Amphetamine

In the first experiment, which used the same experimental protocol as in Taylor and Robbins' (1984) study (see above for details), surgical manipulations were performed after the training phase and before the testing phase. During four consecutive test sessions, each animal was assigned to receive four counterbalanced injections into the nucleus accumbens, including three doses of d-amphetamine (3, 10, 30 μg/μl in 1 μl saline) and saline (1 μl).

Postoperatively, but prior to any pharmacological manipulations, additional training sessions were given to measure the effects of amygdala lesions on training performance. The percentage of time pushing the panel during the CS and NCS periods was similar for the sham and NMDA-lesioned animals, and was, respectively, 92 per cent (CS), 26 per cent (NCS), and 93 per cent (CS) and 23 per cent (NCS). Figure 5 shows the dose-related responses made on the CR and NCR levers during the testing phases when the two levers were introduced into the chambers, but water was no longer made available.

Amygdala-lesioned animals showed a selective reduction in the number of responses made on the CR lever, which was independent of the action of d-amphetamine into the nucleus accumbens (the two curves being parallel). Several control experiments addressed the behavioral specificity of the deficit observed, and showed that experimental animals were neither hyperdipsic or hypodipsic nor hyperactive or hypoactive, either spontaneously or after peripheral injection of d-amphetamine (Table 3).

Furthermore, the deficits could not be the result of differences in extinction processes since no deficit was observed in responding to the CS in a control experiment in which the unconditioned reinforcer (water delivery) was extinguished (Cador et al., 1989). Similarly, a deficit in motor function

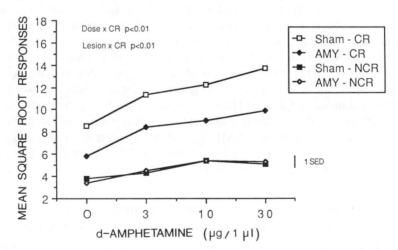

Figure 5. Effect of d-amphetamine (3, 10, 30 μg/μl) or saline infused into the nucleus accumbens in sham-lesioned animals (Sham) or excitotoxic-lesioned animals in the basolateral part of the amygdala (AMY), on responding for conditioned reinforcer. (Modified from Cador et al., 1989)

Table 3. Effect of excitotoxic lesion of the basolateral part of the amygdala on drinking behavior and on intra-accumbens saline- and amphetamine-induced locomotor activity

Group	Water consumption (ml)*	Spontaneous motor activity†	Amphetamine-induced locomotor activity†
Sham	5.37	42.6	90.6
AMY	5.6	41.2	98.8

*The amount of water consumed was measured for 15 minutes after 18 hours of water deprivation.
†Locomotor activity was measured in activity cages for 2 hours immediately after either intra-accumbens saline (1 µl) or amphetamine (10 µg/µl) infusions.

could not explain the deficit reported above since no differences between the two groups were observed in the acquisition of a new motor task such as pressing a lever under a fixed or variable schedule of reinforcement of water presentation (Cador et al., 1989). These results seem to indicate that amygdala lesions attenuate the selective difference in responding between the CR lever and the NCR lever observed in control animals, without impairing the effect of intra-accumbens amphetamine. Amygdala lesions appear to affect primarily mechanisms which determine the choice (sampling) between the CR lever and the NCR lever, whereas facilitation of DA transmission multiplies the behavioral expression of this choice by a constant factor. Accordingly, in the Taylor and Robbins experiments, DA depletion in the ventral striatum prevents the 'gain amplifying' effect of intra-accumbens d-amphetamine without altering the choice between the two levers. Thus, amygdala lesions seem to impair specifically the processing of the rewarding properties of the CS but not its discriminative properties, since in retention of the training phase, amygdala-lesioned animals directed their behavior towards the panel as often as controls (Cador et al., 1989). These experiments lead to the conclusion that an excitotoxic lesion of the amygdala reduces the strength of effect of CS-reward associations on behavior without affecting the discriminative properties of the CS, drinking, or spontaneous or amphetamine-induced locomotor activity. These results are consistent with the hypothesis that the basal and lateral parts of the amygdala are involved in mediating the effects of conditioned or secondary reinforcement on behavior.

Interaction between the Amygdala and the Ventral Striatum using a Second-Order Schedule with Sexual Reinforcement

In the second experiment, the same hypothesis as before was tested using a second-order schedule with sexual reinforcement.

Male rats were placed in an operant chamber above which a trapdoor box containing a receptive female was situated; the female was presented to the male by falling down into the operant chamber. Male rats were trained to press a lever to obtain the female; the CS+ was a light situated above the lever. A fixed ratio (FR) second-order schedule was first implemented, of the type FRx(FRy:S): for every y responses on the lever, the CS+ was presented and after x such ratios were completed, the primary reinforcer (the female) was presented to the male automatically via the trapdoor. After several sessions of this schedule, a fixed interval-fixed ratio was introduced such that the first ratio of 10 responses performed on the lever after a fixed interval of 15 minutes elicited the presentation of the female. The male was then allowed to copulate with the female and the first ejaculation terminated the session. Responding on the lever during the interval was maintained by the presentation of the light stimulus (the CS+) which had been previously paired with the primary reward. This conditioned stimulus is formally equivalent to a conditioned reinforcer, and it has been shown to be very important for the maintenance of the behavior (Everitt et al., 1987). At the beginning of the interval (the first 5 minutes) the animals hardly responded. Their response rate then increased gradually until 15 minutes, at which time the female was presented. Lever press rate as well as the unconditioned behavior after the female was delivered were recorded. Once operant behavior was stable, surgical manipulations were performed.

As shown in Table 4, in a first postoperative session, both groups showed a decrease in responding. In a second postoperative session, this deficit was no longer apparent in the control group, whereas amygdala-lesioned animals still showed a marked reduction in lever pressing which lasted across the whole experiment. D-amphetamine administration in the ventral striatum dose-dependently allowed a recovery of this deficit in amygdala-lesioned animals such that their level of responding no longer differed from the

Table 4. Effect of excitotoxic lesion of the basolateral part of the amygdala on responding in a second-order schedule for sexual reinforcement during a 15-minute session. Preoperative responding from the to-be-lesioned (AMY) and the to-be-sham-operated (Sham) groups; postoperative 1 and postoperative 2, first and second postoperative sessions. Values are means ± SEM

	Preoperative	Postoperative 1	Postoperative 2
Sham	159 ± 8	113 ± 14*	130 ± 13
AMY	175 ± 14	67 ± 14*	86 ± 13*

*$P < 0.05$ significantly different from respective preoperative session.

controls (Figure 6). No difference was observed in unconditioned sexual behavior between the two groups of animals, either in the latency to copulate or to ejaculate (Everitt et al., 1989a).

These results indicate that amygdala-lesioned animals exhibited less responding for conditioned reinforcers whereas their behavior in the presence of the primary reward was intact. To test the extent to which their behavior was dependent on the presentation of the conditioned reinforcer we recorded the level of responding of the two groups in several consecutive sessions in which the CR was not presented. Results are presented in Figure 7 and show that the level of responding in controls dramatically declined, demonstrating the importance of the presentation of the CR in the maintenance of instrumental behavior. In contrast, amygdala-lesioned animals showed no change at all in their levels of responding after removal of the CR, suggesting that their behavior is under relatively weak control by the presentation of the CR.

We then tested to determine whether this deficit was reversed by injecting amphetamine into the nucleus accumbens. Amphetamine (1 μg/μl) or saline was injected into the nucleus accumbens, either in the presence or absence of the conditioned reinforcer. Results presented in Figure 8 show clearly that when the CR is removed, amphetamine infused into the ventral striatum induced a very small increase in responding in both groups compared to the increase observed when the CR is presented. These results indicated once

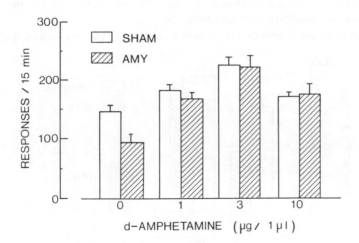

Figure 6. Effect of intra-accumbens d-amphetamine infusion (1, 3, 10 μg/μl) or saline, in sham-operated or excitotoxic-lesioned animals at the level of the basolateral amygdala, upon instrumental responding for sexual reinforcement under a second-order schedule of reinforcement. Means ± SEM. (Modified from Everitt et al., 1989a)

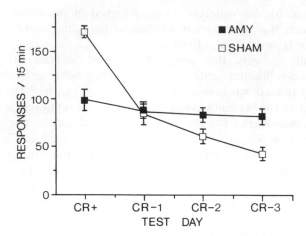

Figure 7. Effects upon instrumental responding of omitting the presentation of the CR during sessions in sham-operated (Sham) and amygdala-lesioned (AMY) rats. CR+, Last session in which CR was presented; CR-1, CR-2, CR-3, three consecutive sessions in which the presentation of the CR was omitted. The estrous female was still earned on completion of the first ratio after the 15-minute fixed interval had elapsed. Means ± SEM. (Reproduced with permission from Everitt et al., 1989)

more that the presence of the CR is crucial for the potentiation of responding induced by d-amphetamine injection into the nucleus accumbens. However, much of the difference between the groups was removed by this intra-accumbens administration of amphetamine.

In summary, these results are in accordance with the previous experiment

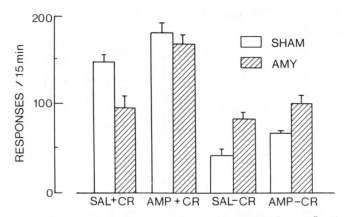

Figure 8. Effects upon instrumental responding of d-amphetamine (AMP, 1 µg/1 µl) or saline (SAL, 1 µl) infused bilaterally into the ventral striatum of rats, during sessions in which CR was (+CR) or was not (−CR) presented. Means ± SEM. (Modified from Everitt et al., 1989a)

in that responding under the second-order schedule maintained by the CR was markedly suppressed following axon sparing-excitotoxic amino acid lesions of the amygdala. Furthermore, the amygdala appears to interact functionally with DA-dependent processes in the ventral striatum since increasing DA transmission at this level restored normal behavior in amygdala-lesioned animals. As previously, there was no significant effect on unconditioned behavior elicited by primary reward. Again, the impairment induced by amygdala lesion was incomplete. Nevertheless, it is clear that the presentation of the CR is crucial for maintaining responding in control animals, and to allow the expression of the potentiating effect of intra-accumbens amphetamine. In contrast, amygdala-lesioned animals appear to rely on components other than the CR for the observed residual level of responding. One of these may be the stimulus associated with the presence of the female in the trapbox such as odor (which is intrinsically associated, therefore, with the primary reward). Gaffan and Harrison (1987) were able to dissociate in the monkey a specific effect of amygdala lesion on stimulus–reward association rather than on the association between intrinsic incentive stimuli associated with the primary reward (such as smell, taste or sight).

DISCUSSION

These experiments have established a definite interaction between the amygdala and DA-dependent processes in the ventral striatum for the effectiveness of CR in controlling behavior. Clearly, it appears that a lesion of the amygdala attenuates the control exerted by such CR on behavior. Increasing DA transmission at the level of the nucleus accumbens enabled some recovery from the deficit produced by amygdala lesions. It seems that the efficacy of the recovery is proportional to the residual effect left after amygdala lesion. We could hypothesize that if no difference were left between the two levers, amelioration of the deficit would not have been evidenced following d-amphetamine. It is difficult to explain the residual effect observed after amygdala lesion in both experiments. One explanation could be that the lesions were not total, but no obvious correlation was observed between the extent of amygdala damage and the size of the deficit. Alternatively, additional structures such as the hippocampus or the frontal cortex, which are both limbic structures and project onto the ventral striatum, may contribute to conditioned reinforcement (Krettek and Price, 1978; Carter and Pycock, 1980; Kelley et al., 1982). This is particularly relevant since it has previously been demonstrated in monkeys that combined but not separate lesions of the hippocampus and the amygdala are necessary to induce a global anterograde amnesia (Mishkin, 1978).

The interaction between amygdala- and DA-dependent processes in the ventral striatum demonstrated here appears to be behaviorally specific. In both experiments, amygdala lesions appear to leave intact unconditioned behavior maintained by the primary reward (water consumption or sexual behavior), but rather showed a marked effect when conditioned or secondary reinforcers controlled the behavior. Furthermore, a general motor impairment cannot explain the results obtained here, since amygdala-lesioned animals performed adequately in new motor tasks and no gross difference between the two groups in amphetamine-induced hyperactivity was evidenced. Moreover, in the second experiment an increase in responding after removal of the CR would have been expected if a non-specific effect of amphetamine was the cause of the reversal of the deficit. In fact, these results demonstrate that d-amphetamine does not always induce non-specific general increases in locomotor activity, but rather that this hyperactivity can be influenced by more selective interaction with contingencies of the environment. The specific effect of the lesions of the basolateral part of the amygdala on conditioned reinforcers as distinct from its discriminative properties is particularly interesting. Indeed, there are several ways through which a representation of the CS may come to control behavior. The CS may act as a CR as a result of a prior stimulus–reward association, which then motivates learning of a new response by evoking a mental representation of the reward, even in the absence of the latter. Alternatively, a CS may act as a pure discriminative stimulus to 'set the occasion' (Skinner, 1938) to perform an instrumental response (such as pushing the panel) via a prior stimulus–response association. These considerations suggest that different representations of the CS may be mediated through different neuronal mechanisms. The present findings, showing that amygdala-lesioned animals responded identically to controls in pushing the panel appropriately (when the CS was presented) but were none the less impaired when required to perform a new response to obtain the CS, indicate a specific impairment of the effectiveness of the CS in controlling behavior via stimulus–reward associations. These findings have been extended recently by a study in which an amygdala lesion has been shown to produce a reduction in food-induced place preference which can be considered as another expression of conditioned reinforcement (Everitt et al., 1989b). Recent specific studies with DA agonists and antagonists provided evidence for a more specific implication of the D1 rather than the D2 receptor. For example, in the behavioral paradigm used here, a D1 agonist injected into the nucleus accumbens more effectively increased responding on the CR lever than a D2 agonist, and the D1 antagonist specifically reduced responding for the CR lever whereas the D1 antagonist induced a non-specific reduction in behavioral output (Wolterink et al., 1989).

Amygdala–Ventral Striatum Interaction

Functional interactions between the amygdala and the ventral striatum have been demonstrated previously. Most often, manipulation of the amygdala has been shown to induce changes in DA transmission in the nucleus accumbens. Kindling of the amygdala has been shown to alter DA transmission in the nucleus accumbens (Gee et al., 1979; Post et al., 1981; Csernansky et al., 1985; Ehlers and Koob, 1985). More recently, Yim and Mogenson (1989) demonstrated a functional behavioral interaction between amygdala and the DA innervation of the ventral striatum. They showed that intra-amygdala infusion of NMDA dose-dependently suppressed locomotor activity in a novel environment, and that DA infusions in the nucleus accumbens, at a dose which did not by itself increase locomotor activity, counteracted this inhibition. They concluded that there was a neuromodulatory role of DA at the level of non-DA presynaptic inputs in the nucleus accumbens (see Mogenson and Yim, Chapter 4, this volume). *In vivo* voltammetric studies clarified these interactions between the amygdala and the ventral striatum. Blockade of DA transmission in the amygdala increased the DOPAC signal in the nucleus accumbens (Louilot et al., 1985). In accord with these results, 6-OHDA lesions of the amygdala increased DA turnover in the ventral striatum and increased the locomotor response to a systemic injection of d-amphetamine (Simon et al., 1988) and amphetamine self-administration (Deminière et al., 1988) which depend principally on DA transmission in the nucleus accumbens (see Piazza et al., Chapter 18, this volume).

Amplification and Facilitatory Role of DA

More generally these results indicate that amygdala- and DA-dependent processes in the ventral striatum appear jointly to determine, respectively, response choice and the 'gain-amplifying' effect of enhanced activation on this choice. This interpretation is consistent with previous results using the same behavioral model as used here and showing that DA lesions in the nucleus accumbens prevent the amphetamine-induced potentiation of responding for conditioned reinforcement while leaving intact the basal choice between the CR and NCR levers (Taylor and Robbins, 1984). Similarly, it has been shown that moderate doses of DA antagonists impaired speed of responding without altering response choice (Evenden and Robbins, 1983; Tombaugh et al., 1983; Bowers et al., 1985). These results agree with the conclusions of Salamone following a study on the effect of pimozide on activational versus directional aspects of motivated behaviors. He concluded that: 'Low doses of DA antagonists selectively impair the quantitative features of behavior that are characteristic of response activation, but leave intact the ability to direct behavior in relation to an appetitive or aversive stimulus and to select an appropriate approach or avoidance behavior' (Salamone, 1988).

An even more elaborate distinction related to the role of mesolimbic DA in behavior has been proposed. Based on the consideration that behavior can be divided into preparatory versus consummatory phases, several authors have shown that impairment of DA transmission affects preparatory rather than consummatory components of behavior (see Phillips et al., Chapter 8, this volume). For example, hoarding behavior and food-associated locomotor activity are attenuated by 6-OHDA lesions of the nucleus accumbens without altering quantitatively feeding behavior (Koob et al., 1978; Kelley and Stinus, 1985). Entry into a feeding niche in anticipation of the delivery of a signalled meal is attenuated by pimozide, but consummatory behavior as soon as the food is delivered is left intact (Blackburn et al., 1987). Female rats bearing 6-OHDA lesions of the ventral striatum show a specific loss of proceptive behavior in the presence of the male but exhibit normal lordotic behavior in response to male mounting attempts (Robbins and Everitt, 1982).

The present data are consistent with the notion that the ventral striatum represents a limbic–motor interface which gates the effects of acquired motivational influences on response outputs. Mogenson and co-workers principally placed their emphasis on the motor aspect and, following a series of functional anatomical experiments, proposed a cascade of neuronal events leading to the instrumental performance of behavior. To summarize their findings, they demonstrated the importance in locomotor activity of the ventral striatal projection to the ventral pallidum, and then from the ventral pallidum to the mesencephalic locomotor region (Jones and Mogenson, 1980; Mogenson and Nielsen, 1983, 1984a, b) through a series of inhibitory GABAergic neurons. Whereas it is clear that the mesencephalic locomotor region is important in the generation of motor sequences, other pallidal projections such as those to the frontal cortex via the mediodorsal thalamus might play an important role in more complex control of temporally organized sequential motor outputs. This is specifically relevant when the question of the role of limbic–motor interactions in more cognitive processes such as those described in the above experiments is addressed. These processes are likely to be mediated by much more complex neural interactions than those subserved by direct projections towards the mesencephalic locomotor region.

In summary, the results reported here try to specify the role of DA transmission, particularly at the level of the ventral striatum. The results reviewed support the idea that association formed at the level of the limbic system may be modulated by DA activity at the level of the ventral striatum to facilitate behavioral outputs, including instrumental responding. The DA system is proposed to subserve an activational or facilitatory influence on behavior, whereas limbic structures such as the amygdala help to mediate the directional component of the behavioral outputs.

REFERENCES

Beninger, R.J., Hanson, D.R. and Phillips, A.G. (1981) The acquisition of responding with conditioned reinforcement: effects of cocaine, (+)-amphetamine and pipradrol. *British Journal of Pharmacology* **74**, 149–154.

Berger, B., Verney, C., Alvarez, C., Vigny, A. and Helle, K.B. (1985) New dopaminergic fields in the motor, visual (area 18b) and retrosplenial cortex in the young and adult rat: immunohistochemical and catecholamine histochemical analyses. *Neuroscience* **15**, 983–998.

Bindra, D. (1969) A unified interpretation of emotion and motivation. *Annals of the New York Academy of Sciences* **159**, 1071–1083.

Björklund, A. and Lindvall, O. (1984) Dopamine containing systems in the CNS. In: Björklund, A. and Hökfelt, T (eds) *Handbook of Chemical Neuroanatomy, Vol. 2: Classical Neurotransmitters in the CNS*. Amsterdam: Elsevier, pp. 55–122.

Blackburn, J.R., Phillips, A.G. and Fibiger, H.C. (1987) Dopamine and preparatory behavior: I. Effect of pimozide. *Behavioral Neuroscience* **101**, 352–360.

Bolles, R.C. (1975) *Theory of Motivation*. New York: Harper and Row.

Bowers, W., Hamilton, M., Zacharko, R.M. and Anisman, H. (1985) Differential effects of pimozide on response rate and choice accuracy in a self-stimulation paradigm in mice. *Pharmacology Biochemistry and Behavior* **22**, 521–526.

Brozoski, T.J., Brown, R.M., Rosvold, H.E. and Goldman, P.S. (1979) Cognitive deficits caused by regional depletion of dopamine in prefrontal cortex of rhesus monkey. *Science* **205**, 929–931.

Cador, M., Robbins, T.W. and Everitt, B.J. (1989) Involvement of the amygdala in stimulus-reward associations: interaction with the ventral striatum. *Neuroscience* **30**, 77–86.

Carr, G.D. and White, N. (1983) Conditioned place-preference from intra-accumbens amphetamine but not intra-caudate amphetamine injection. *Life Science* **33**, 2551–2557.

Carter, C.J. and Pycock, C.J. (1980) Behavioral and biochemical effects of dopamine and noradrenaline depletion within the medial prefrontal cortex of the rat. *Brain Research* **192**, 163–176.

Cormier, S.M. (1981) A match-mismatch theory of limbic system function. *Physiological Psychology* **9**, 3–36.

Costall, B., Domeney, A.M. and Naylor, R.J. (1984) Locomotor hyperactivity caused by dopamine infusion into the nucleus accumbens of rat brain: specificity of action. *Psychopharmacology* **82**, 174–180.

Csernansky, J.G., Csernansky, C.A., Bonnet, K.A. and Hollister, L.E. (1985) Dopaminergic supersensitivity following ferric chloride-induced limbic seizures. *Biological Psychiatry* **20**, 723–733.

Dahlström, A. and Fuxe, K. (1964) Evidence for the existence of monoamine-containing neurons in the ventral nervous system. I. Demonstration of monoamines in the cell bodies of brainstem neurons. *Acta Physiologica Scandinavica* **62**, 1–55 (suppl 232).

De France, J.F., Marchand, J.E., Stanley, J.C., Sikes, R.W. and Chronister, R.B. (1980) Convergence of excitatory amygdaloid and hippocampal input in the nucleus accumbens septi. *Brain Research* **185**, 183–186.

Deminière, J.M., Taghzouti, K., Tassin, J.P., Le Moal, M. and Simon, H. (1988) Increased sensitivity to amphetamine and facilitation of self-administration after 6-hydroxydopamine lesion of the amygdala. *Psychopharmacology* **94**, 232–236.

Descarries, L., Lemay, B., Doucet, G. and Berger, B. (1987) Regional and laminar density of the dopamine innervation in adult rat cerebral cortex. *Neuroscience* **21**, 807–824.

Ehlers, C.L. and Koob, G.F. (1985) Locomotor behavior following kindling in three different brain sites. *Brain Research* **326**, 71–79.

Emson, P.C. and Koob, G.F. (1978) The origin and distribution of dopamine-containing afferents to the rat frontal cortex. *Brain Research* **142**, 249–267.

Evans, K.R. and Vaccarino, F.J. (1986) Intra-nucleus accumbens amphetamine: dose-dependent effects on food-intake. *Pharmacology Biochemistry and Behavior* **25**, 1149–1152.

Evenden, J.L. and Robbins, T.W. (1983) Dissociable effects of d-amphetamine, chlordiazepoxide and alpha-flupentixol on choice and rate measures of reinforcement in the rat. *Psychopharmacology* **79**, 180–186.

Everitt, B.J., Fray, P., Kostarczyk, E., Taylor, S. and Stacey, P. (1987) Studies of instrumental behavior with sexual reinforcement in male rats (*Rattus norvegicus*): I. Control by brief visual stimuli paired with a receptive female. *Journal of Comparative Psychology* **101**, 395–406.

Everitt, B.J., Cador, M. and Robbins, T.W. (1989a) Interactions between the amygdala and ventral striatum in stimulus-reward associations: studies using a second order schedule of sexual reinforcement. *Neuroscience* **30**, 63–75.

Everitt, B.J., Morris, K.A., O'Brien, A., Burns, L. and Robbins, T.W. (1989b) The effects of basolateral amygdala and ventral striatum lesions on conditioned place-preference in rats. *Society for Neuroscience Abstracts* **15**, 1251.

Fallon, J.H. and Moore, R.Y. (1978a) Catecholamine innervation of the basal forebrain. III. Olfactory bulb, anterior olfactory nuclei, olfactory tubercle and piriform cortex. *Journal of Comparative Neurology* **180**, 533–544.

Fallon, J.H. and Moore, R.Y. (1987b) Catecholamine innervation of the basal forebrain and neostriatum. IV. Topography of the dopamine projection to the basal forebrain and neostriatum. *Journal of Comparative Neurology* **180**, 545–580.

Fallon, J.H., David, A.K. and Moore, R.Y. (1978) Catecholamine innervation of the basal forebrain. II. Amygdala, suprarhinal cortex and entorhinal cortex. *Journal of Comparative Neurology* **180**, 509–532.

Fuxe, K., Hökfelt, T., Johanson, O., Johnson, G., Lindbrink, P. and Ljundhal, A. (1974) The origin of the dopamine nerve terminals in limbic and frontal cortex. Evidence for mesocorticodopamine neurons. *Brain Research* **82**, 349–355.

Gaffan, D. and Harrison, S. (1987) Amygdalectomy and disconnection in visual learning for auditory secondary reinforcement by monkeys. *Journal of Neuroscience* **7**, 2285–2292.

Gee, K.W., Hollonger, M.A., Bowyer, J.F. and Killam, E.K. (1979) Modification of dopaminergic receptor sensitivity in rat brain after amygdaloid kindling. *Experimental Neurology* **66**, 721–777.

Groenewegen, H.J. and Russchen, F.T. (1964) Organization of the efferent projections of the nucleus accumbens to pallidal, hypothalamic and mesencephalic structures: a tracing and immunohistochemical study in the cat. *Journal of Comparative Neurology* **223**, 347–367.

Groenewegen, H.J., Becker, N.E.H. and Lohman, A.H.M. (1980) Subcortical afferents of the nucleus accumbens septi in the cat, studied with retrograde axonal transport of horseradish peroxidase and bisbenzimid. *Neuroscience* **5**, 1903–1916.

Groenewegen, H.J., Vermeulen-Van Der Zee, E., te Korstschot, A. and Witter,

M.P. (1987) Organization of the projections from the subiculum to the ventral striatum in the rat. A study using anterograde transport of *Phaseolus vulgaris* leucoagglutinin. *Neuroscience* **223**, 103–120.

Heimer, L. and Wilson, R.D. (1975) The subcortical projections of the allocortex: similarities in the neural connections of the hippocampus, the pyriform cortex and the neocortex. In: Santini, M. (ed.) *Golgi Centennial Symposium: Perspectives in Neurobiology*. New York: Raven Press, pp. 177–193.

Herman, J.P., Choulli, K., Geffard, M., Nadaud, D., Taghzouti, K. and Le Moal, M. (1986) Reinnervation of the nucleus accumbens and frontal cortex of the rat by dopaminergic grafts and effects on hoarding behavior. *Brain Research* **372**, 210–216.

Hill, R.T. (1970) Facilitation of conditioned reinforcement as a mechanism of psychomotor stimulation. In: Costa, E. and Garratini, S. (eds) *Amphetamine and Related Compounds*. New York: Raven Press, pp. 781–795.

Hoebel, B.G., Monaco, A.P., Hernandez, L., Avilisi, E.F., Stanley, B.G. and Lenard, L. (1983) Self-injection of amphetamine directly into the brain. *Psychopharmacology* **81**, 158–163.

Isaacson, R.L. (1982) *The Limbic System*. New York: Plenum Press.

Jackson, D.M., Anden, N.E. and Dahlström, A. (1975) A functional effect of dopamine in the nucleus accumbens and in some other dopamine-rich parts of the brain. *Psychopharmacology* **45**, 139–149.

Jones, B. and Mishkin, M. (1972) Limbic lesion and the problem of stimulus-reinforcement association. *Experimental Neurology* **36**, 362–377.

Jones, D.L. and Mogenson, G.J. (1980) Nucleus accumbens to globus pallidus GABA projection subserving ambulatory activity. *American Journal of Physiology* **238**, R65–R69.

Kelley, A.E. and Domesick, V.B. (1982) The distribution of the projections from the hippocampal formation to the nucleus accumbens in the rat; an anterograde and retrograde horseradish peroxydase study. *Neuroscience* **7**, 2331–2335.

Kelley, A.E. and Stinus, L. (1984) The distribution of the projection from the parataenial nucleus of the thalamus to the nucleus accumbens in the rat: an autoradiographic study. *Experimental Brain Research* **54**, 499–512.

Kelley, A.E. and Stinus, L. (1985) Disappearance of hoarding behavior after 6-hydroxydopamine lesions of the mesolimbic dopamine neurons and its reinstatement with L-dopa. *Behavioral Neuroscience* **99**, 531–545.

Kelley, A.E., Domesick, V.B. and Nauta, W.J.H. (1982) The amygdalostriatal projection in the rat. An anatomical study by anterograde and retrograde tracing methods. *Neuroscience* **7**, 615–630.

Kelley, A.E., Winnock, M. and Stinus, L. (1986) Amphetamine, apomorphine and investigatory behavior in the rat: analysis of the structure and pattern of response. *Psychopharmacology* **88**, 66–74.

Kelley, A.E., Lang, C.G. and Gauthier, A.M. (1988) Induction of oral stereotypy following amphetamine microinjection into a discrete subregion of the striatum. *Psychopharmacology* **95**, 556–559.

Kelly, P.H., Seviour, P.W. and Iversen, S.D. (1975) Amphetamine and apomorphine responses in the rat following 6-OHDA lesions of the nucleus accumbens septi and corpus striatum. *Brain Research* **94**, 507–522.

Koob, G.F., Riley, M.S.T., Smith, S.C. and Robbins, T.W. (1978) Effects of 6-hydroxydopamine lesions of the nucleus accumbens septi and olfactory tubercle on feeding, locomotor activity and amphetamine anorexia in the rat. *Journal of Comparative and Physiological Psychology* **92**, 917–927.

Krettek, J.E. and Price, J.L. (1978) Amygdaloid projections to subcortical structures within the basal forebrain and brainstem in the rat and cat. *Journal of Comparative Neurology* 178, 225–254.

Lindvall, O. (1975) Mesencephalic dopaminergic afferents to the lateral septal nucleus of the rat. *Brain Research* 87, 89–95.

Lindvall, O. and Björklund, A. (1974) The organization of the ascending catecholamine neuron systems in the rat brain. *Acta Physiologica Scandinavica* 412, 1–48 (suppl).

Lindvall, O. and Steveni, U. (1978) Dopamine and noradrenaline neurons projecting to the septal area in the rat. *Cell and Tissue Research* 190, 383–407.

Lindvall, O., Björklund, A., Moore, R.Y. and Steveni, U. (1974) Mesencephalic dopamine neurons projecting to neocortex. *Brain Research* 8, 325–331.

Louilot, A., Simon, H., Taghzouti, K. and Le Moal, M. (1985) Modulation of dopaminergic activity in the nucleus accumbens following facilitation or blockade of the dopaminergic transmission in the amygdala. A study by in vivo differential pulse voltammetry. *Brain Research* 346, 141–146.

Louilot, A., Taghzouti, K., Deminière, J.M., Simon, H. and Le Moal, M. (1987) Dopamine and behavior: functional and theoretical considerations. In: Sandler, M., Feuerstein, C. and Scatton, B. (eds) *Neurotransmitter Interactions*. New York: Raven Press, pp. 193–204.

Louilot, A., Le Moal, M. and Simon, H. (1989) Opposite influences of dopaminergic pathways to the prefrontal cortex or the septum on the dopaminergic transmission in the nucleus accumbens. An *in vivo* voltammetric study. *Neuroscience* 29, 45–56.

Lyness, W.H., Friedel, N.M. and Moore, K.E. (1979) Destruction of dopaminergic nerve terminals in nucleus accumbens: effect on d-amphetamine self-administration. *Pharmacology Biochemistry and Behavior* 11, 553–556.

McGeorge, A.J. and Faull, R.L.M. (1989) The organization of the projection from the cerebral cortex to the striatum in the rat. *Neuroscience* 29, 503–537.

Mishkin, M. (1978) Memory in monkeys severely impaired by combined but not by separate removal of amygdala and hippocampus. *Nature* 273, 297–298.

Mogenson, G.J. and Nielsen, M. (1983) Evidence that an accumbens to subpallidal GABAergic projection contributes to locomotor activity. *Brain Research Bulletin* 11, 309–314.

Mogenson, G.J. and Nielsen, M. (1984a) A study of the contribution of hippocampal-accumbens-subpallidal projections to locomotor activity. *Behavioral and Neural Biology* 42, 38–51.

Mogenson, G.J. and Nielsen, M. (1984b) Neuropharmacological evidence to suggest that the nucleus accumbens and subpallidal region contribute to exploratory locomotion. *Behavioral and Neural Biology* 42, 52–60.

Mogenson, G., Jones, D.L. and Yim, C.Y. (1982) From motivation to action: functional interface between the limbic system and the motor system. *Progress in Neurobiology* 14, 69–97.

Nauta, W.J.H., Smith, G.P., Fall, R.L.M. and Domesick, V.B. (1978) Efferent connections and nigral afferents of the nucleus accumbens septi in the rat. *Neuroscience* 3, 385–401.

Phillipson, O.T. and Griffiths, A.C. (1985) The topographic order of inputs to nucleus accumbens in the rat. *Neuroscience* 16, 275–296.

Pijnenburg, A.J.J., Honig, W.M.M., Van der Heyden, J.A.M. and Van Rossum, J.M. (1976) Effects of chemical stimulation of mesolimbic dopamine system upon locomotor activity. *European Journal of Pharmacology* 35, 45–58.

Post, R.M., Squillace, K.M., Pert, A. and Sass, W. (1981) The effect of amygdala kindling on spontaneous and cocaine-induced motor activity and lidocaine seizures. *Psychopharmacology* 72, 189–196.

Robbins, T.W. (1975) The potentiation of conditioned reinforcement by psychomotor stimulant drugs. A test of Hill's hypothesis. *Psychopharmacology* **45**, 103–114.

Robbins, T.W. (1978) The acquisition of responding with conditioned reinforcement: effect of pipradrol, methylphenidate, d-amphetamine and nomifensine. *Psychopharmacology* **58**, 79–87.

Robbins, T.W. and Everitt, B.J. (1982) Functional studies of the central catecholamines. *International Review of Neurobiology* **23**, 303–365.

Robbins, T.W. and Koob, G.F. (1978) Pipradrol enhances reinforcing properties of stimuli paired with brain stimulation. *Pharmacology Biochemistry and Behavior* **8**, 219–222.

Robbins, T.W., Watson, B.A., Gaskin, M. and Ennis, C. (1983) Contrasting interactions of pipradrol, d-amphetamine, cocaine, cocaine analogues, apomorphine and other drugs with conditioned reinforcement. *Psychopharmacology* **80**, 113–119.

Roberts, D.C.S. and Koob, G.F. (1982) Disruption of cocaine self-administration following 6-hydroxydopamine lesions of the ventral tegmental area in rats. *Pharmacology Biochemistry and Behavior* **17**, 901–904.

Roberts, D.C.S., Koob, G.F., Klonoff, P. and Fibiger, H.C. (1980) Extinction and recovery of cocaine self-administration following 6-hydroxydopamine lesions of the nucleus accumbens. *Pharmacology Biochemistry and Behavior* **12**, 781–787.

Salamone, J.D. (1988) Dopaminergic involvement in activational aspects of motivation: effects of haloperidol on schedule-induced activity, feeding, and foraging behavior. *Psychobiology* **16**, 196–206.

Simon, H. (1981) Neurones dopaminergiques A10 et système frontal. *Journal of Physiology* (Lond.) **77**, 81–95.

Simon, H. and Le Moal, M. (1984) Mesencephalic dopaminergic neurons: functional role. In: Usdin, E., Carlsson, A., Dahlström, A. and Engel, J. (eds) *Catecholamines: Neuropharmacology and Central Nervous System. Theoretical Aspects.* New York: Alan R. Liss, Inc., pp. 293–307.

Simon, H., Le Moal, M., Galey, D. and Cardo, B. (1976) Silver impregnation of dopaminergic systems after radiofrequency and 6-OHDA lesions of the rat ventral tegmentum. *Brain Research* **115**, 215–231.

Simon, H., Le Moal, M. and Calas, A. (1979) Efferents and afferents of the ventral tegmental-A10 region studied after the local injection of (3H) leucine and horseradish peroxidase. *Brain Research* **178**, 77–86.

Simon, H., Scatton, B. and Le Moal, M. (1980) Dopaminergic A10 neurones are involved in cognitive functions. *Nature* **286**, 150–151.

Simon, H., Taghzouti, K., Gozlan, H., Studler, J.M., Louilot, A., Hervé, D., Glowinski, J.P. and Le Moal, M. (1988) Lesion of dopaminergic terminals in the amygdala produces enhanced locomotor responses to d-amphetamine and opposite changes in dopaminergic activity in prefrontal cortex and nucleus accumbens. *Brain Research* **447**, 335–340.

Skinner, B.F. (1938) *The Behavior of Organisms.* New York: Appleton-Century Crofts.

Spiegler, B.J. and Mishkin, M. (1981) Evidence for the sequential participation of inferior temporal cortex and amygdala in the acquisition of stimulus-reward associations. *Behavioral Brain Research* **3**, 303–317.

Spyraki, C., Fibiger, H.C. and Phillips, A.G. (1982) Dopaminergic substrates of amphetamine-induced place-preference conditioning. *Brain Research* **253**, 185–193.

Swanson, L.W. (1982) The projections of the ventral tegmental area and adjacent regions: a combined fluorescent retrograde tracer and immunofluorescence study in the rat. *Brain Research Bulletin* **9**, 321–353.

Swanson, L.W. and Cowan, W.M. (1975) A note on the connections and development of the nucleus accumbens. *Brain Research* **92**, 324–330.

Taghzouti, K., Le Moal, M. and Simon, H. (1985a) Enhanced frustrative non-reward effect following 6-OHDA lesions of the lateral septum in the rat. *Behavioral Neuroscience* **99**, 1066–1073.

Taghzouti, K., Louilot, A., Herman, J.P., Le Moal, M. and Simon, H. (1985b) Alternation behavior, spatial discrimination and reversal disturbances following 6-OHDA lesions in the nucleus accumbens of the rat. *Behavioral and Neural Biology* **44**, 354–363.

Taghzouti, K., Simon, H., Louilot, A., Herman, J.P. and Le Moal, M. (1985c) Behavioral study following 6-hydroxydopamine injection in the nucleus accumbens of the rat. *Brain Research* **344**, 9–20.

Taghzouti, K., Simon, H. and Le Moal, M. (1986) Disturbances in exploratory behavior and functional recovery in the Y and radial mazes following dopamine depletion of the lateral septum. *Behavioral and Neural Biology* **45**, 48–56.

Taylor, J.R. and Robbins, T.W. (1984) Enhanced behavioral control by conditioned reinforcers following microinjections of d-amphetamine into the nucleus accumbens. *Psychopharmacology* **84**, 405–412.

Taylor, J.R. and Robbins, T.W. (1986) 6-Hydroxydopamine lesions of the nucleus accumbens but not the caudate nucleus attenuates enhanced responding with reward-related stimuli produced by intra-accumbens d-amphetamine. *Psychopharmacology* **90**, 390–397.

Tombaugh, T.N., Szostak, C. and Mills, P. (1983) Failure of pimozide to disrupt acquisition of light-dark and spatial discrimination problems. *Psychopharmacology* **76**, 161–168.

Weiskrantz, L. (1956) Behavioral changes associated with ablation of the amygdaloid complex in monkeys. *Journal of Comparative and Physiological Psychology* **49**, 381–391.

Winn, P., Williams, S.F. and Herberg, L.J. (1982) Feeding stimulated by very low doses of d-amphetamine administered systemically or by injection into the striatum. *Psychopharmacology* **78**, 336–341.

Wolterink, G., Cador, M., Wolterink, I., Robbins, T.W. and Everitt, B.J. (1989) Involvement of D1 and D2 receptor mechanisms in the processing of reward-related stimuli in the ventral striatum. *Society for Neuroscience Abstracts* **15**, 1252.

Yang, C.R. and Mogenson, G.J. (1984) Electrophysiological responses of neurones in the nucleus accumbens to hippocampal stimulation and the attenuation of the excitatory responses by the mesolimbic system. *Brain Research* **324**, 69–84.

Yim, C.Y. and Mogenson, G.J. (1982) Response of nucleus accumbens neurons to amygdala stimulation and its modification by dopamine. *Brain Research* **239**, 401–415.

Yim, C.Y. and Mogenson, G.J. (1986) Mesolimbic dopamine projection modulates amygdala-evoked EPSP in nucleus accumbens neurons: an in vivo study. *Brain Research* **369**, 347–352.

Yim, C.Y. and Mogenson, G.J. (1989) Low doses of accumbens dopamine modulate amygdala suppression of spontaneous exploratory activity in rats. *Brain Research* **477**, 202–210.

10

Suppression of Rewarded Behaviour by Neuroleptic Drugs: Can't or Won't, and Why?

PAUL WILLNER, GAVIN PHILLIPS AND RICHARD MUSCAT

Department of Psychology, City of London Polytechnic, Old Castle Street, London E1 7NT, UK

INTRODUCTION

Neuroleptic drugs, as well as other treatments that reduce brain dopamine (DA) function, suppress behaviour over a wide range of doses (Beninger, 1983; Iversen, 1977). However, while these empirical observations are extremely well established, their interpretation remains the subject of intense controversy.

According to the anhedonia hypothesis (Wise, 1982; see also Bozarth, Chapter 12, this volume), neuroleptics suppress rewarded behaviours by devaluing the reinforcer. Certainly, neuroleptics suppress behaviours maintained by a wide variety of rewards, including food (Wise et al., 1978), water (Gerber et al., 1981), temperature change (Ettenberg and Carlisle, 1985), brain stimulation (Olds and Travis, 1960), and intravenous drug infusions (Yokel, 1987). However, it is difficult to exclude the alternative explanation that neuroleptics have a direct suppressant effect on the motor system. While some experiments have suggested that motor capacity is unimpaired by neuroleptic pretreatment (Fouriezos and Wise, 1976; Fouriezos et al., 1978; Wise, 1982), other data suggest that motor impairments are

The Mesolimbic Dopamine System: From Motivation to Action.
Edited by P. Willner and J. Scheel-Krüger

© 1991 John Wiley & Sons Ltd

primarily responsible (Rolls et al., 1974; Fibiger et al., 1976; Ahlenius, 1979; Ettenberg et al., 1981).

In the special case of brain stimulation reward, the demonstration that administration of a DA antagonist to the nucleus accumbens suppressed performance only when delivered on the side ipsilateral to the stimulating electrode (Kurimaya and Nakajima, 1988) provides an elegant resolution of this problem. Unfortunately, however, this technique is not available for use with other types of reinforcers. There is little doubt that at high doses, neuroleptic drugs do cause motor impairment. In this review we describe a programme of research in which we have used low doses of neuroleptics in an attempt to confirm without doubt the existence of non-motor impairment in the effects of neuroleptics on behaviour maintained by natural rewards, over and above any motor deficits that might additionally be present.

THE OPERANT 'MATCHING' PARADIGM

The so-called 'matching' paradigm potentially offers an elegant solution to the problem of dissociating neuroleptic-induced motivational and motor impairments by providing quantitative estimates of both. The term 'matching' refers to the empirical observation that if the amount of reinforcement available is varied, rats adjust their behaviour accordingly, and 'match' their rate of responding to the pay-off. Matching experiments are usually conducted using variable or random interval schedules of reinforcement, in which the probability of reinforcement is controlled by the experimenter, and response rates at a given level of reinforcement remain roughly constant. In these conditions, responding rises as a negatively accelerating function of reinforcement density, such that at high levels of reinforcement further increases produce smaller and smaller increases in responding. Herrnstein (1970) first noted that, for individual animals tested at several levels of reinforcement, this function may be fitted to a high degree of precision by a simple hyperbolic equation. The equation includes two constants which may be extracted by curve-fitting procedures. A substantial body of literature confirms that one of the constants, which corresponds to the asymptote of the curve, is sensitive to changes in the experimental procedure that affect the motor requirements of the task, while the other, which corresponds to the degree of curvature, is sensitive to manipulations of motivational variables (Herrnstein, 1970; de Villers and Herrnstein, 1976; Heyman and Monaghan, 1987).

This clear separation of the factors that influence the two parameters of the matching equation suggests that the paradigm should lend itself to pharmacological analysis, based on the assumption that drug-induced changes in asymptotic responding imply changes in motor capacity, while drug-induced changes in curvature (i.e. more potent drug effects on poorly rewarded behaviour) imply changes in motivational processes. Unfortunately, the initial studies of neuroleptic effects within this framework were inconsistent: while all agree that neuroleptics can cause motor disability, there was disagreement concerning the presence of an additional motivational impairment (Heyman, 1983; Morley et al., 1984; Hamilton et al., 1985; Heyman et al., 1986).

As the matching paradigm had been implemented in different ways by different laboratories, we decided to examine the effects of neuroleptics in a variety of matching procedures. An initial, and informative, series of experiments used multiple random interval schedules, in which five different reinforcement frequencies were offered to rats, each for a short period, during the course of a 55-minute session. We were disconcerted to discover that the effects of pimozide were dependent upon the order in which the different reinforcement components were presented. Pimozide apparently caused a motivational impairment when the schedule components were presented in descending order of reinforcement densities, but a motor impairment when the components were presented in the reverse order (Willner et al., 1987). When the components were presented in random order, both types of effect were seen (Willner et al., 1990a).

Clearly, this set of conclusions is almost certainly mistaken, and a potential artifact was immediately apparent: in all cases, the effect of pimozide was greatest towards the end of the experimental session. To investigate the contribution of time-dependent effects, we moved to a 'stripped-down' version of the paradigm, in which only two or three different schedule components were used, and only one component was presented on any one day (Willner et al., 1987, 1990a). While it may seem somewhat unorthodox (though not improper: Dunn et al., 1988) to calculate parameters of an underlying hyperbolic equation from two sets of data points, the parameters so derived respond to motivational and motor manipulations in the same way as those derived from more extensive data sets (Figure 1). In these simpler procedures pimozide had two very obvious effects: suppression of behaviour was substantially greater under reinforcement-lean conditions, and the effect increased dramatically with time (Figure 2). The matching equation parameters calculated from these data suggested that both motor and motivational impairments were present, the latter first appearing at a slightly lower dose. The putative motor impairment was constant across the session, but the putative motivational impairment was time-dependent (Willner et al., 1987). Subsequent experiments using either the specific D2 antagonist sulpiride (Figure 1), or the specific D1 antagonist SCH 23390, found very similar effects, the only difference being that with both of these drugs selective motivational impairments were observed over a somewhat wider dose window (Willner et al., 1990a).

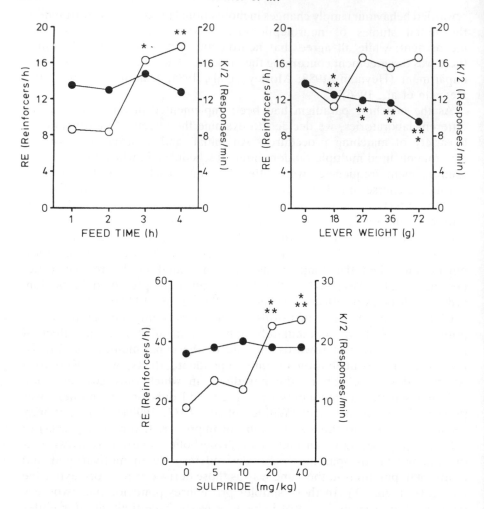

Figure 1. Twenty-four-hour food-deprived rats were trained to lever-press on two random interval (RI) reinforcement schedules, RI 7.5 seconds and RI 120 seconds, presented on alternate days. The parameters K and RE were calculated from the formulae $P_1 = KR_1/(R_1+R_E)$ and $P_2+KR_2(R_2+R_E)$, where P and R represent, respectively, the response rate and reinforcement density in the two schedules (Willner et al., 1987). The top left panel shows that allowing access to food prior to testing increases the parameter RE without affecting K; the top right panel shows that increasing the force required to depress the lever reduces K without affecting RE. Similar results have been obtained when the parameters K and RE are extracted from more extensive data sets (e.g. five-component multiple schedules) by curve-fitting techniques (de Villiers and Herrnstein, 1976). The bottom left panel shows the effects of i.p. injects of sulpiride. $*P<0.05$; $**P<0.01$; $***P<0.001$. (Calculated from data reported in Willner et al., 1990a)

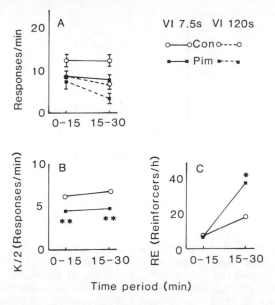

Time period (min)

Figure 2. Effect of pimozide (Pim) (0.25 mg/kg) on performance in each half of a 30-minute session of random interval (VI) operant performance in 21-hour food-deprived rats. The top figure (**A**) shows a constant effect of pimozide on reinforcement-rich (VI 7.5 seconds) responding, but a time-dependent increase in the effect on reinforcement-lean (VI, 120 seconds) responding; in proportional terms, the effect was substantially greater at VI, 120 seconds in the second half of the session. The lower panels show that these effects correspond to a time-independent decrease in the calculated parameter K (**B**) and a time-dependent increase in the calculated parameter RE (**C**). See legend to Figure 1 for the interpretation of K and RE. *$P<0.05$; **$P<0.01$ (From Willner et al., 1987)

To demonstrate that time dependency in the effect of neuroleptics really does introduce an artifact into the multiple schedule procedure, we devised a pair of novel multiple schedules which contained both ascending and descending sequences of reinforcement densities in different temporal locations. The results confirmed the earlier conclusions: both pimozide and SCH 23390 selectively suppressed poorly rewarded responding, and the effects increased according to whether that schedule component was located at the beginning, in the middle, or at the end of the session. Amphetamine provided a mirror image of the neuroleptics: poorly rewarded responding was selectively increased, again in a time-dependent manner (Figure 3). Parameter calculation confirmed that, as in the earlier experiments, the neuroleptics caused a time-dependent motivational impairment together with a time-independent motor impairment at higher doses (Willner et al., 1989; Phillips et al., 1990).

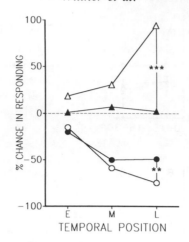

Figure 3. Effects of amphetamine (0.5 mg/kg: △, upper part of figure) and pimozide (0.25 mg/kg: ○, lower part of figure) on reinforcement-rich (VI 7.5 seconds: white) and reinforcement-lean (VI 120 seconds: black) operant responding, in 21-hour food-deprived rats. The two schedules were presented as components of five-component multiple schedules, in which they appeared in the early (E, first component), middle (M, third component) or late (L, fifth component) part of the session. Values are proportional changes relative to vehicle treatment. **$P<0.01$; ***$P<0.001$. (From Phillips et al., 1990)

One implication of these studies is that the elegant and sophisticated matching paradigm is in fact very poorly suited for analysing the behavioural processes underlying the effects of neuroleptics, because any calculations are confounded by time-dependent response decrements. Nevertheless, experiments using implementations of the paradigm that take response decrements into account confirm that neuroleptics do produce some form of motivational impairment over and above the time-independent motor impairment that appears at higher doses.

EFFECTS OF NEUROLEPTICS ON VERY SWEET REWARD

We return below to the problem of neuroleptic-induced response decrements, and turn now to a series of studies which confirm in a dramatic and surprising way that neuroleptics can cause non-motor impairments. In brief, response rates fall when the sweetness of reinforcers is increased beyond an optimal concentration, and in this supramaximal region, neuroleptics actually increase rewarded behaviour.

In one series of experiments, consumption of sucrose and water was measured in two-bottle tests in three groups of rats tested with different concentrations of sucrose (0.7, 7 and 34 per cent). Sucrose consumption was highest at intermediate concentrations. Pimozide, sulpiride and raclopride all dose-dependently decreased consumption of, and preference for, the weakest solution. However, at the highest sucrose concentration, the neuroleptics increased sucrose consumption and preference (Figure 4, left) (Muscat and Willner, 1989; Phillips et al., 1989a; Willner et al., 1990b). Similar effects were observed using continuously reinforced (CRF) food-rewarded operant performance. In initial experiments, lever pressing in food-deprived rats was reinforced with standard (10 per cent sucrose) pellets or with 95 per cent sucrose pellets. Response rates were lower with 95 per cent pellets, and rats failed to consume a proportion of the pellets earned. Both pimozide and raclopride decreased responding for bland pellets, but increased responding for (and consumption of) sweet pellets. A subsequent experiment using three types of pellet (1, 10 and 95 per cent) showed that the concentration/performance function is bell-shaped, as it is for sucrose drinking; again, raclopride increased responding for 95 per cent sucrose pellets (Figure 4, right) (Phillips et al., 1989b, 1990).

A simple empirical account of these two sets of experiments is that neuroleptics shift the concentration/intake curve to the right; in other words, the animal behaves as though it were consuming a weaker reward. There could be an almost trivial explanation for these effects: neuroleptics could act to suppress sensory input and inhibit the perception of sweetness. This seems a rather remote possibility. Nevertheless, it seems important that it be excluded, and we have done this by using sucrose solutions as discriminative stimuli (Willner et al., 1990b). Rats were trained to perform

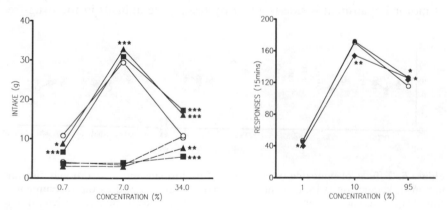

Figure 4. Raclopride increases performance maintained by very sweet rewards. Left panel: consumption of sucrose solutions (full lines, above) and water (broken lines, below) in two-choice tests. Right panel: lever pressing for pellets varying in sucrose content. White circles, vehicle. Black symbols, raclopride: circles 50 μg/kg, diamonds 100 μg/kg, triangles 200 μg/kg, squares 400 μg/kg. Three separate groups of rats were used in each experiment. *$P<0.05$; **$P<0.01$; ***$P<0.001$

a conditional discrimination in a T-maze. A correct response was rewarded by access to a 10 per cent sucrose solution; an incorrect response was punished by confinement in the non-rewarded arm. In the first part of the experiment, the discriminative stimulus, located at the choice point of the T maze, was either water or sucrose, initially a 10 per cent solution, but reduced gradually to 0.0003 per cent. In the second part of the experiment, the discriminative stimulus was either a 1 per cent sucrose or a weaker solution, which was initially 0.0001 per cent, and was raised gradually to 0.5 per cent. In both experiments, performance was stable at around 80 per cent correct over a wide concentration range, but eventually fell to chance. Administration of pimozide at the most difficult but still discriminable sucrose concentrations decreased running speed but had no effect on discrimination accuracy (Figure 5).

As pimozide affected neither the threshold for sweetness perception nor the discrimination of a just noticeable difference, the decreased responsiveness of neuroleptic-treated rats to sweet rewards cannot be explained by a change in the perception of sweetness. After neuroleptic treatment the reward is correctly perceived, but its control over behaviour is attenuated. The observation that the effects of neuroleptics resemble those of dilution is not new (Xenakis and Sclafani, 1981; Gramling et al., 1984; Geary and Smith, 1985; Bailey et al., 1986; Schneider et al., 1986), but the present data certainly make the point more dramatically and less ambiguously than previous studies.

The conclusion that neuroleptics reduce the perceived intensity of sweet rewards is consistent with data derived from procedures in which the question of motor impairment is side-stepped by testing the animals in the drug-free

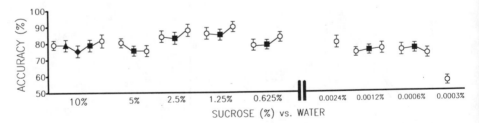

Figure 5. Effects of pimozide on accuracy of performance in a conditional discrimination task. Sucrose (various concentrations) or water served as the discriminative stimulus at the choice point of a T-maze; correct responses were rewarded with 10 per cent sucrose; incorrect responses were punished by confinement in the non-rewarded arm. Vehicle treatments are shown in open circles and pimozide treatment in black symbols: triangle, 0.125 mg/kg; diamond, 0.25 mg/kg; squares, 0.5 mg/kg. The lower doses of pimozide were administered at the 10 per cent sucrose concentration only. Pimozide had no effect on discrimination accuracy, but increased response latency (not shown) in every trial. (From Willner et al., 1990b)

state. For example, the effect of intermittent haloperidol treatment on animals performing on a CRF schedule has been found to resemble the effect of intermittent reward omission: in both cases the animals subsequently emitted more responses during extinction (Ettenberg and Camp, 1986a, b). Although interpretations of the partial reinforcement extinction effect are complex (Mackintosh, 1974), these data are certainly consistent with a reward-attenuating effect of haloperidol. More direct evidence comes from a paradigm in which the presentation of a single reward after prolonged extinction led to a reinstatement of responding on the following day: this effect was not seen in animals receiving haloperidol prior to the rewarded trial (Horvitz and Ettenberg, 1988).

The concept of reward dilution provides a simple means of understanding the effects of neuroleptics on the biphasic sweetness/performance function. However, to interpret the neuroleptic-induced increases in behaviour maintained by very sweet rewards, it is essential also to understand why it is that very sweet rewards support lower rates of behaviour. Very sweet rewards are potentially satiating and possibly aversive: either of these properties could explain why very sweet rewards inhibit behaviour. However, neither explanation is successful. First, the sweetness/performance functions retain their essential biphasic shape in satiated (i.e. non-deprived) animals (Figure 6). In any case, the effects of neuroleptics could not result from an inhibition of satiety: in both drinking and food-rewarded operant paradigms, neuroleptics increased the consumption of very sweet rewards throughout the session, and the effect was present at the start (Phillips et al., 1989a, b). Second, very sweet rewards are not aversive, as first demonstrated by Young and Greene (1953). Although response rates for 95 per cent sucrose

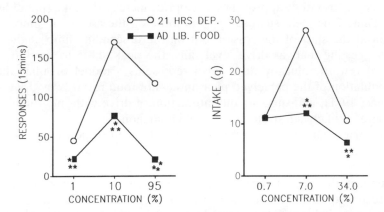

Figure 6. Effect of removing food deprivation on lever pressing for food pellets varying in sucrose content (left), and on intake of sweetened solutions (right). Separate groups of rats were used at each concentration

pellets are lower than for 10 per cent sucrose, the 95 per cent pellets gave rise to higher response rates than standard pellets on the first day of extinction. Similarly, for sweet solutions, 34 per cent sucrose was preferred to 7 per cent or 0.7 per cent in a three-bottle test. In this three-bottle paradigm, raclopride again increased consumption of the 34 per cent solution (Phillips et al., 1989a, b).

The preference data show unequivocally that the reward value of sucrose is monotonically related to concentration. This relationship appears to hold also for other sugars, such as maltose and glucose, which show similar bell-shaped concentration/intake curves (Sclafani and Clyne, 1987); however, it is not true of saccharin, which in rats, as in humans, has clear aversive effects (a bitter taste) at high concentrations (unpublished observations). At present, the descending limb of the sucrose function seems best explained by the common-sense notion that it is possible to have 'too much of a good thing'. While we have not yet succeeded in translating this concept into more respectable terminology, the concentration/performance function provides an empirical distinction between preference and acceptability, with the peak of the function representing maximum acceptability.

It is interesting to note that acceptability is to some extent controlled by drive state: the maximal intake is achieved at a lower concentration in non-deprived than in deprived animals (Figure 6). A similar effect is apparent in the time course of the effects of raclopride on consumption of sweet solutions. Raclopride suppressed consumption of a weak (0.7 per cent) solution throughout the experimental session, and increased consumption of a strong (34 per cent) solution throughout the session. However, in rats consuming an intermediate (7 per cent) sucrose concentration, raclopride suppressed intake during the early part of the session, but towards the end of the session, as satiety approaches, raclopride increased intake (unpublished data). Thus, 7 per cent sucrose appears to be on the ascending limb of the function at the start of the session but on the descending limb at the end, again suggesting that, as drive level falls, the peak shifts to the left. This gating of reward value by drive level represents a model of alliaesthesia, the modulation of the perceived pleasantness of food rewards by drive state (Cabanac, 1971), and suggests the interaction of drive with mesolimbic DA function as a likely substrate for this phenomenon.

An inverse relationship between reward value and response rate is found not only at high concentrations of sucrose, but is also characteristically observed in experiments using drugs as reinforcers (Wise, 1987). Animals self-administering drugs typically respond to increases in dosage by decreasing their response rate to maintain a constant level of the drug in the bloodstream, and, if short-acting drugs are used, this 'titration' can be extremely precise (Yokel, 1987; Wise, 1987; Finlay et al., 1989). As in the present experiments, however, higher drug concentrations are preferred, at least in monkeys (Yokel, 1987). (Rats show no preference between different doses of cocaine, but this may simply reflect their inability to integrate information over the long time interval between infusions (Wise, 1987).)

The simplest explanation of these paradoxical effects would seem to be that, in some sense, intense reinforcers saturate a component of an underlying reward system and introduce a refractory period during which further responding is ineffective. The rate-increasing effects of neuroleptics, both in the present experiments and, under some circumstances, in drug self-administration studies (reviewed by Wise, 1987), suggest strongly that the saturable component is either the ability of the mesolimbic system itself to release DA, or the transmission of information in a system postsynaptic to, and modulated by, mesolimbic DA. It will clearly be of great importance to test directly which of these hypotheses is correct, using *in vivo* voltammetric monitoring of DA release.

NEUROLEPTIC-INDUCED RESPONSE DECREMENTS

While these experiments strongly imply that neuroleptics blunt the impact of rewards, as first suggested by Wise (1982; Wise et al., 1978), not all of the effects of neuroleptics on rewarded behaviour can be explained in this way. This is seen most clearly in the literature on time dependency in the effects of neuroleptics, to which we now return.

Gradual response decrements, both within sessions and across sessions, have been described extensively in neuroleptic-treated animals in a variety of rewarded paradigms, including continuously reinforced, variable and random interval, and fixed-ratio operant performance (Fouriezos and Wise, 1976; Franklin and McCoy, 1979; Gray and Wise, 1980; Tombaugh et al., 1980; Wise et al., 1978; Willner et al., 1988; Fowler, 1989). A progressive onset of neuroleptic action is also seen in behaviours maintained by contingencies other than reward, including exploratory behaviour, avoidance behaviour and treadmill running (Sanger, 1986; Hillegaert et al., 1987; Fowler, 1989). A number of potential explanations of these effects may be ruled out relatively easily. For example, the hypotheses that neuroleptics might enhance fatigue (Fibiger et al., 1976) or satiety would both predict greater drug effects on richly reinforced responding, whereas in fact the opposite is the case (see Figures 2 and 4).

Neuroleptic-induced response decrements have frequently been referred to as 'extinction-like'. The use of this terminology amounts, in effect, to a hypothesis that the reward-attenuating effect of neuroleptics can explain the response decrements. This account appeared to receive support from an initial experiment in which operant response decrements generated by extinction persisted when animals were tested with reward once more available, but pretreated with pimozide (Wise et al., 1978). This effect has been replicated many times. However, equivalence between neuroleptic treatment and non-reward requires that the response decrements transfer in both directions, and neuroleptic-induced response decrements do not transfer to extinction: when neuroleptic-treated animals are tested drug-free, response rates return to their original level, even though now, no rewards are delivered (Mason et al., 1980; Tombaugh et al., 1980; Beninger, 1982). The notion that responding extinguishes in neuroleptic-treated animals appears not to be correct.

It has been argued (Wise, 1982; Martin-Iverson et al., 1987) that the transfer paradigm does not provide an appropriate test of the neuroleptic/non-reward hypothesis, as there are a number of important differences between the presence of a devalued reward and the absence of any reward. This point is well taken. However, there is no way in which reward attenuation can explain a response decrement in non-appetitive paradigms. Response decrements are observed, for example, in animals running on a treadmill, or performing avoidance tasks (Sanger, 1986; Hillegaert et al., 1987). Of course, different principles may operate in these paradigms that do not use rewards to maintain behaviour. However, the same principle may be demonstrated in a rewarded paradigm. In our laboratory, the omission of reinforcement rarely leads to a complete cessation of operant responding, even after prolonged extinction; rather the animals reach a new steady-state of responding at around 20–40 per cent of their rewarded rate. (This effect has been widely reported (Morgan, 1974) but is rarely discussed.) In an experiment carried out during sessions 9–12 of extinction of continuously reinforced lever pressing, raclopride caused a typical within-session response decrement in the absence of both the original food reinforcer and also of the secondary cues originally associated with the delivery of reward (Figure 7).

Fowler (1990) has recently suggested that the very concept of 'neuroleptic-induced response decrement' may be incorrect. Instead, it is proposed that response decrements may reflect a constant motor impairment which is not apparent early in the session because it is masked by the activating effects of handling and initial exposure to the apparatus. We have carried out two tests of this hypothesis (Willner and Phillips, 1989). In the first experiment, animals were returned to the operant chambers 2 minutes after the end of their first session. This procedure reinstates the activational cues present at the start of the first session, so that, according to the motor activation hypothesis, the effect of pimozide should diminish at the start of the second session. In the second experiment, animals were confined in the operant chambers for 30 minutes before the start of the session; the motor activation hypothesis predicts that the initial effect of pimozide should be enhanced, as many of the activational cues normally present at the start of the session are now absent. Neither of these predictions was confirmed (Figure 8); we

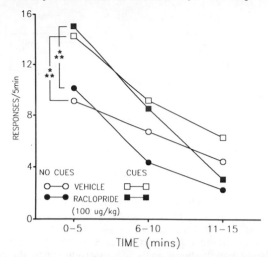

Figure 7. Within-session response decrements following raclopride treatment. The experiment was carried out on days 9–12 of extinction; the behaviour had previously been maintained by CRF. Performance was tested in the presence and absence of cues previously associated with reinforcement (tray light and feeder noise). The effect of raclopride was equivalent under the two conditions. (Interactions: raclopride × time, $F(2,126)=4.4$, $P<0.05$; raclopride × time × cues, $F(2,26)=0.5$, n.s.)

conclude that even this more sophisticated type of motor impairment cannot explain neuroleptic-induced response decrements.

By contrast, Gallistel et al. (1982), using brain stimulation reward, found that the pimozide response decrement generated in an operant chamber was not apparent if the animals were subsequently tested in a runway. This manipulation is superficially similar to the removal/replacement procedure used in the Willner and Phillips (1989) study. However, Franklin and McCoy (1979), also using brain stimulation reward, found that operant responding in response-decremented, pimozide-treated animals could be reinstated simply by presenting a flashing light that had previously been paired with reward, and Fouriezos and Wise (1976) reported spontaneous recovery of intracranial self-stimulation in a single pimozide-treated animal following a period in which access to the lever was prevented by a barrier. Together with the present observations, these data suggest that the crucial feature in the reinstatement of a neuroleptic-induced response decrement is a change in the stimulus conditions, rather than a motor arousal.

How, then, are we to explain the observation that neuroleptics can cause a further suppression of responding in the absence of reward (see Figure 7)? Presumably raclopride acts in this experiment by blocking the process

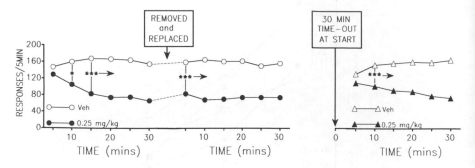

Figure 8. Lack of effect of 'activation' (left panel) or 'deactivation' (right panel) on the within session response decrement induced by pimozide (○, vehicle; ●, pimozide, 0.25 mg/kg). Left panel: following a 30-minute session at RI, 30 seconds, the animals were removed to their home cage, then replaced in the chamber for a second 30-minute session. Right panel: the animals were introduced to the operant chambers 30-minutes before the start of the session

responsible for maintaining responding. What is this process? During extinction, animals are usually maintained under conditions of food deprivation. In an experiment carried out to examine the relevance of this factor in animals trained under continuous reinforcement it was found that by the fourth daily 15-minute extinction session, response rates had fallen to 50 per cent in animals maintained under food deprivation, but to 22 per cent in animals given free access to food during extinction; in the final 5 minutes of the session, the discrepancy was even greater: 37 per cent in deprived animals as compared to only 6 per cent in non-deprived animals (unpublished data). It is interesting to note that the effects on rewarded responding of removing food deprivation in some respects resemble those of neuroleptic treatment. Like pimozide-treated animals, non-deprived animals also showed gradual within- and between-session response decrements. More significantly, we have reported that there was symmetrical transfer of response decrement between pimozide treatment and free feeding: responding remained low not only when non-deprived animals were transferred to pimozide and deprivation, but also when pimozide-treated, deprived animals were transferred to free feeding (and no drug) (Willner et al., 1988).

Despite these marked similarities between neuroleptic treatment and drive reduction in the response decrement paradigm, it is clear that the parallel is of limited value as these two manipulations have opposite effects in the sweet reward paradigm: as described above, the consumption of very sweet rewards is decreased by drive reduction (see Figure 6), but increased by neuroleptics (see Figure 4). One approach that can potentially reconcile these two effects is to see the effects of drive in the response decrement paradigm as being mediated through incentive mechanisms. Learning theory accounts of incentive motivation make exactly this assumption: in the classical model, an increase in drive facilitates responding indirectly by increasing the incentive value of reward-associated cues (Spence, 1956; Bindra, 1972). In the sweet reward paradigm, behaviour at low levels of sweetness is controlled primarily by the incentive value of the sweet reward; however, at high levels of sweetness, the direct suppressant effects of satiating the animal might outweigh the tendency to increase intake associated in this situation with a decrease in incentive.

The position that neuroleptic-induced response decrements reflect the extinction of an incentive process has been adopted in a number of accounts of neuroleptic drug action (Beninger, Chapter 11; Salamone, Chapter 23, this volume). Given the theoretical burden carried by this concept, it is somewhat surprising that there has been almost no attempt to test empirically the degree of equivalence between neuroleptic treatment and incentive devaluation. The failure to address this issue stands in stark contrast to the rigour applied to the question of equivalence between neuroleptic treatment and reward omission (see above). To our knowledge, the only study to make a direct comparison between performance following an incentive manipulation and following neuroleptic treatment is that illustrated in Figure 7. Contrary to the incentive devaluation hypothesis, the effects of removing incentive cues (feeder noise and tray light), in animals performing under extinction conditions, were not equivalent to those of neuroleptic treatment. While raclopride caused a response decrement with a gradual onset, the effect of removing incentive cues was immediately apparent, but decreased during the session. Clearly, it would be inappropriate to read too much into a single study; the parallels between incentive devaluation and neuroleptic treatment require — and deserve — systematic study. However, these initial data are not encouraging.

An alternative account of neuroleptic-induced response decrements places them within the motor domain. Using an operant chamber in which the lever is connected to a force transducer, it has been shown that neuroleptics increase the duration of the operant response. The onset of the response was relatively normal, but the peak force emitted during the response was elevated by neuroleptics and the termination of the response was slower (Fowler et al., 1986a, b; Ettenberg, 1989). Together, these observations suggest that responding is less well controlled after neuroleptic treatment. Clearly, an increase in the duration of each response would tend to reduce the overall rate of responding, and significantly, the delay in terminating the response increases during the course of the session (Skjoldager and Fowler, 1988; Fowler and Kirkpatrick, 1989). While still not explaining why the neuroleptic effect is time-dependent, this account does, potentially, explain why the effect is seen in such a diversity of behavioural paradigms. However, it is not without problems: the effect of response slowing would be expected to increase at higher rates of responding, whereas the time dependency in the action of neuroleptic effects is more apparent at lower response rates (see Figures 2 and 4). However, in the random interval schedules that we have used, rates of responding are confounded with reinforcement density, and it may be that time dependency would be more apparent at higher response rates, as predicted, if reinforcement density were held constant.

CONCLUDING REMARKS

The original objective of this research programme was to devise a methodology to determine conclusively whether neuroleptic drugs impair performance by mechanisms unrelated to their ability to disrupt motor performance. The demonstration that neuroleptics can increase behaviour when very sweet rewards are used provides a clear and unequivocal affirmative answer. As noted above, these results are consistent with data from other paradigms. Nevertheless, this said, a number of perplexing questions remain unresolved. We do not yet have an acceptable account of why performance declines at high levels of sweetness (though the effects of neuroleptics under these conditions reveal the important principle that under neuroleptic treatment, stimuli are functionally less intense in their control over behaviour). We also do not understand why neuroleptic action in behavioural tests has a gradual onset. The notion of a functional equivalence between neuroleptic treatment and the withdrawal of incentive stimuli is attractive, not least because it can encompass neuroleptic effects in both the appetitive and aversive domains (Sanger, 1986), but it requires testing, and our initial efforts in this direction are disappointing. The response slowing account (Skjoldager and Fowler, 1988; Ettenberg, 1989) is also attractive for the same reason, though it too requires testing, and at present does not actually provide an explanation for time dependency.

It is also far from clear that a single principle will suffice to explain both the performance-enhancing effects of neuroleptics in the sweet reward paradigm, and the gradual onset of neuroleptic action in the response decrement paradigm (Ettenberg, 1989). Perhaps a unitary explanation should not be expected. Dopaminergic fibres innervate a variety of structures, and it is clear from studies in which a subset of terminals have been manipulated that different projection systems subserve different functions which are determined by the structure innervated (Cador et al., Chapter 9, this volume). Almost inevitably, therefore, systemic neuroleptic treatment will have multiple effects on behaviour which can be teased apart only using intracranial drug administration. The dopaminergic projection to the amygdala, a structure known to be involved in the process of stimulus evaluation (Cador et al., Chapter 9, this volume), and the nucleus accumbens are two candidates for the site at which neuroleptics have their 'stimulus-diluting' effect on sweet rewards. The gradual onset of neuroleptic-induced response decrement, on the other hand, which is seen in both conditioned and unconditioned behaviours (Hillegaert et al., 1987), might originate in a structure closer to the motor system, such as the dorsal striatum. In fact, in recent studies (unpublished) using local administration of sulpiride to the nucleus accumbens and dorsal striatum we have observed exactly this dissociation.

Finally, it is important to emphasize that studies of neuroleptic drug effects are neutral with respect to the question of whether the DA system constitutes a reward pathway (Wise, 1982). Studies of this type cannot, in principle, distinguish between a reward/incentive effect transmitted along the DA axon, and a modulating effect of DA on information transmitted through the structure(s) that receive a dopaminergic innervation (Mogenson and Yim, Chapter 4, this volume): the deleterious effects of neuroleptic, or 6-hydroxydopamine, treatment would be the same in either case. The question of whether DA neurons transmit or modulate reward-related information can only be answered by techniques that measure directly their level of activity. Although such techniques are still in their infancy, the answers are clear. First, preliminary evidence suggests that mesolimbic DA neurons are activated in anticipation of reward, but their activity does not appear to increase markedly when rewards are delivered (Phillips et al., Chapter 8, this volume): therefore, they do not appear to transmit reward information directly. Second, mesolimbic DA neurons are activated not only by positive affective states, but also by stress (Blanc et al., 1980; Tassin et al., Chapter 7; Zacharko and Anisman, Chapter 16, this volume): therefore, they do not code the instruction to approach or avoid incentive stimuli. It would appear rather, that release of DA modulates the intensity at which the instructions to approach or avoid incentive stimuli are transmitted through the mesolimbic structures in which the DA axons terminate.

REFERENCES

Ahlenius, S. (1979) An analysis of behavioural effects produced by drug-induced changes of dopaminergic neurotransmission in the brain. *Scandinavian Journal of Psychology* **20**, 59–64.

Bailey, C.S., Hsiao, S. and King, J.E. (1986) Hedonic reactivity to sucrose in rats: modification by pimozide. *Physiology and Behavior* **38**, 447–452.

Beninger, R.S. (1982) A comparison of the effects of pimozide and non-reinforcement on discriminated operant responding in rats. *Pharmacology Biochemistry and Behavior* **16**, 667–669.

Beninger, R.S. (1983) The role of dopamine in locomotor activity and learning. *Brain Research Reviews* **6**, 173–196.

Bindra, D. (1972) A unified account of classical conditioning and operant training. In: Black, A.H. and Prokasy, W.F. (eds) *Classical Conditioning II: Current Research and Theory.* New York: Appleton-Century-Crofts, pp. 453–481.

Blanc, G., Hervé, D., Simon, H., Lisoprawski, A., Glowinski, J. and Tassin, J.-P. (1980) Response to stress of mesocortical frontal dopaminergic neurons in rats after long-term isolation. *Nature* **284**, 265–276.

Cabanac, M. (1971) Physiological role of pleasure. *Science* **173**, 1103–1107.

de Villiers, P.A. and Herrnstein, R.J. (1976) Toward a law of response strength. *Psychological Bulletin* **83**, 1131–1153.

Dunn, G., Koshikawa, N., Durcan, M.J. and Campbell, I.C. (1988) An examination of experimental design in relation to receptor binding assays. *British Journal of Pharmacology* **94**, 693–698.

Ettenberg, A. (1989) Dopamine, neuroleptics and reinforced behavior. *Pharmacology Biochemistry and Behavior* **13**, 105–111.

Ettenberg, A. and Camp, C.H. (1986a) Haloperidol induces a partial reinforcement extinction effect in rats: implications for a dopamine involvement in food reward. *Pharmacology Biochemistry and Behavior* **25**, 818–821.

Ettenberg, A. and Camp, C.H. (1986b) A partial reinforcement extinction effect in water-reinforced rats intermittently treated with haloperidol. *Pharmacology Biochemistry and Behavior* **25**, 1231–1235.

Ettenberg, A. and Carlisle, H. (1985) Neuroleptic-induced deficits in operant responding for temperature reinforcement. *Pharmacology Biochemistry and Behavior* **22**, 761–767.

Ettenberg, A., Koob, G.F. and Bloom, F.E. (1981) Response artifact in the measurement of neuroleptic-induced anhedonia. *Science* **209**, 357–359.

Fibiger, H.C., Carter, D.A. and Phillips, A.G. (1976) Decreased intracranial self-stimulation after neuroleptics or 6-hydroxydopamine: evidence for mediation by motor deficits rather than reduced reward. *Psychopharmacology* **47**, 21–27.

Finlay, J.M., Szostak, C. and Fibiger, H.C. (1989) Further characterization of intravenous self-administration of midazolam in the rat. *Behavioural Pharmacology* **1**, 13–24.

Fouriezos, G. and Wise, R.A. (1976) Pimozide-induced extinction of intra-cranial self-stimulation: response patterns rule out motor performance deficits. *Brain Research* **103**, 377–380.

Fouriezos, G., Hansson, P. and Wise, R.A. (1978) Neuroleptic-induced attenuation of brain stimulation reward. *Journal of Comparative and Physiological Psychology* **92**, 659–669.

Fowler, S.C. (1990) Neuroleptics produce within-session response decrements: facts and theories. *Drug Development Research* **20**, 101–116.

Fowler, S.C. and Kirkpatrick, M.A. (1989) Behavior-decrementing effects of low doses of haloperidol result from disruptions in response force and duration. *Behavioural Pharmacology* **1**, 123–132.

Fowler, S.C., LaCerra, M.M. and Ettenberg, A. (1986a) Effects of haloperidol on the biophysical characteristics of operant responding: implications for motor and reinforcement processes. *Pharmacology Biochemistry and Behavior* **25**, 791–796.

Fowler, S.C., Gramling, S.E. and Laio, R.M. (1986b) Effects of pimozide on emitted force, duration and rate of operant responding maintained at high and low levels of required force. *Pharmacology Biochemistry and Behavior* **25**, 615–622.

Franklin, K.B. and McCoy, S.H. (1979) Pimozide-induced extinction in rats: stimulus control of responding rules out motor deficit. *Pharmacology Biochemistry and Behavior* **11**, 71–75.

Gallistel, C.R., Boytim, M., Gomita, Y. and Klebanoff, L. (1982) Does pimozide block the rewarding effect of brain stimulation. *Pharmacology Biochemistry and Behavior* **17**, 769–781.

Geary, N. and Smith, G.P. (1985) Pimozide decreases the reinforcing effect of sham-fed sucrose in the rat. *Pharmacology Biochemistry and Behavior* **22**, 787–790.

Gerber, G.J., Sing, J. and Wise, R.A. (1981) Pimozide attenuates lever pressing for water in rats. *Pharmacology Biochemistry and Behavior* **14**, 201–205.

Gramling, S.E., Fowler, S.C. and Collins, K.R. (1984) Some effects of pimozide on nondeprived rats licking sucrose solutions in an anhedonia paradigm. *Pharmacology Biochemistry and Behavior* **21**, 617–624.

Gray, T. and Wise, R.A. (1980) Effects of pimozide on lever-pressing behaviour maintained on an intermittent reinforcement schedule. *Pharmacology Biochemistry and Behavior* **12**, 931–935.

Hamilton, A.L., Stellar, J.R. and Hart, E.B. (1985) Reward, performance, and the response-strength method in self-stimulating rats: validation and neuroleptics. *Physiology and Behavior* **35**, 897–904.

Herrnstein, R.J. (1970) On the law of effect. *Journal of the Experimental Analysis of Behavior* **13**, 243–266.

Heyman, G.M. (1983) A parametric evaluation of the hedonic and motoric effects of drugs: pimozide and amphetamine. *Journal of the Experimental Analysis of Behavior* **40**, 113–122.

Heyman, G.M. and Monaghan, M.M. (1987) Effects of changes in response requirement and deprivation on the parameters of the matching law equation: new data and review. *Journal of Experimental Psychology: Animal Behavior Processes* **13**, 384–394.

Heyman, G.M., Kinzie, D.L. and Seiden, L.S. (1986) Chlorpromazine and pimozide alter reinforcement efficacy and motor performance. *Psychopharmacology* **88**, 346–353.

Hillegaert, V., Ahlenius, S., Magnusson, O. and Fowler, C.J. (1987) Repeated testing of rats markedly enhances the duration of effects produced by haloperidol on treadmill locomotion, catalepsy and a conditional avoidance response. *Pharmacology Biochemistry and Behavior* **27**, 159–164.

Horvitz, J.C. and Ettenberg, A. (1988) Haloperidol blocks the response-reinstating effects of food reward: a methodology for separating neuroleptic effects on reinforcement and motor processes. *Pharmacology Biochemistry and Behavior* **31**, 861–865.

Iversen, S.D. (1977) Brain dopamine systems and behaviour. In: Iversen, L.L., Iversen, S.D. and Snyder, S.H. (eds) *Handbook of Psychopharmacology, Vol. 8.* New York: Plenum, pp. 333–384.

Kurimaya, S. and Nakajima, S. (1988) Dopamine D1 receptors in the nucleus accumbens: involvement on the reinforcing effect of tegmental stimulation. *Brain Research* **448**, 1–6.

Mackintosh, N.J. (1974) *The Psychology of Animal Learning.* London: Academic Press.

Martin-Iverson, M.T., Wilkie, D. and Fibiger, H.C. (1987) Effects of haloperidol and d-amphetamine on perceived quantity of food and tones. *Psychopharmacology* **93**, 374–381.

Mason, S.T., Beninger, R.J., Fibiger, H.C. and Phillips, H.C. (1980) Pimozide induced suppression of responding: evidence against a block of food reward. *Pharmacology Biochemistry and Behavior* **12**, 917–923.

Morgan, M.J. (1974) Resistance to extinction. *Animal Behavior* **22**, 449–466.

Morley, M.J., Bradshaw, C.M. and Szabadi, E. (1984) The effects of pimozide on variable-interval performance: a test of the anhedonia hypothesis of the mode of action of neuroleptics. *Psychopharmacology* **84**, 531–536.

Muscat, R. and Willner, P. (1989) Effects of selective dopamine receptor antagonists on sucrose consumption and preference. *Psychopharmacology* **99**, 98–102.

Olds, J. and Travis, R.P. (1960) Effects of chlorpromazine, meprobamate, pentobarbital and morphine on self-stimulation. *Journal of Pharmacology and Experimental Therapeutics* **128**, 397–404.

Phillips, G., Muscat, R. and Willner, P. (1989a) Dopamine blockade can increase rewarded behaviour. I. Consumption of very sweet solutions. *Behavioural Pharmacology* ? 14 (suppl 1).

Phillips, G., Muscat, R. and Willner, P. (1989b) Dopamine blockade can increase rewarded behaviour. II. Operant responding for very sweet pellets. *Behavioural Pharmacology* **1**, 14 (suppl 1).

Phillips, G., Willner, P., Sampson, D., Nunn, J. and Muscat, R. (1990) Time-, schedule- and reinforcer-dependent effects of pimozide and amphetamine. *Psychopharmacology* (in press).

Rolls, E.T., Rolls, B.J., Kelly, P.H., Shaw, S.G., Wood, R.J. and Dale, R.I. (1974) The relative attenuation of self-stimulation, eating and drinking produced by dopamine-receptor blockade. *Psychopharmacologia* **38**, 219–230.

Sanger, D.J. (1986) Response decrement patterns after neuroleptic and non-neuroleptic drugs. *Psychopharmacology* **89**, 125–130.

Schneider, L.H., Gibbs, J. and Smith, G.P. (1986) Selective D1 or D2 antagonists inhibit sucrose sham feeding in rats. *Appetite* **7**, 294–295.

Sclafani, A. and Clyne, A.E. (1987) Hedonic responses of rats to polysaccharide and sugar concentrations. *Neuroscience and Biobehavioral Reviews* **11**, 173–180.

Skjoldager, P. and Fowler, S.C. (1988) Effects of pimozide, across doses and within sessions, on discriminated lever release performance in rats. *Psychopharmacology* **96**, 21–28.

Spence, K.W. (1956) *Behavior Theory and Conditioning*. New Haven: Yale University Press.

Tombaugh, T.N., Anisman, H. and Tombaugh, J. (1980) Extinction and dopamine receptor blockade after intermittent reinforcement training: failure to find functional equivalence. *Psychopharmacology* **70**, 19–28.

Willner, P., Towell, A. and Muscat, R. (1987) Effects of amphetamine and pimozide on reinforcement and motor parameters in variable interval performance. *Journal of Psychopharmacology* **1**, 140–153.

Willner, P. and Phillips, G. (1989) Two tests of the motor activation hypothesis of neuroleptic-induced response deficit. *Behavioural Pharmacology* **1**, 20 (suppl. 1).

Willner, P., Chawla, K., Sampson, D., Sophokleous, S. and Muscat, R. (1988) Tests of functional equivalence between pimozide pretreatment, extinction and free feeding. *Psychopharmacology* **95**, 423–426.

Willner, P., Phillips, G. and Muscat, R. (1989) Time-dependent and schedule-dependent effects of dopamine receptor blockade. *Behavioural Pharmacology* **1**, 169–176.

Willner, P., Sampson, D., Phillips, G. and Muscat, R. (1990a) A matching law analysis of the effects of dopamine receptor antagonists. *Psychopharmacology* **101**, 560–567.

Willner, P., Papp, M., Phillips, G., Maleeh, M. and Muscat, R. (1990b) Pimozide does not impair sweetness discrimination. *Psychopharmacology* **102**, 278–282.

Wise, R.A. (1982) Neuroleptics and operant behavior: the anhedonia hypothesis. *Behavioral and Brain Sciences* **5**, 39–87.

Wise, R.A. (1987) Intravenous drug self-administration: a special case of positive reinforcement. In: Bozarth, M.A. (ed.) *Methods of Assessing the Reinforcing Properties of Abused Drugs*. New York: Springer, pp. 117–141.

Wise, R.A., Spindler, J., De Wit, H. and Gerber, G.J. (1978) Neuroleptic-induced 'anhedonia' in rats: pimozide blocks the reward quality of food. *Science* **201**, 262–264.

Xenakis, S. and Sclafani, A. (1981) The effects of pimozide on the consumption of a palatable saccharin-glucose solution in the rat. *Pharmacology Biochemistry and Behavior* **15**, 435–442.

Yokel, R.A. (1987) Intravenous self-administration: response rates, the effects of pharmacological challenges, and drug preferences. In: Bozarth, M.A. (ed.) *Methods of Assessing the Reinforcing Properties of Abused Drugs*. New York: Springer, pp. 1–33.

Young, P.T. and Greene, J.T. (1953) Quantity of food ingested as a measure of relative acceptability. *Journal of Comparative and Physiological Psychology* **46**, 288–294.

11

Receptor Subtype-Specific Dopamine Agonists and Antagonists and Conditioned Behaviour

RICHARD J. BENINGER

Department of Psychology, Queen's University, Kingston,
Canada K7L 3N6

INTRODUCTION

There is good evidence that dopamine (DA) may play a critical role in reward-related incentive learning (Beninger, 1983). This type of learning involves the acquisition of the ability to elicit approach and other responses by reward-associated stimuli. For example, when a rat receives a food reward for pressing a lever, an increase in lever pressing is observed. This can be understood as a consequence of the effects of food reward on the lever-associated stimuli, increasing their ability to elicit responses. Such conditioned stimuli are defined as incentive stimuli. Many data implicate DA in this learning process.

In recent years, the availability of pharmacological compounds that are relatively specific for subtypes of the DA receptor has progressively increased to the point where there are several agonists and antagonists to choose from for both the D1 and the D2 receptor (Clark and White, 1987; Waddington and O'Boyle, 1989). This has made possible the evaluation of the role of receptor subtypes in functions previously found to be mediated by DA, including reward-related learning (Beninger, 1983; Wise, 1982, 1989a).

Interpretation of the results of behavioural studies of the possible involvement of DA in reward has been widely debated (Ettenberg, 1989; Liebman and Cooper, 1989; Willner et al., Chapter 10, this volume). This

The Mesolimbic Dopamine System: From Motivation to Action.
Edited by P. Willner and J. Scheel-Krüger

© 1991 John Wiley & Sons Ltd

debate reflects the historical problem of distinguishing between performance versus learning effects in physiological psychology (Beninger, 1989a), and the fact that DA is clearly involved in the control of unconditioned locomotor activity (Beninger, 1983). However, there have been numerous convincing demonstrations that DA is involved in the rewarding effects of brain stimulation reward (Phillips and Fibiger, 1989; Schizgal and Murray, 1989; Steller and Rice, 1989), drugs (Carr et al., 1989; Hoffman, 1989; Katz, 1989; Koob and Goeders, 1989) and natural reinforcers such as food (Ettenberg, 1989; Bradshaw and Szabadi, 1989; Willner et al., Chapter 10, this volume). The following review will include studies of behavioural paradigms previously shown to allow a dissociation of reward from performance effects.

This chapter will be concerned with a review of the results of behavioural studies that report the effects of D1 or D2 receptor-specific compounds in paradigms assessing reward-related learning. This will be followed by a review of a range of data from the neurosciences which suggest the hypothesis that the D1 receptor may be critically involved in this type of learning (Miller et al., 1990). The hypothesis will then be evaluated in the light of the behavioural data.

D1 ANTAGONISTS AND REWARD-RELATED LEARNING

It has been shown the the D1 antagonist SCH 23390 blocks the rewarding effects of self-administered cocaine in rats; rates were elevated in a dose-related manner similar to the elevations in rate seen following decreases in the concentration of cocaine (Koob et al., 1987). Woolverton (1986) failed to see a similar elevation of rate of self-administration following treatment with SCH 23390 in three of four monkeys tested. However, only three of five monkeys given the D2 receptor blocker pimozide showed the typical pattern of dose-dependent increases in responding. The reasons for the discrepancies between the results of these two studies are not clear and further studies are needed. It has been reported that rats will self-administer cocaine or amphetamine directly into the frontal cortex (Phillips et al., 1981; Goeders et al., 1986) and Goeders et al. (1986) have reported that this effect was not blocked by co-administration of SCH 23390 although it was blocked by a D2 antagonist. This result may reflect a differential involvement of D1 receptors in the frontal cortex versus elsewhere in mediating the effects of reward on behaviour. However, additional studies are clearly needed.

In place-preference studies it has recently been shown that SCH 23390 dose-dependently blocked learning produced by amphetamine (Figure 1) (Leone and DiChiara, 1987; Hoffman and Beninger, 1989a). Hoffman and Beninger (1989a) reported that SCH 23390 produced no place-preference or aversion when administered on its own; others, however, have reported

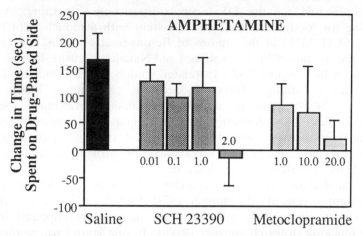

Figure 1. The effects of SCH 23390 or metoclopramide on place conditioning produced by (+)-amphetamine. The experiments consisted of three phases. During the pre-exposure phase, male Wistar rats explored two distinctive compartments (38 × 27 × 36 cm) joined by a small tunnel for 15 minutes on each of 3 days. The compartments differed in brightness, pattern and floor texture, and the amount of time spent in each compartment was recorded. During the 8-day conditioning phase, separate groups of rats were treated (i.p.) with amphetamine (2.0 mg/kg) preceded 1 hour earlier with saline, SCH 23390 (0.01, 0.1, 1.0, or 2.0 mg/kg) or metoclopramide (1.0, 10.0 or 20.0 mg/kg), and were confined to one compartment for 30 minutes. On alternate days rats received saline and were placed in the opposite compartment. The postconditioning test occurred on the following day during which drug-free animals explored both compartments for 15 minutes and the time spent on each side was recorded. The mean (±SEM) difference score for each group is presented. The difference scores were calculated by subtracting the time spent on the drug-paired side during the pre-exposure session (averaged over the 3 days) from the test-day. Thus, a positive score suggests a preference, whereas a negative score suggests an aversion for the drug-paired environment. Doses are indicated in mg/kg under each bar. From Hoffman and Beninger (1989a)

place aversions with SCH 23390 alone (Shippenberg and Herz, 1987). In studies of opiate receptor subtypes in place conditioning, SCH 23390 blocked the reward effects of the μ-opiate agonist morphine (Leone and DiChiara, 1987; Shippenberg and Herz, 1987), and, furthermore, also blocked place aversions produced by a κ-opiate agonist (Shippenberg and Herz, 1987). As opiate-mediated incentive learning has been shown to involve DA in the brain (Bozarth, 1986; Wise, 1989a, b; Wise and Rompre, 1989; Cooper, Chapter 13, this volume), these data suggest that DA may produce its learning effects, at least in part, via the D1 receptor.

Treatments with SCH 23390 of animals performing operant responses for various rewards (Nakajima, 1989) have quite consistently produced results supporting a role for the D1 receptor in incentive learning. Animals responding for food showed effects consistent with a reduction of reward following SCH 23390 in the studies of Beninger et al. (1987) (Figure 2), Willner et al. (Chapter 10, this volume) and Nakajima (1986), but this effect was not seen by Sanger (1987). In related studies, SCH 23390 significantly reduced the rewarding effects of saccharin (Nakajima, 1986), water (Nakajima, 1986) or brain stimulation (Nakajima and McKenzie, 1986). In a well-controlled study, Kurumiya and Nakajima (1988) recently reported that brain stimulation reward from the region of the dopaminergic cell bodies in the ventral tegmentum was reduced by intra-accumbens injections of SCH 23390 ipsilateral to the electrode.

Conditioned avoidance learning is a classic paradigm for studying negative reinforcement or reward (Mackintosh, 1974; Hineline, 1977). This is another paradigm that involves incentive learning and that is impaired by DA receptor blocking drugs (Beninger, 1989b). In one study, where the intra- or inter-session effects of SCH 23390 on the maintenance of a pretrained avoidance response were investigated, no evidence of a reduction in reward

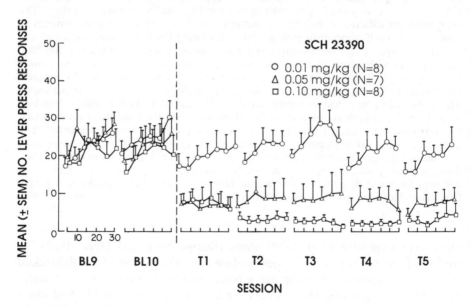

Figure 2. Effects of SCH 23390 on lever pressing for food reward. Data show the mean (±SEM) responses per minute for 5-minute segments of the last two of ten 30-minute baseline training sessions (BL9 and BL10) on a variable interval 30-second schedule, and five test sessions (T1–T5). Two hours before each test-session groups received injections of SCH 23390 in doses of 0.01, 0.05 or 0.1 mg/kg s.c. SCH 23390 produced a significant dose-dependent decrease in responding, and the high doses produced a significant within session effect on responding. From Beninger et al. (1987)

was observed although response reductions consistent with a motor effect of the drug were seen (Sanger, 1987). This was the only study to have specifically investigated possible reward-reducing effects of a D1 antagonist in an avoidance paradigm. Others have reported that SCH 23390 or the D1 antagonist SCH 39166 impaired pretrained avoidance in rats or monkeys (Iorio et al., 1983; Gerhardt et al., 1985; Chipkin et al., 1988). In these studies it was reported that avoidance responding was reduced at some doses that minimally affected escape responding, suggesting that the effects of the drugs may not have been simply motor. However, further studies are needed before any conclusions can be drawn about the effects of D1 antagonists on negative reward in avoidance paradigms.

It has been argued previously that conditioned activity effects seen in animals injected with saline and placed in an environment previously associated with injections of a stimulant drug, e.g. amphetamine, can be understood as an example of incentive learning (Beninger, 1983; Beninger et al., 1989). The establishment of these effects has been shown to depend on DA (Beninger and Hahn, 1983; Beninger and Herz, 1986); it has also been found that the establishment of amphetamine-produced conditioned activity is blocked by co-treatment with SCH 23390 during conditioning sessions (Mazurski and Beninger, in preparation). When sensitization to a stimulant effect can be shown to follow repeated injections in a particular environment (Stewart and Vezina, 1988; Post et al., Chapter 17, this volume), this phenomenon, like conditioned activity, can also be understood as an example of incentive learning. Thus, stimuli associated with the test environment become conditioned incentive stimuli which acquire an enhanced ability to elicit approach and other responses, and this effect adds to the unconditioned effects of the drug producing the sensitized response. Note that the sensitized response to the drug is only seen in the test environment, supporting this analysis. Recently, Vezina and Stewart (1989) reported that sensitization produced by amphetamine was blocked by co-administration of SCH 23390. This result, and the finding that the D1 antagonist blocked the establishment of conditioned activity, suggest that D1 receptors may participate in the establishment of incentive learning.

An additional finding that may be relevant to the current discussion is the recent report by Koechling et al. (1988) that SCH 23390 increased latencies to initiate feeding. Food was periodically presented on a small automated platter. Latencies increased progressively over testing with the drug but there were still instances when latencies of the drugged rats were as fast as those seen in undrugged animals. The authors argued from this that the drug was not simply reducing performance capacity. From an incentive learning point of view, during training of this task, stimuli associated with the food presentation (e.g. the platter, click of the automated equipment, etcetera) would become conditioned incentive stimuli, acquiring an enhanced ability to elicit approach responses in the (undrugged) animals. During testing with the D1 antagonist, if the usual reward effects of the food were blocked, these incentive stimuli would gradually lose their ability to elicit approach responses, and latencies would lengthen progressively. The elegant approach of the authors, allowing the observation of some peak latencies in the drugged rats and the progressive nature of the drug effect, makes simple motor interpretations of the data difficult to support.

In summary, the effects of D1 receptor antagonists have been assessed in a number of paradigms that may involve reward-related DA-mediated incentive learning. These include stimulant self-administration, place-preference conditioning, operant conditioning rewarded with food, water, saccharin or brain stimulation, conditioned activity or sensitization, avoidance conditioning and conditioned approach to a feeder. In every case, perhaps with the exception of avoidance conditioning where more studies are needed, good evidence that a D1 antagonist could block reward-related learning was found.

D1 AGONISTS AND REWARD-RELATED LEARNING

It is perhaps worth noting here that all studies reviewed in this section use the partial D1 agonist, SKF 38393. Although a full D1-specific agonist is now available (Waddington and O'Boyle, 1989), no studies evaluating its effects in conditioning paradigms have yet appeared. However, preliminary studies of the effects of this new compound on unconditioned behaviours reveal results similar to those of SKF 38393 (Waddington et al., 1988). It will be especially interesting to compare the results of studies with full D1 agonists eventually to those reviewed here.

In self-administration studies it has been reported that the D1 agonist SKF 38393 was not self-administered by monkeys (Woolverton et al., 1984). This can be contrasted with agonists such as cocaine or D2-specific agonists that were self-administered (Woolverton et al., 1984; Woolverton 1986). The D2 agonists are discussed below.

In place conditioning studies it has been reported that SKF 38393 did not produce place-preferences in experiments where significant effects were seen with non-specific or D2 agonists (Gilbert et al., 1986; Hoffman and Beninger, 1988). In fact, Hoffman and Beninger (1988) found that SKF 38393 produced a significant place aversion (Figure 3)!

Animals trained in an operant learning situation for food reward showed a disruption of responding when injected with SKF 38393 (Hoffman and Beninger, 1989b). However, in the same study, animals treated with amphetamine or a D2 agonist showed a similar disruption. It is unclear how to interpret these data in the present context.

Using a different approach, Beninger (in preparation) investigated the

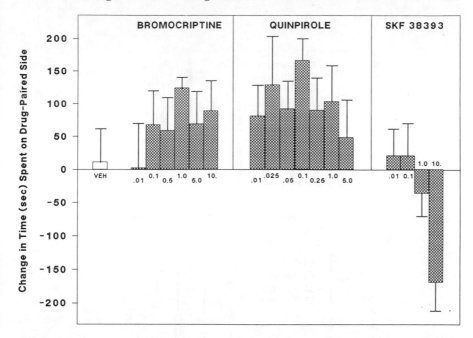

Figure 3. Place conditioning with bromocriptine, quinpirole and SKF 38393. The details of the place conditioning experiment are described in the caption for Figure 1. On conditioning days, individual groups of rats received injections (i.p.) of saline (VEH) or drug in the doses (mg/kg) indicated below or above each bar. The mean difference score for each group is presented. The calculation of these scores is described in the caption for Figure 1. Adapted from Hoffman and Beninger (1988) and Hoffman et al. (1988)

effects of D1- or D2-specific DA agonists on the acquisition of responding for conditioned reward. A lights-off stimulus was repeatedly paired with food when the animals were drug-free, and was then subsequently used to reward acquisition of pressing one of two levers in conditioned reward tests carried out when the animals were drugged. Whereas amphetamine or D2 agonists differentially enhanced responding on the lever producing conditioned reward, SKF 38393 did not enhance responding and impaired, in a dose-related fashion, differential responding on the lever producing conditioned reward. Apomorphine, although producing an overall enhancement in responding, also led to an impairment in differential responding for conditioned reward (Figures 4 and 5) (for further discussion see Beninger et al., 1989).

One recent result might be seen to be inconsistent with these data. Mazurski and Beninger (in preparation) observed conditioned activity in rats having received a number of pairings of SKF 38393 with a particular

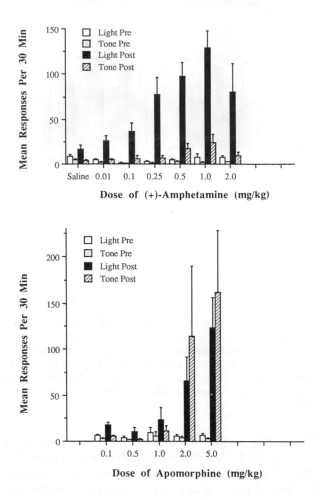

Figure 4. Differential effects of amphetamine and apomorphine on the acquisition of responding for conditioned reward. Rats received three phases of training in a two-lever chamber. The pre-exposure phase measured the rates of pressing the levers; one produced a 3-second tone and the other turned the lights off for 3 seconds. In the conditioning phase, with the levers absent, the light-off stimulus was paired with food for four sessions. The test phase again measured the rate of pressing the levers. Conditioned reward was shown by a relative increase in responding on the light-off lever during the test. Separate groups of male Wistar rats were treated (i.p.) with amphetamine or apomorphine before the test-session. The mean (±SEM) number of responses on each lever during the pre-exposure and test-phases are presented

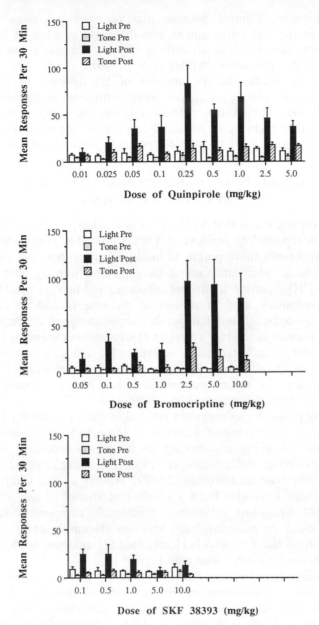

Figure 5. Effects of quinpirole, bromocriptine and SKF 38393 on the acquisition of responding for conditioned reward. The mean (±SEM) number of presses on the tone and light-off lever during the pre-exposure and test-phases are presented. For a description of the procedure, see the caption of Figure 4.

test environment. Control animals that received the same number of exposures to the test environment and the same number of injections of drug did not show conditioned activity. This effect was replicated several times. It awaits explanation (Miller et al., 1990).

In summary, studies of the abilities of D1 agonists to support self-administration or place-preferences were consistent in finding that these compounds were not effective. These findings are in agreement with the observation that SKF 38393 impaired responding for conditioned reward. On the other hand, a D1 agonist did produce conditioned activity.

D2 AGONISTS AND ANTAGONISTS AND REWARD-RELATED LEARNING

The basis for the claim that SCH 23390 is a selective D1 antagonist is the observation, reported by Iorio et al. (1983), that this compound was in the order of 1000 times more potent in inhibiting by 50 per cent the ability of DA to stimulate adenylate cyclase than in inhibiting by 50 per cent the binding of [^{3}H]spiperone to striatal membranes. Many of the DA receptor blockers extensively used in studies of the role of DA in reward, e.g. pimozide, spiroperidol and haloperidol, over the past 20 years have the opposite potencies in the two assays of DA receptors (Seeman, 1981). Thus, if SCH 23390 is accepted as a selective D1 antagonist it would seem appropriate to identify pimozide, spiroperidol and haloperidol as selective D2 antagonists. In recent papers, this has become common practice (Woolverton, 1986; Koechling et al., 1988).

Accepting pimozide, spiroperidol and haloperidol as selective D2 antagonists makes an undertaking of a review of the effects of D2 antagonists on reward-related learning unnecessary as it has been done many times in recent years (Wise, 1982; Beninger, 1983; Ettenberg, 1989; Liebman and Cooper, 1989; Wise and Rompre, 1989; Willner et al., Chapter 10, this volume). There have also been a number of studies of the effects of the selective D2 antagonist substituted benzamide compounds (Jenner and Marsden, 1981) on reward-related learning (Beninger et al., 1989). The conclusion from these reviews is clearly that D2 antagonists block the usual effects of reward on behaviour (see Figure 1).

Some studies have investigated the possibility that D2 agonists may have rewarding effects. In general, results have shown that they do. Thus, the D2 agonists piribedil and bromocriptine were self-administered by monkeys (Woolverton et al., 1984; Woolverton, 1986). Place-preference conditioning has been reported following pairings of the D2 agonists bromocriptine, quinpirole or N-0437 with a specific environment (see Figure 3) (Gilbert et al., 1986; Hoffman and Beninger, 1988, 1989a; Hoffman et al., 1988), and Morency and Beninger (1986) reported this effect following intracerebroventricular injections of bromocriptine in rats. Quinpirole decreased operant responding (Hoffman and Beninger, 1989b); however, as already discussed, the same effect was seen with amphetamine or SKF 38393, making interpretation of these results in the present context difficult. When the effects of quinpirole or bromocriptine on the acquisition of operant responding for conditioned reward were assessed, a dose-dependent enhancement was seen (Figure 5) (Beninger, in preparation). Finally, quinpirole produced conditioned activity (Mazurski and Beninger, in preparation). In general, these effects are suggestive of a role for D2 receptors in reward.

D1 RECEPTOR AS A POSSIBLE MEDIATOR OF INCENTIVE LEARNING

There may be good reason for suspecting that the D1 receptor subtype is specifically involved in reward-related learning (Miller et al., 1990). D1 receptors activate the enzyme adenylate cyclase that, in turn, stimulates the formation of the cyclic nucleotide, cyclic 3′, 5′ adenosine monophosphate (AMP) (Kebabian et al., 1972). There has been considerable interest in the possibility that second messengers, including cyclic AMP, may be involved in the storage of information that underlies learning and memory (Greengard and Kuo, 1970: for a recent review see Matthies, 1989).

In recent years, huge advances in our understanding of the possible molecular mechanisms underlying memory have been made. In a recent review, for example, Schwartz and Greenberg (1987) discussed three protein kinases that may participate in memory formation. The cascade of events that follows the binding of DA to the D1 receptor leads to the activation of cyclic AMP-dependent protein kinase; this kinase, in turn, leads to protein modifications that may participate in the molecular mechanisms underlying the consolidation of memory (Schwartz and Greenberg, 1987). The actual proteins involved in the formation of memory remain to be specified. However, there is intense research activity directed at identifying changes in proteins associated with stimulation of D1 receptors, and steady advances are being made. For example, the studies of Greengard and his associates (Walaas et al., 1983; Hemmings et al., 1984, 1987) have revealed a DA- and cAMP-regulated phosphoprotein in the brain. Researchers studying long-term potentiation of the hippocampus have similarly identified a protein kinase and membrane protein associated with memory in this model (Akers et al., 1986; Lovinger et al., 1986). Results to date strongly suggest that activation of D1 receptors may lead to a cascade of molecular events which eventually produce the structural basis of memory.

There is a related line of study that also points to the D1 receptor as the possible mediator of learning produced by DA. In a now classic paper, Libet et al. (1975) demonstrated that DA could produce lóng-term enhancement of the muscarinic cholinergic response in the rabbit superior cervical ganglion. They suggested that this constituted a form of memory (for further discussion see Libet, 1984). In more recent studies, Libet and his co-workers have shown that this DA-mediated memory effect required the stimulation of D1 receptors; thus the effect was blocked by the D1 antagonist SCH 23390, but not by the D2 antagonists sulpiride or domperidone (Mochida et al., 1987). Using a hippocampal slice preparation, Gribkoff and Ashe (1984) and Stein and Belluzzi (1989) have shown a similar DA-mediated modulation of the excitability of CA1 cells. Although the substrate proteins mediating the changes in these models remain to be identified, the results combine with those of molecular studies to point to the D1 receptor as a good candidate for mediating DA-related learning.

Some theorists have recognized the potential of the results of Libet et al. (1975) in the understanding of the neuronal organization that may underlie the action of DA in memory consolidation. As early as 1978, Routtenberg and Kim proposed that nigroneostriatal dopaminergic projections may modulate muscarinic synaptic effectiveness via DA receptors linked to adenylate cyclase. Beninger (1983) similarly drew on the findings of Libet et al. (1975) to suggest that, when reward-related learning occurs, it might be the action of DA at D1 receptors in the striatum (i.e. the caudate, putamen, nucleus accumbens and olfactory tubercle; Heimer and Wilson, 1975) that may mediate changes in cholinergic synaptic effectiveness that form the substrate of the memory. D1 receptor stimulation would presumably lead to the formation of cyclic AMP, the activation of protein kinases, and the eventual phosphorylation of proteins leading to changes in synaptic effectiveness.

One aspect of the model developed by Beninger (1983) involved the assumption that DA would act to modify only muscarinic synapses that were most recently active. According to the model, specific stimuli, for example from the environment, would lead to the activation of specific subsets of cortical cells and therefore specific subsets of corticostriatal fibres (see Grofova (1979) for a review of the extrinsic connections of the striatum and Viaud and White (1989) for a related discussion; see also Groenewegen et al., Chapter 2, this volume). These fibres would, in turn, activate specific subsets of cholinergic neurons intrinsic to the striatum. When reward occurs and the dopaminergic neurons are activated (Keller et al., 1983; Phillips et al., 1989), there would be a fairly diffuse release of DA (the DA signal) in the striatum (McGeer et al., 1978). However, only the synapses of the most recently active neurons, representing the most recently encountered stimuli, would undergo the DA-mediated modification in synaptic effectiveness. Thus, a diffuse DA signal would effectively select the most recently active synapses to modify.

The results of recent highly sophisticated studies using *in vivo* voltammetry to assess the effects of reward on DA levels in the striatum (including the nucleus accumbens) bear importantly on the model under development (Phillips et al., Chapter 8, this volume). Perhaps the most crucial finding is that DA levels have not been observed to rise immediately after unsignalled food reward but only after a considerable delay. In fact, in one of the experiments reported by Phillips et al. (this volume), the first presentation of a palatable liquid diet was not followed by increases in DA levels at all, even after a delay! Do these results indicate that there is not a DA signal associated with reward?

Such a conclusion may not be necessary for the following reasons. There is a wealth of data, some of which is reviewed here, showing that the establishment of reward-related incentive learning fails to occur in animals undergoing conditioning trials while dopaminergic neurotransmission is blocked; this has been seen, for example, in lever pressing for food (Tombaugh et al., 1979; Wise and Schwartz, 1981), avoidance learning (Beninger et al., 1980), place conditioning based on food (Spyraki et al., 1982), establishment of conditioned reward based on food (Beninger and Phillips, 1980; Hoffman and Beninger, 1985), and establishment of conditioned activity (Beninger and Hahn, 1983; Beninger and Herz, 1986), all examples of incentive learning (Beninger, 1983). Thus, DA seems to play an important role in the establishment of incentive learning.

A reconciliation of these findings with the *in vivo* voltammetric data reported by Phillips et al. (Chapter 8, this volume), showing a delayed onset of action of feeding on DA levels, may be possible. In this regard it may be useful to note the differential rate of acquisition in some tasks involving incentive learning. Thus, responding for brain stimulation reward (BSR) is acquired extremely rapidly, especially with electrodes in the ventral tegmental area (VTA). Similarly, responding in one-way conditioned avoidance paradigms is acquired extremely rapidly, usually in less than five trials (Levis, 1989). By comparison, acquisition of lever pressing for food is slow; usually a session of magazine training precedes one or two sessions of response shaping. Results of *in vivo* voltammetric experiments have shown that the increases in DA levels following VTA BSR are very rapid (Phillips et al., 1989), and electric shock has been shown to produce rapid onset of increased DA levels (D'Angio et al., 1988; Keller et al., 1983), but, as already mentioned, the onset of effects of unsignalled food on DA levels is slow (Phillips et al., Chapter 8, this volume). Perhaps this apparent relationship between the rate of acquisition of tasks involving incentive learning, and the immediacy of the effects of different types of reward on increases in DA levels, may provide a basis for reconciling the observation that, while DA appears to play an important role in the establishment of incentive learning, food reward has a delayed effect on DA release (Phillips et al., Chapter 8, this volume). The data reported here by Phillips et al. clearly show that delayed increases in DA levels follow unsignalled food, and that immediate increases occur during conditioned stimuli that signal food. As the acquisition of responding for food is relatively slow, perhaps during the period of acquisition, the peak increase in DA levels slowly shifts from some time during the postingestive period of the meal towards the onset of the meal, and is finally elicited by the stimuli that signal food. Such a pattern was seen in some experiments described by Phillips et al. (Phillips, personal communication).

Why was no DA increase seen on the first day of eating the palatable liquid diet? Only speculation is possible. Perhaps, on the first occasion of a novel food, no reward mechanism is engaged until the postprandial effects of the meal are assessed, assuring that the food is not toxic. The well-documented observation of taste aversion learning following a substantial delay between ingestion and illness is consistent with this suggestion. If no toxic effects ensue, the next ingestion of the food may lead to a delayed increase in DA levels that may act to produce incentive learning to taste cues, for example, and, as acquisition continues, other preingestion cues may become conditioned incentive stimuli. (The results of Koechling et al. (1988), discussed above, may reflect the gradual loss of this conditioning with repeated exposure to food while DA receptors are blocked.)

Whether or not the mechanisms being proposed here eventually prove correct, it is important to note that the acquisition by neutral stimuli of conditioned incentive properties, and of the ability to stimulate increases in DA levels (Phillips et al., Chapter 8, this volume), involves a plastic change in the brain. The mechanism proposed here provides a means by which this learning might take place. Thus, a diffuse DA signal associated with the presentation of rewarding stimuli might alter synapses most recently activated by environmental stimuli signalling reward.

The notion of selective modification by a diffuse signal has been suggested by others. For example, in a recent paper, Miller (1988) suggested that the most recently active synapses go into a 'state of readiness' whereby they are primed for modification if the appropriate signal arrives. He credited Hebb (1949) with the origin of this basic idea. From a somewhat different orientation, researchers interested in computational models of learning have developed the concept of a diffusely projecting reward system that would only strengthen connections that happen to be active at that moment (Donahoe and Palmer, 1989).

The hypothesis that a diffuse DA signal might modify only the most recently active synapses has, at least, heuristic value for understanding some of the behavioural effects of D1 agonists, as reviewed below. How might the most recently active synapses be selected for modification? A number of investigators have reported that electrically- or K^+-evoked DA release is modulated by presynaptic muscarinic (de Belleroche and Gardiner, 1982; Lehmann and Langer, 1982; Raiteri et al., 1982) or perhaps nicotinic cholinergic receptors (Giorguieff-Chesselet et al., 1979). Such a modulation could have the effect of producing a relatively greater increase in the local concentrations of DA when diffuse dopaminergic activity putatively increases as a result of a rewarding stimulus being encountered. This might enhance the local stimulation of cyclic AMP formation and thus produce the largest modification in cholinergic synaptic effectiveness at the cholinergic synapses that have been most recently active.

The model for DA-mediated learning proposed by Beninger (1983) hypothesized that the locus of synaptic modifications was muscarinic cholinergic synapses in the striatum. This was a direct application of the elements of the Libet et al. (1975) finding in the peripheral nervous system to the central nervous system. It was appealing because the main elements of the Libet et al. (1975) model, namely, efferent cells receiving both cholinergic and dopaminergic afferents, and having both muscarinic and D1 receptors, could be found in the striatum. However, cholinergic cells in the striatum are relatively rare (Bolam, 1984). Although I know of no current data supporting this suggestion, another possible locus for the DA-mediated synaptic change in the striatum is the glutamatergic corticostriatal synapses themselves (Wickens, 1990). They, like cholinergic synapses, are found on striatal efferent cells along with dopaminergic afferents, and the activity of cortical glutamatergic cells would change with changing environmental stimuli. Previous studies have shown that glutamate, like acetylcholine, can modulate striatal DA release (Chéramy et al., 1986; Romo et al., 1986). Furthermore, a DA- and cyclic AMP-regulated striatal phosphoprotein may influence glutamate neurotransmission (Hemmings et al., 1987).

Clearly, more work is needed before the mechanisms underlying the structural changes associated with DA-mediated learning can be specified. However, from this brief review it can be seen that results from a number of areas of neuroscience converge on the possibility that DA-mediated reward-related learning could involve the D1 receptor.

CONSIDERATION OF THE BEHAVIOURAL DATA FROM THE POINT OF VIEW OF THE D1 HYPOTHESIS

If D1 receptors are critical for DA-mediated reward-related learning to occur, D1 antagonists should block the usual response acquisition and maintenance effects of rewarding stimuli. Many data support this hypothesis. As reviewed above, D1 antagonists have been reported to produce effects consistent with a block of reward in self-administration, place-preference, operant responding for various rewards, avoidance responding, conditioned activity, sensitization and conditioned approach to a feeder. These results provide strong support for the hypothesis that the D1 receptor may be involved in mediating learning produced by reward.

As discussed in the previous section, there is theoretically a diffuse DA signal associated with reward, and the effect of this putative signal may be to modify the strength of the striatal synapses most recently activated by the particular environmental stimuli encountered by the organism. One mechanism suggested for this selective action of DA at only a subset of synapses was the possible local enhancement of DA release by adjacent synapses activated by the most recently encountered stimuli (see above). From this point of view, the administration of D1 agonists would not be expected to produce a reward effect because they would act not only at the synapses activated in association with the pre-reward stimuli but, rather, indiscriminately at many synapses in DA terminal regions; i.e. they would create noise that would interfere with the usual selective action of the DA signal. As a consequence, environmental stimuli associated with reward might not uniquely undergo a change in their ability to elicit approach and other responses in the future. Therefore, little or no stimulus control of responding would be seen.

In general, the few results that are available provide some support for this point of view. Thus the partial D1 agonist SKF 38393 was not self-administered, perhaps because the D1 noise created by the postsynaptic action of the self-administered D1 agonist did not lead to the specific enhancement of the ability of lever-associated stimuli to control responding. The failure of SKF 38393 to support place-preference conditioning or to enhance responding for conditioned reward can be similarly understood. SKF 38393 also produced a place aversion. It is not clear how this result can be understood from the present point of view. However, this result and the failure of a D1 agonist to be self-administered might suggest that the putative state of indiscriminate incentive learning may be undesirable (Miller et al., 1990).

If D1 receptors mediate learning associated with reward, as the data suggest, how might the apparent reward effects of D2 agonists and reward-blocking effects of D2 antagonists be understood? It should be pointed out that the results with D2-specific compounds do not negate the hypothesis being developed in this chapter; the observation of reward effects related to manipulations of the D2 receptor does not in itself lead to the conclusion that the D1 receptor is not involved. The D2 effects require explanation, however, but only speculation is possible at this time. The following is an attempt to understand the data within a single explanatory framework.

It now appears clear that the activation of dopaminergic neurons leading to the release of DA at their terminal regions (the DA signal) may form an essential link in the neurocircuitry mediating the effects of reward on behaviour. As discussed in the previous section, there are many data that show that DA is released when animals encounter unconditioned (Heffner et al., 1980; Keller et al., 1983; Blackburn et al., 1986; Damsma et al.,

1989; Phillips et al., 1989, Chapter 8, this volume) or conditioned rewarding stimuli (Schiff, 1982; Blackburn et al., 1989; Phillips et al., Chapter 8, this volume). Additionally, there are many data that suggest that DA is released simply as a consequence of the performance of motor acts, presumably by the influence of striatal efferent systems on mesencephalic DA neurons (Heffner and Seiden, 1980; Heffner et al., 1981, 1984; Yamamoto et al., 1982; Yamamoto and Freed, 1984; Freed and Yamamoto, 1985; Church et al., 1986; Szostak et al., 1986; Speciale et al., 1986; Heyes et al., 1988). It is therefore suggested that, under normal circumstances, reward-related learning may occur as a consequence of the DA signal generated by the combined influence from these two sources on the dopaminergic neurons. The main effect of blocking D2 receptors might be to decrease the motor output of the animal (Clark and White, 1987) or, at least, to decrease the amount of drive on the DA neurons; this would have the effect of reducing the usual stimulation of the DA neurons provided from this source and, therefore, reducing the strength of the DA signal normally associated with reward. As a result, the stimulation of D1 receptors that may mediate reward-related learning may be proportionally reduced. Shifts to the right in the function relating response output to reward magnitude (Willner et al., Chapter 10, this volume) or extinction-like decreases in responding for reward may, therefore, be seen following D2 receptor blockade, perhaps depending on dose. It is noteworthy that such a combined influence may provide a basis for understanding the apparent synergistic action of D1 and D2 receptors on behaviour. See Miller et al. (1990) for further discussion of this point.

Another mechanism may also be involved. It is well known that one of the effects of D2 receptor blockers is to produce an acute increase in *in vivo* DA release in the terminal regions, probably as a consequence of blocking autoreceptors (Nielsen and Moore, 1982; Blaha and Lane, 1984; DiChiara and Imperato, 1985, 1988; Imperato and DiChiara, 1985; Louilot et al., 1985; O'Neill and Fillenz, 1985). Thus, following treatment with D2 antagonists, the level of DA would be high and D1 receptor stimulation would be possible. However, this tonic stimulation of D1 receptors would constitute noise and the DA signal may be lost or, at least, critically attenuated. As a result, the usual D1 receptor stimulation may not occur at a discrete time associated with the presentation of reward (as discussed above), but rather in a more sustained fashion masking any reward-related signal. In this way the noise effects at the D1 receptor produced by D2 antagonists and D1 agonists might be expected to be similar.

Either of these two consequences of D2 receptor blockade, reduced stimulation of the dopaminergic neurons in association with striatal output and the performance of motor acts or increased dopaminergic noise in the terminal regions, could reduce the effectiveness of reward. The two might also sum to lead to the observed reductions in reward-related learning following D2 blockade. Further studies are needed to sort out the possible contribution of these two mechanisms.

From the point of view of the first mechanism, some of the effects of D2 agonists can be understood. In the self-administration paradigm, the performance of the required operant response would lead to an intravenous injection. The resultant pulse of stimulation of D2 receptors might lead to increased stimulation of DA neurons and a strong DA signal that might mediate incentive learning via an action at the D1 receptor; the lever-related stimuli might therefore maintain their ability to control responding. In the case of responding for conditioned reward, increased activity produced by the D2 agonist combined with the presentation of conditioned reward might provide an enhanced DA signal, possibly leading to greater responding for the conditioned reward. Here the putative DA signal at the D1 receptor associated with reward would be intact, only larger than normal, producing the selective enhancement of responding for the conditioned reward. In place conditioning with a D2 agonist, the DA signal at the D1 receptor associated with the performance of motor acts would be intact, only larger as a result of increased stimulation of dopaminergic neurons. This may allow for selective incentive conditioning of stimuli in the drug-associated environment.

The second mechanism suggested that D2 antagonists might produce acute increases in DA release that may have the effect of masking the DA signal at the D1 receptor, leading to a failure of incentive conditioning. If D2 agonists had the complementary effect of decreasing DA release, they might be expected also to lead to a loss of incentive conditioning because the DA signal might be lost. However, D2 agonists produce reward effects, not a block of the reward signal. This apparent contradiction may be resolved by reference to a recent paper by Martin-Iverson et al. (1988). They cited evidence suggesting that the ability of D2 agonists to shut down release in DA neurons was inversely proportional to the level of activity of those neurons. Thus, from the present perspective, the activation of DA neurons in association with the performance of a motor act might release sufficient DA to produce learning effects even in the presence of a D2 agonist. Although this account is clearly speculative, it is supported by the data.

There is a clear prediction from the hypothesis that the D1 receptor may mediate the incentive learning effects of DA. The reward effects of D2 agonists should be blocked by D1 antagonists. There are very few relevant data available at this time and there is a great need for more studies on this specific topic. The available data certainly do not provide a strong case for the model being developed here. Woolverton (1986) reported that only one of four monkeys self-administering the D2 agonist piribedil showed an extinction-like elevation in rate following SCH 23390; five of five monkeys showed this effect with the D2 antagonist pimozide. However, Hoffman and Beninger (1989a) found that some doses of SCH 23390 antagonized the development of place conditioning based on quinpirole. Finally, Mazurski and Beninger (in preparation) found that SCH 23390 failed to antagonize the establishment of conditioned activity based on quinpirole although the same dose was effective in blocking conditioning produced by amphetamine or SKF 38393. The final resolution of this question must await further studies.

SUMMARY AND CONCLUSIONS

There is evidence that DA may play a critical role in reward-related incentive learning. This type of learning involves the acquisition of the ability to elicit approach and other responses by reward-associated stimuli. Learning may involve structural changes in the brain and these changes may be effected through the activation of receptor-linked enzymes that lead to a cascade of intracellular biochemical events. One receptor that is a candidate for producing learning via these mechanisms is the D1 receptor, the one linked in an excitatory fashion to the enzyme adenylate cyclase.

Neuronal organization and events underlying DA-mediated incentive learning might be as follows. Specific subsets of cortical cells may be activated by specific environmental stimuli; as these cells project heavily into the striatum (including the nucleus accumbens), their terminals there may be correspondingly activated. Whenever a corticostriatal terminal is activated, its synapses may be brought into a transient 'state of readiness' during which an appropriate signal may lead to a relatively permanent change in the effectiveness of these synapses. The signal in this case would be the activation of dopaminergic neurons that project into the same target region as the corticostriatal fibres. The DA signal might effect the change in synaptic strength via D1 receptors. A possible mechanism for the 'state of readiness' might be a transient local enhancement of DA release produced by the corticostriatal projections. The usual influence of corticostriatal projections on striatal output cells may be to alter their firing rate, leading to increases in locomotor activity. The consequence of the change in synaptic strength might be to augment the ability of corticostriatal projections to increase locomotor activity, specifically, approach responses, in the future. This would be the basis of DA-mediated incentive learning.

A critical feature of this model is that the reward-related activation of dopaminergic neurons (the DA signal), and the subsequent stimulation of D1 receptors, be a discrete event associated with the most recently encountered environmental stimuli. Treatment either with a D1 agonist leading directly to indiscriminate stimulation of D1 receptors, or with a D2 antagonist leading to increased release of DA, and indirectly to indiscriminate stimulation of D1 receptors, might mask the usual reward signal. Decreases in motor activity produced by D2 antagonists might also reduce the strength of the reward signal by reducing the level of stimulation of dopaminergic neurons provided from this source. D1 antagonists would block the reward signal directly. Finally, D2 agonists might lead to an enhancement of the reward signal by increasing the stimulation of the dopaminergic cell bodies that normally accompanies motor output.

In general, the data fit this scheme. Thus, either D1 or D2 antagonists produce a block of the usual effects of reward on behaviour. D1 agonists do not apparently produce reward effects. D2 agonists appear to produce reward effects in their own right and to augment the acquisition of responding for conditioned rewards. D1 antagonists would also be expected to block reward effects produced by D2 agonists according to this scheme. Additional data are eagerly awaited for a definitive evaluation of this possibility.

ACKNOWLEDGEMENTS

This chapter is dedicated to Lynne and Max. The author was supported by grants from the Natural Sciences and Engineering Research Council of Canada, and the Ontario Ministry of Health.

REFERENCES

Akers, R.F., Lovinger, D.M., Colley, P.A., Linden, D.J. and Routtenberg, A. (1986) Translocation of protein kinase C activity may mediate hippocampal long-term potentiation, *Science* **231**, 587–589.
de Belleroche, J.S. and Gardiner, I.M. (1982) Cholinergic action in the nucleus accumbens: modulation of dopamine and acetylcholine release. *British Journal of Pharmacology* **75**, 359–365.
Beninger, R.J. (1983) The role of dopamine in locomotor activity and learning. *Brain Research Reviews* **6**, 173–196.
Beninger, R.J. (1989a) Dissociating the effects of altered dopaminergic function on performance and learning. *Brain Research Bulletin* **23**, 365–371.
Beninger, R.J. (1989b) The role of dopamine and serotonin in learning to avoid aversive stimuli. In: Archer, T. and Nilsson, L.-G. (eds) *Aversion, Avoidance and Anxiety: Perspectives in Aversively Motivated Behavior*. Hillsdale, New Jersey: Lawrence Erlbaum Associates, pp. 265–284.
Beninger, R.J. and Hahn, B.L. (1983) Pimozide blocks establishment but not expression of amphetamine-produced environment-specific conditioning. *Science* **220**, 1304–1306.
Beninger, R.J. and Herz, R.S. (1986) Pimozide blocks establishment but not expression of cocaine-produced environment-specific conditioning. *Life Sciences* **38**, 1425–1431.
Beninger, R.J. and Phillips, A.G. (1980) The effect of pimozide on the establishment of conditioned reinforcement. *Psychopharmacology* **68**, 147–153.
Beninger, R.J., Mason, S.T., Phillips, A.G. and Fibiger, H.C. (1980) The use of

conditioned suppression to evaluate the nature of neuroleptic-induced avoidance deficits. *Journal of Pharmacology and Experimental Therapeutics* **213**, 623–627.

Beninger, R.J., Cheng, M., Hahn, B.L., Hoffman, D.C., Mazurski, E.J., Morency, M.A., Ramm, P. and Stewart, R.J. (1987) Effects of extinction, pimozide, SCH 23390, and metoclopramide on food-rewarded operant responding of rats. *Psychopharmacology* **92**, 343–349.

Beninger, R.J., Hoffman, D.C. and Mazurski, E.J. (1989) Receptor subtype-specific dopaminergic agents and conditioned behavior. *Neuroscience and Biobehavioral Reviews* **13**, 113–122.

Blackburn, J.R., Phillips, A.G., Jakubovic, A. and Fibiger, H.C. (1986) Increased dopamine metabolism in the nucleus accumbens and striatum following consumption of a nutritive meal but not a palatable non-nutritive saccharine solution. *Pharmacology, Biochemistry and Behavior* **25**, 1095–1100.

Blackburn, J.R., Phillips, A.G., Jakubovic, A. and Fibiger, H.C. (1989) Dopamine and preparatory behavior: II. A neurochemical analysis. *Behavioral Neuroscience* **103**, 15–23.

Blaha, C.D. and Lane, R.F. (1984) Direct in vivo electrochemical monitoring of dopamine release in response to neuroleptic drugs. *European Journal of Pharmacology* **98**, 113–117.

Bolam, J.P. (1984) Synapses of identified neurons in the neostriatum. In: Evered, D. and O'Connor, M. (eds) *Functions of the Basal Ganglia* London: Pitman, pp. 30–42.

Bozarth, M.A. (1986) Neural basis of psychomotor stimulant and opiate reward: evidence suggesting the involvement of a common dopaminergic system. *Behavioural Brain Research* **22**, 107–116.

Bradshaw, C.M. and Szabadi, E. (1989) Central neurotransmitter systems and the control of operant behaviour by 'natural' positive reinforcers. In: Liebman, J.M. and Cooper, S.J. (eds) *The Neuropharmacological Basis of Reward*. Oxford: Oxford University Press, pp. 320–376.

Carr, G.D., Fibiger, H.C. and Phillips, A.G. (1989) Conditioned place preference as a measure of drug reward. In: Liebman, J.M. and Cooper, S.J. (eds) *The Neuropharmacological Basis of Reward* Oxford: Oxford University Press, pp. 264–319.

Chéramy, A., Romo, R., Godeheu, G., Baruch, P. and Glowinski, J. (1986) In vivo presynaptic control of dopamine release in the cat caudate nucleus—II. Facilitatory or inhibitory influence of L-glutamate. *Neuroscience* **19**, 1081–1090.

Chipkin, R.E., Iorio, L.C., Coffin, V.L., McQuade, R.D., Berger, J.G. and Barnett, A. (1988) Pharmacological profile of SCH 39166: a dopamine D1 selective benzonaphthazepine with potential antipsychotic activity. *Journal of Pharmacology and Experimental Therapeutics* **247**, 1093–1102.

Church, W.H., Sabol, K.E., Justice, Jr., J.B. and Neill, D.B. (1986) Striatal dopamine activity and unilateral barpressing in rats. *Pharmacology, Biochemistry and Behavior* **25**, 865–871.

Clark, D. and White, F.J. (1987) Review: D1 dopamine receptor—the search for a function: a critical evaluation of D1/D2 dopamine receptor classification and its functional implications. *Synapse* **1**, 347–388.

Damsma, G., Yoshida, M., Wendstern, D., Nomikos, G.G., Phillips, A.G. and Fibiger, H.C. (1989) Dopamine transmission in the rat striatum, nucleus accumbens and pre-frontal cortex is differentially affected by feeding, tail pinch and immobilization. *Society for Neuroscience Abstracts* **15**, 557.

D'Angio, M.D., Serrano, A., Driscoll, P. and Scatton, B. (1988) Stressful environmental stimuli increase extracellular DOPAC levels in the prefrontal cortex of hypoemotional (Roman high-avoidance) but not hyperemotional (Roman low-avoidance) rats. An in vivo voltammetric study. *Brain Research* **451**, 237–247.

DiChiara, G. and Imperato, A. (1985) Rapid tolerance to neuroleptic-induced stimulation of dopamine release in freely moving rats. *Journal of Pharmacology and Experimental Therapeutics* **235**, 487–494.

DiChiara, G. and Imperato, A. (1988) Drugs abused by humans preferentially increase synaptic dopamine concentrations in the mesolimbic system of freely moving rats. *Proceedings of the National Academy of Sciences of the United States of America* **85**, 5274–5278.

Donahoe, J.W. and Palmer, D.C. (1989) The interpretation of complex human behavior: some reactions to parallel distributed processing. *Journal of the Experimental Analysis of Behavior* **51**, 399–416.

Ettenberg, A. (1989) Dopamine, neuroleptics and reinforced behavior. *Neuroscience and Biobehavioral Reviews* **13**, 105–112.

Freed, C.R. and Yamamoto, B.K. (1985) Regional brain dopamine metabolism: a marker for the speed, direction, and posture of moving animals. *Science* **229**, 62–65.

Gerhardt, S., Gerber, R. and Liebman, J.M. (1985) SCH 23390 dissociated from conventional neuroleptics in apomorphine climbing and primate acute dyskinesia models. *Life Sciences* **37**, 2355–2363.

Gilbert, D.B., Dembski, J.E., Stein, L. and Belluzzi, J.D. (1986) Dopamine and reward: conditioned place preference induced by dopamine D2 receptor agonist. *Society for Neuroscience Abstracts* **12**, 938.

Giorguieff-Chesselet, M.F., Kemel, M.L., Wandscheer, D. and Glowinski, J. (1979) Regulation of dopamine release by presynaptic nicotinic receptors in rat striatal slices: effect of nicotine in a low concentration. *Life Sciences* **25**, 1257–1262.

Goeders, N.E., Dworkin, S.I. and Smith, J.E. (1986) Neuropharmacological assessment of cocaine self-administration into the medial prefrontal cortex. *Pharmacology, Biochemistry and Behavior* **24**, 1429–1440.

Greengard, P. and Kuo, J.F. (1970) On the mechanism of action of cyclic AMP. *Advances in Biochemical Psychopharmacology* **3**, 287–306.

Gribkoff, V.K. and Ashe, J.H. (1984) Modulation by dopamine of population responses and cell membrane properties of hippocampal CA1 neurons in vitro. *Brain Research* **292**, 327–338.

Grofova, I. (1979) Extrinsic connections of the neostriatum. In: Divac, I. and Oberg, G.E. (eds) *The Neostriatum*. London: Pergamon, pp. 37–51.

Hebb, D.O. (1949) *Organization of Behavior*. New York: John Wiley and Sons.

Heffner, T.G. and Seiden, L.S. (1980) Synthesis of catecholamines from [^{3}H]tyrosine in brain during the performance of operant behavior. *Brain Research* **183**, 403–419.

Heffner, T.G., Hartman, J.A. and Seiden, L.S. (1980) Feeding increases dopamine metabolism in the rat brain. *Science* **208**, 1168–1170.

Heffner, T.G., Luttinger, D., Hartman, J.A. and Seiden, L.S. (1981) Regional changes in brain catecholamine turnover in the rat during performance on fixed ratio and variable interval schedules of reinforcement. *Brain Research* **214**, 215–218.

Heffner, T.G., Vosmer, G. and Seiden, L.S. (1984) Increased transport of 3,4-dihydroxyphenylacetic acid from brain during performance of operant behavior in the rat. *Brain Research* **293**, 85–91.

Heimer, L. and Wilson, R.D. (1975) The subcortical projections of the allocortex: similarities in the neural associations of the hippocampus, piriform cortex, and the neocortex. In: Santini, M. (ed.) *Golgi Centennial Symposium, Proceedings*. New York: Raven Press, pp. 117–193.

Hemmings, Jr, H.C., Greengard, P., Tung, H.Y.L. and Cohen, P. (1984) DARPP-32, a dopamine-regulated neuronal phosphoprotein, is a potent inhibitor of protein phosphatase-1. *Nature* **310**, 503–508.

Hemmings Jr, H.C., Walaas, S.I., Ouimet, C.C. and Greengard, P. (1987) Dopaminergic regulation of protein phosphorylation in the striatum: DARPP-32. *Trends in Neuroscience* **10**, 377–383.

Heyes, M.P., Garnett, E.S. and Coates, G. (1988) Nigrostriatal dopaminergic activity is increased during exhaustive exercise stress in rats. *Life Sciences* **42**, 1537–1542.

Hineline, P.N. (1977) Negative reinforcement and avoidance. In: Honig, W.K. and Staddon, J.E.R. (eds) *Handbook of Operant Behavior*. Englewood Cliffs, New Jersey: Prentice Hall, pp. 364–414.

Hoffman, D.C. (1989) The use of place conditioning in studying the neuropharmacology of drug reinforcement. *Brain Research Bulletin* **23**, 373–387.

Hoffman, D.C. and Beninger, R.J. (1985) The effects of pimozide on the establishment of conditioned reinforcement as a function of the amount of conditioning. *Psychopharmacology* **87**, 454–460.

Hoffman, D.C. and Beninger, R.J. (1988) Selective D1 and D2 dopamine agonists produce opposing effects in place conditioning but not in conditioned taste aversion learning. *Pharmacology, Biochemistry and Behavior* **31**, 1–8.

Hoffman, D.C. and Beninger, R.J. (1989a) The effects of selective dopamine D1 and D2 receptor antagonists on the establishment of agonist-induced place conditioning in rats. *Pharmacology, Biochemistry and Behavior* **33**, 273–279.

Hoffman, D.C. and Beninger, R.J. (1989b) Preferential stimulation of D1 or D2 receptors disrupts food-rewarded operant responding in rats. *Pharmacology, Biochemistry and Behavior* **34**, 923–925.

Hoffman, D.C., Dickson, P.R. and Beninger, R.J. (1988) The dopamine D2 receptor agonists, quinpirole and bromocriptine produce conditioned place preferences. *Progress in Neuro-Psychopharmacology and Biological Psychiatry* **12**, 315–322.

Imperato, A. and DiChiara, G. (1985) Dopamine release and metabolism in awake rats after systemic neuroleptics as studied by trans-striatal dialysis. *Journal of Neuroscience* **2**, 297–306.

Iorio, L.C., Barnett, A., Leitz, F.H., Houser, V.P. and Korduba, C.A. (1983) SCH 23390, a potential benzazepine antipsychotic with unique interactions on dopaminergic systems. *Journal of Pharmacology and Experimental Therapeutics* **226**, 462–468.

Jenner, P. and Marsden, C.D. (1981) Substituted benzamide drugs as selective neuroleptic agents. *Neuropharmacology* **20**, 1285–1293.

Katz, J.L. (1989) Drugs as reinforcers: pharmacological and behavioral factors. In: Liebman, J.M. and Cooper, S.J. (eds) *The Neuropharmacological Basis of Reward*. Oxford: Oxford University Press, pp. 164–263.

Kebabian, J.W., Petzold, G.L. and Greengard, P. (1972) Dopamine sensitive adenylate cyclase in caudate nucleus of rat brain and its similarity to the dopamine receptor. *Proceedings of the National Academy of Sciences of the United States of America* **69**, 2145–2149.

Keller, Jr, R.W., Stricker, E.M. and Zigmond, M.J. (1983) Environmental stimuli but not homeostatic challenges produce apparent increases in dopaminergic activity in the striatum: an analysis by in vivo voltammetry. *Brain Research* **279**, 159–170.

Koechling, U., Colle, L.M. and Wise, R.A. (1988) Effects of SCH 23390 on motivational aspects of deprivation-induced feeding. *Psychobiology* **16**, 207–212.

Koob, G.F. and Goeders, N.E. (1989) Neuroanatomical substrates of drug self-administration. In: Liebman, J.M. and Cooper, S.J. (eds) *The Neuropharmacological Basis of Reward*. Oxford: Oxford University Press, pp. 214–263.

Koob, G.F., Le, H.T. and Creese, I. (1987) The D_1 dopamine receptor antagonist SCH 23390 increases cocaine self-administration in the rat. *Neuroscience Letters* **79**, 315–320.

Kurumiya, S. and Nakajima, S. (1988) Dopamine D_1 receptors in the nucleus accumbens: involvement in the reinforcing effect of tegmental stimulation. *Brain Research* **448**, 1–6.

Lehmann, J. and Langer, S.Z. (1982) Muscarinic receptors on dopamine terminals in the cat caudate nucleus: neuromodulation on [^{3}H]dopamine release in vitro by endogenous acetylcholine. *Brain Research* **248**, 61–69.

Leone, P. and DiChiara, G. (1987) Blockade of D-1 receptors by SCH 23390 antagonizes morphine- and amphetamine-induced place preference conditioning. *European Journal of Pharmacology* **135**, 251–254.

Levis, D.J. (1989) The case for a return to a two-factor theory of avoidance: the failure of non-fear interpretations. In: Klein, S.B. and Mower, R.R. (eds) *Contemporary Learning Theories: Pavlovian Conditioning and the Status of Traditional Learning Theory*. Hillsdale, New Jersey: Lawrence Erlbaum, pp. 227–278.

Libet, B. (1984) Heterosynaptic interaction at a sympathetic neuron as a model for induction and storage of a postsynaptic memory trace. In: Lynch, G., McGaugh, J.L. and Weinberger, N.M. (eds) *Neurobiology of Learning and Memory*. New York: Guilford Press, pp. 405–430.

Libet, B., Kobayashi, H. and Tanaka, T. (1975) Synaptic coupling into the production and storage of a neuronal memory trace. *Nature* **258**, 155–157.

Liebman, J.M. and Cooper, S.J. (eds) (1989) *The Neuropharmacological Basis of Reward*. Oxford: Oxford University Press.

Louilot, A., Buda, M., Gonon, F., Simon, H., LeMoal, M. and Pujol, J.F. (1985) Effect of haloperidol and sulpiride on dopamine metabolism in nucleus accumbens and olfactory tubercle: a study by in vivo voltammetry. *Neuroscience* **14**, 775–782.

Lovinger, D.M., Colley, P.A., Akers, R.F., Nelson, R.B. and Routtenberg, A. (1986) Direct relation of long-term synaptic potentiation to phosphorylation of membrane protein F_1, a substrate for membrane protein kinase C. *Brain Research* **399**, 205–211.

Mackintosh, J.J. (1974) *The Psychology of Animal Learning*. New York: Academic Press.

Martin-Iverson, M.T., Iversen, S.D. and Stahl, S.M. (1988) Long-term motor stimulant effects of (+)-4-propyl-9-hydronaphthoxazine (PHNO), a dopamine D-2 receptor agonist: interactions with a dopamine D-1 receptor antagonist and agonist. *European Journal of Pharmacology* **149**, 25–31.

Matthies, H. (1989) Neurobiological aspects of learning and memory. *Annual Reviews of Psychology* **40**, 381–404.

McGeer, P.L., Eccles, J.C. and McGeer, E.G. (1978) *Molecular Neurobiology of the Mammalian Brain*. New York: Plenum Press.

Miller, R. (1988) Cortico-striatal and cortico-limbic circuits: a two-tiered model of learning and memory functions. In: Marcowitsch (ed.) *Information Processing by the Brain: Views and Hypotheses from a Cognitive-Physiological Perspective*. Bern: Hans Huber Press, pp. 179–198.

Miller, R., Wickens, J.R. and Beninger, R.J. (1990) Dopamine D-1 and D-2 receptors in relation to reward and performance: a case for the D-1 receptor as a primary site of therapeutic action of neuroleptic drugs. *Progress in Neurobiology* **34**, 143–183.

Mochida, S., Kobayashi, H. and Libet, B. (1987) Stimulation of adenylate cyclase in relation to dopamine-induced long-term enhancement (LTE) of muscarinic depolarization in the rabbit superior cervical ganglion. *Journal of Neuroscience* **7**, 311–318.

Morency, M.A. and Beninger, R.J. (1986) Dopaminergic substrates of cocaine-induced place conditioning. *Brain Research* **399**, 33–41.

Nakajima, S. (1986) Suppression of operant responding in the rat by dopamine D1 receptor blockade with SCH 23390. *Physiological Psychology* **14**, 111–114.

Nakajima, S. (1989) Subtypes of dopamine receptors involved in the mechanism of reinforcement. *Neuroscience and Biobehavioral Reviews* **13**, 123–128.

Nakajima, S. and McKenzie, G.M. (1986) Reduction of the rewarding effect of brain stimulation by a blockade of dopamine D1 receptor with SCH 23390. *Pharmacology, Biochemistry and Behavior* **24**, 919–923.

Nielsen, J.A. and Moore, K.E. (1982) Measurement of ·metabolites of dopamine and 5-hydroxytryptamine in cerebroventricular perfusates of unanesthetized, freely-moving rats: selective effects of drugs. *Pharmacology, Biochemistry and Behavior* **16**, 131–137.

O'Neill, R.D. and Fillenz, M. (1985) Detection of homovanillic acid *in vivo* using microcomputer-controlled voltammetry: simultaneous monitoring of rat motor activity and striatal dopamine release. *Neuroscience* **14**, 753–763.

Phillips, A.G. and Fibiger, H.C. (1989) Neuroanatomical bases of intracranial self-stimulation: untangling the Gordian knot. In: Liebman, J.M. and Cooper, S.J. (eds) *The Neuropharmacological Basis of Reward*. Oxford: Oxford University Press, pp. 66–105.

Phillips, A.G., Mora, F. and Rolls, E.T. (1981) Intracranial self-administration of amphetamine by rhesus monkeys. *Neuroscience Letters* **24**, 81–86.

Phillips, A.G., Blaha, C.D. and Fibiger, H.C. (1989) Neurochemical correlates of brain-stimulation reward measured by ex vivo and in vivo analyses. *Neuroscience and Biobehavioral Reviews* **13**, 99–104.

Raiteri, M., Marchi, M. and Maura, G. (1982) Presynaptic muscarinic receptors increase striatal dopamine release evoked by 'quasi-physiological' depolarization. *European Journal of Pharmacology* **83**, 127–129.

Romo, R., Chéramy, A., Godeheu, G. and Glowinski, J. (1986) *In vivo* presynaptic control of dopamine release in the cat caudate nucleus—III. Further evidence for the implication of corticostriatal glutamatergic neurons. *Neuroscience* **19**, 1091–1099.

Routtenberg, A. and Kim, H.-J. (1978) The substantia nigra and neostriatum: substrates for memory consolidation. In: Butcher, L.L. (ed.) *Cholinergic-Monoaminergic Interactions in the Brain*. New York: Academic Press, pp. 305–331.

Sanger, D.J. (1987) The actions of SCH 23390, a D1 receptor antagonist, on operant and avoidance behavior in rats. *Pharmacology, Biochemistry and Behavior* **26**, 509–513.

Schiff, S.R. (1982) Conditioned dopaminergic activity. *Biological Psychiatry* **17**, 135–154.

Schizgal, P. and Murray, B. (1989) Neuronal basis of intracranial self-stimulation. In: Liebman, J.M. and Cooper, S.J. (eds) *The Neuropharmacological Basis of Reward*. Oxford: Oxford University Press, pp. 106–163.

Schwartz, J.H. and Greenberg, S.M. (1987) Molecular mechanisms for memory: second-messenger induced modifications of protein kinases in nerve cells. *Annual Review of Neuroscience* **10**, 459–476.

Seeman, P. (1981) Brain dopamine receptors. *Pharmacological Reviews* **32**, 229–313.

Shippenberg, T.S. and Herz, A. (1987) Place preference conditioning reveals the involvement of D_1-dopamine receptors in the motivational properties of μ- and κ-opioid agonists. *Brain Research* **436**, 169–172.

Speciale, S.G., Miller, J.D., McMillen, B.A. and German, D.C. (1986) Activation of specific central dopamine pathways: locomotion and footshock. *Brain Research Bulletin* **16**, 33–38.

Spyraki, C., Fibiger, H.C. and Phillips, A.G. (1982) Attenuation by haloperidol of place preference conditioning using food reinforcement. *Psychopharmacology* **77**, 379–382.

Stein, L. and Belluzzi, J.D. (1989) Cellular investigations of behavioral reinforcement. *Neuroscience and Biobehavioral Reviews* **13**, 69–80.

Stellar, J.R. and Rice, M.B. (1989) Pharmacological basis of intracranial self-stimulation. In: Liebman, J.M. and Cooper, S.J. (eds) *The Neuropharmacological Basis of Reward*. Oxford: Oxford University Press, pp. 14–65.

Stewart, J. and Vezina, P. (1988) Conditioning and behavioral sensitization. In: Kalivas, P.W. and Barnes, C.D. (eds) *Sensitization in the Nervous System*. Caldwell, New Jersey: Telford Press, pp. 207–224.

Szostak, C., Jakubovic, A., Phillips, A.G. and Fibiger, H.C. (1986) Bilateral augmentation of dopaminergic and serotonergic activity in the striatum and nucleus accumbens induced by conditioned circling. *Journal of Neuroscience* **6**, 2037–2044.

Tombaugh, T.N., Tombaugh, J. and Anisman, H. (1979) Effects of dopamine receptor blockade on alimentary behaviour: home cage food consumption, magazine training, operant acquisition, and performance. *Psychopharmacology* **66**, 219–225.

Vezina, P. and Stewart, J. (1989) The effects of dopamine receptor blockade on the development of sensitization to the locomotor effects of amphetamine and morphine. *Brain Research* **449**, 108–120.

Viaud, M.D. and White, N.M. (1989) Dissociation of visual and olfactory conditioning in the neostriatum of rats. *Behavioural Brain Research* **32**, 31–42.

Waddington, J.L. and O'Boyle, K.M. (1989) Drug actions on brain dopamine receptors: a conceptual re-evaluation five years after the first selective D-1 antagonist. *Pharmacology and Therapeutics* **43**, 1–52.

Waddington, J.L., Murray, A.M. and O'Boyle, K.M. (1988) New selective D-1 and D-2 dopamine receptor agonists as further probes for behavioural interaction between D-1 and D-2 systems. In: Beart, P., Woodruff, G. and Jackson, D. (eds) *Pharmacology and Functional Regulation of Dopaminergic Neurons*. London: MacMillan Press, pp. 117–123.

Walaas, S.I., Aswad, D.W. and Greengard, P. (1983) A dopamine- and cyclic AMP-regulated phosphoprotein enriched in dopamine-innervated brain regions. *Nature* **301**, 69–71.

Wickens, J.R. (1990) Striatal dopamine in motor activation and reward-mediated learning: steps towards a unifying model. *Journal of Neural Transmission* **80**, 9–31.

Wise, R.A. (1982) Neuroleptics and operant behavior: the anhedonia hypothesis. *Behavioral and Brain Sciences* **5**, 39–88.

Wise, R.A. (1989a) The brain and reward. In: Liebman, J.M. and Cooper, S.J. (eds) *The Neuropharmacological Basis of Reward*. Oxford: Oxford University Press, pp. 377–424.

Wise, R.A. (1989b) Opiate reward: sites and substrates. *Neuroscience and Biobehavioral Reviews* **13**, 129–134.

Wise, R.A. and Rompré, P.-P. (1989) Brain dopamine and reward. *Annual Reviews of Psychology* **40**, 191–225.

Wise, R.A. and Schwartz, H.V. (1981) Pimozide attenuates acquisition of lever-pressing for food in rats. *Pharmacology, Biochemistry and Behavior* **15**, 655–656.

Woolverton, W.L. (1986) Effects of a D_1 and a D_2 dopamine antagonist on the self-administration of cocaine and piribedil by rhesus monkeys. *Pharmacology, Biochemistry and Behavior* **24**, 531–535.

Woolverton, W.L., Goldberg, L.I. and Ginos, J.Z. (1984) Intravenous self-administration of dopamine receptor agonists by rhesus monkeys. *Journal of Pharmacology and Experimental Therapeutics* **230**, 678–683.

Yamamoto, B.K. and Freed, C.R. (1984) Asymmetric dopamine and serotonin metabolism in nigrostriatal and limbic structures of the trained circling rat. *Brain Research* **297**, 115–119.

Yamamoto, B.K., Lane, R.F. and Freed, C.R. (1982) Normal rats trained to circle show asymmetric caudate dopamine release. *Life Sciences* **30**, 2155–2162.

12

The Mesolimbic Dopamine System as a Model Reward System

MICHAEL A. BOZARTH

Department of Psychology, State University of New York at Buffalo,
Buffalo, NY 14260, USA

INTRODUCTION

Brain dopamine (DA) systems have been the focus of considerable research since their initial identification almost three decades ago. Dahlström and Fuxe (1964) identified several clusters of catecholamine-containing cell bodies and traced the primary axonal projections of these cell groups to various brain regions. Subsequent work (Andén, et al., 1966; Lindvall and Björklund, 1974; Palkovits and Jacobowitz, 1974; Ungerstedt, 1971a) provided more precise anatomical localization of central DA-containing cells and their projections. Two major systems emerged from this work—the nigrostriatal and the mesolimbic/mesocortical DA systems—and several shorter neural projections were also described. These DA systems have been implicated in a wide variety of behavioral actions, including locomotor activity, stereotypy, feeding and drinking, drug reinforcement, and brain stimulation reward (BSR) as well as in human psychopathology. The fact that these behaviors appear to share a common neuropharmacological and neuroanatomical basis has prompted numerous attempts to develop an integrative theoretical model (Mogenson and Phillips, 1976; Mogenson et al., 1980; Beninger, 1983; Depue and Iacono, 1989).

This chapter will describe some of the motivational functions of the mesolimbic DA system with an emphasis on appetitive motivation and reward processes. Literature supporting the involvement of this system in the rewarding effects of electrical brain stimulation, psychomotor stimulants

The Mesolimbic Dopamine System: From Motivation to Action.
Edited by P. Willner and J. Scheel-Krüger

© 1991 John Wiley & Sons Ltd

and opiates will be reviewed, and additional data suggesting the possible involvement of the mesolimbic DA system in other behaviors will be briefly surveyed. No attempt will be made to review the literature exhaustively; rather, a specific model is described that integrates much of the empirical data, and the heuristic value of this model is explored.

PRELUDE TO THE STUDY OF BRAIN REWARD SYSTEMS

Before proceeding with a description of the motivational function of the mesolimbic DA system, two general issues need to be addressed. The first involves the concept of brain reward systems and briefly examines both the empirical and theoretical basis of their existence. The second concerns the approach to studying brain reward function and an examination of several factors important in evaluating the empirical database.

Specialized Brain Function

There are numerous examples of specialized neural functioning. Specific sensory pathways have been identified and many can be traced from their peripheral transducer organs to their central nervous system (CNS) representation (e.g. retinal activation from light stimulus to neural representation at the occipital cortex). Similarly, motor pathways can be traced from their CNS origin (e.g. motor cortex), through their efferent outputs, to the effector organ (e.g. neuromuscular junction). The exact anatomical linkages, stimulus coding information, and neurochemical mediation of many sensory and motor events have been described in fine detail. The linkage that has been evasive is that between the sensory input and the motor output. Except for a few examples of reflexive behavior, the exact nature of CNS mediation between sensory input and motor output remains obscure.

The nature of mechanisms mediating between stimulus input and motor output is a topic long considered by motivational psychologists. In general, their approach has used molar units of stimuli and behavior; intervening variables have been postulated to account for the variability in responding to constant stimulus conditions, and to describe when a given antecedent condition will yield a specific response (e.g. determining when a food stimulus is associated with an eating response). Physiological psychologists, however, have specifically addressed the CNS mediation of these processes and have attempted to identify specific neurophysiological conditions that influence responding. Few, though, have attempted to integrate these CNS processes with general motivational theory just as relatively few motivational psychologists have attempted to describe specific physiological processes underlying motivated behavior. (The theories of Hull (1943, 1952) and of Bindra (1976) have implications regarding the nature of neurophysiological mechanisms mediating their models, but little empirical work has been generated by these formulations.)

The work of Hess (1949) demonstrated that electrical activation of certain CNS sites can modulate the organism's responses to various stimulus conditions (e.g. elicit attack behavior, feeding). Subsequent work has shown that a variety of behaviors can be evoked by appropriate stimulus conditions concomitant with electrical activation of CNS sites. For examples, feeding behavior, sexual behavior and attack behavior can all be elicited by hypothalamic stimulation. This work suggests a possible CNS focus for gating stimulus-response phenomena, and the hypothalamus has emerged as a possible center for these motivational effects.

The report by Olds and Milner (1954) that rats would work to electrically stimulate certain parts of their brains opened a new dimension in the conceptualization of CNS mediation of behavior. Arbitrarily selected responses could be reinforced by electrical stimulation of the lateral hypothalamus and other brain sites, despite the absence of any appropriate goal object or pre-existing biological need. The finding that animals will work to activate specific CNS pathways directly was initially met with skepticism by some motivational psychologists; apparent differences in the way that electrical stimulation and the way that natural rewards controlled behavior were emphasized by some learning theorists, and BSR was suggested to represent a special case of motivated behavior. However, subsequent work revealed that electrical brain stimulation could control behavior in much the same fashion as conventional rewards (Reid, 1967; Trowill et al., 1969: Olds, 1977), and the notion that electrical stimulation could activate reward systems involved in the control of natural behavior gained widespread acceptance.

The demonstration of rewarding effects from electrical brain stimulation along with the concurrent discovery that electrical stimulation of other brain regions produced intense aversive effects (Delgado et al., 1954) suggested that goal-directed behavior might be guided and maintained by simple approach and avoidance systems. Separate neural systems were identified that elicited approach and avoidance behavior, and naturally occurring motivational conditions were postulated to be mediated by the activation of these systems (Olds, 1962; Olds and Olds, 1963; Stein, 1964). This line of investigation specifically addressed what happens between stimulus presentation and response emission. Neutral stimuli (e.g. a lever) can develop motivational significance and engender approach responding (e.g. lever manipulation) contingent upon electrical activation of brain reward pathways. The study of motivation, from this perspective, starts with what happens in the middle (the 'organismic' variable) and then precedes backward to stimulus input and forward to response output.

Approaches to Studying Brain Reward Function

There are three dimensions to be considered in the study of brain reward systems. The first consideration is the use of a correlative versus a functional approach to the study of brain reward systems (Bozarth, 1987a). The correlative approach observes behavior and measures changes in CNS activity that are associated with specific behaviors. The putative mediation of function is inferred by high correlations between specific neural events and the occurrence of the behavior being studied. In contrast, the functional approach uses direct experimental manipulation to determine the role of various CNS events in reward processes. A specific neural system can be stimulated chemically or electrically, or the function of the neural system can be disrupted by the use of selective lesioning or pharmacological procedures. The functional role of the neural system is determined by causing the occurrence of the behavior through stimulation or by the disruption of the behavior through selectively blocking the activity of the system. The strongest demonstration that a given neural system mediates a behavior comes from the functional approach where the behavior can be directly elicited or inhibited by experimental manipulation. The correlative approach is most useful for preliminary exploratory studies that suggest possible neural events involved in the behavior, and for providing corroborative evidence that the neural events identified by the functional approach behave according to the predictions derived from the experimental model.

A second consideration is specification of the conditions identified by the functional approach. The activity of a neural system may be sufficient to produce the behavior, it may be necessary for the expression of the behavior, or it may be both necessary and sufficient for the occurrence of the behavior (Bozarth, 1983, 1987a). These three cases represent separate conditions that can be identified using the functional approach. If the behavioral response is elicited by activation of the neural system, then activation of that system is sufficient for elicitation of the behavioral response. There is no reason, however, to presuppose that the same neural system is necessary for the behavioral response following activation by other response-eliciting stimuli. Similarly, a specific neural system may be necessary for the occurrence of a behavior, but the activation of the same neural system may fail to evoke a behavioral response. The case where a stimulus is sufficient but not necessary to elicit a behavior merits special consideration. Some important neural functions may be overdetermined, having several independent systems that can produce a behavioral response. For example, drinking behavior can be elicited by activating one of two independent physiological mechanisms— intracellular or extracellular processes (Fitzsimons, 1971). Interestingly, the normal control of water intake in *ad libitum* conditions probably does not involve either mechanism. Nonetheless, drinking can be elicited by intracellular or extracellular fluid loss despite the apparent unimportance of these mechanisms in the control of *ad libitum* drinking.

The last consideration involves the level of study. With few exceptions, rewarding effects are measured by the behavioral response of the intact organism. This necessitates a molar approach to the study of reward processes (but see Olds, 1962; Stein and Belluzzi, 1987). Until the relevant neurological events are identified, it is necessary to anchor studies of reward processes with behavioral measures that indicate when reward processes are operative. Attempts to determine molecular events linked with reward are futile without proper reference to behavioral indices of reward. An understanding of basic motivational theory is just as important as an understanding of basic neuropharmacology and neuroanatomy in the elucidation of reward mechanisms. Most psychopharmacologists have at least an elementary understanding of operant conditioning theory, but many have no training in the broader field of motivational psychology. This creates three types of difficulties: (1) problems discerning the necessary control procedures for behavioral studies; (2) problems determining the significance of the observed behaviors; and (3) problems identifying the relevant behavioral processes to study. During the past several decades, scientists studying reward processes have become more sophisticated in their knowledge of neuroscientific techniques, but they have concomitantly become less sophisticated in their understanding of basic motivational processes.

The model developed in this chapter emphasizes the *functional approach* and determines what events are *sufficient* to activate reward processes described in *molar* units of behavior. This perspective is important in understanding how the neural elements are assembled in the present model and in understanding how specific predictions are derived from the model.

INVOLVEMENT OF DA IN BRAIN REWARD FUNCTION

The terms 'reward' and 'reinforcement' have various meanings. Some authors use these terms interchangeably (e.g. Stellar and Stellar, 1985), while others emphasize important differences based on the histories of the two terms (e.g. White, 1989). Reinforcement suffers from less ambiguity in its usage, largely because of the general acceptance of the empirical law of effect which describes reinforcement as a process whereby certain events (i.e. reinforcing stimuli) increase the probability of behaviors with which they are associated (e.g. Spence, 1956). Wise (1989) presents arguments that behaviors described as involving reward or reinforcement may have the same underlying neural mechanism and therefore represent manifestations of the same phenomenon; by implication, the terms reward and reinforcement may be used interchangeably according to this view (c.f. Wise and Rompré, 1989).

In the context of the present chapter, there is a subtle but important difference in reward and reinforcement processes. Reward refers to the tendency of certain events to direct behavior; specifically, to elicit and reinforce approach behavior. The term connotes a pleasant hedonic impact of rewarding stimuli, and the argument of Bindra (1969) that the motivational and hedonic attributes of stimuli are inherently related will be adopted. Reward and reinforcement can frequently be used interchangeably, but there are circumstances where the difference in the appropriate usage of these terms becomes apparent. A common observation made by workers studying BSR or intravenous drug self-administration illustrates this point. If a well-trained subject is placed in the test apparatus and does not immediately initiate responding for BSR, a single priming stimulus is usually sufficient to elicit responding. Consider the situation where the subject is sitting in the corner of the operant chamber grooming. According to a strict interpretation of reinforcement theory, a non-contingent rewarding stimulus should reinforce the grooming response. But the subject's response to that non-contingent reward is much different. Approach and vigorous lever pressing behavior immediately follow the priming stimulation. Similar effects are noted by those working with intravenous drug self-administration; non-contingent, experimenter-delivered drug infusions usually elicit lever pressing behavior in trained subjects, and priming infusions seldom effectively reinforce the behavior that the animal was emitting during the experimenter-delivered reward (e.g. grooming, rearing in the opposite corner of the test apparatus; see Stewart and de Wit, 1987).

The difference between reward and reinforcement processes can be very important when studying basic motivational processes. The case where a reward does not reinforce behavior (in the traditional operant sense) identifies an important attribute of reward mechanisms—they increase behaviors associated with their activation. Brain reward function thus describes processes that elicit approach behavior and processes that the subject 'seeks' to activate. Reward functions to direct the animal's behavior toward whatever stimulus or response is most strongly associated with reward expectancy; reinforcement refers to the process where these expectancies are developed, frequently through simple contiguity. Behavior, in this view, becomes purposive in the sense described by Tolman (1932), and reward processes are neural events that direct the subject toward stimuli associated with activation of these reward processes.

Brain Stimulation Reward

Although electrical stimulation at many different brain sites is rewarding (see Phillips and Fibiger, 1989), electrode placements along the medial forebrain bundle (MFB) extending from the lateral hypothalamus to the ventral tegmental area (VTA) have been the focus of considerable research. Electrical stimulation of this region produces the strongest rewarding effects, demonstrated by the highest lever pressing rates, lowest stimulation thresholds, and the least sensitivity to disruption by aversive contingencies (Olds, 1962, 1977; Mogenson and Phillips, 1976). There is evidence that several independent systems can support BSR (Phillips, 1984; Robertson, 1989), but the rewarding effects from electrode placements along the MFB probably represent activation of a common reward substrate.

Disruption of DA synthesis (Cooper et al., 1971; Stinus and Thierry, 1973) or blockade of DA receptors (Wauquier and Niemegeers, 1972; Lippa et al., 1973) attenuates the rewarding effects of MFB stimulation. Several behavioral measures have been developed that distinguish motor impairment from reward attenuation (Mora et al., 1975; Fouriezos and Wise, 1976; Fouriezos et al., 1978; Franklin and McCoy, 1979; Phillips and Fibiger, 1979; Gallistel et al. 1982), and most studies have reported that DA receptor blockade disrupts the rewarding impact of electrical stimulation at doses that do not produce significant impairment in the animal's ability to respond (Fibiger, 1978; Wise 1978, 1982). Microinjections of DA receptor antagonists directly into the nucleus accumbens attenuate BSR (Broekkamp and van Rossum, 1975; Mora et al., 1975; Mogenson et al., 1979; Stellar and Corbett, 1989), suggesting that this DA terminal field is critically involved in the rewarding effects of MFB stimulation. DA-depleting lesions of the mesolimbic system have been less successful in disrupting BSR, but many of the lesion studies failed to test adequate DA depletions. Several studies (Koob, et al., 1978; Fibiger and Phillips, 1979) suggest that severe DA depletions disrupt the rewarding effects of MFB stimulation.

Although the lesion data are less clear, the pharmacological data suggest an important role for DA in the rewarding effects of electrical brain stimulation. The simplest hypothesis suggests that DA neurons are directly activated by the electrical stimulation, and manipulations that interfere with the resulting enhancement of dopaminergic neurotransmission disrupt the rewarding impact of this stimulation. Studies investigating the activation of DA neurons by rewarding stimulation have used three general approaches: anatomical mapping which determines the effectiveness of electrical stimulation along the DA systems, electrophysiological characterization of the neural population directly activated by rewarding stimulation, and neurochemical evidence for activation of the ascending DA systems.

German and Bowden (1974) compared the distribution of electrode placements effective in supporting BSR with the distribution of catecholamines. Their review showed a close correspondence between sites supporting BSR and brain regions containing catecholamine fibers, cell bodies and terminal fields. Using a movable stimulation electrode combined with fluorescence histochemical visualization of DA-containing cell bodies,

Corbett and Wise (1980) reported that rewarding effects were produced by electrical stimulation within the ventral tegmental and substantia nigra–pars compacta DA-containing cell layers but not at placements adjacent to these sites. The anatomical mapping studies seemed to provide strong support for the notion that rewarding stimulation directly activated DA neurons (Wise, 1980a).

Experimental procedures developed from cellular electrophysiology have been adapted to determine the characteristics of the behaviorally relevant neurons directly activated by electrical stimulation. Electrical stimulation non-selectively activates heterogeneous neural populations, but methods have been developed that can determine the electrophysiological characteristics of the neurons that mediate the behavioral effect being studied (Gallistel et al., 1981; Shizgal, 1989). Studies using stimulation pulse pairs have determined the refractory periods (Yeomans, 1979), the conduction velocities (Bielajew and Shizgal, 1982), and the direction of conduction (Bielajew and Shizgal, 1986) for the neural population directly activated by rewarding stimulation in the lateral hypothalamus. These studies have revealed that the neurons directly activated by rewarding lateral hypothalamic stimulation are primarily fast-conducting, myelinated neurons that descend from the lateral hypothalamus to the VTA. This electrophysiological characterization eliminates the ascending DA systems as candidates for direct activation by rewarding stimulation. The DA neurons are unmyelinated and have substantially slower conduction velocities. The direction of impulse conduction is also opposite for the first-stage neurons directly activated by lateral hypothalamic stimulation and the ascending DA systems. Thus, DA neurons do not appear to be directly activated by lateral hypothalamic stimulation (but see Yeomans, 1989).

The simplest model integrating the pharmacological data (namely those that implicate DA in BSR) and the electrophysiological data (namely those that rule out DA neurons as the system directly activated by the rewarding stimulation) proposes that the ascending DA system is trans-synaptically activated by the descending system traversing the lateral hypothalamus (Wise, 1980b; Yeomans, 1982; Wise and Bozarth, 1984; Stellar and Stellar, 1985; Bozarth, 1987a). Arbuthnott et al. (1970) showed a decline in catecholamine fluorescence following lateral hypothalamic and ventral tegmental stimulation; this was attributed to the activation of dopaminergic and noradrenergic systems by the electrical stimulation. Other studies using electrical stimulation of the VTA have shown an activation of the mesolimbic DA system (for reviews see Fibiger and Phillips, 1987; Phillips et al., 1989): DA levels in the nucleus accumbens are reduced while metabolite levels are increased following rewarding stimulation. A preliminary study (M. Bozarth, unpublished observations cited in Bozarth, 1987a) suggested that rewarding lateral hypothalamic stimulation may produce bilateral activation of the mesolimbic DA system, although changes on the stimulated side corresponded better with manipulation of stimulation intensity. If bilateral activation does result from unilateral electrical stimulation, this effect could explain the apparent difficulty in disrupting BSR with unilateral DA-depleting lesions. Further work is needed to document this effect fully.

The data suggest a circuitous pathway: lateral hypothalamic stimulation along the MFB appears to activate a descending pathway that trans-synaptically activates the ascending mesolimbic DA system. The myelin sheath on the first-stage neurons functions as an electrical insulator concentrating the electrical charge at the nodes of Ranvier. This increased charge density probably permits electrical stimulation at parameters that are insufficient to activate the ascending DA neurons directly. Thus, even if electrode placements are proximal to the unmyelinated DA neurons, the electrical stimulation would preferentially activate the descending myelinated system. The neurotransmitter system comprising the descending pathway is probably heterogeneous which explains why manipulations of other neurotransmitters are not as effective as dopaminergic manipulations in altering BSR. One component of this descending system appears to be cholinergic (Gratton and Wise, 1985; Yeomans et al., 1985; Kofman and Yeomans, 1989), although non-cholinergic and perhaps even some DA neurons are also involved (see Yeomans, 1989).

Psychomotor Stimulant Reward

Two lines of evidence have converged to identify independently the neural substrate of psychomotor stimulant reward. The first involves the study of the neural basis of BSR, and the second involves the study of the neural basis of direct reinforcement from psychomotor stimulants. Early studies showed that amphetamine (Stein, 1962) and cocaine (Crow, 1970) enhanced BSR. These data were interpreted as supporting the proposed role of catecholamines in the rewarding effects of electrical stimulation. Later studies identified the nucleus accumbens as the site of action for the reward-enhancing effects of amphetamine (Broekkamp et al., 1975; Broekkamp, 1976). With the demonstration that morphine also facilitates BSR, a general model was proposed which suggested that the facilitatory effect of drugs on BSR was related to the drugs' intrinsic rewarding properties (namely, addiction liability; Broekkamp, 1976; Esposito and Kornetsky, 1978; Reid and Bozarth, 1978; Kornetsky et al., 1979; Esposito et al., 1987; Reid, 1987). This hypothesis had appreciable appeal to some groups but was not generally accepted by others who advocated study of direct reinforcing effects of drugs by using self-administration techniques. If the model is valid (i.e. that the intrinsically rewarding effect of a drug can be assessed by its facilitatory action on BSR), then studies localizing the site of the facilitation of BSR of amphetamine concurrently determined the site of its rewarding action.

Another approach to determining the neural basis of psychomotor stimulant reward examines the direct reinforcing action of these compounds. Although a number of approaches have been developed to study drug reward (Bozarth, 1987b), the most popular method uses animals prepared with intravenous catheters and allowed to self-administer drugs intravenously (Yokel, 1987). Drugs that are self-administered (and hence rewarding) in humans are generally self-administered by animals, and most drugs that are not self-administered by animals are not self-administered by humans (e.g. Deneau et al., 1969; Weeks and Collins, 1987; Yokel, 1987). The intravenous self-administration method provides an accepted paradigm for assessing drug reward and reinforcement processes, and it has been widely used to study the neuropharmacological and neuroanatomical basis of drug reinforcement (e.g. Roberts and Zito, 1987; Yokel, 1987).

Psychomotor stimulants enhance catecholaminergic neurotransmission (Axelrod, 1970; Carlsson, 1970; Heikkila et al., 1975), but only the dopaminergic enhancement is critical for the rewarding action of these drugs. Specific DA receptor blockers attenuate the rewarding impact of cocaine (de Wit and Wise, 1977; Ettenberg et al., 1982) and amphetamine (Yokel and Wise, 1975, 1976), while noradrenergic receptor-blockers are ineffective or decrease drug intake by impairing motor performance. DA-depleting lesions of the mesolimbic system at the level of the nucleus accumbens disrupt cocaine (Roberts et al., 1977, 1980) and amphetamine (Lyness et al., 1979) self-administration. Lesions in the striatum and lesions of the noradrenergic systems do not affect cocaine intake (Roberts and Zito, 1987). Destruction of the mesolimbic system by neurotoxin injections into the VTA also disrupts intravenous cocaine self-administration (Roberts and Koob, 1982). Further support for the role of the nucleus accumbens in psychomotor stimulant reward comes from the demonstration that animals will self-administer amphetamine (Hoebel et al., 1983) and DA (Dworkin et al., 1986) directly into this brain region. Other projections of the mesolimbic DA system have also been suggested to play a role in psychomotor stimulant reward (Goeders and Smith, 1983; Phillips et al., 1981; but see Martin-Iverson et al., 1986), but the importance of the nucleus accumbens terminal field is well established (Roberts and Zito, 1987).

Opiate Reward

If the facilitatory action of opiates on BSR does in fact reflect the intrinsic rewarding impact of these drugs, then the site of opiate reward was initially identified by BSR studies. Microinjection of morphine (Broekkamp, 1976; Broekkamp et al., 1976) and other opioids (Broekkamp et al., 1979) into the VTA facilitates lateral hypothalamic BSR, while injections into other brain regions do not enhance the rewarding impact of electrical stimulation. Because the significance of these data was not widely appreciated, recognition of the importance of the mesolimbic DA system in opiate reward waited for independent corroboration from more direct tests of opiate reward. Indeed, the predominant view of the 1970s and early 1980s was that opiates inhibited dopaminergic neurotransmission (e.g. Eidelberg, 1976; Schwartz et al., 1978), and that psychomotor stimulants and opiates generally produced opposite pharmacological effects. Data were reported suggesting that opiate reward was produced by an inhibition of dopaminergic neurotransmission (e.g. Glick and Cox, 1977), although the DA-enhancing effects of psychomotor stimulants were widely appreciated. Early reviews of the role of DA in reward processes did not attempt to reconcile these seemingly conflicting data and simply omitted opiate reward processes from consideration (e.g. Fibiger, 1978; Wise, 1978; c.f. Wise, 1980b; Wise and Bozarth, 1982). However, adherents to the hypothesis that the effects of addictive drugs on BSR reflect their intrinsic rewarding properties suggested that opiates, psychomotor stimulants and BSR shared a common dopaminergic substrate (Broekkamp, 1976; Bozarth, 1978).

Opiates enhance DA cell firing (Gysling and Wang, 1983; Matthews and German, 1984) and increase metabolic indices of DA release in the nucleus accumbens (Westerink, 1978; Wood, 1983). Behavioral data also suggest that opiate administration activates the mesolimbic DA system; increased locomotor activity follows bilateral morphine injections into the VTA (Joyce and Iversen, 1979), and circling behavior is produced by unilateral morphine application at the ventral tegmentum (Holmes et al., 1983; Bozarth, 1983). These studies provide electrophysiological, neurochemical and behavioral data suggesting an enhancement of the mesolimbic DA system following opiate administration.

Animals quickly learn to self-administer morphine (Bozarth and Wise, 1981a; Welzl et al., 1989) or fentanyl (van Ree and de Wied, 1980) directly into the VTA. Opiate injections into this region also produce a conditioned place preference (Phillips and LePiane, 1980; Bozarth and Wise, 1982), and the rostrocaudal boundaries of the reward-relevant opiate receptor field correspond to the approximate location of the ventral tegmental DA-containing cell bodies (Bozarth, 1987c). DA receptor blockers attenuate the rewarding impact of systemically administered opiates (Schwartz and Marchok, 1974; Bozarth and Wise, 1981b; Phillips et al., 1982), and DA-depleting lesions of the mesolimbic system disrupt the initial rewarding impact of opiates (Spyraki et al., 1983; Bozarth and Wise, 1986). Marked differences, however, are apparent in the sensitivity of opiate and psychomotor stimulant self-administration to nucleus accumbens lesions in animals previously trained to self-administer drugs (M. Bozarth and R. Wise, unpublished observation; Pettit et al., 1984). This suggests that repeated opiate administration may involve other reward processes mediated by brain regions outside the mesolimbic DA system (Bozarth, 1988; Bozarth and Wise, 1983). Nonetheless, ventral tegmental morphine infusions partially substitute for intravenous cocaine reward (Bozarth and Wise, 1986).

Other Drug Rewards

These data suggest a common dopaminergic basis for electrical brain stimulation, psychomotor stimulation and opiate rewards (see Bozarth, 1986, 1987a; Wise and Bozarth, 1984 for reviews). The fact that two distinctively different pharmacological drug classes derive at least part of their rewarding impact by activating the mesolimbic DA system prompts investigation of the possibility that other rewarding drugs may also activate this system. Data have been reported suggesting that ethanol, nicotine and barbiturates may all activate the mesolimbic DA system (DiChiara and Imperato, 1988; see also Di Chiara et al., Chapter 14, this volume). Although the importance of this effect in mediating the rewarding impact of these compounds has not been established, a general theory of addiction has been proposed that attributes the rewarding properties of various drugs to activation of the mesolimbic DA system (Wise and Bozarth, 1987). Further empirical work is needed to determine the merit of this proposal.

Other Rewards

DA has been suggested to be involved in several other appetitive behaviors, most notably feeding and drinking, sexual and maternal behavior. The role of DA in feeding behavior is well established, although the specific role of the mesolimbic DA system is less clear. The importance of DA in other motivated behaviors is more speculative, and considerable work remains to be done in these areas.

Feeding and Drinking Behavior

Specific DA-depleting lesions of the nigrostriatal system have been shown to disrupt regulation of food and water intake (Ungerstedt, 1971b; Fibiger et al., 1973; Marshall and Teitelbaum, 1973). Animals do, however, eventually resume intake of food and water, although enduring deficits persist. Lesions of the mesolimbic DA system do not attenuate food or water intake (Le Moal, et al., 1977; Bozarth and Wise, 1986; Kelley and Stinus, 1985), but they have been reported to disrupt food hoarding behavior (Kelley and Stinus, 1985). This latter measure may reflect non-regulatory food acquisition. Systemic administration of DA receptor blockers attenuates various instrumental responses maintained by food and water rewards; as with BSR studies, specific procedures have been devised to eliminate motor impairment as a factor in this effect (for review, see Wise, 1982). The DA system involved in this effect has not been established, and it is possible that either the nigrostriatal or the mesolimbic (or perhaps both) systems can influence responding for food and water.

Electrical stimulation of the lateral hypothalamus can elicit eating in food-satiated animals (for review, see Wise, 1974), and stimulation-induced feeding is attenuated by DA receptor blockade (Phillips and Nikaido, 1975; Jenck et al., 1986; Streather and Bozarth, 1987). Opioid microinjections into the VTA facilitate stimulation-induced feeding (Jenck et al., 1987), and opioid microinjections into this region also elicit feeding in non-stimulated animals (Mucha and Iversen, 1986; Hamilton and Bozarth, 1988).

It appears that activation of the mesolimbic DA system is a sufficient but not a necessary condition for feeding. The dissociation of neural systems that constitute necessary and sufficient conditions for feeding is interesting and illustrates the importance of separate consideration of these two factors in the study of brain reward systems. The integrity of the nigrostriatal DA system appears to be necessary for the normal regulation of food intake, but electrical stimulation of the substantia nigra does not elicit feeding (Phillips and Fibiger, 1973; Cioé and Mogenson, 1974). In contrast, the integrity of the mesolimbic DA system is not necessary for the normal regulation of food intake, but activation of this system does appear to elicit feeding.

Sexual Behavior

DA agonists enhance and DA antagonists attenuate male sexual behavior (Bitran and Hull, 1987). These effects are generally considered to be mediated by mechanisms in the preoptic area of the hypothalamus, but recent data suggest that the mesolimbic DA system may also be involved. Male sexual behavior is associated with increased DA release in the nucleus accumbens (Pfauss et al., 1989; see also Phillips et al., Chapter 8, this volume), and opioid microinjections into the ventral tegmentum elicit sexual behavior in castrated male rats (Mitchell and Stewart, 1990). The potential involvement of DA in opioid modulation of sexual behavior has not been determined, but the fact that ventral tegmental opioid application enhances nucleus accumbens DA function makes this possibility viable. As in the case of feeding behavior, however, the mesolimbic DA system does not appear to be necessary for normal sexual behavior, but activation of this system may be sufficient to enhance sexual responsiveness.

Maternal Behavior

Numan (1988) has reviewed evidence that neural projections from the preoptic area to the ventral tegmentum are important in maternal behavior, and that bilateral ventral tegmental lesions disrupt maternal behavior. Although the effects of DA-depleting lesions of the mesolimbic system have not been evaluated, systemic administration of a DA receptor antagonist also disrupts maternal behavior. Furthermore, prolactin, which appears to be involved in the induction of maternal behavior (Numan, 1988; Stern, 1989), has been reported to increase DA turnover in the nucleus accumbens (Fuxe et al., 1977).

GENERAL MODELS OF MOTIVATION

Two general models that have dominated motivational theory will be briefly described here. Drive-reduction theory asserts that organisms are motivated by drives which 'push' the animal toward the goal object; the behavioral objective is to reduce the drive. Incentive motivational theory asserts that organisms are motivated by the incentive value of various stimuli (namely, attraction to the goal object) which 'pull' the animal toward the goal object; motivation is generated by the expectancy of reward. Both theories recognize the relevance of drive (or at least organismic conditions that may function as a drive-like process), but the role ascribed to drive is markedly different. Drive-reduction theory specifically asserts that drive states provide motivational energy and the organism seeks to diminish drive stimulation. Incentive motivational theory asserts that organismic conditions (e.g. drive-like stimuli) modulate the incentive value of various stimuli; for example, food deprivation (producing what is classically defined as a food drive) enhances the incentive attraction of various stimuli associated with food. The increased incentive value of these stimuli, in turn, functions to energize and direct the organism's behavior toward the goal object. The primary motivation, however, is not to reduce the drive, but rather to increase and maintain contact with the incentive stimuli. Drive-reduction (e.g. food satiation) is associated with the termination of goal-directed behavior but only because the incentive stimuli are no longer able to motivate the organism without the appropriate drive-like condition.

Drive-reduction Theory

The Hullian (1943, 1952) derivation of drive-reduction theory postulated that separate energizing and directional mechanisms govern behavior. The independence of these mechanisms is illustrated by the various equations used to describe an organism's behavior. For example:

$$_sE_r = f\ (D \times\ _sH_r)\ \text{(functional equation from Hull, 1951)}$$

The organism's tendency to engage in a particular behavior ($_sE_r$, effective reaction potential) is a function of drive level (D, typically the number of hours deprivation) and habit strength ($_sH_r$, number of reinforced trials); drive provides the motivational energy, while habit strength is a primary determinant of response direction. The variables drive and habit strength are independent, except that (*1*) the reduction of drive (Hull, 1943) or the reduction of drive-related stimuli (Hull, 1952) on previous trials reinforces stimulus-response associations (i.e. increases habit strength), and (*2*) specific stimuli associated with a particular drive can increase the probability of certain behavioral responses. Nonetheless, separate mechanisms provide motivational energy and directionality for goal-directed behavior.

There are two features that must be present in the neural substrate mediating this version of drive-reduction theory—separate energizing and directional mechanisms, and a drive process that is active when the organism is motivated and whose diminished activity reinforces responding. For the drive mechanism itself, neural substrate activity is decreased during the reward process, but this reduced drive-substrate activity maintains responding until satiation.

Incentive Motivational Theory

Although Hull's drive-reduction theory also recognized the influence of incentive factors on behavior, the behavioral objective of the organism remained the reduction of drive (Hull, 1943) or drive stimuli (Hull, 1952). The incentive properties of the goal object were viewed as modulating the organism's behavior, but incentive was considered neither a primary source of motivational energy nor an important factor in governing directionality.

Incentive motivational theory permits consideration of a unitary energizing and directional mechanism. Stimuli associated with the goal object energize behavior, and the organism is motivated to increase contact with these stimuli (through approach behavior) until the motivational condition is terminated by satiation. The neural substrate mediating reward is activated by the joint action of the incentive stimulus and the internal organismic condition (i.e. central motive state; Bindra, 1974, 1978). The behavioral objective of the organism is to enhance or maintain activation of the reward substrate, not to reduce its activity as specified by drive-reduction theory.

Motivational Function of Reward Systems

The notion that organisms are motivated to decrease drive states produced by various biological needs is generally untenable. Most motivational theorists favor incentive motivational explanations of appetitive motivation (Bolles, 1967, 1972, 1975; Bindra, 1969, 1974, 1976, 1978; Toates, 1981), although aversively motivated tasks (e.g. avoidance and escape behavior) may be adequately explained by drive-reduction theory (Spence, 1956, 1960). The reward substrate mediating this incentive motivational process could both energize and direct behavior: the organism is simply motivated to maximize activation of this reward substrate. Approach behavior would increase contact with relevant incentive stimuli, and this model postulates that forward locomotion is elicited by various appetitive stimuli.

A distinctive feature of this motivational model is that animals work to maximize activation of the reward substrate. Normally, this can only be achieved by increasing contact with relevant incentive stimuli; however, if the animal could modify its own organismic condition (which in turn can increase the central motive state and enhance reward substrate activation by incentive stimuli), then the animal would perform various tasks to increase this drive-like condition. Indeed, support for this notion has been obtained from studies showing that animals will perform an instrumental response to receive lateral hypothalamic stimulation (that elicits feeding) if food is concurrently available (Mendelson, 1966; Coons and Cruce, 1968; Streather et al., 1982). This is the converse of drive-reduction theory, which states that animals work to decrease organismic conditions with drive-like properties.

Incentive stimuli operate in concert with the organism's internal state to engender approach behavior. When forward locomotion of the organism no longer continues to increase (or even maintain) activation of the reward system, then goal-directed movement ceases and the organism is functionally satiated. This condition may be associated with one of two extremely different situations—maximum-level or zero-level reward activation. The hedonic state associated with the former condition is gratification, while the hedonic state associated with the latter condition is amotivational satisfaction. Appetitive external stimuli will continue to add to (or enhance) intrinsic reward substrate activation until satiation is reached; thus the organism will continue to be motivated to approach appetitive stimuli up to the point of maximum reward. Non-contingent activation of the reward system in the absence of relevant appetitive stimuli will elicit forward locomotion similar to Hull's innate response tendencies ($_sU_r$): the organism is essentially seeking relevant stimuli. When the organism comes into contact with a relevant appetitive stimulus (e.g. food), further contact with that stimulus (e.g. consummatory response of eating) will enhance the reward activation. In this fashion, non-contingent/non-selective activation of certain reward processes can increase the effective incentive value of some appetitive stimuli, thereby broadening the stimulus–generalization gradient. This permits marginally effective stimuli to direct behavior until more salient stimuli are available. Throughout this process, the behavioral objective of the organism is to maximize activation of the reward system. One simple mechanism that could direct behavior in this manner has been described by Milner (1970).

THE MESOLIMBIC DA SYSTEM AS A MODEL REWARD SYSTEM

Research on brain reward mechanisms has developed to a stage where large amounts of empirical data appear to be explained by relatively few neural elements. Three distinct rewarding events—opioids, psychomotor stimulants and BSR—all seem to derive a major part of their reinforcing impact by the activation of a common brain reward system. This same brain system also appears to be involved in feeding, maternal behavior and forward locomotion. A specific model reward system has been formulated on the basis of these data, and the following section will describe some of the characteristics of the proposed model.

Biological Modeling of Brain Reward Systems

The concept of biological modeling is an extension of the use of model systems to study various neurological and neurobehavioral events as well as phenomena in the natural sciences. A readily identifiable system is intensely studied, and the principles elucidated by the use of the model are later tested for generalization to other applications. Whether brain reward systems actually exist is a moot point: neural elements have been identified that behave like a brain reward system, and that fulfil the criteria of a brain reward system. Specifically, activation of these neural elements, either by electrical or chemical stimulation, can selectively direct and reinforce behavior. Several distinct events can activate this system, and each appears to derive an important part of its rewarding impact through its action in this system. In addition, other, naturally motivated behaviors, such as feeding and sexual behavior, may be modulated by the activation of this system.

The use of the term biological modeling denotes that this model is not synthetically assembled *in vitro*, but rather makes use of neural elements functioning normally *in situ*. Selective activation or inhibition of these neural elements can produce reward or *may* blunt the rewarding impact of some stimuli, respectively. The utility of model construction is appreciated by the model builders, but other scientists, who are seemingly content with collecting and cataloging apparently unrelated sets of empirical observations, may be puzzled and ask 'Why build a model?' In addition to the obvious use in organizing empirical observations, a model serves as a representative testing device that can direct research aimed at determining the underlying mechanisms of behavior.

Intervening variables can be used to describe the relationship between unobservable events and behavior without exceeding the empirical database. Model construction, however, relies more heavily on hypothetical constructions that attempt to describe the underlying mechanisms mediating the behavior; this process exceeds the directly observed empirical relationships and postulates the existence of specific events not presently observed. The primary use of model construction is in its heuristics. Seemingly disparate events can sometimes be shown to share an underlying basis, when analysis supersedes the often superficial abstractive phase. For example, the marked differences in the general CNS effects of psychomotor stimulants and opiates obscured for most scientists the common basis of their rewarding effects. Adherents to the model that the effect on BSR of a drug could reveal its rewarding action had sufficient reason to probe beyond the superficial dissimilarities and question whether a common neural basis might mediate these events. This tenacity (or naïveté) may have prompted an important breakthrough in the study of drug addiction.

Many models are formulated *post hoc* and a new model is seemingly fabricated with each new experiment. This approach fails to test critically the derivations of any model and voids the primary usefulness of model construction: the model is reduced to a convenient form of data summary and loses its most important attribute for directing new research.

Application of the Hypothetico-deductive Method

One of the most rigorous attempts to develop a unifying theory of behavior based on an experimental analysis was that of Clark Hull (1943, 1952). The influence of Hull's work on contemporary motivational psychology is unclear, and little survives from Hull's extensive formulations and mathematical models. Several features of this approach to the study of behavior, however, may merit resurrection: in particular, his use and popularization of the hypothetico-deductive method of investigation.

This method begins 'with a set of explicitly stated postulates accompanied by specific or "operational" definitions of the critical terms employed' (Hull, 1937). Theorems are then derived from the postulates, and specific empirical tests are conducted to determine the validity of these predictions. This approach emphasizes deductive logic and the systematic construction of a theoretical system based on empirically substantiated theorems. 'If the theorems agree with the observed facts, the system is probably true; if they disagree, the system is false' (Hull, 1937). Although space does not permit presentation of a formal system, this approach can be used to direct model construction.

Three factors must be borne in mind when reviewing the system described in the following section. First, the model addresses only appetitive motivation;

considerable literature suggests an involvement of similar mechanisms in behavior governed by aversive stimuli, but no attempt has been made to integrate these data. Second, the mesolimbic DA system is postulated to function as a reward system, but a more comprehensive treatment of the available data would also consider other terminal projections of the ventral tegmental DA system as well as the nigrostriatal system. Restriction to the mesolimbic system will suffice to illustrate the basic approach, summarize much of the data, and postulate specific elements in a reward system. Third, the following section omits considerable data that are relevant to the system being described for brevity. The current application of this method is only illustrative and it is not intended to delineate a complete system. Rather, it is intended to show the direction dictated by this approach to theory development and scientific research.

Model Construction

Model construction proceeds by summarizing a series of empirical observations linking reward processes to mesolimbic DA function. Several distinctively different rewarding events appear to activate the mesolimbic DA system. Other, undefined commonalities may also exist, but these rewarding events are generally acknowledged as being dissimilar except for two properties: they are rewarding and they enhance mesolimbic DA function. This provides a convenient starting point for model construction as shown in Figure 1.

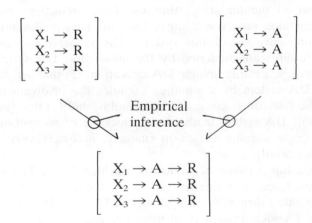

Figure 1. Model construction. X_1, Electrical brain stimulation (from LH-MFB electrode placements); X_2, psychomotor stimulant administration; X_3, opiate administration; R, reward process; A, functional activation of mesolimbic DA system

Specific neural events can be identified that are sequentially related to enhancement of mesolimbic DA function by these three stimulus events. Anatomical/functional linkages in the reward activation process include:

$$A_1 \rightarrow R$$
$$A_2 \rightarrow A_1 \rightarrow R$$
$$A_3 \rightarrow A_2 \rightarrow A_1 \rightarrow R$$
$$A_4 \rightarrow A_3 \rightarrow A_2 \rightarrow A_1 \rightarrow R$$

where R, reward; A_1, activation of postsynaptic DA receptors in the nucleus accumbens; A_2, functional release/enhancement of DA from presynaptic neurons in the nucleus accumbens DA terminal field; A_3, accelerated cell firing of ventral tegmental neurons producing an increase in impulse-coupled DA release; and A_4, stimulation of descending MFB neurons that trans-synaptically activate A10 cell bodies. This delineation provides the initial test of the model's internal validity; specific manipulations of these various linkages should produce reward. For example, the demonstration that amphetamine (Hoebel et al., 1983; White et al., 1987) and DA (Dworkin et al., 1986) microinjections into the nucleus accumbens are rewarding provides empirical confirmation for unit A_2 and unit A_1, respectively. Numerous other tests can be easily derived from the model, many of which have already received empirical support.

Model Predictions

To disrupt the reward process, substrate activation can be inhibited at any point efferent to the initiating stimulus. This 'prediction' has a single restrictive condition—the rewarding effects of the stimulus must depend exclusively on activation of this system. The model does *not* postulate (*1*) that all rewards are mediated by the mesolimbic DA system or even that all rewards necessarily involve DA activation, (*2*) that activation of the mesolimbic DA system by a stimulus excludes the involvement of other systems in the rewarding action of that stimulus, and (*3*) that disruption of the mesolimbic DA system leads to the blockade of motivational effects, even for a single stimulus condition (namely, necessary versus sufficient condition for reward).

The relationship between activation of the mesolimbic DA system and reward is postulated as a simple conditional function. *If* the mesolimbic system is activated *then* reward is produced ($A \rightarrow R$). It is not, however, biconditional ($A \Leftrightarrow R$): reward is produced *if and only if* the mesolimbic system is activated. The conclusion that reward is not produced if the mesolimbic system is not activated accepts the contrapositive of the above postulate; this is a logical fallacy (namely $A \rightarrow R$, therefore $\sim A \rightarrow \sim R$). The model readily acknowledges that activation of the mesolimbic DA system may not be a necessary condition for reward.

Some of the theorems readily derived from this model include: (*1*) drugs activating the mesolimbic DA system are rewarding (Wise and Bozarth, 1987); (*2*) drugs activating the mesolimbic DA system produce conditioned incentive effects (Beninger, 1983; Stewart and de Wit, 1987); (*3*) drugs activating the mesolimbic DA system produce forward locomotion (Wise and Bozarth, 1987); and (*4*) activation of the descending myelinated system (that trans-synaptically activates the mesolimbic DA system) specifically enhances approach behaviors associated with appetitive stimuli (Stellar et al., 1979). Each of these predictions has received partial empirical confirmation.

CONCLUSION

The model reward system developed in this chapter is obviously not intended to represent a complete system. Rather, an attempt is made to integrate a small segment of motivated behavior and to illustrate application of this method in behavioral neurobiology. The primary objective of this work is to establish a functional relationship between reward processes and activation of the mesolimbic DA system; the current objective is *not* to postulate the exact neural mechanisms underlying specific behaviors. Too much emphasis is sometimes placed on describing complex neural networks that *could* explain the relationship between two events *if* such a relationship were shown to exist.

In many respects there seems to have been very little theoretical progress in the past 30 years. The basic formulations outlined in this chapter have been previously suggested by various authors, although not necessarily assembled in the context used in this paper (Bindra, 1969, 1974, 1976; Bolles, 1972, 1975; Hull, 1943, 1952; Mendelson, 1966; Milner, 1970). However, considerable progress has been achieved in the empirical realm; specific neural mechanisms are postulated to mediate the motivational processes previously described in vague terms. The hypothetical constructs of the 1940s and 1950s are being replaced with specific neural elements, and the black box has become translucent. The heuristic value of such specification and integration with basic motivational theory can only be established by further empirical work.

REFERENCES

Andén, N.E., Dahlström, A., Fuxe, K., Larsson, K. Olson, L. and Ungerstedt, U. (1966) Ascending monoamine neurons to the telencephalon and diencephalon. *Acta Physiologica Scandinavica* **67**, 313–326.
Arbuthnott, G.W., Crow, T.J., Fuxe, K., Olson, L. and Ungerstedt, U. (1970)

Depletion of catecholamines *in vivo* induced by electrical stimulation of central monoamine pathways. *Brain Research* **24**, 471–483.

Axelrod, J. (1970) Amphetamine: metabolism, physiological disposition and its effects on catecholamine storage. In: Costa, E. and Garattini, S. (eds) *Amphetamine and Related Compounds*. New York: Raven Press, pp. 207–216.

Beninger, R.J. (1983) The role of dopamine in locomotor activity and learning. *Brain Research Reviews* **6**, 173–196.

Bielajew, C. and Shizgal, P. (1982) Behaviorally derived measures of conduction velocity in the substrate for rewarding medial forebrain bundle stimulation. *Brain Research* **237**, 107–119.

Bielajew, C. and Shizgal, P. (1986) Evidence implicating descending fibers in self-stimulation of the medial forebrain bundle. *Journal of Neuroscience* **6**, 919–929.

Bindra, D. (1969) The interrelated mechanisms of reinforcement and motivation and the nature of their influence on response. In: Arnold, W.J. and Levine, D. (eds) *Nebraska Symposium on Motivation*. Lincoln: University of Nebraska Press, pp. 1–33.

Bindra, D. (1974) A motivational view of learning, performance, and behavior modification. *Psychological Review* **81**, 199–213.

Bindra, D. (1976) *A Theory of Intelligent Behavior*. New York: John Wiley and Sons.

Bindra, D. (1978) How adaptive behavior is produced: a perceptual-motivational alternative to response-reinforcement. *Behavioral and Brain Sciences* **1**, 41–91.

Bitran, D. and Hull, E.M. (1987) Pharmacological analysis of male rat sexual behavior. *Neuroscience and Biobehavioral Reviews* **11**, 365–389.

Bolles, R.C. (1967) *Theory of Motivation*. New York: Harper and Row.

Bolles, R.C. (1972) Reinforcement, expectancy, and learning. *Psychological Review* **79**, 394–409.

Bolles, R.C. (1975) *Theory of Motivation*, 2nd ed. New York: Harper and Row.

Bozarth, M.A. (1978) Intracranial self-stimulation as an index of opioid addiction liability: an evaluation. Unpublished master's thesis, Rensselaer Polytechnic Institute.

Bozarth, M.A. (1983) Opiate reward mechanisms mapped by intracranial self-administration. In: Smith, J.E. and Lane, J.D. (eds) *Neurobiology of Opiate Reward Processes*. Amsterdam: Elsevier/North Holland Biomedical Press, pp. 331–359.

Bozarth, M.A. (1986) Neural basis of psychomotor stimulant and opiate reward: evidence suggesting the involvement of a common dopaminergic substrate. *Behavioral Brain Research* **22**, 107–116.

Bozarth, M.A. (1987a) Ventral tegmental reward system. In: Oreland, L. and Engel, J. (eds) *Brain Reward Systems and Abuse*. New York: Raven Press, pp. 1–17.

Bozarth, M.A. (ed.) (1987b) *Methods of Assessing the Reinforcing Properties of Abused Drugs*. New York: Springer-Verlag.

Bozarth, M.A. (1987c) Neuroanatomical boundaries of the reward-relevant opiate-receptor field in the ventral tegmental area as mapped by the conditioned place preference method in rats. *Brain Research* **414**, 77–84.

Bozarth, M.A. (1988) Opioid reinforcement processes. In: Rodgers, R.J. and Cooper, S.J. (eds) *Endorphins, Opiates and Behavioral Processes*. London: John Wiley and Sons, pp. 53–75.

Bozarth, M.A. and Wise, R.A. (1981a). Intracranial self-administration of morphine into the ventral tegmental area in rats. *Life Sciences* **28**, 551–555.

Bozarth, M.A. and Wise, R.A. (1981b) Heroin reward is dependent on a dopaminergic substrate. *Life Sciences* **28**, 557–562.

Bozarth, M.A. and Wise, R.A. (1982) Localization of the reward-relevant opiate receptors. In: Harris, L.S. (ed.) *Problems of Drug Dependence 1981.* Washington, DC: U.S. Government Printing Office, pp. 158–164.

Bozarth, M.A. and Wise, R.A. (1983) Neural substrates of opiate reinforcement. *Progress in Neuro-Psychopharmacology and Biological Psychiatry* 7, 569–575.

Bozarth, M.A. and Wise, R.A. (1986) Involvement of the ventral tegmental dopamine system in opioid and psychomotor stimulant reinforcement. In: Harris, L.S. (ed.) *Problems of Drug Dependence, 1985.* Washington, DC: U.S. Government Printing Office, pp. 190–196.

Broekkamp, C.L.E. (1976) The modulation of rewarding systems in the animal brain by amphetamine, morphine, and apomorphine. Druk, The Netherlands: Stichting Studentenpers Nijmegen.

Broekkamp, C.L.E. and van Rossum, J.M. (1975) The effect of microinjections of morphine and haloperidol into the neostriatum and the nucleus accumbens on self-stimulation behaviour. *Archives Internationales de Pharmacodynamie et de Therapie* 217, 110–117.

Broekkamp, C.L.E., Pijnenburg, A.J.J., Cools, A.R. and van Rossum, J.M. (1975) The effect of microinjections of amphetamine into the neostriatum and the nucleus accumbens on self-stimulation behavior. *Psychopharmacology* 42, 179–183.

Broekkamp, C.L.E., van den Bogaard, J.H., Heynen, H.J., Rops, R.H., Cools, A.R. and van Rossum, J.M. (1976) Separation of inhibiting and stimulating effects of morphine on self-stimulation behavior by intracerebral microinjection. *European Journal of Pharmacology* 36, 443–446.

Broekkamp, C.L.E., Phillips, A.G. and Cools, A.R. (1979) Facilitation of self-stimulation behavior following intracerebral microinjections of opioids into the ventral tegmental area. *Pharmacology Biochemistry and Behavior* 11, 289–295.

Carlsson, A. (1970) Amphetamine and brain catecholamines. In: Costa, E. and Garattini, S. (eds) *Amphetamine and Related Compounds.* New York: Raven Press, pp. 289–300.

Cioé, J. and Mogenson, G.J. (1974) Effects of electrical stimulation and lesions in the region of the dorsal noradrenergic (NA) pathway on feeding behavior. *Federation Proceedings* 33, 342.

Coons, E.E. and Cruce, J.A.F. (1968) Lateral hypothalamus: food and current intensity in maintaining self-stimulation of hunger. *Science* 159, 1117–1119.

Cooper, B.R., Black, W.C. and Paolino, R.M. (1971) Decreased septal-forebrain and lateral hypothalamic reward after alpha-methyl-p-tyrosine. *Physiology and Behavior* 6, 425–429.

Corbett, D. and Wise, R.A. (1980) Intracranial self-stimulation in relation to the ascending dopamine systems of the midbrain: a moveable electrode mapping study. *Brain Research* 185, 1–15.

Crow, T.J. (1970) Enhancement by cocaine of the intra-cranial self-stimulation in the rat. *Life Sciences* 9, 375–381.

Dahlström, A. and Fuxe, K. (1964) Evidence for the existence of monoamine-containing neurons in the central nervous system. I. Demonstration of monoamines in the cell bodies of brain stem neurons. *Acta Physiologica Scandinavica* 62, 1–55, (suppl 232).

Delgado, J.M.R., Roberts, W.W. and Miller, N.E. (1954) Learning motivated by electrical stimulation of the brain. *American Journal of Physiology* 179, 587–593.

Deneau, G., Yanagita, T. and Seevers, M.H. (1969) Self-administration of psychoactive substances by the monkey. *Psychopharmacologia* 16, 30–48.

Depue, R.A. and Iacono, W.G. (1989) Neurobehavioral aspects of affective disorders. *Annual Review of Psychology* 40, 457–492.

de Wit, H. and Wise, R.A. (1977) Blockade of cocaine reinforcement in rats with the dopamine receptor blocker pimozide, but not with the noradrenergic blockers phentolamine or phenoxybenzamine. *Canadian Journal of Psychology* **31**, 195–203.

DiChiara, G. and Imperato, A. (1988) Drugs abused by humans preferentially increase synaptic dopamine concentrations in the mesolimbic system of freely moving rats. *Proceedings of the National Academy of Sciences* **85**, 5247–5278.

Dworkin, S.I., Goeders, N.E. and Smith, J.E. (1986) The reinforcing and rate effects of intracranial dopamine administration. In: Harris, L.S. (ed.) *Problems of Drug Dependence, 1985*. Washington, DC: U.S. Government Printing Office, pp. 242–248.

Eidelberg, E. (1976) Possible actions of opiates upon synapses. *Progress in Neurobiology* **6**, 81–102.

Esposito, R.U. and Kornetsky, C. (1978) Opioids and rewarding brain stimulation. *Neuroscience and Biobehavioral Reviews* **2**, 115–122.

Esposito, R.U., Porrino, L.J. and Seeger, T.F. (1987) Brain stimulation reward: measurement and mapping by psychophysical techniques and quantitative 2-[^{14}C] deoxyglucose autoradiography. In: Bozarth, M.A. (ed.) *Methods of Assessing the Reinforcing Properties of Abused Drugs*. New York: Springer-Verlag, pp. 421–445.

Ettenberg, A., Pettit, H.O., Bloom, F.E. and Koob, G.F. (1982) Heroin and cocaine intravenous self-administration in rats: mediation by separate neural systems. *Psychopharmacology* **78**, 204–209.

Fibiger, H.C. (1978) Drugs and reinforcement mechanisms: a critical review of the catecholamine theory. *Annual Review of Pharmacology and Toxicology* **18**, 37–56.

Fibiger, H.C. and Phillips, A.G. (1979) Dopamine and the neural mechanisms of reinforcement. In: Horn, A.S., Westerink, B.H.C. and Korf, J. (eds) *The Neurobiology of Dopamine*. New York: Academic Press, pp. 597–615.

Fibiger, H.C. and Phillips, A.G. (1987) Role of catecholamine transmitters in brain reward systems: implications for the neurobiology of affect. In: Engel, J. and Oreland, L. (eds) *Brain Reward Systems and Abuse*. New York: Raven Press, pp. 61–74.

Fibiger, H.C., Zis, A.P. and McGeer, E.G. (1973) Feeding and drinking deficits after 6-hydroxydopamine administration in the rat: similarities to the lateral hypothalamic syndrome. *Brain Research* **55**, 135–148.

Fitzsimons, J.T. (1971) The physiology of thirst: a review of the extraneural aspects of the mechanisms of drinking. In: Stellar, E. and Sprague, J.M. (eds) *Progress in Physiological Psychology, Vol. 4*. New York: Academic Press, pp. 119–201.

Fouriezos, G. and Wise, R.A. (1976) Pimozide-induced extinction of intracranial self-stimulation: response patterns rule out motor or performance deficits. *Brain Research* **103**, 377–380.

Fouriezos, G., Hansson, P. and Wise, R.A. (1978) Neuroleptic-induced attenuation of brain stimulation reward in rats. *Journal of Comparative and Physiological Psychology* **92**, 661–671.

Franklin, K.B.J. and McCoy, S.N. (1979) Pimozide-induced extinction in rats: stimulus control of responding rules out motor deficit. *Pharmacology Biochemistry and Behavior* **11**, 71–75.

Fuxe, K., Eneroth, P., Gustafsson, J.-A., Lofstrom, A. and Skett, P. (1977) Dopamine in the nucleus accumbens: preferential increase of DA turnover by rat prolactin. *Brain Research* **122**, 177–182.

Gallistel, C.R., Shizgal, P. and Yeomans, J.S. (1981) A portrait of the substrate for self-stimulation. *Psychological Review* **88**, 228–273.

Gallistel, C.R., Boytim, M., Gomita, Y. and Klebanoff, L. (1982) Does pimozide block the reinforcing effect of brain stimulation? *Pharmacology Biochemistry and Behavior* **17**, 769–781.

German, D.C. and Bowden, D.M. (1974) Catecholamine systems as the neural substrate for intracranial self-stimulation: a hypothesis. *Brain Research* 73, 381–419.

Glick, S.D. and Cox, R.D. (1977) Changes in morphine self-administration after brainstem lesions in rats. *Psychopharmacology* 52, 151–156.

Goeders, N.E. and Smith, J.E. (1983) Cortical dopaminergic involvement in cocaine reinforcement. *Science* 221, 773–775.

Gratton, A. and Wise, R.A. (1985) Hypothalamic reward mechanism: two first-stage fiber populations with a cholinergic component. *Science* 227, 545–548.

Gysling, K. and Wang, R.Y. (1983) Morphine-induced activation of A10 dopamine neurons in the rat. *Brain Research* 277, 119–127.

Hamilton, M.E. and Bozarth, M.A. (1988) Feeding elicited by dynorphin 1-13 microinjections into the ventral tegmental area in rats. *Life Sciences* 43, 941–946.

Heikkila, R.E., Orlansky, H. and Cohen, G. (1975) Studies on the distinction between uptake inhibition and release of [^{3}H]dopamine in rat brain tissue slices. *Biochemical Pharmacology* 24, 847–852.

Hess, W.R. (1949) *Das Zwischenhirn*. Basel: Schwabe.

Hoebel, B.G., Monaco, A.P., Hernandez, L., Aulisi, E.F., Stanley, B.G. and Lenard, L. (1983) Self-injection of amphetamine directly into the brain. *Psychopharmacology* 81, 158–163.

Holmes, L.J., Bozarth, M.A. and Wise, R.A. (1983) Circling from intracranial morphine applied to the ventral tegmental area in rats. *Brain Research Bulletin* 11, 295–298.

Hull, C.L. (1937) Mind, mechanism, and adaptive behavior. *Psychological Review* 44, 1–32.

Hull, C.L. (1943) *Principles of Behavior: An Introduction to Behavior Theory*. New York: Appleton-Century-Crofts.

Hull, C.L. (1951) *Essentials of Behavior*. New Haven: Yale University Press.

Hull, C.L. (1952) *A Behavior System*. New Haven: Yale University Press.

Jenck, F., Gratton, A. and Wise, R.A. (1986) Effects of pimozide and naloxone on latency for hypothalamically induced eating. *Brain Research* 375, 329–337.

Jenck, F., Quirion, R. and Wise, R.A. (1987) Opioid receptor subtypes associated with ventral tegmental facilitation and periaqueductal gray inhibition of feeding. *Brain Research* 423, 39–44.

Joyce, E.M. and Iversen, S.D. (1979) The effect of morphine applied locally to mesencephalic dopamine cell bodies on spontaneous motor activity in the rat. *Neuroscience Letters* 14, 207–212.

Kelley, A.E. and Stinus, L. (1985) Disappearance of hoarding behavior after 6-hydroxydopamine lesions of the mesolimbic dopamine neurons and its reinstatement with L-dopa. *Behavioral Neuroscience* 99, 531–545.

Kofman, O. and Yeomans, J.S. (1989) Cholinergic antagonists in ventral tegmentum elevate thresholds for lateral hypothalamic and brainstem self-stimulation. *Pharmacology Biochemistry and Behavior* 31, 547–559.

Koob, G.F., Fray, P.J. and Iversen, S.D. (1978) Self-stimulation at the lateral hypothalamus and locus coeruleus after specific unilateral lesions of the dopamine system. *Brain Research* 146, 123–140.

Kornetsky, C., Esposito, R.U., McLean, S. and Jacobson, J.O. (1979) Intracranial self-stimulation thresholds: a model for the hedonic effects of drugs of abuse. *Archives of General Psychiatry* 36, 289–292.

Le Moal, M., Stinus, L., Simon, H., Tassin, J.P., Thierry, A.M., Blanc, G., Glowinski, J. and Cardo (1977) Behavioral effects of a lesion in the ventral mesencephalic tegmentum: evidence for involvement of A10 dopaminergic neurons. In: Costa, E. and Gessa, G.L. (eds) *Advances in Biochemical Psychopharmacology*. New York: Raven Press, pp. 237–245.

Lindvall, O. and Björklund, A. (1974) The organization of the ascending catecholamine neuron systems in the rat brain. *Acta Physiologica Scandinavica* **412**, 1–48.

Lippa, A.S., Antelman, S.M., Fisher, A.E. and Canfield, D.R. (1973) Neurochemical mediation of reward: a significant role for dopamine? *Pharmacology Biochemistry and Behavior* **1**, 23–28.

Lyness, W.H., Friedle, N.M. and Moore, K.E. (1979) Destruction of dopaminergic nerve terminals in nucleus accumbens: effect on d-amphetamine self-administration. *Pharmacology Biochemistry and Behavior* **11**, 553–556.

Marshall, J.F. and Teitelbaum, P. (1973) A comparison of the eating in response to hypothermic and glucoprivic challenges after nigral 6-hydroxydopamine and lateral hypothalamic electrolytic lesions in rats. *Brain Research* **55**, 229–233.

Martin-Iverson, M.T., Szostak, C. and Fibiger, H.C. (1986) 6-hydroxydopamine lesions of the medial prefrontal cortex fail to influence intravenous self-administration of cocaine. *Psychopharmacology* **88**, 310–314.

Matthews, R.T. and German, D.C. (1984) Electrophysiological evidence for excitation of rat ventral tegmental area dopamine neurons by morphine. *Neuroscience* **11**, 617–625.

Mendelson, J. (1966) Role of hunger in T-maze learning for food by rats. *Journal of Comparative and Physiological Psychology* **62**, 341–349.

Milner, P.M. (1970) *Physiological Psychology*. New York: Holt, Rinehart and Winston.

Mitchell, J.B. and Stewart, J. (1990) Facilitation of sexual behaviors in the male rat associated with intra-VTA injections of opiates. *Pharmacology Biochemistry and Behavior* **33**, 643–650.

Mogenson, G.J. and Phillips, A.G. (1976) Motivation: a psychological construct in search of a physiological substrate. In: Sprague, J.M. and Epstein, A.N. (eds) *Progress in Psychobiology and Physiological Psychology, Vol. 6*. New York: Academic Press, pp. 189–243.

Mogenson, G.J., Takigawa, M., Robertson, A. and Wu, M. (1979) Self-stimulation of the nucleus accumbens and ventral tegmental area of Tsai attenuated by microinjections of spiroperidol into the nucleus accumbens. *Brain Research* **171**, 247–259.

Mogenson, G.J., Jones, D.L. and Yim, C.Y. (1980) From motivation to action: functional interface between the limbic system and the motor system. *Progress in Neurobiology* **14**, 69–97.

Mora, F., Sanguinetti, A.M., Rolls, E.T. and Shaw, S.G. (1975) Differential effects on self-stimulation and motor behavior produced by microintracranial injections of a dopamine-receptor blocking agent. *Neuroscience Letters* **1**, 179–184.

Mucha, R.F. and Iversen, S.D. (1986) Increased food intake after opioid microinjections into nucleus accumbens and ventral tegmental area of rat. *Brain Research* **397**, 214–224.

Numan, M. (1988) Maternal behavior. In: Knobil, E. and Neill, J. (eds) *The Physiology of Reproduction*. New York: Raven Press, pp. 1569–1645.

Olds, J. (1962) Hypothalamic substrates of reward. *Physiological Review* **42**, 554–604.

Olds, J. (1977) *Drives and Reinforcements: Behavioral Studies of Hypothalamic Functions*. New York: Raven Press.

Olds, J. and Milner, P. (1954) Positive reinforcement produced by electrical stimulation of septal area and other regions of rat brain. *Journal of Comparative Physiological Psychology* **47**, 419–427.

Olds, M.E. and Olds, J. (1963) Approach-avoidance analysis of the rat diencephalon. *Journal of Comparative Neurology* **120**, 259–295.

Palkovits, M. and Jacobowitz, D.M. (1974) Topographic atlas of catecholamine and acetylcholinesterase-containing neurons in the rat brain. II. Hindbrain (mesencephalon, rhombencephalon). *Journal of Comparative Neurology* **157**, 29–42.

Pettit, H.O., Ettenberg, A., Bloom, F.E. and Koob, G.F. (1984) Destruction of dopamine in the nucleus accumbens selectively attenuates cocaine but not heroin self-administration in rats. *Psychopharmacology* **84**, 167–173.

Pfauss, J.G., Newton, T.N., Blaha, C.D., Fibiger, H.C. and Phillips, A.G. (1989) Electrochemical detection of central dopamine efflux during sexual activity in male rats. *Society for Neuroscience Abstracts* **15**, 558.

Phillips, A.G. (1984) Brain reward circuitry: a case for separate systems. *Brain Research Bulletin* **12**, 195–201.

Phillips, A.G. and Fibiger, H.C. (1973) Substantia nigra: self-stimulation and poststimulation feeding. *Physiological Psychology* **1**, 233–236.

Phillips, A.G. and Fibiger, H.C. (1979) Decreased resistance to extinction after haloperidol: implications for the role of dopamine in reinforcement. *Pharmacology Biochemistry and Behavior* **10**, 751–760.

Phillips, A.G. and Fibiger, H.C. (1989) Neuroanatomical bases of intracranial self-stimulation: untangling the Gordian knot. In: Liebman, J.M. and Cooper, S.J. (eds) *The Neuropharmacological Basis of Reward*. Oxford: Oxford University Press, pp. 66–105.

Phillips, A.G. and LePiane, F.G. (1980) Reinforcing effects of morphine microinjection into the ventral tegmental area. *Pharmacology Biochemistry and Behavior* **12**, 965–968.

Phillips, A.G. and Nikaido, R.S. (1975) Disruption of brain stimulation-induced feeding by dopamine receptor blockade. *Nature* **258**, 750–751.

Phillips, A.G., Mora, F. and Rolls, E.T. (1981) Intracerebral self-administration of amphetamine by rhesus monkeys. *Neuroscience Letters* **24**, 81–86.

Phillips, A.G., Spyraki, C. and Fibiger, H.C. (1982) Conditioned place preference with amphetamine and opiates as reward stimuli: attenuation by haloperidol. In: Hoebel, B.G. and Novin, D. (eds) *The Neural Basis of Feeding and Reward*. Brunswick, ME: Haer Institute, pp. 455–464.

Phillips, A.G., Blaha, C.D. and Fibiger, H.C. (1989) Neurochemical correlates of brain-stimulation reward measured by ex vivo and in vivo analyses. *Neuroscience and Biobehavioral Reviews* **13**, 99–104.

Reid, L.D. (1967) Reinforcement from direct stimulation of the brain. Unpublished doctoral dissertation, University of Utah.

Reid, L.D. (1987) Tests involving pressing for intracranial stimulation as an early procedure for screening likelihood of addiction of opioids and other drugs. In: Bozarth, M.A. (ed.) *Methods of Assessing the Reinforcing Properties of Abused Drugs*. New York: Springer-Verlag, pp. 391–420.

Reid, L.D. and Bozarth, M.A. (1978) Addictive agents and intracranial stimulation (ICS): the effects of various opioids on pressing for ICS. *Problems of Drug Dependence*, **1977**, 729–741.

Roberts, D.C.S. and Koob, G.F. (1982) Disruption of cocaine self-administration following 6-hydroxydopamine lesions of the ventral tegmental area in rats. *Pharmacology Biochemistry and Behavior* **17**, 901–904.

Roberts, D.C.S. and Zito, K.A. (1987) Interpretation of lesion effects on stimulant self-administration. In: Bozarth, M.A. (ed.) *Methods of Assessing the Reinforcing Properties of Abused Drugs*. New York: Springer-Verlag, pp. 87–103.

Roberts, D.C.S., Corcoran, M.E. and Fibiger, H.C. (1977) On the role of ascending catecholaminergic systems in intravenous self-administration of cocaine. *Pharmacology Biochemistry and Behavior* **6**, 615–620.

Roberts, D.C.S., Koob, G.F., Klonoff, P. and Fibiger, H.C. (1980) Extinction and recovery of cocaine self-administration following 6-hydroxydopamine lesions of the nucleus accumbens. *Pharmacology Biochemistry and Behavior* **12**, 781–787.

Robertson, A. (1989) Multiple reward systems and the prefrontal cortex. *Neuroscience and Biobehavioral Reviews* **13**, 163–170.

Schwartz, A.S. and Marchok, P.L. (1974) Depression of morphine-seeking behaviour by dopamine inhibition. *Nature* **248**, 257–258.

Schwartz, J.C., Pollard, H., Llorens, C., Malfroy, B., Gros, C., Pradelles, Ph. and Dray, F. (1978) Endorphins and endorphin receptors in striatum: relationships with dopaminergic neurons. *Advances in Biochemical Psychopharmacology* **18**, 245–264.

Shizgal, P. (1989) Toward a cellular analysis of intracranial self-stimulation: contribution of collision studies. *Neuroscience and Biobehavioral Reviews* **13**, 81–90.

Spence, K.W. (1956) *Behavior Theory and Conditioning*. New Haven: Yale University Press.

Spence, K.W. (1960) *Behavior Theory and Learning*. Engelwood Cliffs, New Jersey: Prentice-Hall.

Spyraki, C., Fibiger, H.C. and Phillips, A.G. (1983) Attenuation of heroin reward in rats by disruption of the mesolimbic dopamine system. *Psychopharmacology* **79**, 278–283.

Stein, L. (1962) Effects and interactions of imipramine, chlorpromazine, reserpine and amphetamine on self-stimulation: possible neuro-physiologial basis of depression. In: Wortis, J. (ed.) *Recent Advances in Biological Psychiatry*. New York: Academic Press, pp. 288–308.

Stein, L. (1964) Reciprocal action of reward and punishment mechanisms. In: Heath, R.G. (ed.) *The Role of Pleasure in Behavior*. New York: Harper and Row, pp. 113–139.

Stein, L. and Belluzzi, J.D. (1987) Reward transmitters and drugs of abuse. In: Engel, J. and Oreland, L. (eds) *Brain Reward Systems and Abuse*. New York: Raven Press, pp. 19–33.

Stellar, J.R. and Corbett, D. (1989) Regional neuroleptic microinjections indicate a role for nucleus accumbens in lateral hypothalamic self-stimulation reward. *Brain Research* **477**, 126–143.

Stellar, J.R. and Stellar, E. (1985) *The Neurobiology of Motivation and Reward*. New York: Springer-Verlag.

Stellar, J.R., Brooks, F.H. and Mills, L.E. (1979) Approach and withdrawal analysis of the effects of hypothalamic stimulation and lesions in rats. *Journal of Comparative and Physiological Psychology* **93**, 446–466.

Stern, J.M. (1989) Maternal behavior: sensory, hormonal, and neural determinants. In: Brush, F.R. and Levine, S. (eds) *Psychoendocrinology*. San Diego: Academic Press, pp. 105–226.

Stewart, J. and de Wit, H. (1987) Reinstatement of drug-taking behavior as a method of assessing incentive motivational properties of drugs. In: Bozarth, M.A. (ed.) *Methods of Assessing the Reinforcing Properties of Abused Drugs*. New York: Springer-Verlag, pp. 211–227.

Stinus, L. and Thierry, A.-M. (1973) Self-stimulation and catecholamines. II. Blockade of self-stimulation by treatment with alpha-methylparatyrosine and the reinstatement by catecholamine precursor administration. *Brain Research* **64**, 189–198.

Streather, A. and Bozarth, M.A. (1987) Effect of dopamine-receptor blockade on stimulation-induced feeding. *Pharmacology Biochemistry and Behavior* **27**, 521–524.

Streather, A., Bozarth, M.A. and Wise, R.A. (1982) Instrumental responding in the absence of drive: the role of reward-expectancy. Paper presented to the 43rd Annual Meeting of the Canadian Psychological Association, Montréal.

Toates, F.M. (1981) The control of ingestive behaviour by internal and external stimuli: a theoretical review. *Appetite* **2**, 35–50.

Tolman, E.C. (1932) *Purposive Behavior in Animals and Men*. New York: Century.

Trowill, J.A., Panksepp, J. and Gandelman, R. (1969) An incentive model of rewarding brain stimulation. *Psychological Review* **76**, 264–281.

Ungerstedt, U. (1971a) Stereotaxic mapping of the monoamine pathways in the rat brain. *Acta Physiologica Scandinavica* **367**, 1–48.

Ungerstedt, U. (1971b) Adipsia and aphagia after 6-hydroxydopamine induced degeneration of the nigro-striatal dopamine system. *Acta Physiologica Scandinavica* **367**, 95–122 (suppl).

van Ree, J.M. and de Wied, D. (1980) Involvement of neurohypophyseal peptides in drug-mediated adaptive responses. *Pharmacology Biochemistry and Behavior* **13**, 257–263 (suppl 1).

Wauquier, A. and Niemegeers, C.J.E. (1972) Intracranial self-stimulation in rats as a function of various stimulus parameters. II. Influence of haloperidol, pimozide, and pipamperone on medial forebrain bundle stimulation with monopolar electrodes. *Psychopharmacologia* **27**, 191–202.

Weeks, J.R. and Collins, R.J. (1987) Screening for drug reinforcement using intravenous self-administration in the rat. In: Bozarth, M.A. (ed.) *Methods of Assessing the Reinforcing Properties of Abused Drugs*. New York: Springer-Verlag, pp. 35–43.

Welzl, H., Kuhn, G. and Huston, J.P. (1989) Self-administration of small amounts of morphine through glass micropipettes into the ventral tegmental area of the rat. *Neuropharmacology* **28**, 1017–1023.

Westerink, B.H.C. (1978) Effects of centrally acting drugs on regional dopamine metabolism. In: Roberts, P.J., Woodruff, G.N. and Iversen, L.L. (eds) *Advances in Biochemical Psychopharmacology*. New York: Springer-Verlag, pp. 35–43.

White, N.M. (1989) Reward or reinforcement: what's the difference? *Neuroscience and Biobehavioral Reviews* **13**, 181–186.

White, N.M., Messier, C. and Carr, G.D. (1987) Operationalizing and measuring the organizing influence of drugs on behavior. In: Bozarth, M.A. (ed.) *Methods of Assessing the Reinforcing Properties of Abused Drugs*. New York: Springer-Verlag, pp. 591–617.

Wise, R.A. (1974) Lateral hypothalamic stimulation: does it make animals 'hungry'? *Brain Research* **67**, 187–209.

Wise, R.A. (1978) Catecholamine theories of reward: a critical review. *Brain Research* **152**, 215–247.

Wise, R.A. (1980a) The dopamine synapse and the notion of 'pleasure centers' in the brain. *Trends in Neurosciences* **3**, 91–94.

Wise, R.A. (1980b) Action of drugs of abuse on brain reward systems. *Pharmacology Biochemistry and Behavior* **13**, 213–223.

Wise, R.A. (1982) Neuroleptics and operant behavior: the anhedonia hypothesis.

Behavioral and Brain Sciences **5**, 39–88.

Wise, R.A. (1989) The brain and reward. In: Liebman, J.M. and Cooper, S.J. (eds) *The Neuropharmacological Basis of Reward*. Oxford: Oxford University Press, pp. 377–424.

Wise, R.A. and Bozarth, M.A. (1982) Actions of drug abuse on brain reward systems: an update with specific attention to opiates. *Pharmacology Biochemistry and Behavior* **17**, 239–243.

Wise, R.A. and Bozarth, M.A. (1984) Brain reward circuitry: four elements 'wired' in apparent series. *Brain Research Bulletin* **12**, 203–208.

Wise, R.A. and Bozarth, M.A. (1987) A psychomotor stimulant theory of addiction. *Psychological Review* **94**, 469–492.

Wise, R.A. and Rompré, P.-P. (1989) Brain dopamine and reward. *Annual Review of Psychology* **40**, 191–225.

Wood, P.L. (1983) Opioid regulation of CNS dopaminergic pathways: a review of methodology, receptor types, regional variations and species differences. *Peptides* **4**, 595–601.

Yeomans, J.S. (1979) Absolute refractory periods of self-stimulation neurons. *Physiology and Behavior* **22**, 911–919.

Yeomans, J.S. (1982) The cells and axons mediating medial forebrain bundle reward. In: Hoebel, B.G. and Novin, D. (eds) *The Neural Basis of Feeding and Reward*. Brunswick, ME: Haer Institute, pp. 405–417.

Yeomans, J.S. (1989) Two substrates for medial forebrain bundle self-stimulation: myelinated axons and dopamine axons. *Neuroscience and Biobehavioral Reviews* **13**, 91–98.

Yeomans, J.S., Kofman, O. and McFarlane, V. (1985) Cholinergic involvement in lateral hypothalamic rewarding brain stimulation. *Brain Research* **329**, 19–26.

Yokel, R.A. (1987) Intravenous self-administration: response rates, the effects of pharmacological challenges, and drug preferences. In: Bozarth, M.A. (ed.) *Methods of Assessing the Reinforcing Properties of Abused Drugs*. New York: Springer-Verlag, pp. 1–35.

Yokel, R.A. and Wise, R.A. (1975) Increased lever pressing for amphetamine after pimozide in rats: implications for a dopamine theory of reward. *Science* **187**, 547–549.

Yokel, R.A. and Wise, R.A. (1976) Attenuation of intravenous amphetamine reinforcement by central dopamine blockade in rats. *Psychopharmacology* **48**, 311–318.

13

Interactions between Endogenous Opioids and Dopamine: Implications for Reward and Aversion

STEVEN J. COOPER

School of Psychology, University of Birmingham, Birmingham B15 2TT, UK

INTRODUCTION

The behavioural pharmacology of dopamine (DA) began in the 1960s, ushered in with the discovery of its presence in the brain in the mid-1950s; Carlsson's (1959) insight that DA might be involved in extrapyramidal motor functions; the discovery by Ehringer and Hornykiewicz (1960) that there was an almost complete loss of DA in the caudate and putamen of parkinsonian patients; and the extraordinary visualization of monoamines (including DA) in nerve cell bodies and terminals of the brain, achieved first using the Falck–Hillarp fluorescence method (Andén et al., 1964, 1966; Dahlström and Fuxe, 1964; Fuxe, 1965). Many of the earlier behavioural studies were concerned with the stereotyped responses elicited by the DA agonist apomorphine and the indirectly acting agonist d-amphetamine (Cooper and Dourish, 1990).

It was inevitable that the effects on brain DA of a drug as important to pharmacology and clinical therapy as morphine should be investigated at an early stage. In one of the first studies by Gauchy et al (1973), acute administration of morphine increased the synthesis and release of DA in the striatum. However, the dose of morphine used in this study (60 mg/kg) was exceedingly large. Sugrue (1974) detected an increase in DA turnover in the rat striatum following the administration of a smaller, yet still

The Mesolimbic Dopamine System: From Motivation to Action.
Edited by P. Willner and J. Scheel-Krüger

© 1991 John Wiley & Sons Ltd

substantial, dose of morphine (10 mg/kg). More recently, Kim et al. (1986) reported that acute administration of morphine (16 mg/kg) increased DA metabolism not only in the rat striatum but also in other brain regions that receive DA innervation: the olfactory tubercle, cingulate cortex, prefrontal cortex and pyriform cortex.

The effects of smaller doses of morphine are of more direct interest to behavioural pharmacologists. At doses of 1 or 2 mg/kg of morphine, injected subcutaneously, stimulation of grooming, locomotion, rearing, feeding or drinking occurs in rats (Fog, 1970; Babbini and Davis, 1972; Ayhan and Randrup, 1973; Norton, 1977; Sanger and McCarthy, 1980; Cooper, 1981). At a larger dose (5 mg/kg), rats may appear sedated, while, at 20 mg/kg, morphine can induce a cataleptic state (Fog, 1970). Hence, the early studies on DA metabolism and release appear to relate more to morphine-induced catalepsy rather than to the behavioural stimulant effects which are encountered at much smaller doses. However, Scheel-Krüger and his colleagues (1977b) observed that a small dose of apomorphine inhibited morphine-induced locomotor stimulation. Since small doses of apomorphine preferentially stimulate DA autoreceptors, these authors suggested a role for dopaminergic mechanisms in morphine's stimulant effects. Iwamoto (1981) confirmed the observation and also showed that morphine-induced hypermotility could be blocked by spiperone, a DA receptor antagonist.

By the late 1970s, investigators had turned to the method of direct administration of morphine into selected regions of the brain to explore more fully the effects of the drug on brain DA activity. One group reported that morphine, injected directly into the substantia nigra (a region containing dopaminergic cell bodies), caused hypermotility in rats but induced sedation and catalepsy when injected into the nucleus accumbens or caudate nucleus (regions that are rich in DA terminals) (Di Chiara et al., 1977). Costall et al. (1978) confirmed that the initial effect of morphine injected into the nucleus accumbens was a cataleptic state, but that it was followed, some hours later, by a hyperactivity phase. It is interesting to note that, earlier, Lorens and Mitchell (1973) had reported a biphasic effect of morphine on the rate of intracranial brain stimulation in rats. They administered morphine systemically, finding that an initial complete inhibition of responding was followed, some hours later, by a substantial increase. Broekkamp and his colleagues (1976, 1979b) demonstrated that it was possible to obtain increased rates of self-stimulation (in the absence of any depressant effects), when morphine was injected directly into the posterior hypothalamus, ventral tegmental area (VTA) or substantia nigra. The inference they drew from their results was that purely stimulant effects of morphine can be obtained, provided that the drug is injected in the vicinity of DA-containing cell bodies, located in the ventral midbrain.

Subsequent electrophysiological studies indicated that morphine, either administered systemically or injected directly into the VTA or into the substantia nigra, excited the activity of dopaminergic neurones (Gysling and Wang, 1983; Hommer and Pert, 1983; Matthews and German, 1984). *In vivo* dialysis experiments have also demonstrated that morphine and methadone increase the extracellular concentration of DA in the nucleus accumbens, consistent with increased activity of mesolimbic DA pathways (Di Chiara and Imperato, 1988a, b). Measurements of tissue 3-methoxytyramine (a metabolite of DA formed after DA release) also indicate that opioids increase DA release in mesolimbic and mesocortical terminal areas (Wood and Altar, 1988).

Understandably, behavioural pharmacologists were drawn to the effects of morphine, and of related drugs, in the ventral mesencephalon, and to the idea that purely stimulant effects may depend upon the excitation of DA-containing neurons. Attention, for a time at least, was largely diverted away from the effects of these drugs within brain regions that are rich in DA terminals.

This brief, historical introduction sets the stage for a more detailed discussion of behavioural experiments involving opioid–DA interactions. However, we must first consider certain momentous discoveries of the 1970s and early 1980s which created an entirely new climate in which to understand not only opioid pharmacology, but also novel features of brain function itself.

OPIOID SYSTEMS OF THE BRAIN

Multiple Opioid Receptors

The first significant discovery was the detection within the brain of specific receptors for morphine and other narcotic analgesics (Pert and Snyder, 1973; Simon et al., 1973; Terenius, 1973). Morphine produces its pharmacological effects by its action as an agonist at these sites. Using autoradiographic methods, the localization of opioid receptors throughout the brain and spinal cord has been described in great detail (Atweh and Kuhar, 1977a, b, c). Opioid receptors are found in many regions of the central nervous system, but these regions include the caudate nucleus and nucleus accumbens, as well as the ventral mesencephalon (Pollard et al., 1977, 1978; Llorens-Cortes et al., 1979; Murrin et al., 1980).

Pharmacological studies by Martin and his colleagues (1976) in the dog indicated that subtypes of the opioid receptor exist: their work distinguished between the μ type (after morphine), and the κ type (after the benzomorphan ketocyclazocine). Lord and his colleagues (1977) then identified the δ type (after the mouse vas deferens preparation). A specific receptor for β-endorphin (the ε receptor) has also been proposed (Schulz et al., 1979), but its presence in the central nervous system is uncertain. It was realized, therefore, that opioid drugs might interact with one or more of the receptor subtypes, which then led to the idea that different neuropharmacological effects of opioids may depend upon the relative potencies of the drugs at each of the subtypes (Zukin and Zukin, 1981). More recently, details of the distribution of μ, κ and δ opioid receptors within the rat brain have been published (Mansour et al., 1986, 1987). *Mu* opioid receptors are present in high concentrations in the amygdala, nucleus accumbens, caudate-putamen and substantia nigra zona compacta. *Delta* receptors are found in DA terminal regions, e.g. amygdala, olfactory tubercle, nucleus accumbens and caudate-putamen, but appear to be largely absent from midbrain structures. *Kappa* receptors are also found in the DA terminal regions, and in high concentrations in the interpeduncular nucleus of the midbrain. In general terms, therefore, brain regions rich in DA terminals contain all three types of opioid receptor, whereas in the mesencephalon, μ receptors predominate and δ receptors are poorly represented.

Multiple Opioid Peptides

The second major discovery was the presence of endogenous ligands for opioid receptors within the brain. Two pentapeptides were identified: leu- and met-enkephalin (Hughes et al., 1975). Thereafter, the potent analgesic peptide β-endorphin was discovered, and was found to be distributed within the brain in ways that were quite different from those of the two enkephalins (Bloom et al., 1978; Watson et al., 1978). More endogenous opioid peptides followed, including dynorphin (Goldstein et al., 1979), and α-neo-endorphin (Kangawa et al., 1981). By 1982, it was realized that endogenous opioid peptides are cleavage products derived from three large precursor molecules: *pro-opiomelanocortin* (POMC), which gives rise to β-endorphin as well as the non-opioid peptide hormone adrenocorticotrophic hormone (ACTH); *proenkephalin*, which contains multiple copies of met-enkephalin and a single copy of leu-enkephalin; and *prodynorphin*, which contains neo-endorphin, dynorphin A and dynorphin B (Akil et al., 1988).

Is there a relationship between multiple opioid receptors and multiple opioid peptides? Table 1 shows that peptides show some degree of selectivity for opioid receptors; however, as Akil and her colleagues (1988) have clarified, opioid peptides may interact with other opioid receptors for which they have lower affinity under physiological conditions.

The discovery of endogenous opioid peptides, and of multiple receptors, has given new directions to our thinking about DA–opioid interactions. Above, the possible effects of a drug, morphine, on DA activity are discussed. Are its effects shared by other drugs that bind with different affinities to the several opioid receptors? If not, then there may be several

Table 1. Relationships between multiple opioid receptors and opioid receptor ligands. Modified from Herz and Shippenberg (1989) with permission

Receptor type	Endogenous ligand	Exogenous ligand	Antagonist
μ	β-Endorphin?	Morphine DAGO	Naloxone (low dosage) CTOP
δ	Enkephalins	DPDPE DTLET	ICI 174,864
κ	Dynorphins	U-50,488H U-69593	Norbinaltorphimine
ε	β-Endorphin	—	(β-Endorphin$_{1-27}$)

β-Endorphin may interact with the ε receptor in the periphery, but does not appear to exert its central effects through this receptor sub-type; the specificity of β-endorphin$_{1-27}$ as a β-endorphin antagonist is unclear (Shippenberg, personal communication). CTOP, D-Pen-Cys-Tyr-D-Trp-Orn-Thr-Pen-Thr-NH$_2$; DPDPE, D-Pen^2-D-Pen^5-enkephalin; U-50,488H, trans-3,4-dichloro-N-methyl-N(2-(1-pyrolidinyl)-cyclohexyl)-benzeneacetamide; U-69593, [5,7,8]-(+)-methyl-N-[7-(1-pyrrolidinyl)1-oxa-spiro(4,5)dec-8-yl]benzeneacetamide; ICI 174,864, Allyl$_2$-Tyr-Aib-Phe-Leu-OH; DAGO, D-Ala^2-N-Phe^4-Gly-ol^5 enkephalin; DTLET, D-Thr^2-Leu^5-enkephanyl-Thr^6

differing types of effects of opioid compounds on DA activity. As far as brain function is concerned, a fundamental question is whether or not endogenous opioid peptides affect DA transmission.

At present there are insufficient data to answer each of these questions in full, and certainly not so far as behavioural data are concerned. Nevertheless, they are questions which must be borne in mind, not only to help in the assessment and interpretation of existing data but also to indicate what remains to be ascertained. In the next section, I shall concentrate on the ventral mesencephalon and review behavioural experiments, in which attempts have been made to analyse opioid effects on DA activity, mediated (it is assumed) by opioid receptors located on, or near, DA cell bodies and their dendrites. As discussed above, by the late 1970s, the notion that morphine acts in the VTA and substantia nigra to excite dopaminergic neurons was current. In the following examples, investigators examined the effects of direct injections of morphine, or other opioid compounds, into ventral midbrain regions.

VTA AND SUBSTANTIA NIGRA

Circling Responses

Iwamoto and Way (1977) described the effects of morphine in the substantia nigra of naïve rats. Unilateral injection of morphine produced continuous circling behaviour that was contralateral to the site of injection. The induced circling could be blocked either by the opioid antagonist naloxone or by the DA antagonist haloperidol. The circling response could also be obtained with unilateral microinjection of β-endorphin, methadone and other opioid agonists. These authors suggested that the contralateral circling arose as a result of a unilateral stimulation of ascending DA pathways. Jacquet (1983) confirmed that unilateral injection of morphine into the rat substantia nigra produced contralateral rotation. A similar effect was observed when met[5]-encephalin was injected into the same site.

Dynorphin-containing neurons originate in the striatum and project to the substantia nigra zona reticulata (Vincent et al., 1982; Fallon et al., 1985; McLean et al., 1985). When dynorphins are injected unilaterally into this division of the substantia nigra, marked contralateral rotation is obtained and the effect is blocked by naloxone (Herrera-Marschitz et al., 1984). Morelli and Di Chiara (1985) confirmed that dynorphins and morphine stimulated contralateral circling after unilateral injection into the substantia nigra. While naltrexone antagonized the circling response to the opioid treatments, 6-hydroxydopamine (6-OHDA) lesions of the medial forebrain bundle (MFB) (which contains ascending dopaminergic fibres) did not. Morelli and Di Chiara (1985) came to a conclusion quite different from that of previous authors; they proposed that the circling response elicited by opioids occurred independently of the DA nigrostriatal projection, and reflected, instead, an inhibition of non-DA 'output' neurons from the substantia nigra. They also noted the similarity between opioid and GABAergic stimulation of the substantia nigra in producing circling responses (Scheel-Krüger et al., 1977a; Arnt and Scheel-Krüger, 1979a) for effects of GABA agonists in the substantia nigra.

Confirmation of these interesting data has been furnished by Matsumoto and colleagues (1988a). Their results indicate that unilateral injection of rimorphin, an opioid peptide derived from prodynorphin (Kilpatrick et al., 1982), into the substantia nigra zona reticulata, produced contralateral rotation, but that 6-OHDA lesions of midbrain DA cells did not reduce the effect. Matsumoto et al. (1988a) concluded that rimorphin acts at opioid receptors that are not linked to DA neurons, but affects GABAergic efferents in the substantia nigra.

Morphine also induces contralateral turning when it is injected unilaterally into the VTA (Holmes et al., 1983). Since its effect was blocked by a DA antagonist, pimozide, Holmes and Wise (1985) concluded that the circling response was mediated by DA neurons in the VTA. Hence, there appear to be two opposing views on the involvement of DA in opioid-induced rotational behaviour: the principal issue is whether or not ascending DA neurons are involved in the circling response to opioid treatments. Moreover, while some investigators have concentrated upon the substantia nigra, Wise and his collaborators have turned their attention to the VTA. A resolution, at least in part, of the main issue comes from experiments in which various agonists, selective for the several opioid receptor subtypes, have been used.

Matsumoto and colleagues (1988b) compared the effects of unilateral injections of selective agonists into the substantia nigra pars reticulata: they chose the selective μ receptor ligand DAGO ([D-Ala^2,MePhe^4,Gly-ol^5]-enkephalin) (Handa et al., 1981), the δ receptor ligand DPDPE ([D-Pen^2, D-Pen^5]-enkephalin) (Corbett et al., 1984; Cotton et al., 1985), and the κ receptor ligand U-50,488H (trans-3,4-di-chloro-N-methyl-N-[2-(1-pyrolidinyl)-cyclohexyl]-benzeneacetamide) (von Voigtlander et al., 1983). All three produced dose-dependent contralateral turning, and, in each case, the effect was blocked by naloxone. However, unilateral 6-OHDA lesions of the MFB decreased the circling produced by DAGO and DPDPE, but enhanced the response to U-50,488H. Systemic administration of amphetamine increased the circling response to DAGO and DPDPE, but had no effect on the response to U-50,488H. From these results, Matsumoto et al. (1988b) concluded that nigrostriatal DA neurons are involved to some extent in the rotational responses elicited by selective stimulation of μ and δ receptors. However, they excluded a role for DA pathways in the response to selective κ stimulation. Instead, these authors propose that inhibition of GABAergic efferents in the pars reticulata is responsible for the motor effects of κ stimulation. Since the products of prodynorphin are endogenous opioid peptides with high affinity for κ receptors (Chavkin et al., 1982; Young et al., 1986), their suggestion would account for the DA-independent effects of dynorphins on circling, reported earlier by Morelli and Di Chiara (1985).

Jenck et al. (1988) reported that unilateral injections of morphine and DPDPE into the VTA elicited circling, whereas injection of U-50,488H into the same region had no effect. Their data also implicate μ and δ receptors in the circling response to opioids, and it is possible that both the VTA and the substantia nigra are sites of action for this effect. Cannula placements are, of course, not an exact guide to the sites of action of intracranially administered drugs; structures adjacent to target sites can also be affected.

Behavioural Stimulant Effects

Iwamoto and Way (1977) also noted that bilateral injection of either morphine or β-endorphin resulted in intense stereotyped behaviour: continuous sniffing, biting and gnawing were seen. They proposed that morphine can act at opioid receptors located in the substantia nigra and hence bring about stimulation of the dopaminergic nigrostriatal pathway. Morelli and colleagues (1989) have recently confirmed and extended these observations. When the selective opioid agonist N-MePhe^3,-D-Pro^4 morphiceptin (Blanchard et al., 1987) was injected bilaterally into the substantia nigra zona reticulata, stereotyped sniffing and gnawing were elicited. These effects were blocked by naloxone and the μ-selective irreversible antagonist β-funaltrexamine. They also showed that bilateral administration of DPDPE elicited exploratory activity and rearing, but not gnawing. Its effects were reduced by the selective δ receptor antagonist ICI 174,864 (Cotton et al., 1984). Stimulation of μ- and δ-opioid receptors in the zona reticulata appears therefore to give rise to distinguishable behavioural effects. Morelli et al. (1989) went further and suggested that, in both cases, activation of dopaminergic neurons occurs since the effects of the opioid agonists were blocked by the DA antagonists haloperidol and the selective DA D1 antagonist SCH 23990.

Arnt and Scheel-Krüger (1979b) also observed several effects of morphine when it was injected bilaterally into the caudal region of the VTA in rats: increased locomotion, rearing, licking and sniffing were seen. They suggested that the DA projection from the VTA to the nucleus accumbens (the mesolimbic projection) may underlie the stimulant effects of morphine. Joyce and Iversen (1979) reached a similar conclusion. Rats exhibited increased locomotor activity following bilateral injection of morphine into the VTA. The effect was blocked either by naloxone or by haloperidol.

Later studies confirmed that bilateral injection of opioids into the VTA leads to stimulation of locomotor activity and other behavioural responses. Thus, injection of the stabilized enkephalin analogue, [D-Ala^2]-Met^5-enkephalinamide (DALA) resulted in increased locomotion, rearing and sniffing (Broekkamp et al., 1979a; Kalivas et al., 1983; Kelley et al., 1980). Stimulation of locomotor activity was also reported when either β-endorphin or [D-Ala^2,D-Leu^5]-enkephalin (DADLE) was injected bilaterally into the VTA (Stinus et al., 1980; Joyce et al., 1981). Latimer et al. (1987) attempted to identify the type of opioid receptor that mediates these effects. They reported that the specific μ receptor agonist DAGO was more potent than the δ receptor agonist DPDPE in stimulating locomotor activity, and also in increasing DA metabolism in the nucleus accumbens, striatum, septum and prefrontal cortex. They proposed, therefore, that μ receptors are largely responsible for the activation of VTA DA neurons by morphine and other opioid agonists.

The relationship between behavioural stimulant effects and activation of DA pathways may not be completely straightforward, however. Thus, Cador and her colleagues (1989) showed that, when DALA was injected into the VTA, there were dose-related increases in the DOPAC:DA ratio in DA terminal regions, namely the nucleus accumbens, striatum and septum. However, the behavioural effects of DALA injected into the VTA showed a biphasic relationship to dose (Cador et al., 1988). Small doses of DALA (0.05 and 0.1 μg/ul) had stimulant effects, but larger doses (1.0 and 2.5 μg/ul) suppressed behaviour. Hence, increased DA metabolism does correlate with behavioural stimulation for smaller doses of DALA, but with larger doses the increased DA metabolism is apparently associated with behavioural depression.

I have dealt with circling, stereotyped behaviour and locomotor responses in some detail to highlight the major problems which confront investigators of the functional effects of opioid–DA interactions. First, there is the pharmacological issue of which of the several types of opioid receptors mediate the behavioural response: μ, δ or κ? Second, there is the critical question of establishing whether the response to opioid stimulation is indeed dependent upon DA activity. If it is dependent, then the next question to consider is whether or not a subdivision of the ascending DA pathways from the ventral midbrain is primarily responsible for the opioid effects.

With regard to the circling data, it appears that all three types of opioid receptor in the ventral midbrain are capable of mediating opioid-inducing circling. However, while the rotational responses to μ and δ receptor stimulation appear to involve dopaminergic mechanisms, the circling responses to κ receptor stimulation do not. The evidence for the neuroanatomical identity of the DA pathways which mediate the μ and δ effects is divided: one group (Matsumoto et al., 1988b) proposes that the nigrostriatal projection is critical for the opioid-induced circling, whereas another (Jenck et al., 1988) suggests that the mesolimbic DA projection from the VTA area is more importantly involved. Bilateral stimulation of μ receptors in the substantia nigra zona reticulata elicits stereotyped gnawing, whereas stimulation of δ receptors elicited sniffing and exploratory locomotor activity. Both types of responding appear to be DA-dependent, since they are blocked by DA antagonists.

In the case of locomotor activity, the evidence consistently shows that stimulation of opioid receptors in the VTA produces marked increases in locomotor activity. The opioid receptors are probably μ and δ types, although μ receptors may be more influential for the activating effect of the opioid stimulation (Latimer et al., 1987). Furthermore, the behavioural effect is associated with stimulation of ascending DA pathways to a number of forebrain regions.

Feeding

Sanger and McCarthy (1980) have shown that small doses of morphine, systemically administered, increase food intake in non-deprived rats. More recently, Mucha and Iversen (1986) obtained a similar result when they injected morphine into the VTA. Two further studies suggest that the VTA is a site for opioid receptors involved in feeding responses. Cador et al. (1986) reported that the bilateral infusion of DALA (0.1 and 1.0 μg/ul) increased food intake in both non-deprived and food-deprived animals.

Hamilton and Bozarth (1988) have shown that dynorphin$_{1-13}$ is considerably more potent than morphine in eliciting feeding when injected into the VTA.

The last result is interesting since dynorphins are selective for κ receptors (Table 1). Selective κ agonists, when administered systemically, increase food consumption in rats (Cooper et al., 1985). Therefore, κ receptors may mediate the response to dynorphin$_{1-13}$ in the VTA. Nevertheless, dynorphins are also effective μ ligands (Akil et al., 1988), and therefore one cannot exclude the possibility that μ receptors in the VTA mediate the feeding responses. Whatever the opioid receptor, there is no direct evidence, as yet, that the feeding response to opioids injected into the VTA depends on the DA cells located there. Neither is it clear that the feeding response is related to the stimulant effects described in the previous section. Comparisons with the effects of the peptide neurotensin are instructive. When neurotensin is injected into the VTA, there is a marked increase in DA turnover in the nucleus accumbens and a DA-dependent increase in locomotor activity (Kalivas et al., 1983). Nevertheless, neurotensin has a pronounced inhibitory effect on feeding when it is injected into the VTA (Cador et al., 1986). Hence, there is no simple relationship between feeding responses on the one hand and locomotor stimulation with increased DA activity on the other.

Brain Stimulation Reward

In this, and the next two sections, the evidence for opioid–DA interactions in the VTA and their relevance to reward processes will be considered.

As discussed above, Broekkamp and his colleagues (1979b) found that morphine strongly facilitated the rate of self-stimulation when injected directly into the VTA. In addition, it has been shown that both DALA and DPDPE have the same effect (Broekkamp et al., 1979b; Jenck et al., 1987). The κ agonist U-50,488H, however, has no effect on brain self-stimulation (Jenck et al., 1987).

If DA pathways are involved in these facilitatory effects, then it would be expected that self-stimulation in the VTA itself would lead to increased activity in these pathways. Indeed, it has been shown that increases in the DOPAC:DA ratio occur in the nucleus accumbens, striatum and olfactory tubercle as a result of VTA self-stimulation (Simon et al., 1979; Fibiger et al., 1987). Nevertheless, a critical issue left unresolved by these data is the extent to which the 'reward' of the brain stimulation is associated with the increased DA turnover. There is some evidence which leaves this question open. First, yoked-stimulation of the VTA (on a non-contingent basis) in a second animal produced the same neurochemical effects as self-stimulation (Fibiger et al., 1987). Since non-contingent brain stimulation can be aversive (Steiner et al., 1969), the relationship between increased DA turnover and reward is left ambiguous. Second, responding for food reward on an FR8 schedule of reinforcement had no effect on DA metabolism (Fibiger et al., 1987). Hence, the primary reward of food may not require the involvement of mesolimbic DA activity (Phillips et al., Chapter 8, this volume).

Intracranial Drug Self-administration

Bozarth and Wise (1981a) reported that naïve rats would learn a response which led to infusion of morphine directly into the VTA. Other brain regions were found not to support morphine self-administration (Bozarth and Wise, 1982). Furthermore, injection of an opioid antagonist into the VTA resulted in a compensatory increase in the rate of intravenous heroin self-stimulation (Britt and Wise, 1983). The conclusion drawn by these authors was that the VTA is the most important site for the reward of opioid administration. As such, these data have provided key support for the hypothesis that the mesolimbic DA system is responsible, at least in part, for opioid-induced reward, and, more generally, for the reward of all drugs of abuse (Bozarth, 1986; Wise and Bozarth, 1987).

Other work had shown that in animals previously trained to self-administer heroin intravenously, responding could be reinstated after a period of extinction by a non-contingent, 'priming' injection of heroin (de Wit and Stewart, 1983). Stewart (1984) then showed that the VTA was a site of action for an opioid 'priming' effect. Injection of morphine into the VTA reinstated both heroin and cocaine self-administration in previously trained rats. Stewart suggested that the morphine acted at opioid receptors to stimulate mesolimbic DA activity and thereby engaged appetitive motivational systems of the brain.

It is apparent that the types of opioid receptors involved in intracranial drug self-stimulation or in the priming effect have not yet been identified. More importantly, there is no direct evidence that the reward and priming effects of opioids within the VTA are DA-dependent, as postulated. Identifying sites of action within the VTA remains insufficient evidence, in itself, for the underlying hypothesis that the reward effect of opioids depends upon actions at opioid receptors, followed by stimulation of mesolimbic DA neurons.

Conditioned Place Preference

Conditioning of place preference, as a result of pairings with drug treatments, is an increasingly popular method of assessing the rewarding effects of such treatments (Carr et al., 1989). In an early study, Schwartz and Marchok (1974) demonstrated that morphine-dependent rats acquired a preference for a distinctive environment that had been repeatedly paired with morphine.

Rossi and Reid (1976) then provided evidence for a place preference conditioning effect when morphine was administered to naïve rats. This was followed by a study of Katz and Gormezano (1979), who reported conditioning of a place preference when morphine was administered into the lateral ventricles of naïve rats.

However, it was Phillips and LePiane (1980) who first demonstrated that bilateral administration of morphine into the VTA could serve as a reinforcer in the conditioning of a place preference. The same authors then demonstrated that a conditioned place preference could be obtained when DALA was injected directly into the VTA (Phillips and LePiane, 1982), and that its effect could be blocked either by haloperidol or by 6-OHDA lesions of ascending DA pathways (Phillips et al., 1983). As a result, Phillips et al. (1983) proposed that the reinforcing effects of opioids, at least when injected directly into the VTA, depend upon ascending DA pathways. Bozarth (1987) mapped the neuroanatomical boundaries for morphine-reinforced place preference conditioning, and showed that they corresponded with the distribution of dopaminergic cell bodies in the VTA. Glimcher et al. (1984) reported that not only was DALA effective in the VTA, but also that the enkephalinase inhibitor thiorphan, injected into the same region, would serve as a reinforcer.

Taken together, these studies indicate quite strongly that stimulation of opioid receptors within the VTA gives rise to an appetitive motivational effect which determines conditioning of specific place preferences. There is also evidence to suggest that opioid action leads to the activation of ascending dopaminergic pathways. In a later section, the involvement of opioid receptor subtypes, not only in reward processes, but also in relation to aversion will be considered in detail. Furthermore, the involvement of DA receptor subtypes in the effects of opioids will be discussed.

NUCLEUS ACCUMBENS

Opioids may interact with dopaminergic activity not only by their actions at receptors located in the ventral mesencephalon, but also through their actions at receptors located within the terminal fields (Pollard et al., 1977). The material in this section is organized so that comparisons can be drawn between the effects of opioids injected into the nucleus accumbens and those of indirectly acting DA agonists, e.g. d-amphetamine, or directly acting agonists, e.g. DA, apomorphine, injected into the same brain region. The similarities between the effects of the two categories of drugs (opioids or DA agonists) can be quite striking. Nevertheless, the data will also be scrutinized to determine whether there is evidence for interactions between the effects of the two types of drugs. Does opioid activity in the nucleus accumbens modulate or mediate dopaminergic function? Alternatively, are there two separate systems, with little interaction between them, and which act in parallel fashion?

Locomotor Activity

Several groups have reported that injection of DA (given together with nialamide, a monoamine oxidase inhibitor) into the nucleus accumbens increases locomotor activity and induces intense sniffing in rats (Pijnenburg and van Rossum, 1973; Costall and Naylor, 1975; Jackson et al., 1975; Makanjuola et al., 1980). These effects of DA could be blocked by DA antagonists, including haloperidol, pimozide and sulpiride (Jackson et al., 1975; Pijnenburg et al., 1975a; Costall and Naylor, 1976). Injections of d-amphetamine into the nucleus accumbens also produced locomotor stimulant effects which were blocked by DA antagonists (Jackson et al., 1975; Pijnenburg et al., 1975b). The situation, so far as opioids are concerned, is more complicated. Pert and Sivit (1977) reported that the injection of either morphine or DALA into the nucleus accumbens induced hyperactivity in rats. Other authors, however, observed that an immediate effect of morphine in the nucleus accumbens was the induction of akinesia and catalepsy (Di Chiara et al., 1977; Costall et al., 1978; Winkler et al., 1982; Havemann and Kuschinsky, 1985). One resolution to this apparent discrepancy is provided by Daugé et al. (1988). These authors demonstrated that injection of DTLET, a selective δ agonist, into the nucleus accumbens produced locomotor hyperactivity which could be blocked by naloxone and by ICI 174,864, a selective δ receptor antagonist (Cotton et al., 1984). Hyperactivity was also induced by injection of kelatorphan, an enkephalinase inhibitor (Fournié-Zaluski et al., 1984). Thus, endogenous enkephalins acting at δ receptors in the nucleus accumbens may stimulate locomotor activity. In contrast, injection of the μ agonist DAGO into the nucleus accumbens produced initial suppression of activity (Daugé et al., 1988). Longoni and colleagues (1989) also reported that intra-accumbens injection of MePhe³-DPRO⁴ morphiceptin, a selective μ receptor agonist, produced catalepsy followed by behavioural depression. Hence, stimulation of μ receptors appears to be responsible for the akinetic and cataleptic effects of opioids in the nucleus accumbens.

Do the behavioural activating effects of opioids in the nucleus accumbens depend upon dopaminergic transmission? Pert and Sivit (1977) reported that haloperidol did not block the hypermotility response to injection of morphine into the nucleus accumbens. Likewise, the increase in locomotion and rearing produced by injection of DALA into the nucleus accumbens was not affected by DA receptor blockade, or by 6-OHDA lesions of mesolimbic DA pathways (Kalivas et al., 1983). Indeed, lesions of the mesolimbic DA system actually enhanced the locomotor activity response to intra-accumbens injections of DALA (Kalivas and Bronson, 1985). Similarly, thioproperazine (a DA antagonist) had no effect on the behavioural responses to the administration of kelatorphan, or of selective μ and δ agonists, into the nucleus accumbens (Daugé et al., 1989).

Nevertheless, Longoni et al. (1989) have reported that the behavioural stimulant effects of ala-deltorphin, a selective δ receptor agonist, injected into the nucleus accumbens could be blocked by the selective DA D1 receptor antagonist, SCH 23390. It seems possible, therefore, that δ receptor stimulation in the nucleus accumbens produces hypermotility that depends on D1 receptor stimulation. It would be interesting to determine whether the locomotor stimulant effects of DA agonists injected into the nucleus accumbens also depend upon the stimulation of D1 receptors. If they do, a common mechanism may underlie the responses to the two classes of drugs (receptor agonists and DA agonists). Activity at opioid receptors must precede the stimulation of DA receptors (and not vice versa) since the stimulant effects of DA in the nucleus accumbens are unaffected by naloxone (Pert and Sivit, 1977; Swerdlow et al., 1987).

Feeding

Injection of small doses of d-amphetamine (2–2.5 μg bilaterally) into the nucleus accumbens has a facilitatory effect on feeding responses (Evans and Vaccarino, 1986; Colle and Wise, 1988). In larger doses, however, an anorectic effect is obtained (Carr and White, 1986; Evans and Vaccarino, 1986; Colle and Wise, 1988). Whether or not this facilitatory effect on feeding is DA-dependent remains to be determined.

Bilateral injection of morphine into the nucleus accumbens also increases food consumption in rats (Mucha and Iversen, 1986). A more detailed pharmacological analysis has been reported by Majeed and co-workers (1986). They confirmed the hyperphagic response to morphine, but also provided evidence that stimulation of either μ or δ receptors may underlie the effect. Thus, morphine, DADLE and β-endorphin were effective in stimulating food consumption, and so too was the selective δ receptor agonist DPDPE. β-Funaltrexamine, a selective μ antagonist, blocked the response to morphine but not that to DADLE. It seems unlikely that κ opioid receptors are implicated since injections of U-50,488H or bremazocine (both are κ agonists) into the nucleus accumbens were ineffective. Nevertheless, hyperphagic effects of α-neo-endorphin and dynorphin were detected although it remains possible that these were mediated by non-κ receptors.

At the present time, the relationship between amphetamine-induced feeding and opioid-induced feeding, involving the nucleus accumbens, remains open for further investigation.

Brain Stimulation Reward

Positive sites for intracranial self-stimulation are found in the main terminal regions of the mesolimbic and mesocortical DA pathways, namely the nucleus accumbens (Phillips et al., 1975), striatum (Phillips et al., 1976) and prefrontal cortex (Routtenberg and Sloan, 1972; Rolls and Cooper, 1974). With regard to the nucleus accumbens, Broekkamp (1975) reported that bilateral injections of amphetamine into this region increased rate of lever pressing in rats with electrodes in the VTA. This result is consistent with data that self-stimulation of the VTA activates ascending DA pathways (Phillips and Fibiger, 1978). However, 6-OHDA lesions of mesolimbic DA pathways have little effect on intra-accumbens self-stimulation (Phillips and Fibiger, 1978). The reward effects of nucleus accumbens stimulation may therefore depend upon non-dopaminergic mechanisms.

De Witte and colleagues (1989) reported that rates of self-stimulation at sites in the MFB were decreased by intra-accumbens injections of kelatorphan and DAGO, but slightly increased by DTLET. However, Daugé et al. (1988) found that intra-accumbens injections of DAGO decreased locomotor activity, whereas DTLET stimulated activity. Hence, changes in the rates of self-stimulation may have been due to non-specific increases in activity, as distinct from any change in the reward value of the brain stimulation. The results for kelatorphan appear to be discrepant, since intra-accumbens injection produced a slight increase in locomotor activity (Swerdlow et al., 1987; Daugé et al., 1988). Nevertheless, intraventricular administration of kelatorphan increased the rate of self-stimulation (De Witte et al., 1989), so that the discrepancy may be more apparent than real.

Kurumiya and Nakajima (1988) reported that injection of the selective DA D1 antagonist SCH 23390 into the nucleus accumbens reduced the rate of responding for rewarding stimulation of the VTA. Whether or not the effects of opioids injected into the VTA, or into the nucleus accumbens, on responding for rewarding brain stimulation are dependent upon D1 receptors in the accumbens remains to be determined.

Intracranial Drug Self-Administration

Rats will self-administer DA and indirectly acting DA agonists into forebrain regions that are rich in DA terminals. Rats learn to self-administer DA (Guerin et al., 1984) or d-amphetamine (Hoebel et al., 1983) into the nucleus accumbens. Rhesus monkeys self-administer amphetamine into the orbitofrontal cortex (Phillips and Rolls, 1981), while rats have been shown to self-administer cocaine into the medial prefrontal cortex (Goeders and Smith, 1983). These data suggest that activation of forebrain DA mechanisms underlies the reinforcing effects of intracranial administration of stimulants. 6-OHDA lesions of the nucleus accumbens have been reported to abolish intravenous d-amphetamine self-administration (Lyness et al., 1979), and to disrupt intravenous cocaine self-administration (Roberts et al., 1980). Such lesions would be expected to reduce or prevent the increased release of DA in the nucleus accumbens caused by d-amphetamine or cocaine (Di Chiara and Imperato, 1988a; Carboni et al., 1989). However, the response to a directly acting DA agonist should not be impaired, and indeed could be enhanced, as a result of the development of postsynaptic DA receptor supersensitivity. Roberts (1989) has recently shown that supersensitivity does develop and that intravenously administered apomorphine becomes a more effective reinforcer in rats with 6-OHDA lesions of the nucleus accumbens.

Opioids acting at opioid receptors in the nucleus accumbens are also effective as reinforcers. Olds (1982) reported that rats self-administer morphine into the nucleus accumbens, while Goeders and colleagues (1984) showed that rats self-administer met-enkephalin into the same region. Administration of an opioid antagonist (methyl naloxonium chloride) into the nucleus accumbens increased intravenous self-administration of heroin in rats (Vaccarino et al., 1985; Corrigall and Vaccarino, 1988). This effect was interpreted in terms of a decrease in the reinforcement provided by the heroin injections, leading to an increase in the rate of responding. Thus, blockade of opioid receptors in the nucleus accumbens may be sufficient to reduce the reward value of self-administered opioids.

Are the reward effects of psychomotor stimulants and opioids in the nucleus accumbens related? One approach to this question has been to lesion the nucleus accumbens with kainic acid, an excitotoxin which selectively destroys cell bodies (Schwarcz and Coyle, 1977). Bilateral infusions of kainic acid into the nucleus accumbens decreases the reinforcing efficacy of morphine, and also disrupts intravenous self-administration of apomorphine, cocaine and heroin (Zito et al., 1985; Dworkin et al., 1988). One interpretation of these data is that destruction of cell bodies in the nucleus accumbens damages neural systems, postsynaptic to dopaminergic afferents which are involved in mediating the reward of opioids and psychomotor stimulants. Nevertheless, these studies do not identify the sites of action of the reinforcing drugs and it would be of considerable interest to repeat these experiments with intra-accumbens self-administration of opioids and stimulants.

The kainic acid lesion results suggest that neurons intrinsic to the nucleus accumbens are involved in the reinforcing effects of opioid and stimulant drugs. However, they do not provide evidence that the *same* neurons are involved in mediating the effects of both classes of drugs. There is some evidence, in fact, that intravenous cocaine self-administration is DA-dependent, whereas heroin self-administration is not. Thus, α-flupenthixol (a DA antagonist) and 6-OHDA lesions of the nucleus accumbens disrupted cocaine self-administration but not heroin self-administration (Ettenberg et al., 1982; Pettit et al., 1984). The neural systems underlying the reinforcing effects of heroin and cocaine may be independent (Bozarth, Chapter 12, this volume).

Conditioned Place Preferences

Carr and White (1983) obtained conditioned place preferences in rats with intra-accumbens injections of d-amphetamine (10 μg). The reward effect of amphetamine may depend on both dopaminergic and serotonergic innervations of the nucleus accumbens (Spyraki et al., 1982, 1988). Van der Kooy et al. (1982) showed that conditioned place preferences can be obtained when morphine is injected into the nucleus accumbens (or into the lateral hypothalamus or periaqueductal grey). While 6-OHDA lesions of mesolimbic DA neurons, or DA antagonists, disrupt place preferences conditioned with systemically administered heroin (Bozarth and Wise, 1981b; Spyraki et al., 1983), there is as yet no direct evidence that the reward effects of intra-accumbens opioid stimulation are dependent on DA.

OPIOID PRODUCED REWARD AND AVERSION

Considerable efforts have gone into identifying central opioid receptors that mediate place conditioning effects. (The evidence that stimulation of peripheral opioid receptors produces aversive effects will not be considered in this chapter; see Bechara and Van der Kooy, 1985.) An interesting and fundamental distinction which emerges is that conditioned place *preferences* can be obtained with drugs selective for either μ or δ opioid receptors. In contrast, conditioned place *aversions* are obtained with ligands selective for κ receptors. These results have led to the view that the rewarding, euphoric effects of opioids depend upon stimulation of either μ or δ receptors, whereas stimulation of κ receptors produces aversive, dysphoric effects.

Mu and Delta Receptor-mediated Reward

As discussed above, the μ ligand morphine, whether injected subcutaneously, intravenously or intracerebroventricularly, reliably conditions place preference in rats (Table 2). Intracerebroventricular administration of DAGO, a selective μ receptor ligand, also produces a conditioned place preference (Bals-Kubik et al., 1988). Morphine also produces conditioned place preferences when injected either into the VTA or nucleus accumbens. Its reward effects, determined using the place preference conditioning paradigm, are blocked by naloxone, but not by the selective δ receptor antagonist ICI 174,864 (Shippenberg et al., 1987). The selective δ agonist DPDPE is also effective in conditioning a place preference, which is blocked by ICI 174,

Table 2. A summary of the evidence of μ receptor agonists and δ receptor agonists condition place preferences in rats

Drug	Action	Routes of administration	Place preference blocked by:	Place preference unaffected by:	References
Morphine	μ Agonist	s.c. i.c.v. VTA NAS	Naloxone SCH 23390 (DA D1 antagonist) Ritanserin (a 5-HT$_2$ antagonist) 5-HT lesions of nucleus accumbens	D2 antagonists Inflammatory pain ICI 174,864 (selective δ opioid antagonist)	Rossi and Reid, 1976 Katz and Gormezano, 1979 Stapleton et al., 1979 Phillips and LePiane, 1980 Mucha et al., 1982 Van der Kooy et al., 1982 Mucha and Iversen, 1984 Mucha and Herz, 1985 Iwamoto, 1986 Mucha and Herz, 1986 Nomikos and Spyraki, 1988 Shippenberg and Herz, 1987 Shippenberg et al., 1987 Shippenberg and Herz, 1988 Shippenberg et al., 1988 Spyraki et al., 1988 Acquas et al., 1989
DAGO	Selective μ agonist	i.c.v.	i.c.v. injection of β-endorphin$_{1-27}$		Bals-Kubik et al., 1988
DPDPE	selective δ agonist	i.c.v.	ICI 174,854 (selective δ opioid antagonist) i.c.v. injection of β-endorphin$_{1-27}$		Shippenberg et al., 1987 Bals-Kubik et al. 1988.

s.c., Subcutaneous; i.c.v., intraventricular; VTA, intraventral tegmental area; NAS, intra-accumbens

864 (Shippenberg et al., 1987). Hence, stimulation of either receptor subtype is sufficient to produce a reward effect, but the effects appear to be independent of each other.

Conversely, selective antagonism of central μ receptors has aversive consequences. The aversive effects of naloxone treatments are well documented (Table 3); however, recently it has been reported that the selective μ receptor antagonist, CTOP (Pelton et al., 1986), also produces a conditioned place aversion (Bals-Kubik et al., 1989). Since the aversive effect of naloxone can be blocked by lesions of the arcuate nucleus (the region of the origin of β-endorphin neural pathways) it seems probable that the effect results from the antagonism of central β-endorphinergic activity. Herz and Shippenberg (1989) noted that β-endorphin-containing fibres innervate the VTA (Figure 1), and suggested that stimulation of either μ or δ opioid receptors could activate DA fibres from the VTA to produce a reward effect.

Stimulation of central κ opioid receptors, however, has aversive consequences (Table 3). The aversion is not blocked by experimental manipulations which affect conditioned place preferences produced by selective μ and δ agonists (Mucha et al., 1985; Bals-Kubic et al., 1988). However, prolonged inflammatory pain does abolish the aversive effect of κ receptor stimulation (Shippenberg et al., 1988) without affecting morphine-induced conditioned place preference. Interestingly, the κ agonist MR 2033 ([2α,3(S*),6α, 11(R*)](±)1,2,3,4,5,5-hexahydro-6,11-dimethyl-3 [(tetrahydro-2-furanyl)-methyl]-2,6-methano-3-benzazocin-8-01) has psychotomimetic and dysphoric effects in male volunteer subjects (Pfeiffer et al., 1986). The conditioned place aversions produced by κ agonists in rats may therefore provide a model for the untoward effects of these drugs in people. It may be significant that tolerance to the aversive effects of opioid treatments develops in rats (Shippenberg et al., 1988).

Recent experiments by Shippenberg and her colleagues (1989) were designed to identify the sites of action of selective μ and κ agonists, either in the VTA or in several DA terminal fields. They reported that conditioned place preferences were obtained when either the μ selective agonist DAGO or the delta selective agonist DPDPE was injected into the VTA, but these were ineffective in the medial prefrontal cortex, nucleus accumbens or caudate (Figure 2a). However, conditioned place aversions were obtained when U-50,488H was microinjected into the VTA, nucleus accumbens and medial prefrontal cortex (Figure 2b). Hence, μ- or δ-related reward effects were found associated with the point of origin of DA neurons, whereas κ-related aversive effects were found associated with both the VTA and limbic/cortical terminal regions.

Table 3. A summary of the evidence that μ receptor antagonists and κ receptor agonists condition place aversions in rats: both effects are blocked by a DA D1 antagonist

Drug	Action	Routes of administration	Place aversion blocked by:	Place aversion unaffected by:	References
Naloxone	Opioid antagonist	s.c. i.c.v.	Lesions of arcuate nucleus SCH 23390 (DA D1 antagonist)	D2 antagonists	Mucha et al., 1982 Mucha and Iversen, 1984 Mucha et al., 1985 Iwamoto, 1986 Shippenberg and Herz, 1988 Acquas et al., 1989 Bals-Kabik et al., 1989
CTOP	Selective μ antagonist	i.c.v.			Bals-Kubik et al., 1989
U-50,488H	κ agonist	s.c. i.c.v.	SCH 23390	Lesions of arcuate nucleus i.c.v. Injection of β-endorphin$_{1-27}$	Mucha and Herz, 1985 Mucha et al., 1985 Iwamoto, 1986 Shippenberg and Herz, 1987 Bals-Kubik et al., 1988 Bals-Kubik et al., 1989
(−)-Bremazocine	κ agonist	s.c.			Mucha and Herz, 1985 Iwamoto, 1986
U-69593	κ agonist	s.c.	SCH 23390 Inflammatory pain	D2 antagonists	Shippenberg and Herz, 1987 Shippenberg and Herz, 1988 Shippenberg et al., 1988
Dynorphin derivative E-2078	κ agonist	i.c.v.			Bals-Kubik et al., 1989

s.c., Subcutaneous; i.c.v., intracerebroventricular. See text and Table 1 for further details of the drugs used in these studies

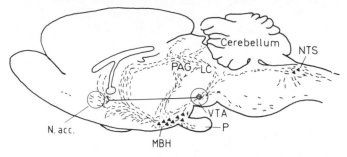

Figure 1. The β-endorphin system of the brain and its relationship to DA pathways ascending from the VTA. The system originates in the mediobasal hypothalamus (MBH), and projects to many regions in the diencephalon and midbrain. Some β-endorphin fibres arise from cells located in the nucleus of the solitary tract (NTS). Fibres connect with the DA system originating in the VTA, ascending to mesolimbic regions, e.g. nucleus accumbens (N.acc.). PAG, periaqueductal gray; LC, locus coeruleus; P, pituitary. Reproduced by kind permission of the authors (Herz and Shippenberg, 1989) and the publisher, Springer-Verlag, New York, Inc.

DA D1 Receptors and Opioid-Induced Reward and Aversion

While the role of DA in opioid self-administration remains controversial (Bozarth, Chapter 12, this volume), the rewarding effects of opioids in the place conditioning paradigm do appear to be DA-dependent. Shippenberg and Herz (1987, 1988), and Leone and Di Chiara (1987), have found that the selective D1-antagonist SCH 23390, but not D2 antagonists, blocked the reward effect of morphine in a place conditioning test. Acquas et al. (1989) showed that SCH 23390 blocked the conditioned place preferences obtained not only with morphine, but also with nicotine and diazepam. These data appear to suggest, therefore, that stimulation of D1 receptors, but not D2 receptors, mediates the reward effects of opioids and other drugs of abuse (Shippenberg and Herz, 1988; Acquas et al., 1989; Herz and Shippenberg, 1989).

Nevertheless, there are problems with data for SCH 23390. First, administration of SCH 23390 itself produces a conditioned place aversion (selective D2 antagonists do not) (Shippenberg and Herz, 1987, 1988). Hence, the effect of SCH 23390, in combination with that of an opioid drug, may simply be a matter of functional opposition, i.e. an aversive effect balancing out a reward effect. Steps should be taken to control for potential aversive effects of SCH 23390 (Shippenberg and Herz, 1987; Acquas et al., 1989).

Second, SCH 23390 is not only a D1 antagonist, but is also effective as a putative 5-HT$_1$ receptor agonist (Skarsfeldt and Larsen, 1988), and as a 5-HT$_2$ receptor ligand (Bischoff et al., 1986; McQuade et al., 1988). Thus,

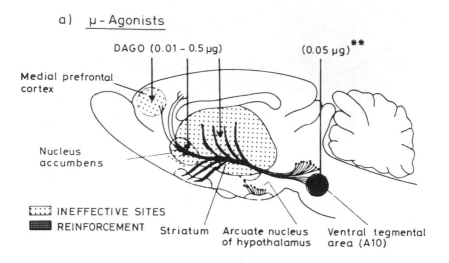

a) μ - Agonists

DAGO (0.01 - 0.5 μg)   (0.05 μg)**

Medial prefrontal
cortex

Nucleus
accumbens

INEFFECTIVE SITES
REINFORCEMENT   Striatum   Arcuate nucleus   Ventral tegmental
                             of hypothalamus   area (A10)

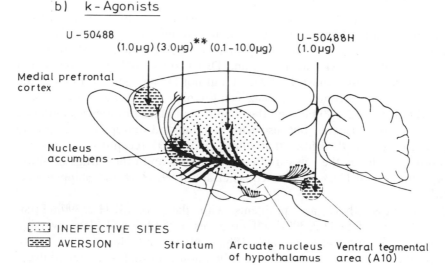

b) k - Agonists

U - 50488   U - 50488H
        (1.0 μg) (3.0 μg)** (0.1 - 10.0 μg)   (1.0 μg)

Medial prefrontal
cortex

Nucleus
accumbens

INEFFECTIVE SITES
AVERSION   Striatum   Arcuate nucleus   Ventral tegmental
                             of hypothalamus   area (A10)

Figure 2 (a). The selective μ opioid agonist DAGO produced a conditioned place preference (reward) when injected into the VTA, but not when injected into the medial prefrontal cortex, nucleus accumbens or striatum. **(b)** The selective κ opioid agonist U-50488 produced conditioned place aversions when injected into the medial prefrontal cortex, nucleus accumbens and VTA, but not in the striatum. Reproduced by kind permission of Dr Toni Shippenberg there could be a serotonergic component to its effects in place conditioning experiments. In view of this possibility, it is interesting to note that Spyraki and her colleagues have demonstrated a serotonergic component in the rewarding effects of morphine and diazepam. Thus, lesions of the serotonergic innervation of the nucleus accumbens with 5,7-dihydroxytryptamine attenuated the conditioned place preference of morphine and blocked that of diazepam completely (Spyraki et al., 1988). Moreover, the selective 5-HT$_2$ antagonist ritanserin attenuated and abolished, respectively, morphine- and diazepam-conditioned place preferences (Nomikos and Spyraki, 1988). Hence, serotonergic mechanisms may offer an explanation for the effects of SCH 23390, as an alternative to DA D1 receptor antagonism.

While morphine increases DA release in the nucleus accumbens, the selective κ opioid agonists U-50,488H, tifluadom and bremazocine, decrease DA output (Di Chiara and Imperato, 1988a, b). At the same time, as reviewed above, κ agonists produce conditioned place aversions. Unexpectedly, SCH 23390 not only blocks the reward effect of morphine but also antagonizes the conditioned place aversions obtained with U-50, 488 or with naloxone (D2 antagonists are ineffective) (Shippenberg and Herz, 1987, 1988; Acquas et al., 1989). In response to these data, it has been proposed that D1 receptors are critically involved in both rewarding and aversive states (Herz and Shippenberg, 1989), or that D1 receptor blockade produces a state of apathy (Acquas et al., 1989). A loss of drive or incentive, so that neither rewards nor punishments have much effect, is a well established description of the effects of neuroleptic drugs (Iversen and Iversen, 1975).

The recent experiments of Shippenberg and colleagues (1989) draw many of these themes together. The conditioned place preference obtained with the μ receptor agonist DAGO injected into the VTA was blocked by injection of SCH 23390 into the nucleus accumbens. Blockade of D2 receptors was ineffective. Furthermore, antagonism of D1 receptors in the nucleus accumbens blocked the aversive effects of κ agonists.

Summary

The place conditioning paradigms have furnished a great deal of important information concerning DA–opioid interactions with regard to drug-induced reward and aversion. Several significant points have emerged: (*1*) μ and δ opioid peptides produce reward effects, as reflected in conditioned place preferences; (*2*) the VTA is confirmed as an important site of action for these reward effects; (*3*) blockade of μ receptors produces aversion, as reflected in conditioned place aversions; (*4*) κ agonists acting in the VTA and in forebrain DA terminal regions produce aversions; (*5*) most interestingly, both rewarding and aversive effects of opioid peptide treatments can be blocked by the D1 receptor antagonist SCH 23390 (but not by D2 antagonists); (6) an important site of action for SCH 23390 is the nucleus accumbens.

Hence it appears that D1 receptors located in the nucleus accumbens are involved in transducing both the reward and aversive effects of opioid receptor agonists. How this is achieved remains unclear at the present time, but it should be emphasized that the nucleus accumbens D1 receptors are not concerned exclusively either with reward processes or with aversion. On the other hand, stimulation of opioid receptors does preserve the distinction since reward is coupled with agonist effects at μ and δ receptors, whereas effects at κ receptors result in aversion.

CONCLUSIONS

The purpose of this chapter has been to review evidence for potential opioid–DA interactions in relation to reward and aversion. The available evidence to address these important issues is certainly incomplete, but some major insights are emerging. It is necessary to take account of the sites of actions linked to the anatomy of central DA pathways, of the varieties of opioid peptidergic systems and multiple opioid receptors, and of the distinction between D1 and D2 DA receptors.

Within the VTA and substantia nigra, selective μ and δ agonists have behaviourally activating effects, measured, for example, in terms of increases in locomotor activity. These activating effects appear to be linked to increased activity of ascending dopaminergic neurons. In addition, selective μ and δ agonists can act in the VTA to produce reward effects, measured, for example, in terms of conditioned place preferences. In contrast, κ receptor stimulation in the VTA produces aversive effects, which in turn appear to be linked to the inhibition of dopaminergic activity. Modulation of DA activity, through opioid receptors located in the VTA, can affect behavioural responses and produce either rewarding or aversive effects. It seems likely that the behaviourally activating effects of μ and δ agonists are closely linked to their reward effects.

A most interesting set of findings to emerge recently is that both the rewarding and aversive consequences of opioid receptor stimulation can be blocked by the selective DA D1 antagonist SCH 23390 (Di Chiara et al., Chapter 14, this volume). Furthermore, the relevant D1 receptors appear to be located within the nucleus accumbens. Thus, both rewarding and aversive consequences of opioid receptor stimulation are diminished by antagonism of nucleus accumbens D1 receptors.

Within the nucleus accumbens, opioid peptides also have mixed effects. Compounds selective for δ receptors bring about a hyperactivity response which is antagonized by SCH 23390. Stimulation of μ receptors, however, produces catalepsy and akinesia, while the κ-selective drug U-50,488H produces an aversive effect. There are also reports that stimulation of opioid receptors in the nucleus accumbens produces reward effects. At the present time, the relationships between these various behavioural responses are far from clear, and future experiments should determine whether the responses are related or are distinguishable. Moreover, the extent to which these responses can be attributed to various modulations of DA activity remains to be fully investigated.

The evidence that D1 receptors in the nucleus accumbens mediate several of the significant responses to opioid receptor agonists is particularly interesting. Further work involving direct injection of not only the antagonist SCH 23390, but also selective D1 agonists, into the nucleus accumbens should contribute significantly to our understanding of the functions of the neural connections of the nucleus accumbens in respect to observable behaviour, and inferred motivational and reinforcement processes.

ACKNOWLEDGEMENTS

I wish to express my deep gratitude to Beverly Conlon and Barbara Hudson for the preparation of the manuscript, and to Ruth Weissenborn for many visits to the Medical Library. I should also like to thank Professor G. Di Chiara and Dr T. Shippenberg for their informative discussions, and to thank Professor A. Herz and Dr Shippenberg for provision of figures used in this chapter.

REFERENCES

Acquas, E., Carboni, E., Leone, P. and Di Chiara, G. (1989) SCH 23390 blocks drug-conditioned place-preference and place-aversion; anhedonia (lack of reward) or apathy (lack of motivation) after dopamine-receptor blockade? *Psychopharmacology* **99**, 151–155.
Akil, H., Bronstein, D. and Mansour, A. (1988) Overview of the endogenous opioid systems. Anatomical, biochemical and functional issues. In: Rodgers, R.J. and Cooper, S.J. (eds) *Endorphins, Opiates and Behavioural Processes*. Chichester: John Wiley, pp. 1–23.
Andén, N.E., Carlsson, A., Dahlström, A., Fuxe, K., Hillarp, N.A. and Larsson, K. (1964) Demonstration and mapping out of nigro-striatal dopamine neurons. *Life Sciences* **3**, 523–530.
Andén, N.E., Dahlström, A., Fuxe, K., Larsson, K., Olson, L. and Ungerstedt, U. (1966) Ascending monoamine neurones to the telecephalon and diencephalon. *Acta Physiologica Scandinavica* **67**, 313–326.
Arnt, J. and Scheel-Krüger, J. (1979a) GABAergic and glycinergic mechanisms within the substantia nigra: pharmacological specificity of dopamine-independent contralateral turning behavior and interactions with other transmitters. *Psychopharmacology* **62**, 267–277.
Arnt, J. and Scheel-Krüger, J. (1979b) GABA in the ventral tegmental area:

differential regional effects on locomotion, aggression and food intake after microinjection of GABA agonists and antagonists. *Life Sciences* **25**, 1351–1360.

Atweh, S.F. and Kuhar, M.J. (1977a) Autoradiographic localization of opiate receptors in rat brain. I. Spinal cord and lower medulla. *Brain Research* **124**, 53–68.

Atweh, S.F. and Kuhar, M.J. (1977b) Autoradiographic localization of opiate receptors in rat brain. II. The brainstem. *Brain Research* **129**, 1–12.

Atweh, S.F. and Kuhar, M.J. (1977c) Autoradiographic localization of opiate receptors in rat brain. III. The telecephalon. *Brain Research* **134**, 393–405.

Ayhan, I.H. and Randrup, A. (1973) Behavioural and pharmacological studies of morphine-induced excitation of rats. Possible relation to brain catecholamines. *Psychopharmacologia* **29**, 317–328.

Babbini, M. and Davis, W.M. (1972) Time-dose relationships for locomotor activity effects of morphine after acute or repeated treatment. *British Journal of Pharmacology* **46**, 213–224.

Bals-Kubik, R., Herz, A. and Shippenberg, T.S. (1988) Endorphin-(1–27) is a naturally occurring antagonist of the reinforcing effects of opioids. *Naunyn-Schmiedeberg's Archives of Pharmacology* **338**, 392–396.

Bals-Kubik, R., Herz, A. and Shippenberg, T.S. (1989) Evidence that the aversive effects of opioid antagonists and κ-agonists are centrally mediated. *Psychopharmacology* **98**, 203–206.

Bechara, A. and Van der Kooy, D. (1985) Opposite motivational effects of endogenous opioids in brain and periphery. *Nature* **314**, 533–534.

Bischoff, S., Heinrich, M., Sonntag, J.M. and Krauss, J. (1986) The D-1 dopamine receptor antagonist SCH 23390 also interacts potently with brain serotonin (5-HT$_2$) receptors. *European Journal of Pharmacology* **129**, 367–370.

Blanchard, S.G., Lee, P.H.K., Pugh, W.W., Hong, J.S. and Chang, K.-J. (1987) Characterization of the binding of a morphine (mu) receptor-specific ligand: Tyr-Pro-NMePhe-D-Pro-NH$_2$, ^{3}H-PLO 17. *Molecular Pharmacology* **31**, 326–333.

Bloom, F., Battenberg, E., Rossier, J., Ling, N. and Guillemin, R. (1978) Neurons containing beta-endorphin in rat brain exist separately from those containing enkephalin: immunocytochemical studies. *Proceedings of the National Academy of Sciences USA* **75**, 1591–1595.

Bozarth, M.A. (1986) Neural basis of psychomotor stimulant and opiate reward: evidence suggesting the involvement of a common dopaminergic system. *Behavioural Brain Research* **22**, 107–116.

Bozarth, M.A. (1987) Neuroanatomical boundaries of the reward-relevant opiate-receptor field in the ventral tegmental area as mapped by the conditioned place preference method in rats. *Brain Research* **414**, 77–84.

Bozarth, M.A. and Wise, R.A. (1981a) Intracranial self-administration of morphine into the ventral tegmental area in rats. *Life Sciences* **28**, 551–555.

Bozarth, M.A. and Wise, R.A. (1981b) Heroin reward is dependent on a dopaminergic substrate. *Life Sciences* **29**, 1881–1886.

Bozarth, M.A. and Wise, R.A. (1982) Localization of the reward-relevant opiate receptors. In: Harris, L.S. (ed.) *Problems of Drug Dependence, 1981*. Washington DC: U.S. Government Printing Office, pp. 158–164.

Britt, M.D. and Wise, R.A. (1983) Ventral tegmental site of opiate reward: antagonism by a hydrophilic opiate receptor blockade. *Brain Research* **258**, 105–108.

Broekkamp, C.L.E. (1975) The effects of manipulations with the dopaminergic system on self-stimulation behavior. In: Wauquier, A. and Rolls, E.T. (eds) *Brain-Stimulation Reward*. Amsterdam: North Holland, pp. 194–195.

Broekkamp, C.L., van den Bogaard, J.H., Heijnen, H.J., Rops, R.H., Cools, A.R. and van Rossum, J.M. (1976) Separation of inhibiting and stimulating effects of morphine on self-stimulation behaviour by intracerebral microinjections. *European Journal of Pharmacology* **36**, 443–446.

Broekkamp, C.L.E., Phillips, A.G. and Cools, A.R. (1979a). Stimulant effects of enkephalin microinjection into the dopaminergic A10 area. *Nature* **278**, 560–562.

Broekkamp, C.L., Phillips, A.G. and Cools, A.R. (1979b) Facilitation of self-stimulation behavior following intracerebral microinjections of opioids into the ventral tegmental area. *Pharmacology Biochemistry and Behavior* **11**, 289–295.

Cador, M., Kelley, A.E., Le Moal, M. and Stinus, L. (1986) Ventral tegmental area infusion of substance P, neurotensin and enkephalin: differential effects on feeding behavior. *Neuroscience* **18**, 659–669.

Cador, M., Kelley, A.E., Le Moal, M. and Stinus, L. (1988) *d*-Ala-met-enkephalin injection into the ventral tegmental area: effect on investigatory and spontaneous motor behaviour in the rat. *Psychopharmacology* **96**, 332–342.

Cador, M., Rivet, J-M., Kelley, A.E., Le Moal, M. and Stinus, L. (1989) Substance P, neurotensin and enkephalin injections into the ventral tegmental area: comparative study on dopamine turnover in several forebrain structures. *Brain Research* **486**, 357–363.

Carboni, E., Imperato, A., Perezzani, L. and Di Chiara, G. (1989) Amphetamine, cocaine, phencyclidine and nomifensine increase extracellular dopamine concentrations preferentially in the nucleus accumbens of freely moving rats. *Neuroscience* **28**, 653–661.

Carlsson, A. (1959) The occurrence, distribution and physiological role of catecholamines in the nervous system. *Pharmacological Reviews* **11**, 490–493.

Carr, G.D. and White, N.M. (1983) Conditioned place preference from intra-accumbens but not intra-caudate amphetamine injections. *Life Sciences* **33**, 2551–2557.

Carr, G.D. and White, N.M. (1986) Contributions of dopamine terminals areas to amphetamine-induced anorexia and adipsia. *Pharmacology Biochemistry and Behavior* **25**, 17–22.

Carr, G.D., Fibiger, H.C. and Phillips, A.G. (1989) Conditioned place preference as a measure of drug reward. In: Liebman, J.M. and Cooper, S.J. (eds) *The Neuropharmacological Basis of Reward*. Oxford: Oxford University Press, pp. 264–319.

Chavkin, C., James, I.F. and Goldstein, A. (1982) Dynorphin is a specific endogenous ligand of the kappa opioid receptor. *Science* **215**, 413–415.

Colle, L.N. and Wise, R.A. (1988) Facilitatory and inhibitory effects of nucleus accumbens amphetamine on feeding. *Annals of the New York Academy of Sciences* **537**, 491–492.

Cooper, S.J. (1981) Behaviourally-specific hyperdipsia in the non-deprived rat following acute morphine treatment. *Neuropharmacology* **20**, 469–472.

Cooper, S.J. and Dourish, C.T. (1990) An introduction to the concept of stereotypy and a historical perspective on the role of brain dopamine. In: Cooper, S.J. and Dourish, C.T. (eds) *Neurobiology of Stereotyped Behaviour*. Oxford: Clarendon Press, pp. 1–24.

Cooper, S.J., Jackson, A. and Kirkham, T.C. (1985) Endorphins and food intake: *kappa* opioid receptor agonists and hypherphagia. *Pharmacology Biochemistry and Behavior* **23**, 889–901.

Corbett, A.D., Gillan, M.G.C., Kosterlitz, H.W., McKnight, A.T., Paterson, S.J. and Robson, L.E. (1984) Selectivities of opioid peptide analogues as agonists and antagonists at the delta receptor. *British Journal of Pharmacology* **83**, 271–279.

Corrigall, W.A. and Vacarino, F.J. (1988) Antagonist treatment in nucleus accumbens or periaqueductal grey affects heroin self-adminstration. *Pharmacology Biochemistry and Behavior* **30**, 443–450.

Costall, B. and Naylor, R.J. (1975) The behavioural effects of dopamine applied intracerebrally to areas of the mesolimbic system. *European Journal of Pharmacology* **32**, 87–92.

Costall, B. and Naylor, R.J. (1976) Antagonism of the hyperactivity induced by dopamine applied intracerebrally to the nucleus accumbens septi by typical neuroleptics and by clozapine, sulpiride and thioridazine. *European Journal of Pharmacology* **35**, 161–168.

Costall, B., Fortune, D.H. and Naylor, R.J. (1978) The induction of catalepsy and hyperactivity by morphine administered directly into the nucleus accumbens of rats. *European Journal of Pharmacology* **49**, 49–64.

Cotton, R., Giles, M.G., Miller, L., Shaw, J.S. and Timms, D. (1984) ICI 174,864: a highly selective antagonist for the opioid receptor. *European Journal of Pharmacology* **97**, 331–332.

Cotton, R., Kosterlitz, H.W., Paterson, S.J., Rance, M.J. and Traynor, J.R. (1985) The use of [^{3}H]-[D-Pen^2, D-Pen^5] enkephalin as a highly selective ligand for the delta binding site. *British Journal of Pharmacology* **84**, 927–932.

Dahlström, A. and Fuxe, K. (1964) Evidence for the existence of monoamine-containing neurons in the central nervous system. I. Demonstration of monoamines in the cell bodies of brain stem neurons. *Acta Physiologica Scandinavica* **62**, 1–55 (suppl 232).

Daugé, V., Rossignol, P. and Roques, B.P. (1988) Comparison of the behavioural effects induced by administration of rat nucleus accumbens or nucleus caudatus of selective μ and δ opioid peptides or kelatorphan an inhibitor of enkaphalin-degrading-enzymes. *Psychopharmacology* **96**, 343–352.

Daugé, V., Rossignol, P. and Roques, B.P. (1989) Blockade of dopamine receptors reverses the behavioral effects of endogenous enkephalins in the *Nucleus caudatus* but not in the *Nucleus accumbens*: differential involvement of μ and δ opioid receptors. *Psychopharmacology* **99**, 168–175.

De Wit, H. and Stewart, J. (1983) Drug reinstatement of heroin-reinforced responding in the rat. *Psychopharmacology* **79**, 29–31.

De Witte, P., Heidbreder, C. and Roques, B.P. (1989) Kelatorphan, a potent enkephalinases inhibitor, and opioid receptor agonists DAGO and DTLET, differentially modulate self-stimulation behaviour depending on the site of administration. *Neuropharmacology* **28**, 667–676.

Di Chiara, G. and Imperato, A. (1988a) Drugs abused by humans preferentially increase synaptic dopamine concentrations in the mesolimbic system of freely moving rats. *Proceedings of the National Academy of Sciences USA* **85**, 5274–5278.

Di Chiara, G. and Imperato, A. (1988b) Opposite effects of μ and κ-opiate agonists on dopamine-release in the nucleus accumbens and in the dorsal caudate of freely moving rats. *Journal of Pharmacology and Experimental Therapeutics* **244**, 1067–1080.

Di Chiara, G., Vargiu, L., Porceddu, M.L., Longoni, R., Mulas, A. and Gessa, G.L. (1977) Indirect activation of the DA system as a possible mechanism for the stimulatory effects of narcotic analgesics. In: Costa, E. and Gessa, G.L. (eds) *Advances in Biochemical Psychopharmacology, Vol. 16*. New York: Raven Press, pp. 571–575.

Dworkin, S.I., Guerin, G.F., Goeders, N.E. and Smith, J.E. (1988) Kainic acid lesions of the nucleus accumbens selectively attenuate morphine self-administration. *Pharmacology Biochemistry and Behavior* **29**, 175–181.

Ehringer, H. and Hornykiewicz, O. (1960) Verteilung von Noradrenalin und Dopamin (3-hydroxytyramin) in Gehirn des Menschen und ihr Verhalter bei Erkrankungen des extrapyramidalen systems. *Klinisches Wochenschrift* **38**, 1236–1239.

Ettenberg, A., Pettit, H.O., Bloom, F.E. and Koob, G.F. (1982) Heroin and cocaine intravenous self-administration in rats: mediation by separate neural systems. *Psychopharmacology* **78**, 204–209.

Evans, K.R. and Vaccarino, F.J. (1986) Intra-nucleus accumbens amphetamine: dose-dependent effects on food intake. *Pharmacology Biochemistry and Behavior* **25**, 1149–1151.

Fallon, J.H., Leslie, F.M. and Cone, R.I. (1985) Dynorphin-containing pathways in the substantia nigra and ventral tegmentum: a double labeling study using combined immunofluorescence and retrograde tracing. *Neuropeptides* **5**, 457–460.

Fibiger, H.C., LePiane, F.G., Jakubovic, A. and Phillips, A.G. (1987) The role of dopamine in intracranial self-stimulation of the ventral tegmental area. *Journal of Neuroscience* **7**, 3888–3896.

Fog, R. (1970) Behavioural effects in rats of morphine and amphetamine and of a combination of the two drugs. *Psychopharmacologia* **16**, 305–312.

Fournié-Zaluski, M.C., Chaillet, P., Bouboutou, R., Coulard, A., Cherot, P., Waksman, G., Costentin, J. and Roques, B.P. (1984) Analgesic effects of kelatorphan, a new highly potent inhibitor of multiple enkephalin degrading enzymes. *European Journal of Pharmacology* **102**, 525–528.

Fuxe, F. (1965) Evidence for the existence of monoamine neurons in the central nervous system. IV. Distribution of monoamine nerve terminals in the central nervous system. *Acta Physiologia Scandinavica* **64**, 39–85 (suppl 247).

Gauchy, C., Agid, Y., Glowinski, J. and Cheramy, A. (1973) Acute effects of morphine on dopamine synthesis and release and tyrosine metabolism in the rat striatum. *European Journal of Pharmacology* **22**, 311–319.

Glimcher, P.W., Giovino, A.A., Margolin, D.H. and Hoebel, B.G. (1984) Endogenous opiate reward induced by an enkephalinase inhibitor, thiorphan, injected into the ventral midbrain. *Behavioral Neuroscience* **98**, 262–268.

Goeders, N.E. and Smith, J.E. (1983) Cortical dopaminergic involvement in cocaine reinforcement. *Science* **221**, 773–775.

Goeders, N.E., Lane, J.D. and Smith, J.E. (1984) Self-administration of methionine enkephalin into the nucleus accumbens. *Pharmacology Biochemistry and Behavior* **20**, 451–455.

Goldstein, A., Tochibana, S., Lownwey, L.I., Hunkapiller, M. and Hood, L. (1979) Dynorphin (1–13), an extraordinary potent opioid peptide. *Proceedings of the National Academy of Sciences USA* **76**, 6666–6670.

Guerin, G.F., Goeders, N.E., Dworkin, S.I. and Smith, J.E. (1984) Intracranial self-administration of dopamine into the nucleus accumbens. *Society for Neuroscience Abstracts* **10**, 1072.

Gysling, K. and Wang, R.Y. (1983) Morphine-induced activation of A10 dopamine neurons in the rat. *Brain Research* **277**, 119–127.

Hamilton, M.E. and Bozarth, M.A. (1988) Feeding elicited by dynorphin (1–13) microinjections into the ventral tegmental area in rats. *Life Sciences* **43**, 941–946.

Handa, B.K., Lane, A.C., Lord, J.A.H., Morgan, B.A., Rance, M.J. and Smith, C.F.C. (1981) Analogues of beta-LPH$_{61-64}$ possessing selective agonists activity at mu-opiate receptors. *European Journal of Pharmacology* **70**, 531–540.

Havemann, U. and Kuschinsky, K. (1985) Locomotor activity of rats after injection of various opioids into the nucleus accumbens and the septum mediale. *Naunyn-Schmiedeberg's Archives of Pharmacology* **331**, 175–180.

Herrera-Marschitz, M., Hökfelt, T., Ungerstedt, U., Terenius, L. and Goldstein, M. (1984) Effect of intranigral injections of dynorphin, dynorphin fragments and α-neoendorphin on rotational behaviour in the rat. *European Journal of Pharmacology* **102**, 213–227.

Herz, A. and Shippenberg, T.S. (1989) Neurochemical aspects of addiction: opioids and other drugs of abuse. In: Goldstein, A. (ed.) *Molecular and Cellular Aspects of Drug Addictions*. Berlin: Springer-Verlag, pp. 111–141.

Hoebel, B.G., Monaco, A.P., Hernandez, L., Aulisi, E.F., Stanley, B.G. and Lenard, L. (1983) Self-injection of amphetamine directly into the brain. *Psychopharmacology* **81**, 158–163.

Holmes, L.J. and Wise, R.A. (1985) Contralateral circling induced by tegmental morphine: anatomical localization, pharmacological specificity, and phenomenology. *Brain Research* **326**, 19–26.

Holmes, L.J., Bozarth, M.A. and Wise, R.A. (1983) Circling from intracranial morphine applied to the ventral tegmental area in rats. *Brain Research Bulletin* **11**, 295–298.

Hommer, D.W. and Pert, A. (1983) The actions of opiates in the rat substantial nigra: an electrophysiological analysis. *Peptides* **4**, 603–608.

Hughes, J., Smith, T.W., Kosterlitz, H.W., Fothergill, L.A., Morgan, M.A. and Morris, H.R. (1975) Identification of two related pentapeptides from the brain with potent opiate agonist activity. *Nature* **258**, 577–579.

Iversen, S.D. and Iversen, L.L. (1975) *Behavioural Pharmacology*. New York: Oxford University Press.

Iwamoto, E.T. (1981) Locomotor activity and antinociception after putative *mu*, *kappa* and *sigma* opioid receptor agonists in the rat: influence of dopaminergic agonists and antagonists. *Journal of Pharmacology and Experimental Therapeutics* **217**, 451–460.

Iwamoto, E.T. (1986) Place-conditioning properties of mu, kappa, and sigma opioid agonists. *Alcohol and Drug Research* **6**, 327–339.

Iwamoto, E.T. and Way, E.L (1977) Circling behavior and stereotypy induced by intranigral opiate micro-injections. *Journal of Pharmacology and Experimental Therapeutics* **203**, 347–359.

Jackson, D.M., Andén, N.-E. and Dahlström, A. (1975) A functional effect of dopamine in the nucleus accumbens and in some other dopamine-rich parts of the rat brain. *Psychopharmacologia* **45**, 139–149.

Jacquet, Y.F. (1983) Met[5]-enkephalin: potent contraversive rotation after microinjection in rat substantia nigra. *Brain Research* **264**, 340–343.

Jenck, F., Gratton, A. and Wise, R.A. (1987) Opioid receptor subtypes associated with ventral tegmental facilitation of lateral hypothalamic brain stimulation reward. *Brain Research* **423**, 34–38.

Jenck, F., Bozarth, M. and Wise, R.A. (1988) Contraversive circling induced by tegmental microinjections of moderate doses of morphine and [D-Pen[2], D-Pen[5]] enkephalin. *Brain Research* **450**, 382–386.

Joyce, E.M. and Iverson, S.D. (1979) The effect of morphine applied locally to mesencephalic dopamine cell bodies on spontaneous motor activity in the rat. *Neuroscience Letters* **14**, 207–212.

Joyce, E.M., Koob, G.F., Strecker, R., Iversen, S.D. and Bloom, F.E. (1981) The behavioural effects of enkephalin analogues injected into the ventral tegmental area and globus pallidus. *Brain Research* **221**, 359–370.

Kalivas, P.W. and Bronson, M. (1985) Mesolimbic dopamine lesions produce an augmented behavioral response to enkephalin. *Neuropharmacology* **24**, 931–936.

Kalivas, P.W., Widerlov, E., Stanley, D., Breese, G. and Prange, A.J. (1983) Enkephalin action on the mesolimbic dopamine system: a dopamine-dependent and a dopamine-independent increase in locomotor activity. *Journal of Pharmacology and Experimental Therapeutics* **227**, 229–237.

Kangawa, K., Minamino, N., Chino, N., Sakakibara, S. and Matsuo, H. (1981) The complete amino acid sequence of alpha-neo-endorphin. *Biochemical Biophysical Research Communications* **99**, 871–878.

Katz, R.J. and Gormezano, G. (1979) A rapid and inexpensive technique for assessing the reinforcing effects of opiate drugs. *Pharmacology Biochemistry and Behavior* **11**, 231–233.

Kelley, A.E., Stinus, L. and Iversen, S.D. (1980) Interactions between D-Ala-Met-enkephalin, A10 dopaminergic neurones, and spontaneous behaviour in the rat. *Behavioural Brain Research* **1**, 3–24.

Kilpatrick, D.L., Wahlstrom, A., Lahm, H.W., Blacher, R. and Udenfriend, S. (1982) Rimorphin, a unique, naturally occurring (Leu)enkephalin-containing peptide found in association with dynorphin and α-neo-endorphin. *Proceedings of the National Academy of Sciences USA* **79**, 6480–6483.

Kim, H.S., Iyengar, S. and Wood, P.L. (1986) Opiate actions on mesocortical dopamine metabolism in the rat. *Life Sciences* **39**, 2033–2036.

Kurumiya, S. and Nakajima, S. (1988) Dopamine D_1 receptors in the nucleus accumbens: involvement in the reinforcing effect of tegmental stimulation. *Brain Research* **448**, 1–6.

Latimer, L.G., Duffy, P. and Kalivas, P.W. (1987) *Mu* opioid receptor involvement in enkephalin activation of dopamine neurons in the ventral tegmental area. *Journal of Pharmacology and Experimental Therapeutics* **241**, 328–337.

Leone, P. and Di Chiara, G. (1987) Blockade of D-1 receptors by SCH 23390 antagonizes morphine- and amphetamine-induced place preference conditioning. *European Journal of Pharmacology* **135**, 251–254.

Llorens-Cortes, C., Pollard, H. and Schwartz, J.C. (1979) Localization of opiate receptors in substantia nigra evidence by lesion studies. *Neuroscience Letters* **12**, 165–170.

Longoni, R., Mulas, A., Spina, L., Melchiorri, P. and Di Chiara, G. (1989) Stimulation of delta opioid receptors in the accumbens elicits D-1 dependent stimulation of motor activity and stereotypes. *Behavioural Pharmacology* **1**, 38 (suppl 1).

Lord, J.A.H., Waterfield, A.A., Hughes, J. and Kosterlitz, H.W. (1977) Endogenous opioid peptides: multiple agonists and receptors. *Nature* **267**, 495–499.

Lorens, S.A. and Mitchell, C.L. (1973) Influence of morphine on lateral hypothalamic self-stimulation in the rat. *Psychopharmacologia* **32**, 271–277.

Lyness, W.H., Friedle, N.M. and Moore, K.E. (1979) Destruction of dopaminergic nerve terminals in nucleus accumbens: effect on *d*-amphetamine self-administration. *Pharmacology Biochemistry and Behavior* **11**, 553–556.

McLean, S., Bannon, M.J., Zamir, N. and Peret, C.B. (1985) Comparison of the Substance P- and Dynorphin-containing projections to the substantia nigra: a radioimmunocytochemical and biochemical study. *Brain Research* **361**, 185–192.

McQuade, R.D., Ford, D., Duffy, R.A., Chipkin, R.E., Iorio, L. and Barnett, A. (1988) Serotonergic component of SCH 23390: in vitro and in vivo binding analyses. *Life Sciences* **43**, 1861–1869.

Majeed, N.H., Przewłocka, B., Wędzony, K. and Przewłocki, R. (1986) Stimulation of food intake following opioid microinjection into the nucleus accumbens septi in rats. *Peptides* **7**, 711–716.

Makanjuola, R.O.A., Dow, R.C. and Ashcroft, G.W. (1980) Behavioural responses to stereotactically controlled injections of monoamine neurotransmitters into the accumbens and caudate-putamen nuclei. *Psychopharmacology* **71**, 227–235.

Mansour, A., Lewis, M.E., Khachaturian, H., Akil, H. and Watson, S.J. (1986) Pharmacological and anatomical evidence of selective μ, δ and κ opioid receptor binding in rat brain. *Brain Research* **399**, 69–79.

Mansour, A., Khachaturian, H., Lewis, M.E., Akil, H. and Watson, S.J. (1987) Autoradiographic differentiation of mu, delta, and kappa opioid receptors in the rat forebrain and midbrain. *Journal of Neuroscience* **7**, 2445–2464.

Martin, W.R., Eades, G.G., Thompson, J.A., Huppler, R.F. and Gilbert, P. (1976) The effects of morphine and nalorphine-like drugs in the nondependent and morphine-dependent chronic spinal dog. *Journal of Pharmacology and Experimental Therapeutics* **197**, 518–532.

Matsumoto, R.R., Lohof, A.M., Patrick, R.L. and Walker, J.M. (1988a) Dopamine-independent motor behavior following microinjection of rimorphin in the substantia nigra. *Brain Research* **444**, 67–74.

Matsumoto, R.R., Brinsfield, K.H., Patrick, R.L. and Walker, J.M. (1988b) Rotational behavior mediated by dopaminergic and nondopaminergic mechanisms after intranigral microinjection of specific mu, delta and kappa opioid agonists. *Journal of Pharmacology and Experimental Therapeutics* **246**, 196–203.

Matthews, R.T. and German, D.C. (1984) Electrophysiological evidence for excitation of rat ventral tegmental area dopamine neurons by morphine. *Neuroscience* **11**, 617–625.

Morelli, M. and Di Chiara, G. (1985) Non-dopaminergic mechanisms in the turning behavior evoked by intranigral opiates. *Brain Research* **341**, 350–359.

Morelli, M., Fenu, S. and Di Chiara, G. (1989) Substantia nigra as a site of origin of dopamine-dependent motor syndromes induced by stimulation of μ and δ opioid receptors. *Brain Research* **487**, 120–130.

Mucha, R.F. and Herz, A. (1985) Motivational properties of kappa and mu opioid receptor agonists studied with place and taste preference conditioning. *Psychopharmacology* **86**, 74–280.

Mucha, R.F. and Herz, A. (1986) Preference conditioning produced by opioid active and inactive isomers of levorphanol and morphine in the rat. *Life Sciences* **38**, 241–249.

Mucha, R.F. and Iversen, S.D. (1984) Reinforcing properties of morphine and naloxone revealed by conditioned place preferences: a procedural examination. *Psychopharmacology* **82**, 241–247.

Mucha, R.F. and Iversen, S.D. (1986) Increased food intake after opioid microinjections into nucleus accumbens and ventral tegmental area of rat. *Brain Research* **397**, 214–224.

Mucha, R.F., van der Kooy, D., O'Shaughnessy, M. and Bucenieks, P. (1982) Drug reinforcement studied by the use of place conditioning in rat. *Brain Research* **243**, 91–105.

Mucha, R.F., Millan, M.J. and Herz, A. (1985) Aversive properties of naloxone in non-dependent (naive) rats may involve blockade of central β-endorphin. *Psychopharmacology* **86**, 281–285.

Murrin, L.C., Coyle, J.T. and Kuhar, M.J. (1980) Striatal opiate receptors: pre- and postsynaptic localization. *Life Sciences* **27**, 1175–1183.

Nomikos, G.C. and Spyraki, C. (1988) Effects of ritanserin on the rewarding properties of d-amphetamine, morphine and diazepam revealed by conditioned place preference in rats. *Pharmacology Biochemistry and Behavior* **30**, 853–858.

Norton, S. (1977) The structure of behavior of rats during morphine-induced hyperactivity. *Communications in Psychopharmacology* **1**, 333–341.

Olds, M.E. (1982) Reinforcing effects of morphine in the nucleus accumbens. *Brain Research* **237**, 429–440.

Pelton, J.T., Kazmierski, W., Gulya, K., Amamura, H.I. and Hruby, V.J. (1986) Design and synthesis of conformationally constrained somatostatin analogues with high potency and specificy for opioid receptors. *Journal of Medicinal Chemistry* **29**, 2370–2375.

Pert, A. and Sivit, C. (1977) Neuroanatomical focus for morphine and enkephalin-induced hypermotility. *Nature* **265**, 645–647.

Pert, C.B. and Snyder, S.H. (1973) Opiate receptor: demonstration in nervous tissue. *Science* **179**, 1011–1014.

Pettit, H.O., Ettenberg, A., Bloom, F.E. and Koob, G.F. (1984) Destruction of dopamine in the nucleus accumbens selectively attenuates cocaine but not heroin self-administration in rats. *Psychopharmacology* **84**, 167–173.

Pfeiffer, A., Brantl, V., Herz, A. and Emrich, H.M. (1986) Psychotomimesis mediated by κ opiate receptors. *Science* **233**, 774–776.

Phillips, A.G. and Fibiger, H.C. (1978) The role of dopamine in maintaining intracranial self-stimulation in the ventral tegmentum, nucleus accumbens and medial prefrontal cortex. *Canadian Journal of Psychology* **32**, 58–66.

Phillips, A.G. and LePiane, F.G. (1980) Reinforcing effects of morphine microinjection into the ventral tegmental area. *Pharmacology Biochemistry and Behavior* **12**, 965–968.

Phillips, A.G. and LePiane, F.G. (1982) Reward produced by microinjection of (D-Ala²), Met⁵-enkephalinamide into the ventral tegmental area. *Behavioural Brain Research* **5**, 225–229.

Phillips, A.G. and Rolls, E.T. (1981) Intracerebral self-administration of amphetamine by rhesus monkeys. *Neuroscience Letters* **24**, 81–86.

Phillips, A.G., Brooke, S.M. and Fibiger, H.C. (1975) Effects of amphetamine isomers and neuroleptics on self-stimulation from the nucleus accumbens and dorsal noradrenergic bundle. *Brain Research* **85**, 13–32.

Phillips, A.G., Carter, D.A. and Fibiger, H.C. (1976) Dopaminergic substrates of intracranial self-stimulation in the caudate-putamen. *Brain Research* **104**, 221–232.

Phillips, A.G., LePiane, F.G. and Fibiger, H.C. (1983) Dopaminergic mediation of reward produced by direct injection of enkephalin into the ventral tegmental area of the rat. *Life Sciences* **33**, 2205–2511.

Pijnenburg, A.J.J. and van Rossum, J.M. (1973) Stimulation of locomotor activity following injection of dopamine into the nucleus accumbens. *Journal of Pharmacy and Pharmacology* **25**, 1003–1005.

Pijnenburg, A.J.J., Honig, W.M.M. and van Rossum, J.M. (1975a) Effects of antagonists upon locomotor stimulation induced by injection of dopamine and noradrenaline into the nucleus accumbens of nialamide-pretreated rats. *Psychopharmacologia* **41**, 175–180.

Pijnenburg, A.J.J., Honig, W.M.M. and van Rossum, J.M. (1975b) Inhibition of *d*-amphetamine-induced locomotor activity by injection of haloperidol into the nucleus accumbens of the rat. *Psychopharmacologia* **41**, 87–95.

Pollard, H., Llorens, C., Bonnet, J.J., Costentin, J. and Schwartz, J.C. (1977) Opiate receptors on mesolimbic dopaminergic neurons. *Neuroscience Letters* **7**, 295–299.

Pollard, H., Llorens, C., Schwartz, J.C., Gros, C. and Dray, F. (1978) Localization of opiate receptors and enkephalins in the rat striatum in relationship with the nigrostriatal dopaminergic system: lesion studies. *Brain Research* **151**, 392–398.

Roberts, D.C.S. (1989) Breaking points on a progressive ratio schedule reinforced by intravenous apomorphine increase daily following 6-hydroxydopamine lesions of the nucleus accumbens. *Pharmacology Biochemistry and Behavior* **32**, 43–47.

Roberts, D.C.S., Koob, G.F., Klonoff, P. and Fibiger, H.C. (1980) Extinction and recovery of cocaine self-administration following 6-hydroxydopamine lesions of the nucleus accumbens. *Pharmacology Biochemistry and Behavior* **12**, 781–787.

Rolls, E.T. and Cooper, S.J. (1974) Anaesthetization and stimulation of the sulcal prefrontal cortex and brain-stimulation reward. *Physiology and Behavior* **12**, 563–571.

Rossi, N.A. and Reid, L.D. (1976) Affective states associated with morphine injections. *Physiological Psychology* **4**, 269–274.

Routtenberg, A. and Sloan, M. (1972) Self-stimulation in the frontal cortex in *Rattus norvegicus*. *Behavioral Biology* **7**, 567–572.

Sanger, D.J. and McCarthy, P.S. (1980) Differential effects of morphine on food and water intake in food deprived and freely feeding rats. *Psychopharmacology* **72**, 103–106.

Scheel-Krüger, J., Arnt, J. and Magelund, G. (1977a) Behavioural stimulation induced by muscimol and other GABA agonists injected into the substantia nigra. *Neuroscience Letters* **4**, 351–356.

Scheel-Krüger, J., Golembiowska, K. and Mogilnicka, E. (1977b) Evidence for increased apomorphine-sensitive dopaminergic effects after acute treatment with morphine. *Psychopharmacology* **53**, 55–63.

Schulz, R., Faase, E., Wuster, M. and Herz, A. (1979) Selective receptors for beta-endorphin on the rat vas deferens. *Life Sciences* **24**, 843–850.

Schwarcz, R. and Coyle, J.T. (1977) Neurochemical sequelae of kainate injections in corpus striatum and substantia nigra of the rat. *Life Sciences* **20**, 431–436.

Schwartz, A.S. and Marchok, P.L. (1974) Depression of morphine seeking behaviour by dopamine inhibition. *Nature* **248**, 257–258.

Shippenberg, T.S. and Herz, A. (1987) Place preference conditioning reveals the involvement of D_1-dopamine receptors in the motivational properties of μ- and κ-opioid agonists. *Brain Research* **436**, 169–172.

Shippenberg, T.S. and Herz, A. (1988) Motivational effects of opioids: influence of D-1 versus D-2 receptor antagonists. *European Journal of Pharmacology* **151**, 233–242.

Shippenberg, T.S., Bals-Kubik, R. and Herz, A. (1987) Motivational properties of opioids: evidence that an activation of δ-receptors mediates reinforcement processes. *Brain Research* **436**, 234–239.

Shippenberg, T.S., Stein, C., Huber, A., Millan, M.J. and Herz, A. (1988) Motivational effects of opioids in an animal model of prolonged inflammatory pain: alteration in the effects of κ- but not of μ-receptor agonists. *Pain* **35**, 179–186.

Shippenberg, T., Bals-Kubik, R., Spanagel, R. and Herz, A. (1989) Reinforcing and aversive effects of opioid agonists: involvement of the mesolimbic dopamine system. *Behavioural Pharmacology* **1**, 18 (suppl 1).

Simon, E.G., Hiller, J.M. and Edelman, I. (1973) Stereospecific binding of the potent narcotic analgesic [^{3}H] etorphine to rat-brain homogenate. *Proceedings of the National Academy of Sciences* **70**, 1947–1949.

Simon, H., Stinus, L., Tassin, J.P., Lavielle, S., Blanc, G., Thierry, A.-M., Glowinski, J. and Le Moal, M. (1979) Is the dopaminergic mesocorticolimbic system necessary for intracranial self-stimulation? Biochemical and behavioral studies from A10 cell bodies and terminals. *Behavioral and Neural Biology* **27**, 125–145.

Skarsfeldt, T. and Larsen, J.-J. (1988) SCH 23390—a selective dopamine D-1 receptor antagonist with putative 5-HT$_1$ receptor agonist activity. *European Journal of Pharmacology* **148**, 389–395.

Spyraki, C., Fibiger, H.C. and Phillips, A.G. (1982) Dopaminergic substrates of amphetamine-induced place preference conditioning. *Brain Research* **253**, 185–193.

Spyraki, C., Fibiger, H.C. and Phillips, A.G. (1983) Attenuation of heroin reward in rats by disruption of the mesolimbic dopamine system. *Psychopharmacology* **79**, 278–283.

Spyraki, C., Nomikos, G.C., Galanopoulou, P. and Daifotis, Z. (1988) Drug-induced place preference in rats with 5,7-dihydroxytryptamine lesions of the nucleus accumbens. *Behavioural Brain Research* **29**, 127–134.

Stapleton, J.M., Lind, M.D., Merriman, V.J., Bozarth, M.A. and Reid, L.D. (1979) Affective consequences and subsequent effects on morphine self-administration of d-ala^2-methionine enkephalin. *Physiological Psychology* **7**, 146–152.

Steiner, S.S., Beer, B. and Shaffer, M.M. (1969) Escape from self-produced rates of brain stimulation. *Science* **163**, 90–91.

Stewart, J. (1984) Reinstatement of heroin and cocaine self-administration behavior in the rat of intracerebral application of morphine in the ventral tegmental area. *Pharmacology Biochemistry and Behavior* **20**, 917–923.

Stinus, L., Koob, G.F., Ling, N., Bloom, F.E. and Le Moal, M. (1980) Locomotor activation induced by infusion of endorphins into the ventral tegmental area: evidence for opiate-dopamine interactions. *Proceedings of the National Academy of Sciences* **77**, 2323–2327.

Sugrue, M.F. (1974) The effects of acutely administered analgesics on the turnover of noradrenaline and dopamine in various regions of the rat brain. *British Journal of Pharmacology* **52**, 159–162.

Swerdlow, N.R., Amalric, M. and Koob, G.F. (1987) Nucleus accumbens opiate-dopamine interactions and locomotor activation in the rat: evidence for a pre-synaptic locus. *Pharmacology Biochemistry and Behavior* **26**, 765–769.

Terenius, L. (1973) Characteristics of the 'receptor' for narcotic analgesics in synaptic plasma membrane fraction from rat brain. *Acta Pharmacologica Toxicologia* **33**, 377–384.

Vaccarino, F.J., Bloom, F.E. and Koob, G.F. (1985) Blockade of nucleus accumbens opiate receptors attenuates intravenous heroin reward in the rat. *Psychopharmacology* **86**, 37–42.

Van der Kooy, D., Mucha, R.F., O'Shaughnessy, M. and Bucenieks, P. (1982) Reinforcing effects of brain microinjections of morphine revealed by conditioned place preference. *Brain Research* **243**, 107–117.

Vincent, S., Hökfelt, T., Christensson, I. and Terenius, L. (1982) Immunohistochemical evidence for a dynorphin immunoreactive striatonigral pathway. *European Journal of Pharmacology* **85**, 251–252.

Von Voigtlander, P.F., Lahti, R.A. and Ludens, J.H. (1983) U-50,488H: a selective and structurally novel non-mu (kappa) opioid agonist. *Journal of Pharmacology and Experimental Therapeutics* **224**, 7–12.

Watson, S.J., Akil, H., Richard, C.W. and Barchas, J.D. (1978) Evidence for two separate opiate peptide neuronal systems. *Nature* **275**, 226–228.

Winkler, M., Havemann, U. and Kuschinsky, K. (1982) Unilateral injection of morphine into the nucleus accumbens induces akinesia and catalepsy, but no spontaneous muscular rigidity in rats. *Naunyn-Schmiedeberg's Archives of Pharmacology* **318**, 143–147.

Wise, R.A. and Bozarth, M.A. (1987) A psychomotor stimulant theory of addiction. *Psychological Review* **94**, 469–492.

Wood, P.L. and Altar, C.A. (1988) Dopamine release in vivo from nigrostriatal, mesolimbic, and mesocortical neurons: utility of 3-methoxy-tyramine measurements. *Pharmacological Reviews* **40**, 163–187.

Young, E., Walker, J.M., Lewis, M.E., Houghten, R.A., Woods, J.H. and Akil, H. (1986) [^{3}H]dynorphin A binding and kappa selectivity of prodynorphin peptides in rat, guinea-pig and monkey brain. *European Journal of Pharmacology* **121**, 355–365.

Zito, K.A., Vickers, G. and Roberts, D.C.S. (1985) Disruption of cocaine and heroin self-administration following kainic acid lesions of the nucleus accumbens. *Pharmacology Biochemistry and Behavior* **23**, 1029–1036.

Zukin, R.S. and Zukin, S.R. (1981) Multiple opiate receptors: emerging concepts. *Life Sciences* **29**, 2681–2690.

14

Role of Mesolimbic Dopamine in the Motivational Effects of Drugs: Brain Dialysis and Place Preference Studies

GAETANO DI CHIARA, ELIO ACQUAS AND
EZIO CARBONI

Institute of Experimental Pharmacoloy and Toxicology, University of
Cagliari, 09100 Cagliari, Sardinia, Italy

INTRODUCTION

Although the role of dopamine (DA) in motivated behaviour is supported by a wealth of experimental studies involving pharmacological manipulations and brain lesions, how this role takes place in relation to behaviour is still obscure. Indeed, we still do not know the quantitative time course of DA neurotransmission in specific brain areas during motivated behaviour.

Neurotransmission consists of at least two integrated aspects: a presynaptic aspect which can be related, in biochemical terms, to the amount of transmitter released in the time unit; and a postsynaptic aspect, which relates to the responsivity of the target element to the released transmitter. In recent years, much effort has been dedicated to the development of quantitative methodologies for monitoring neurotransmitter release in specific brain areas of behaving animals. These methods include the cup technique, push–pull cannula, voltammetry and, more recently, brain dialysis. It should be clear, however, that, given the dual nature of neurotransmission, it is unlikely that a study of the quantitative time course of DA release *in vivo* will be sufficient to describe DA neurotransmission fully in the behaving

The Mesolimbic Dopamine System: From Motivation to Action.
Edited by P. Willner and J. Scheel-Krüger

© 1991 John Wiley & Sons Ltd

animal. One should, therefore, be aware that the study of DA release *in vivo* provides only a first approximation to the integrated function of DA synapses. Only with these limitations in mind can one fully exploit the potential of the most recent technique for the *in vivo* study of central neurotransmission: brain dialysis.

BRAIN DIALYSIS

Brain dialysis involves implantation of a dialysis probe into selected brain areas, perfusion with a physiological fluid, and collection and analysis of the fluid for specific substances. The fluid, while flowing inside the probe, extracts from the extracellular brain compartment low molecular weight substances which diffuse across the dialytic membrane along their concentration gradient. Using this principle, virtually every substance present in the extracellular fluid can be monitored, provided that a sensitive method of analysis is available. The advantages of brain dialysis over other techniques for *in vivo* monitoring of chemical changes in the brain (e.g. cup technique and push–pull cannula) were clearly realized when this system first came into use, and were indicated in the 'closed' characteristic of the system, which avoids direct contact of the superfusion fluid with the tissue, thus reducing local tissue damage and providing relatively clean samples for direct chemical analysis.

Probes for Brain Dialysis

Existing dialysis probes fall into three categories: transcerebral (Figure 1), U-shaped and concentric. Concentric probes consist of an internal rigid cannula and an external dialysis fiber or membrane. The earliest example of this type of probe is Delgado's dialytrode, developed in the early 1970s (Delgado et al., 1972). This original dialysis probe, which consisted of a push–pull cannula closed at the tip by a dialysis membrane, is conceptually not much different from present-day commercial dialysis probes (Carnegie, Stockholm, Sweden: outer diameter 0.5 mm).

Transcerebral probes and U-shaped probes were initially developed by Ungerstedt in the early 1980s using 0.25–0.30-mm outer diameter dialysis fibers. Transcerebral probes, initially used in anesthetized rats (Imperato and Di Chiara, 1984; Zetterstrom and Ungerstedt, 1984), were later applied to freely moving animals (Imperato and Di Chiara, 1985). U-shaped·probes (outer diameter 0.6–0.8 mm) can be simply made of a long U-folded dialysis fiber carried by a removable rigid wire (Zetterstrom et al., 1983). Alternatively, the U-fiber is at the tip of two parallel cannulae (Westerink and De Vries, 1988). Dialysis membranes can be cellulosic (Dow) (Zetterstrom et al., 1983), polycarbonate (Carnegie), acrylic co-polymer (Amicon Vitafiber)

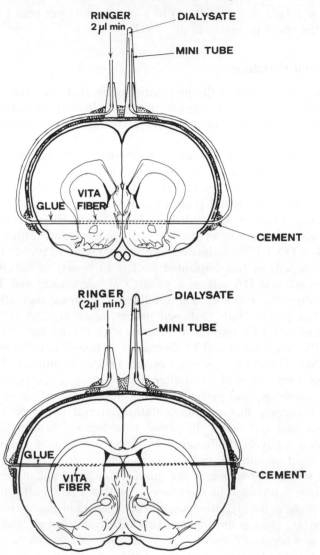

Figure 1. Two dialysis probes implanted at the level of the nucleus accumbens (top) and the dorsal caudate (bottom)

(Imperato and Di Chiara, 1984), or polyacrilonitrile co-polymer (AN.69-HOSPAL) (Consolo et al., 1987), differing in molecular weight cut-off (5000–50 000 daltons) and permeability to solutes. Perfusion rates vary from 0.2 to 4.0 μl/minute, but in most studies 2.0 μl/minute is used. At this rate, non-equilibrium dialysis is performed and relative recoveries in the dialysate range from 10 per cent (cellulose) to as much as 45 per cent (AN.69) using 10 mm-long fibers (Consolo et al., 1987).

Experimental Variables

A comparative analysis of the literature reveals that the results provided by brain dialysis are critically dependent upon at least three variables: type of probe, post-implantation interval and use of either anesthetized or freely moving rats.

A 20 times difference has been demonstrated in the ability to recover acetylcholine (ACh) from the caudate between transverse and U-shaped probes (Damsma et al., 1988). Thus, basal ACh could be detected in dialysates obtained from transcerebral probes but not from U-shaped probes unless a cholinesterase inhibitor was added to the perfusion Ringer (Damsma et al., 1988). Direct comparison of the Ca^{2+} dependency and tetrodotoxin (TTX) sensitivity of DA release estimated with the two types of probes (transcerebral versus U-shaped) in rats implanted acutely (3 hours) or subchronically (24 hours), reveals that DA release is mostly Ca^{2+}-dependent and TTX-sensitive 3 hours after the implant, and totally so 24 hours thereafter, with the transcerebral probe. With U-shaped probes, however, DA release is Ca^{2+}-independent and TTX-insensitive 3 hours after the implant while becoming partially Ca^{2+}-dependent and TTX-sensitive 24 hours later (Westerink and De Vries, 1988). Therefore, U-shaped probes in acutely implanted rats seem to detect only an overflow of transmitter, independent of neuronal firing activity and neurosecretion, and probably arising from damaged nerve terminals. It appears, therefore, that post-implantation interval and type of probe can interact so that differences in probe type become critical at early post-implantation intervals. Differences in probe size and in the related tissue damage might account in part for these differences.

A clue to the explanation of the influence of post-implantation interval on brain dialysis is provided by the observation that 2 hours after the implant of a dialysis probe in the hippocampus, marked changes in glucose metabolism and blood flow take place in the implanted area (Benveniste et al., 1987); moreover, probably as a result of massive K^+ release from damaged elements, 'spreading depression' and depolarization inactivation of intact neurons take place (Benveniste et al., 1989). Recovery from the above changes appears complete 24 hours after implantation of the probe (Benveniste et al., 1987).

Finally, anesthesia can drastically influence the effect of drugs that depend on an intact neuronal excitability and firing activity for their effects. Since stimulation of DA release by drugs like neuroleptics is firing-dependent (Imperato and Di Chiara, 1985), it is not unexpected that these drugs fail to stimulate DA release consistently in anesthetized rats (Di Chiara and Waldmeier, 1984).

Criteria for Brain Dialysis

The above examples indicate the necessity of establishing specific criteria for the evaluation of the nature of neurotransmitter output as estimated by any given dialysis technique. In particular, these criteria should be applied to the characterization of basal neurotransmitter output which is the basic reference for any experimentally induced change. Owing to the 'macro' size of the probes and to their spatial relationship with nerve terminals, brain dialysis is not expected to measure neurotransmitter released at synaptic sites, but rather neurotransmitter diffused into the extracellular space after its release. None the less, basal output of DA, noradrenaline (NA), ACh and 5-HT is Ca^{2+}-dependent and TTX-sensitive to an extent which ranges from 60 per cent for NA (L'Heureux et al., 1986) to 85–100 per cent for DA (Imperato and Di Chiara, 1984; Westerink and De Vries, 1988), ACh (Damsma et al., 1987) and 5-HT (Carboni and Di Chiara, 1989). Thus, basal output of DA, ACh, 5-HT and NA seems to result from the following sequence: action potential, terminal depolarization, activation of voltage-dependent fast Na^+ channels, activation of voltage-dependent Ca^{2+} channels, Ca^{2+} influx, exocytosis, transmitter release. In agreement with this, γ-butyrolactone, an agent known to block the firing activity of DA neurons, abolishes basal DA release (Imperato and Di Chiara, 1984), and prevents impulse-dependent stimulation of DA release (Imperato and Di Chiara, 1985; Imperato and Di Chiara, 1986; Carboni et al., 1989c).

Given these premises, experimental conditions which are unable to demonstrate Ca^{2+}-dependence and TTX-sensitivity for the above transmitters cast serious doubts on the possibility of using neurotransmitter output in dialysates as an estimate of *in vivo* neurotransmitter release under those conditions.

Another criterion currently used for testing the physiological nature of neurotransmitter output in dialysates is the ability of high potassium concentrations (30–100 mM) to stimulate transmitter release (Imperato and Di Chiara, 1984; Westerink et al., 1987; Kalén et al., 1988). This criterion, however, simply indicates that depolarization of neural structures (not only neuronal but also glial) is capable of releasing the transmitter, but tells us little about the nature of basal transmitter release. Thus, with striatal U-probes, 5-HT release is strongly stimulated by K^+ in spite of the fact that it is only partially (50 per cent) TTX-sensitive (Kalén et al., 1988). Basal amino acid release is also stimulated by K^+ but is virtually TTX-insensitive and Ca^{2+}-independent (Westerink et al., 1987). Similar considerations apply to the use of electrical or chemical stimulation of specific neural pathways as a criterion for characterizing basal neurotransmitter release *in vivo* (Imperato and Di Chiara, 1984).

Another criterion currently used for *in vivo* release is the effectiveness of drugs with neurotransmitter-releasing properties such as amphetamine (Zetterstrom et al., 1983; Imperato and Di Chiara, 1984), fenfluramine (Carboni and Di Chiara, 1989) or *p*-chloroamphetamine (Sharp et al., 1986; Kalén et al., 1988). However, the releasing action of these drugs is TTX-insensitive and Ca^{2+}-independent, in agreement with a direct displacing action on intraneuronal amine pools, and in contrast with reuptake blockers such as cocaine and chlorimipramine (Carboni and Di Chiara, 1989; Carboni et al., 1989c). Thus, the effect of these drugs is not a criterion for physiological *in vivo* transmitter release. Similar considerations apply to criteria utilizing drugs which interfere with the synthesis, metabolism or compartmentalization of the transmitter (Imperato and Di Chiara, 1984).

ACTIVE ROLE OF MESOLIMBIC DA IN MOTIVATION

Many centrally acting drugs have motivational properties. Thus, in appropriate experimental conditions, narcotic analgesics, psychostimulants, nicotine, ethanol, benzodiazepines and barbiturates can be shown to act as positive reinforcers. On the other hand, drugs like naloxone, picrotoxin, phencyclidine, lithium and κ opiate agonists show aversive properties.

The evidence that DA is involved in the motivational properties of psychostimulants such as amphetamine, which releases DA, and cocaine, which inhibits DA reuptake, is overwhelming. Given the role of DA in the basic mechanism of action of these drugs, this might even appear obvious. The role of DA in the case of most other drugs, however, has been uncertain and debated for at least two reasons: lack of studies on the effect of these drugs on *in vivo* dopaminergic transmission, and lack of unequivocal experimental evidence in a variety of behavioral paradigms.

With regard to the first issue, the advent of brain dialysis has enabled for the first time the monitoring of DA release in specific brain areas of the freely moving rat and the correlation of DA release with behavior. In a series of studies from our laboratory (Di Chiara and Imperato, 1988a), it was shown that many drugs which possess rewarding properties, such as morphine and narcotic analgesics (methadone and fentanyl) (Di Chiara and Imperato, 1988b), ethanol (Imperato and Di Chiara, 1986) and nicotine (Imperato et al., 1986), increase the extracellular concentration of DA preferentially in the nucleus accumbens as compared to the dorsal striatum. This effect was shared by classic psychostimulants such as amphetamine and cocaine (Carboni et al., 1989c). An analysis of the time and dose relationships between the biochemical and the behavioral effects of morphine and its analogs (Di Chiara and Imperato, 1988b), and of ethanol (Imperato and Di Chiara, 1986), showed that even for these drugs which produce biphasic effects on behavior (stimulant at low doses, inhibitory at high doses), there is, at low doses, a good correlation between stimulation of motor activity and stimulation of DA release in the nucleus accumbens. As the dose of narcotic or ethanol is increased, DA release further increases, but motor stimulation is replaced by motor inhibition (rigidity, frozen postures and catalepsy after narcotics; sedation after ethanol). Thus, after higher doses of narcotic analgesics and ethanol, an action on neural systems located beyond DA neurons can interfere with the behavioural expression of increased DA transmission.

The possible mechanism by which the various drugs investigated preferentially augment extracellular DA concentration in the accumbens as compared to the dorsal caudate is worth discussion. One possibility is that the preferential effect of the drugs studied is an artifact of the technique utilized for estimating the release of DA *in vivo*. Because brain dialysis estimates DA diffused into the extracellular compartment from its release sites, the results provided are influenced to a large extent by the processes of disposition of released DA. Given this, one might envision the possibility that the effect of the drugs on the amount of DA released in the two areas (accumbens versus caudate) is similar, but that the areas differ quantitatively in a process which takes place away from release sites (uptake, degradation etcetera), and makes a major contribution to the level of DA in the extracellular fluid. Indeed, we have suggested (Carboni et al., 1989c) that one factor contributing to the preferential effects of drugs on DA output in the accumbens might be a lower efficiency of the DA reuptake mechanism in the accumbens as compared to the caudate, which, in turn, might be related to differences in the density of DA terminals in the two areas (Abercrombie et al., 1989b). While such mechanisms might contribute to the preferential effect in the accumbens observed with brain dialysis, further results indicate that other factors also operate. Thus, a simple relationship with the density of DA terminals is excluded by the observation that morphine and ethanol fail to stimulate DA release in the prefrontal cortex, an area with the lowest density of DA terminals, at doses which consistently stimulate DA release in the accumbens (Carboni et al., in preparation). Furthermore, electrophysiological studies from different laboratories indicate that systemic morphine (Matthews and German, 1984), ethanol (Gessa et al., 1985) and nicotine (Mereu et al., 1987) preferentially stimulate the firing activity of A10 as compared to A9 dopaminergic neurons. Since the accumbens is innervated mainly by A10 and the dorsal caudate by A9 neurons, these results suggest that the differential effects of morphine, ethanol and nicotine on DA release *in vivo* are directly related to a differential sensitivity to their stimulant action of mesolimbic as compared to mesostriatal DA neurons.

Electrophysiological studies on psychostimulants indicate that systemic cocaine inhibits the firing of dopaminergic neurons and, again, this action is more pronounced on A10 than A9 neurons (Einhorn et al., 1988). Since inhibition of dopaminergic firing activity by cocaine is likely to be a negative feedback response to stimulation of presynaptic or postsynaptic DA receptors, these results are consistent with the idea that cocaine increases synaptic DA concentrations preferentially in the terminal areas of the mesolimbic system.

Further studies on other drug classes confirm the hypothesis that stimulation of DA release in the accumbens is related to the psychostimulant properties of the drugs under study. Thus, κ opiate agonists such as U50, 488H and bremazocine reduce DA release in the accumbens and caudate at doses which reduce motor activity and are aversive in animals (Di Chiara and Imperato, 1988b). Neuroleptics stimulate DA release in the accumbens and caudate to a similar extent, but this effect is a feedback response to their DA receptor blocking properties (Di Chiara and Imperato, 1988a); accordingly, neuroleptics reduce motor activity and disrupt the rewarding properties of primary reinforcers. Acute administration of other drugs, such as anti-muscarinics, anti-depressants (apart from nomifensine which stimulates DA release and is psychostimulant in animals), and anti-histaminics, which do not possess psychostimulant properties, failed to affect DA release (Di Chiara and Imperato, 1988a).

Therefore, brain dialysis in freely moving rats suggests the existence of a relationship between stimulation of DA transmission in the mesolimbic system and behavioral activation. It might be argued that activation of behavior is the cause rather than the result of stimulation of DA release in the accumbens, and, in fact, arousing the stressful stimuli do activate DA release in the mesolimbic system (Abercrombie et al., 1989a). However, pharmacologic and lesion studies point to the contrary as they show that various stimuli (including stress and drugs) which activate behavior, depend on DA for their behavioral stimulant properties. Thus, studies on the effects of narcotic analgesics, ethanol, nicotine, amphetamine and cocaine on unconditioned, as well as on conditioned (place preference) and operant (self-administration), behavior show that the motor stimulant (Longoni et al., 1987) as well as the acquisition phase of motivated behavior induced by these drugs is effectively disrupted by blockade of DA transmission, particularly at D1 receptors (Leone and Di Chiara, 1987; Koob et al., 1987; Acquas et al., 1989) (Figure 2A). Based on these results, we conclude that motivation is related to an active change of DA transmission in the mesolimbic system with reward or aversion depending on the sign of this change. Accordingly, stimulation of DA transmission would be rewarding while its inhibition would be aversive. Stress, which is likely to be aversive, stimulates DA release in the mesolimbic system (Abercrombie et al., 1989a) rather than reducing it, as our hypothesis would predict. However, it is possible that stimulation of DA release by stress could be a homeostatic reaction which tends to withdraw the animal from the stressful stimulus by

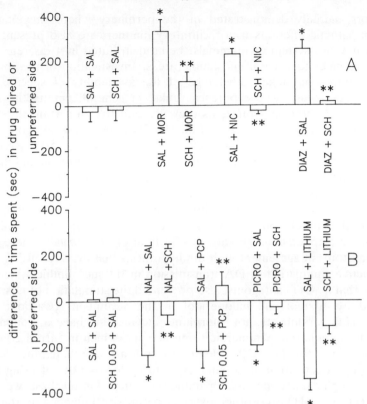

Figure 2. Effect of SCH 23390 (0.05 mg/kg s.c.) on side-preference shift induced by morphine (MOR) (1.0 mg/kg s.c.), nicotine (NIC) (0.6 mg/kg s.c.) and diazepam (DIAZ) (1.0 mg/kg i.p.), paired with the unpreferred compartment (**A**), and by naloxone (NAL) (0.8 mg/kg s.c.), phencyclidine (PCP) (2.5 mg/kg s.c.), picrotoxin (PICRO) (2.0 mg/kg i.p.) and lithium chloride (LITHIUM) (40 mg/kg s.c.), paired with the preferred compartment (**B**). Results are the mean (±SEM) side-preference shift (expressed in seconds). *$P<0.05$ for shift in side-preference (Newman-Keuls); **$P<0.05$ for differences in the shift in side-preference (Newman-Keuls). SAL, saline

promoting motor activity (see also Salamone, Chapter 23, this volume), and to attenuate the aversive impact of stress by providing a pleasurable interoceptive cue.

DA–Serotonin Relationship

Recent brain dialysis and place preference studies with 5-HT$_3$ receptor antagonists support the concept of an active role of DA in reward. 5-HT$_3$

receptors, initially demonstrated in the periphery where they modulate parasympathetic efferents in a facilitatory manner, are also present in the central nervous system of mammals, being distributed in a discrete, highly specific manner to visceral and limbic areas. Investigation of the role of 5-HT_3 receptors has taken advantage of the availability of specific 5-HT_3 receptor antagonists whose potency ranks, in general, among the highest known for receptor antagonists as they are effective in certain tests in the subpicomolar range (Richardson et al., 1985). Using these antagonists (ICS 205–930, MDL 72222), we have shown that blockade of 5-HT_3 receptors specifically prevents the place preference induced by morphine and nicotine, but not that induced by amphetamine (Carboni et al., 1989b) (Figure 3). Subsequently, brain dialysis studies have showed that the 5-HT_3 antagonist ICS 205–930, which fails to modify basal DA release in the accumbens, prevents the stimulation of DA release elicited by morphine and nicotine, but not by amphetamine (Figure 4) (Carboni et al., 1989a). These results are, therefore, in agreement with the hypothesis that drug reward is related to an active stimulation of DA transmission in the mesolimbic system. It is notable that a 5-HT_3 antagonist also prevented the stimulation of DA release induced by ethanol and haloperidol in the accumbens (Carboni et al., 1989a). Haloperidol, ethanol, morphine and nicotine have in common the ability to stimulate dopaminergic firing activity, which in turn accounts for the ability to stimulate DA release; in contrast, amphetamine does not depend upon activation of dopaminergic firing for its DA releasing actions (indeed amphetamine inhibits dopaminergic firing). On this basis we suggest that 5-HT, via 5-HT_3 receptors, exerts a permissive influence on the ability of drugs to stimulate DA release.

The Diazepam Puzzle

Further studies on the relationship between DA release and drugs as motivation stimuli over the last year have indicated the need to modify the initial hypothesis that motivation is related to an active change in DA transmission.

Diazepam is known to be abused by humans and to be self-administered by animals. Diazepam also elicits a conditioned place preference which is blocked by haloperidol (Spyraki and Fibiger, 1988). We have recently found that diazepam fails to stimulate DA release at the threshold doses (1.0 mg/kg i.p.) for place preference; higher doses of diazepam (2.5–5.0 mg/kg i.p.), which induce place preference (Spyraki et al., 1985), consistently reduce DA release (Figure 5). In spite of this, SCH 23390 blocks diazepam-induced place preference (Figure 2A).

Repeated administration of diazepam with the same schedule used for place preference studies also failed to stimulate DA release in the accumbens.

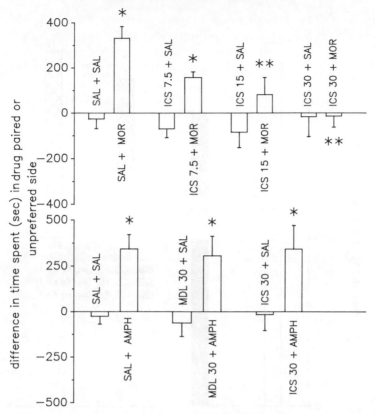

Figure 3. Effect of different doses of ICS 205–930 (ICS) (7.5, 15 and 30 µg/kg s.c.) on place preference induced by morphine (MOR) (1.0 mg/kg s.c.), paired with the unpreferred compartment (top). Effect of MDL 72222 (MDL) (30 µg/kg s.c.) and ICS 205–930 (ICS) (30 µg/kg s.c.) on side-preference shift induced by amphetamine (AMPH) (1.0 mg/kg s.c.), paired with the unpreferred compartment. Results are expressed as the mean (±SEM) of side-preference shift (in seconds) for the drug paired compartment. *$P<0.05$ compared to saline and saline; **$P<0.05$ (top) compared to saline and morphine

This applied also to other dopaminergic areas such as the hippocampus, prefrontal cortex and dorsal caudate. The fact that diazepam elicits reward in spite of its tendency to reduce DA transmission calls for a revision of the hypothesis of an active role of DA transmission in motivation. One might propose, for example, that diazepam reward is related to DA transmission in a manner different from that of other drugs of abuse, and that transmitters other than DA play a role in the rewarding effects of diazepam. Indeed, a 'pluralistic' hypothesis of the neurotransmitter mechan-

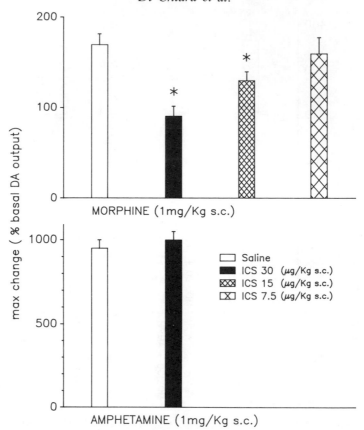

Figure 4. Effect of different doses of ICS 205–930 (7.5, 15 and 30 µg/kg s.c.) on the *in vivo* release of DA from the nucleus accumbens, induced by morphine (1.0 mg/kg s.c.); each column represents the mean (±SEM) of the results from four experiments (top). (The maximal responses are shown.) Effect of ICS 205–930 (30 µg/kg s.c.) on the *in vivo* release of DA from the nucleus accumbens, induced by amphetamine (1.0 mg/kg s.c.); each column represents the mean (±SEM) of the results from four experiments (bottom). (The maximal responses are shown) *$P<0.05$ compared to saline + morphine (top)

ism of reward has been advanced by others on different grounds (Ettenberg et al., 1982; Phillips, 1984).

DUAL ROLE OF DA IN CONDITIONED BEHAVIOR?

Although the primary neurochemical mechanism which confers to the diazepam stimulus its intrinsic rewarding properties might not be DA, it remains to be explained why the diazepam place preference is DA-

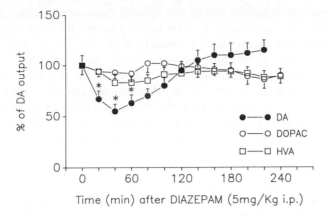

Time (min) after DIAZEPAM (5mg/Kg i.p.)

Figure 5. Effect of diazepam (5.0 mg/kg i.p.) on DA release and metabolism from the nucleus accumbens. Results are expressed as percentage of basal values obtained in four rats. Mean basal values expressed in pmol per 20 minutes ($\pm$SEM) are as follows: DA, 0.12 ± 0.013; DOPAC, 25.8 ± 2.8; HVA, 17.7 ± 1.8. *$P<0.05$ with respect to basal values

dependent. A way out of this paradox is to postulate that DA exerts a dual role in conditioned behavior, first, a stimulus-dependent active role related to the ability of the stimulus (drug or other) to stimulate or to inhibit DA transmission, which determines its intrinsic motivational properties (rewarding or aversive); second, a stimulus-independent role unrelated to the qualitative motivational properties (rewarding or aversive) of the stimulus, but only to a more general role of DA in learning. Accordingly, DA would play an active role in mediating the motivational properties of the stimulus and a permissive role in learning of a conditioned response. If this hypothesis is correct, blockade of DA transmission is expected to interfere with the acquisition of a conditioned response, irrespective of the positive or negative motivational quality of the stimulus and of its ability to act on DA transmission. In fact, we have recently observed that blockade of D1 receptors by SCH 23390 prevents not only place preference elicited by drugs which stimulate DA release, e.g. morphine, nicotine and amphetamine, but also prevents the place aversion induced by drugs which do not have uniform effects on DA transmission, e.g. naloxone, lithium, picrotoxin and phencyclidine (Acquas et al., 1989) (Figure 2B). Naloxone, for example, fails to affect DA transmission in all the areas tested (accumbens, prefrontal cortex, hippocampus and dorsal caudate). Phencyclidine stimulates DA release in all the areas investigated, but none the less elicits aversion. In line with these observations, Shippenberg and Herz (1988) have reported that SCH 23390 also blocks the place aversion induced by κ agonists, which, as we have reported, reduce DA release (Di Chiara and Imperato, 1988b).

An interpretative hypothesis of the present data should take into account current views of the role of DA in motivated behavior and learning. In general, stimuli are operationally defined by their ability to produce biological responses. Natural stimuli have sensory properties (e.g. colour, shape and taste); some stimuli are provided, in addition, with intrinsic motivational properties which make them capable of producing specific motor responses directed to approach and prolong the stimulus (appetitive stimuli), or to terminate and avoid the stimulus (aversive stimuli). Presentation of appetitive stimuli, also called primary incentives, results in positive reinforcement and reward. Presentation of aversive stimuli (punishers) results in negative reinforcement. Repeated temporal association (pairing) of a neutral stimulus with a response-eliciting (unconditioned) stimulus is known to result in transfer (conditioning) to the neutral stimulus of the response-eliciting properties of the unconditioned stimulus.

On the basis of the consideration that natural stimuli (e.g. food) have sensory as well as motivational properties, stimulus–stimulus (S–S) associative learning, as referred to the sensory properties of the stimulus, has been distinguished from incentive (either appetitive or aversive) motivational learning (Bolles, 1972; Mackintosh, 1974). Place conditioning has the characteristics of incentive motivational learning. In this paradigm, neutral environmental stimuli acquire the response eliciting properties of a primary motivational stimulus (e.g. food, electric shock and drug) by being paired with that stimulus.

Various studies indicate that DA is not involved in S–S associative learning; on the other hand, experimental evidence obtained with brain lesions and pharmacological manipulations indicates that DA is essential for incentive motivational learning produced by appetitive, positively reinforcing stimuli (Beninger, 1983). Our results, obtained with drug-induced place preference, are in full agreement with this general conclusion as they show that the acquisition of incentive motivational learning in a place preference paradigm induced by various primary reinforcers (amphetamine, morphine or nicotine) is blocked by the D1 antagonist SCH 23390. Our brain dialysis studies now suggest that the primary appetitive properties of many (though not all) drugs are related to an active stimulation of DA release.

Neuroleptics have been reported to be unable to block negative reinforcement in response to aversive stimuli in the acquisition of avoidance learning; moreover, neuroleptics fail to block acquisition of fear-indicating autonomic responses to the conditioned stimulus in spite of blockade of conditioned avoidance responding (Beninger, 1983). However, our results clearly show that D1 blockade effectively impairs the acquisition of avoidance learning as indicated by the ability of SCH 23390 to block the acquisition of place aversion to aversive stimuli such as naloxone, picrotoxin, phencyclidine and lithium. One might argue that this is due to overshadowing of the effect of the stimulus (drug) by the SCH 23390 cue. We have no evidence for exclusion of this possibility other than the observation that, at the dose used in our studies, SCH 23390 fails to induce significant place preference or aversion when paired with one specific environment. However, because previous studies have been performed with neuroleptics acting preferentially (haloperidol) or specifically (pimozide) on D2 receptors, another possibility is that blockade of D1 receptors impairs either the intrinsic motivational properties of the stimuli or the association of these properties with environmental stimuli (incentive learning). As the motivational properties of the aversive drugs tested, with the exception of κ opiate agonists, do not seem to be related to any specific change of DA transmission, we favour the idea that DA transmission has a non-active (permissive) role in drug-induced aversive motivation, and that DA, acting on D1 receptors, plays a role in aversive learning. It should be mentioned, however, that the aversive properties of certain drugs, such as κ agonists, may be due to an active change (reduction) of DA transmission.

SUMMARY

Psychoactive drugs exert motivational effects by acting on different neurochemical mechanisms; therefore, mesolimbic DA plays an active role in the motivational properties of many, although not all, psychoactive drugs. Thus, stimulation of DA transmission might account for the rewarding effects of amphetamine, cocaine, narcotic analgesics, ethanol and nicotine, while inhibition of DA transmission might result in the aversive properties of κ agonists. Other drugs, e.g. diazepam, naloxone, phencyclidine, lithium and picrotoxin, might exert their primary motivational effects independently from an action on DA transmission. Apart from its primary active role in motivation, DA might have another role which is not intrinsic to the stimulus but to the mechanism of conditioning, being essential for incentive learning elicited by appetitive or aversive stimuli.

The possibility of interfering specifically with one of the two mechanisms is essential to the demonstration of the hypothesis of the dual role of DA in motivated behavior. There is no reason to assume that these two actions involve the same anatomical locus, but, since the stimulus-independent role of DA is located beyond the stimulus-dependent action, any manipulation which would interfere with the first would preclude the possibility of evaluating the effect on the second.

For this reason, D1 antagonists such as SCH 23390, which act on the stimulus-independent process, may be insufficient for dissecting the dual role of DA in conditioned behavior. D2 antagonists might prove more adequate, and such studies are in progress in our laboratory. However, very recent studies have provided evidence that, even when using SCH 23390, an apparently selective effect on the stimulus-dependent process may be demonstrated at low doses. As noted above, a high dose of SCH 23390 (50 μg/kg) was itself without effect in the place conditioning paradigm, but blocked the place preferences and aversions elicited by a range of psychotropic agents (Figure 2). However, at a lower dose (12 μg/kg), SCH 23390 supported a place aversion. At this dose, SCH 23390 blocked the place preference elicited by amphetamine, but failed to affect either the place preference elicited by morphine or the place aversion elicited by naloxone. These results support the suggestion of a dual role for DA in place conditioning, and suggest that, at a sufficiently low dose, SCH 23390 specifically blocks the rewarding effect of amphetamine (stimulus-dependent), while sparing the incentive learning (stimulus-independent) mechanism that is also blocked at higher doses.

REFERENCES

Abercrombie, E.D., Keefe, K.A., DiFrischia, D.S. and Zigmond, M.J. (1989a) Differential effect of stress on in vivo dopamine release in striatum, nucleus accumbens, and medial frontal cortex. *Journal of Neurochemistry* **52**, 1655–1658.

Abercrombie, E., Keefe, K. and Sigmond, M. (1989b) Evidence that nerve terminal density is an important contributor to differences in the activation of central dopamine systems. *Behavioural Pharmacology* **1**, 26, (suppl 1).

Acquas, E., Carboni, E., Leone, P. and Di Chiara, G. (1989) SCH 23390 blocks drug-conditioned place-preference and place-aversion: anhedonia (lack of reward) or apathy (lack of motivation) after dopamine-receptor blockade? *Psychopharmacology* **99**, 151–155.

Beninger, R.J. (1983) The role of dopamine in locomotor activity and learning. *Brain Research Reviews* **6**, 173–196.

Beninger, R.J., Phillips, A.G. and Fibiger, H.C. (1983) Prior training and intermittent retraining attenuate pimozide-induced avoidance deficits. *Pharmacology, Biochemistry and Behavior* **18**, 619–624.

Benveniste, H., Drejer, J., Schousboe, A. and Diemer, N.H. (1987) Regional cerebral glucose phosphorylation and blood flow after insertion of a microdialysis fiber through the dorsal hippocampus in the rat. *Journal of Neurochemistry* **49**, 729–734.

Benveniste, H., Hansen, A.J. and Ottosen, N.S. (1989) Determination of brain interstitial concentrations by microdialysis. *Journal of Neurochemistry* **52**, 1741–1750.

Bolles, R.C. (1972) Reinforcement, expectancy and learning. *Psychological Reviews* **79**, 394–409.

Carboni, E. and Di Chiara, G. (1989) Serotonin release estimated by transcortical dialysis in freely moving rats. *Neuroscience* **32**, 637–645.

Carboni, E., Acquas, E., Frau, R. and Di Chiara, G. (1989a) Differential inhibitory effects of a 5-HT$_3$ antagonist on drug-induced stimulation of dopamine release. *European Journal of Pharmacology* **164**, 515–519.

Carboni, E., Acquas, E., Leone, P. and Di Chiara, G. (1989b) 5HT$_3$ receptor antagonists block morphine- and nicotine- but not amphetamine-induced reward. *Psychopharmacology* **97**, 175–178.

Carboni, E., Imperato, A., Perezzani, L. and Di Chiara, G. (1989c) Amphetamine, cocaine, phencyclidine and nomifensine increase extracellular dopamine concentrations preferentially in the nucleus accumbens of freely moving rats. *Neuroscience* **28**, 653–661.

Consolo, S., Wu, C.F., Fiorentini, F., Ladinsky, H. and Vezzani, A. (1987) Determination of endogenous acetylcholine release in freely moving rats by transtriatal dialysis coupled to a radioenzymatic assay: effect of drugs. *Journal of Neurochemistry* **48**, 1459–1465.

Damsma, G., Westerink, B.H.C., Imperato, A., Rollema, H., De Vries, J.B. and Horn, A.S. (1987) Automated brain dialysis of acetylcholine in freely moving rats: detection of basal acetylcholine. *Life Science* **41**, 873–876.

Damsma, G., Westerink, B.H.C., De Boer, P., De Vries, J.B. and Horn, A.A. (1988) Basal acetylcholine release in freely moving rats detected by on-line transtriatal dialysis: pharmacological aspects. *Life Science* **43**, 1161–1168.

Delgado, J.M.R., DeFeudis, F.V., Roth, R.H., Ryugo, D.K. and Mitruka, B.K. (1972) Dialytrode for long term intracerebral perfusion in awake monkeys. *Archives Internationales de Pharmacodynamie et Therapie* **198**, 9–21.

Di Chiara, G. and Imperato, A. (1988a) Drugs abused by humans preferentially increase synaptic dopamine concentrations in the mesolimbic system of freely moving rats. *Proceedings of the National Academy of Science USA* **85**, 5274–5278.

Di Chiara, G. and Imperato, A. (1988b) Opposite effects of μ and κ-opiate agonists on dopamine-release in the nucleus accumbens and in the dorsal caudate of freely moving rats. *Journal of Pharmacology and Experimental Therapeutics* **244**, 1067–1080.

Di Chiara, G. and Waldmeier, P. (1984) Catecholamine release and metabolism. In: Usdin, E. (ed.) *Progress in Catecholamine Research: Basic and Peripheral Mechanisms.* New York: A.R. Liss, pp. 167–168.

Einhorn, L.C., Johansen, P.A. and White, F.J. (1988) Electrophysiological effects of cocaine in the mesoaccumbens dopamine system: studies in the ventral tegmental area. *Journal of Neuroscience* **8**, 100–112.

Ettenberg, A., Pettit, H.O., Bloom, F.E. and Koob, G.F. (1982) Heroin and cocaine intravenous self-administration in rats: mediation by separate neural systems. *Psychopharmacology* **78**, 204–209.

Gessa, G.L., Muntoni, F., Collu, M., Vargiu, L. and Mereu, G.P. (1985) Low doses of ethanol activate dopaminergic neurons in the ventral tegmental area. *Brain Research* **348**, 201–203.

Imperato, A. and Di Chiara, G. (1984) Trans-striatal dialysis coupled to reverse phase high performance liquid chromatography with electrochemical detection: a new method for the study of the 'in vivo' release of endogenous dopamine and metabolites. *Journal of Neuroscience* **4**, 966–977.

Imperato, A. and Di Chiara, G. (1985) Dopamine release and metabolism in awake rats after systemic neuroleptics as studied by trans-striatal dialysis. *Journal of Neuroscience* **5**, 297–306.

Imperato, A. and Di Chiara, G. (1986) Preferential stimulation of dopamine-release in the accumbens of freely moving rats by ethanol. *Journal of Pharmacology and Experimental Therapeutics* **239**, 219–228.

Imperato, A., Mulas, A. and Di Chiara, G. (1986) Nicotine preferentially stimulates dopamine release in the limbic system of freely moving rats. *European Journal of Pharmacology* **132**, 337–338.

Kalén, P., Strecker, R.E., Rosengren, E. and Bjorklund, A. (1988) Endogenous release of neuronal serotonin and 5-hydroxyindoleacetic acid in the caudate-putamen of the rat as revealed by intracerebral dialysis coupled to high performance liquid chromatography with fluorimetric detection. *Journal of Neurochemistry* **51**, 1422–1435.

Koob, G.F., Le, H.T. and Creese, I. (1987) The D_1 dopamine antagonists SCH 23390 increases cocaine self-administration in the rat. *Neuroscience Letters* **79**, 315–320.

Leone, P. and Di Chiara, G. (1987) Blockade of D-1 receptors by SCH 23390 antagonizes morphine- and amphetamine-induced place preference conditioning. *European Journal of Pharmacology* **135**, 251–254.

L'Heureux, R., Dennis, T., Curet, O. and Scatton, B. (1986) Measurement of endogenous noradrenaline release in the rat cerebral cortex 'in vivo' by transcortical dialysis: effects of drugs affecting noradrenergic transmission. *Journal of Neurochemistry* **46**, 1794–1801.

Longoni, R., Spina, L. and Di Chiara, G. (1987) Dopaminergic D-1 receptors: essential role in morphine-induced hypermotility. *Psychopharmacology* **93**, 401–402.

Mackintosh, J.J. (1974) *The Psychology of Animal Learning*. New York: Academic Press, pp. 222–223.

Matthews, R.T. and German, D.C. (1984) Electrophysiological evidence for excitation of rat ventral tegmental area dopamine neurons by morphine. *Neuroscience* **11**, 617–625.

Mereu, G.P., Woon, P., Boi, V., Gessa, G.L., Naes, L. and Westerfall, T.C. (1987) Preferential stimulation of ventral tegmental area dopaminergic neurons by nicotine. *European Journal of Pharmacology* **141**, 393–395.

Phillips, A.G. (1984) Brain reward circuitry: a case for separate systems. *Brain Research Bulletin* **12**, 195–201.

Richardson, B.P., Engel, G., Donatsch, P. and Stadler, P.A. (1985) Identification of serotonin M-receptor subtypes and their specific blockade by a new class of drugs. *Nature* **316**, 126–131.

Sharp, T., Zetterstrom, T., Christmanson, L. and Ungerstedt, U. (1986) p-Chloroamphetamine releases both serotonin and dopamine into rat brain dialysates 'in vivo'. *Neuroscience Letters* **72**, 320–324.

Shippenberg, T.S. and Herz, A. (1988) Motivational effects of opioids: influence of D-1 versus D-2 receptor antagonists. *European Journal of Pharmacology* **151**, 233–242.

Spyraki, C. and Fibiger, H.C. (1988) A role for the mesolimbic dopamine system in the reinforcing properties of diazepam. *Psychopharmacology* **94**, 133–137.

Spyraki, C., Kazandjian, A. and Varonos, D. (1985) Diazepam-induced place preference conditioning: appetitive and antiaversive properties. *Psychopharmacology* **87**, 225–232.

Westerink, B.H.C. and De Vries, J.B. (1988) Characterization of 'in vivo' dopamine release as determined by brain microdialysis after acute and subchronic implantations: methodological aspects. *Journal of Neurochemistry* **51**, 683–687.

Westerink, B.H.C., Damsma, G., Rollema, H., de Vries, J.B. and Horn, A.S. (1987) Scope and limitation of 'in vivo' brain dialysis: a comparison of its application to various transmitter systems. *Life Science* **41**, 1763–1776.

Zetterstrom, T. and Ungerstedt, U. (1984) Effects of apomorphine on the 'in vivo' release of dopamine and its metabolites, studied by brain dialysis. *European Journal of Pharmacology* **97**, 29–36.

Zetterstrom, T., Sharp, T., Marsden, C.A. and Ungerstedt, U. (1983) 'In vivo' measurement of dopamine and its metabolites by intracerebral dialysis: changes after d-amphetamine. *Journal of Neurochemistry* **41**, 1769–1773.

Part 3

MESOLIMBIC DYSFUNCTION

15

Dopamine, Depression and Anti-Depressant Drugs

PAUL WILLNER, RICHARD MUSCAT, MARIUSZ PAPP
AND DAVID SAMPSON

Department of Psychology, City of London Polytechnic, Old Castle Street,
London E1 7NT, UK

INTRODUCTION

Traditional accounts of the biochemical basis of depression have focused largely on noradrenaline (NA) and serotonin (5-HT), and although most of the evidence that has coalesced into the 'catecholamine hypothesis of depression' (Schildkraut, 1965; Bunney and Davis, 1965) does not distinguish clearly between NA and dopamine (DA), the potential role of DA has until recently been overlooked. Following two influential reviews that drew attention to this oversight (Randrup et al., 1975; Willner, 1983), there has been an upsurge of interest in the DA hypothesis of depression, as evidenced by the inclusion of a symposium on this topic in a number of recent international meetings.

In fact, as will be seen below, there is little in the recent clinical evidence to justify this change in fashion; the pressure to reconsider the role of DA in depression arises almost entirely from preclinical developments. One of these developments is the substantial body of work demonstrating that anti-depressant drugs enhance the functioning of mesolimbic DA synapses. However, the major driving force has undoubtedly been the massive research effort around the involvement of DA in rewarded behaviour. While the precise nature of the signal carried by mesolimbic DA neurons remains controversial, there is now no doubt that the mesolimbic DA system plays a crucial role in the processing of reward-related information, and the selection and elaboration of motivated behaviour (see Part 2 of this volume). These properties make a dysfunction of the mesolimbic system a prime

The Mesolimbic Dopamine System: From Motivation to Action.
Edited by P. Willner and J. Scheel-Krüger

© 1991 John Wiley & Sons Ltd

candidate to mediate the inability to experience pleasure (anhedonia) and loss of motivation (lack of interest) that form the core of endogenous depression (melancholia).

This hypothesis has major aesthetic advantages over its predecessors in that it not only proposes a relationship between a biochemical entity (DA) and a mental disorder (depression), but also defines explicitly the nature of the relationship in terms of the functional properties of the relevant DA neurons (Willner, 1985). The hypothesis also defines certain boundary conditions: it involves a limited set of DA projections (the mesolimbic system), and purports to explain a limited set of depressive symptoms (anhedonia and lack of interest).

This chapter reviews critically the evidence pertinent to this form of the DA hypothesis of depression, focusing on the clinical data, the effects of anti-depressant drugs and studies in a novel animal model of depression.

DA FUNCTION IN DEPRESSION: CLINICAL STUDIES

DA Turnover in Depression

A large number of studies have attempted to assess forebrain DA function in depressed patients by measuring levels of the DA metabolite homovanillic acid (HVA) in the cerebrospinal fluid (CSF). In some studies, patients were pretreated with probenecid to block the transport of HVA out of the CSF; this procedure, which measures the accumulation of HVA, is considered to give a better estimate of DA turnover. Most studies have tended to report a decrease in CSF HVA in depressed patients, and this relationship holds strongly in studies using the probenecid technique. Decreases in CSF HVA are particularly pronounced in patients with marked psychomotor retardation. In fact, a 1983 review of this area concluded that: 'The consistent finding of decreased post-probenecid CSF HVA accumulation in depressed patients, particularly those with psychomotor retardation, is probably the most firmly established observation in the neurochemistry of depression' (Willner, 1983). More recent studies have not altered this conclusion (Jimerson, 1987).

Nevertheless, the interpretation of these data is far from straightforward. Although some studies have reported that CSF HVA was lower in melancholic than in non-melancholic patients (Roy et al., 1985), there is a strong association between low CSF HVA and psychomotor retardation, which tends to be a prominent feature of melancholia. In agitated patients, however, HVA levels are normal or slightly elevated (Banki, 1977; Banki et al., 1981; van Praag et al., 1973). HVA levels are also elevated in delusional patients (Agren and Terenius, 1985; Sweeney et al., 1978). Again, this finding may reflect psychomotor agitation: in a study of psychotic patients, CSF HVA levels were elevated in those with delusions and agitation, but normal in those with delusions but no agitation (van Praag et al., 1975).

These data suggest strongly that CSF HVA levels are related to motor activity rather than mood, and further raise the problem of whether a reduction in HVA level is the primary cause or a secondary reflection of psychomotor retardation. This latter problem has lain dormant since the heroic study in which Post et al. (1973) asked a group of depressed patients to simulate mania: the exercise did increase their DA turnover, but also elevated their mood.

It comes as no surprise that CSF HVA levels are associated with level of motor activity, since CSF HVA derives largely from the caudate nucleus, on account of its large size and its periventricular location (Sourkes, 1973). The contribution of DA release in mesolimbic structures such as the nucleus accumbens and frontal cortex is relatively minor. There is therefore no reason to expect that changes in mesolimbic DA function would be apparent in studies measuring HVA levels in lumbar CSF; it is far more likely that any such changes would be obscured by alterations in nigrostriatal DA function associated with changes in motor output. Thus, although most reviewers have tended to interpret the HVA data as evidence for a DA dysfunction in depression (Randrup et al., 1975; Willner, 1983; Jimerson, 1987), these data are actually silent with respect to the important question of the state of activity in the mesolimbic system.

Reduction of DA function

It is still widely believed that the catecholamine-depleting drug reserpine causes depression, on the basis of a series of reports in the 1950s, despite the findings of Goodwin et al. (1972), on re-analysis of these data, that the great majority of 'reserpine depression' patients had been incorrectly diagnosed. It remains unclear whether the doses of reserpine administered in the 'reserpine depression' studies were sufficient to disable DA transmission. However, it may be significant that in the Goodwin et al. (1972) re-analysis, major depression was the correct diagnosis in almost 50 per cent of patients who developed marked psychomotor retardation.

More convincing evidence that DA depletion can lead to depression is seen in the high incidence of depression in Parkinson's disease (Randrup et al., 1975; Asnis, 1977; Mayeux et al., 1986). Parkinsonian depression is more severe than would be expected from the physical symptoms alone (Robins, 1976), and the onset of depression can precede the physical disabilities (McDowell et al., 1971). However, it is now recognized that Parkinson's disease is in no sense a pure DA deficiency syndrome: NA, 5-HT, acetylcholine (ACh), somatostatin and neurotensin levels are also abnormal (Perry, 1987). Nevertheless, the anti-depressant effect of DOPA in Parkinson's disease (Goodwin, 1972; Randrup et al., 1975) does point towards a dopaminergic substrate of parkinsonian depression. In some cases there is clear evidence that mood improvement precedes the improvement in physical symptoms (Murphy, 1972), suggesting that the anti-depressant effect can not be simply explained away as secondary to an improvement in physical symptoms.

Depression is also frequently encountered as a side-effect of neuroleptic therapy in schizophrenia (Randrup et al., 1975). In this case, there are strong grounds for believing that the effect is caused by antagonism of DA receptors (Creese and Snyder, 1978), but it is difficult to exclude the possibility that by bringing schizophrenic symptoms under control, neuroleptics unmask a pre-existing depression. We are unaware of any study that has formally addressed this issue. Anti-depressant effects on withdrawal of neuroleptics are also well documented, though again, there are few formal studies (Randrup et al., 1975). In a recent trial, del Zompo et al. (1990) treated depressed patients with a haloperidol/chlorimipramine cocktail and reported marked improvement, relative to a group treated with chlorimipramine alone, when the haloperidol component was withdrawn after 3 weeks of treatment. It was assumed that the improvement resulted from the unmasking of DA receptors rendered supersensitive by chronic neuroleptic treatment. Clearly, more trials of this kind are needed, and the proposed mechanism of action requires confirmation.

In sharp contrast, there is also clear evidence that, under certain circumstances, neuroleptics are active as anti-depressants (Robertson and Trimble, 1982; Nelson, 1987). These findings strike at the heart of the DA/anhedonia/depression hypotheses, and therefore require careful consideration. One potential resolution is that neuroleptics are anti-depressant only at low doses which act preferentially as DA autoreceptor antagonists and so increase DA turnover. This hypothesis has been advanced in particular in relation to certain atypical anti-depressants, such as sulpiride, which are said to have 'activating' properties. For example, del Zompo et al. (1990) found that sulpiride, used as an anti-depressant at a dose (75 mg/day) considerably lower than that used in the treatment of psychosis, was superior to placebo and equivalent to amitriptyline in bipolar patients. However, these results provide only weak support for the DA/depression hypothesis, since in anti-depressant screening tests, sulpiride apparently acts through a non-dopaminergic mechanism (Vaccheri et al., 1984).

While an autoreceptor hypothesis might explain some of the data, it is not necessarily the case that low doses are used when neuroleptics are prescribed as anti-depressants. Doses below the anti-psychotic range have usually been prescribed in studies of mild, non-endogenous depression, but in delusional depression, neuroleptics are more commonly prescribed at normal anti-psychotic doses (Nelson, 1987). Again, however, it is not certain that DA antagonism is the mechanism of anti-depressant action: indeed, in one study, anti-depressant effects of cis-flupenthixol were negatively correlated with increase in serum prolactin levels, suggesting that DA blockade might actually antagonize the anti-depressant effect (Robertson and Trimble, 1981).

It is also questionable whether neuroleptics are truly anti-depressant, and examination of the pattern of symptomatic improvement provides the clearest resolution to the paradox of the anti-depressant action of neuroleptics: in brief, there is no evidence that neuroleptics can improve anhedonia. In non-endogenous depressions, neuroleptics and tricyclics appear to be equally effective (Robertson and Trimble, 1982; Nelson, 1987), but, by definition, anhedonia is not a part of these depressions. Neuroleptics also appear to be as effective as tricyclics, or nearly so, in endogenous depressions (Robertson and Trimble, 1982; Nelson, 1987). However, Nelson (1987) suggests that this appearance may be spurious, in so far as the studies in question may have seriously underestimated the true effectiveness of tricyclics (owing to a failure to attain adequate plasma drug levels, and other factors). The anti-depressant potential of neuroleptics is most firmly established in delusional depression, which responds well to combined therapy with a neuroleptic/tricyclic mixture, but responds poorly, if at all, to tricyclics alone. However, neuroleptics alone are also ineffective in delusional depression (Nelson, 1987). Although neuroleptics alone produce a substantial global improvement in delusional depression, this arises almost entirely from a decrease in agitation and delusional thinking; motor retardation, lack of energy and anhedonia do not respond to neuroleptic treatment (Raskin et al., 1970; Nelson and Bowers, 1978; Minter and Mandell, 1979). On the basis of these findings, it seems likely that the global improvement seen in endogenous depressives treated with neuroleptics alone results from the inclusion of agitated and delusional patients. This analysis of the place of neuroleptics in the treatment of depression implies that anhedonia and delusions are mediated by different sets of DA terminals which may be activated independently.

Enhancement of DA function

This conclusion is pertinent to an assessment of the early trials of L-DOPA as an anti-depressant. DOPA produced a modest global improvement, primarily in retarded patients, but the effect was largely one of psychomotor activation with little effect on mood; in bipolar patients, DOPA frequently caused a switch into hypomania (Goodwin and Sack, 1974). These data have been taken as evidence against a prominent role for DA in depression. However, the effects of DOPA were greatest in patients with the lowest pretreatment CSF HVA levels (van Praag and Korf, 1975), suggesting that the primary effect of DOPA is an increase in DA release in the caudate nucleus. We should expect that the untoward consequences of excessive striatal DA activity might mask any underlying beneficial increase in mesolimbic DA release. It follows that the failure to demonstrate anti-depressant efficacy with treatments that cause a global increase in DA activity carries little weight.

More convincing anti-depressant effects have been reported with the directly acting DA agonists piribedil and bromocriptine (Willner, 1983; Jimerson, 1987). These were largely open trials, but two controlled trials found no difference in anti-depressant efficacy between bromocriptine and imipramine (Waehrens and Gerlach, 1981; Theohar et al., 1981). Trials of DA agonists in depression are not currently fashionable, but it is notable that DA uptake inhibition is a prominent feature of a number of newer anti-depressants, including nomifensine, buproprion and amineptine (Danysz et al., 1990). In a particularly interesting development, Mouret and colleagues have described striking and rapid therapeutic effects of piribedil in previously non-responsive patients whose sleep EEG showed signs characteristic for Parkinson's disease; in patients not showing these signs, piribedil was ineffective (Mouret et al., 1987, 1988).

The resurgence of interest in the possibility that stimulation of DA receptors might have anti-depressant potential led to the development of the novel compound GBR-12909, a highly selective DA uptake inhibitor. Unlike buproprion and nomifensine, GBR-12909 did not substitute for amphetamine in the drug discrimination procedure, and substituted only partially for cocaine (Nielsen and Andersen, 1990), suggesting that the pattern of DA stimulation is different from that caused by classical psychostimulants. The results of on-going anti-depressant trials of GBR-12909 are awaited with interest.

Summary of the Clinical Evidence

All in all, the clinical data are far from compelling. The clearest evidence implicating DA in depression, a decrease in DA turnover as measured by CSF HVA accumulation, may in fact be fairly irrelevant, and while there are many suggestive pieces of pharmacological evidence, these are matched by an equally suggestive array of conflicting data and problems of interpretation.

ENHANCEMENT OF DA FUNCTION BY ANTI-DEPRESSANTS

By contrast, the evidence that anti-depressants enhance DA function is far clearer. The major reason that dopaminergic mechanisms were initially considered not to be involved in anti-depressant action was that tricyclics only weakly inhibit the uptake of DA, in contrast to their potent effects on the uptake of NA and 5-HT. However, it is only under conditions of acute treatment that tricyclics are inactive at DA synapses. Following chronic treatment, DA function is clearly enhanced by tricyclics, and also by other types of anti-depressant drugs and by electroconvulsive shock (ECS). Two effects have been described through which anti-depressants enhance DA function: a decrease in the sensitivity of presynaptic autoreceptors and an increase in the sensitivity of postsynaptic D2 receptors.

Presynaptic DA Autoreceptors

In one of the earliest studies to demonstrate an anti-depressant-induced increase in DA function, Serra et al. (1979) reported that imipramine, amitriptyline and mianserin all decreased the sedative effect of a low dose of apomorphine. Since this effect was assumed to be mediated by stimulation of DA autoreceptors, the results were interpreted as a decrease in autoreceptor sensitivity. However, the evidence that anti-depressants desensitize DA autoreceptors is equivocal in the extreme. There are a number of supportive studies using a variety of techniques, but equally, there have been failures to replicate all of these data (Willner, 1983; Jimerson, 1987). In addition, there are certain theoretical difficulties in accepting changes in apomorphine-induced sedation as an index of DA autoreceptor function. First, as high doses of apomorphine cause locomotor stimulation, a decrease in apomorphine-induced sedation might indicate an increase in postsynaptic responsiveness rather than subsensitive autoreceptors. Second, the possibility remains that apomorphine-induced sedation may be mediated postsynaptically (Gessa et al., 1985).

Our own studies of DA autoreceptor sensitivity have used a behavioural assay, based on the ability of apomorphine, applied systemically or in the ventral tegmental area (VTA) (but not in substantia nigra), to reduce the time that food-deprived rats spend eating when given access to food. At low systemic doses of apomorphine, the effect may be blocked by D2 receptor antagonists applied systemically or directly to the VTA. These results confirm that the effects of low systemic doses of apomorphine are mediated by presynaptic DA autoreceptors (Willner et al., 1985; Towell et al., 1986a). Higher doses of apomorphine also reduce feeding time, but apparently by a postsynaptic mechanism: the effect of a low dose, but not that of a high dose, is blocked by tetrabenazine (unpublished data). Thus, this model dissociates the behavioural consequences of autoreceptor subsensitivity (a smaller decrease in feeding time) from those of postsynaptic supersensitivity (a larger decrease in feeding time).

The results of three experiments using this method to investigate the effects of chronic anti-depressant treatment are summarized in Table 1. Only in one group of animals was the action of apomorphine attenuated during the course of anti-depressant treatment, and that effect was small and far from reliable. It should be noted that we failed to observe autoreceptor subsensitivity during anti-depressant treatment even using intracerebral administration of apomorphine, which excludes the possibility of pharmacokinetic interactions. By contrast, all six groups of animals showed clear evidence of DA autoreceptor subsensitivity 3–7 days after withdrawal from chronic anti-depressant treatment (Towell et al., 1986b; Muscat et al., 1988). Similar results were reported by Scavone et al. (1986). In our view, if DA autoreceptor subsensitivity can only be observed reliably following withdrawal from chronic anti-depressant treatment, then this effect is unlikely to contribute significantly to the therapeutic action of anti-depressants.

Postsynaptic DA Receptors

By contrast, a substantial body of literature now demonstrates that, following chronic treatment, anti-depressants increase the responsiveness of postsynaptic D2 receptors in the mesolimbic system (Maj, 1990; Willner, 1989). The majority of studies have examined the locomotor stimulant response to moderate doses of apomorphine or amphetamine; these responses are consistently elevated following chronic administration of anti-depressants. Similar effects were observed using the specific D2 agonist quinpirole (Maj, 1990). Studies using systemic administration of DA agonists are suspect: certain effects of DA agonists are enhanced by acute anti-depressant treatment. The mechanisms by which anti-depressants potentiate apomorphine (Molander and Randrup, 1976; see also Table 1) are as yet unknown,

Table 1. Antidepressant effects on apomorphine anorexia. Results of four separate experiments reported in Towell et al., 1986b and Muscat et al., 1988

| Drug (Dose; mg/kg i.p.) | Apomorphine route | Length of antidepressant treatment | | |
		Subacute (2–7 days)	Chronic (3–7 weeks)	Withdrawal (3–10 days)
DMI (7.5)	s.c.	Enhancement	Variable	Attenuation
DMI (5.0)	s.c.	Enhancement	None	Attenuation
DMI (7.5)	VTA	Enhancement	None	Attenuation
DMI (2.5)	VTA	Not tested	None	Attenuation
Mianserin (2.5)	VTA	Not tested	None	Attenuation
Amitriptyline (2.5)	VTA	Not tested	None	Attenuation

but there are well-known pharmacokinetic interactions between anti-depressants and amphetamine (Sulser et al., 1966). However, anti-depressants also increased the stimulant effect when amphetamine, or DA itself, was administered directly to the nucleus accumbens (Maj and Wedzony, 1985, 1988; Maj et al., 1987), confirming a true pharmacodynamic interaction. Furthermore, these effects were present within a short time (2 hours) of the final anti-depressant treatment, confirming that, unlike DA autoreceptor desensitization, the increase in responsiveness of postsynaptic D2 receptors is not simply a withdrawal effect.

From a functional point of view, the most interesting of these data are experiments showing that chronic administration of imipramine increased the rewarding effects of apomorphine in the place preference paradigm (Papp, 1988). Papp (1989) has also shown that a variety of anti-depressants, and also repeated electroconvulsive therapy, increased the rewarding effect of food in the place preference paradigm. It has not yet been confirmed that changes in mesolimbic DA are responsible for the latter effect; however, in view of the evidence implicating the mesolimbic system in place preference learning (Phillips and Fibiger, 1987), such a mechanism is extremely plausible. The same is true of studies showing that chronic administration of desipramine (DMI) (though not other anti-depressants) can reduce the threshold for brain stimulation reward (Fibiger and Phillips, 1981; McCarter and Kokkinidis, 1988).

The mechanisms by which anti-depressants increase the responsiveness of postsynaptic DA receptors in the nucleus accumbens has until recently been obscure, since receptor binding studies consistently failed to detect any alterations in the binding parameters of DA receptors. Arguably, the majority of these studies were of limited relevance as they assayed DA receptors in samples of caudate nucleus. Nevertheless, no change was detected in D2 receptor number or affinity for DA antagonists, even in the nucleus accumbens (Martin-Iverson et al., 1983; Klimek and Nielsen, 1987). Recently, however, Klimek and Maj (1990) have found that D2 receptors in accumbens (but not striatum) have an increased affinity for the agonist ligand quinpirole following chronic anti-depressant administration. Similar effects have been reported on α-1-adrenergic receptors which also show increased agonist affinity after chronic treatment, but fail to display anti-depressant effects when antagonist ligands are used (Willner, 1989).

In addition to increasing the agonist affinity of D2 receptors, anti-depressants also decrease the number of D1 receptors (Klimek and Nielsen, 1987; de Montis et al., 1990). This effect is associated with a decrease in the ability of DA to stimulate adenyl cyclase (de Montis et al., 1990), and a decreased behavioural response (grooming) to D1 receptor stimulation (Maj et al., 1989) following chronic anti-depressant treatment, consistent with the binding data. The relationship, if any, between anti-depressant effects on D1 and D2 receptors is presently unclear. It is possible that the increase in D2 function could be secondary to the decrease in D1 function: in some circumstances, D1 receptor antagonists can enhance the response to D2 receptor stimulation. For example, the D1 antagonist SCH 23390 enhanced the orectic effect of the D2 agonist quinpirole (Muscat et al., 1989a). However, in the same animals, SCH 23390 antagonized the locomotor stimulant effect of quinpirole (Muscat et al., 1989a), and there are many other instances in which D1 and D2 receptors appear to act synergistically (Clark and White, 1987).

ANIMAL MODELS OF DEPRESSION

Although these data confirm that anti-depressants change the functional status of DA receptors in the nucleus accumbens, they give little insight into the role that these changes play in the clinical action of anti-depressants. Animal models of depression provide one route along which this question may be addressed, albeit as a first approximation.

The mechanisms by which anti-depressants act have been analysed most extensively in the Porsolt swim test. In this model, rats or mice are required to swim in a confined space, and anti-depressants prolong the period in which the animal displays active escape behaviour (Porsolt et al., 1978; Porsolt, 1981). Immobility in the swim test may be reversed by D2 receptor agonists (as well as by drugs acting on a variety of other receptor systems), applied systemically or to the nucleus accumbens (Porsolt et al., 1978; Plaznik and Kostowski, 1987; Borsini et al., 1988; Duterte-Boucher et al., 1988), and a number of studies have addressed the question of whether the action of anti-depressants in the swim test may be reversed by DA antagonists. The data have been mixed. A number of studies have reported that DA antagonists did indeed reverse anti-depressant effects in the swim test (Borsini and Meli, 1990). Particularly cogent are positive studies of this kind in which anti-depressants were administered chronically (Pulvirenti and Samanin, 1986). One important series of experiments demonstrated that the therapeutic effects of imipramine, amitriptyline and DMI were reversed by the administration of sulpiride in the nucleus accumbens, but not in the dorsal striatum (Cervo and Samanin, 1987, 1988). Nevertheless, Borsini and Meli (1990) urge caution in accepting that these data demonstrate a dopaminergic mechanism of anti-depressant action in the swim test: destruction of the VTA is apparently without effect on the anti-immobility effect of DMI (Plaznik et al., 1985); the anti-depressant effects of D2 agonists are confounded by increases in locomotor activity; and there are also a number of anomalous pharmacological data. Borsini and Meli (1990) suggest that the effects of intra-accumbens sulpiride may be related to the presence in the mesolimbic system of non-dopaminergic sulpiride binding sites that also bind anti-depressants (Csernansky et al., 1985).

The swim test has also been criticized on a number of counts, most prominently that it responds to acute administration of anti-depressants, unlike the clinical situation which requires chronic treatment. This criticism is not entirely justified, since the test only responds acutely to extremely high drug doses, but becomes slowly more sensitive with repeated treatment (Willner, 1989). A more cogent critique is that the theoretical rationale of the test as a model of depression is minimal. A further shortcoming is that, even when anti-depressant treatment is chronic, the drugs are administered to normal animals, whereas it is widely believed that anti-depressants do not elevate mood in normal people. Although the evidence that supports this assumption is rather weak (e.g. Hartmann and Cravens, 1973), it would nevertheless be preferable to assess anti-depressant action in animals approximating a depressed state (and also in a model more valid than the swim test).

Chronic Mild Stress Model

The starting point for the model to be described was the study by Katz (1982) in which rats were subjected, over a period of weeks, to a variety of unpredictable stressors, some of them severe. In most of the studies using this model, the effects of the stress regime were evaluated in a test of open field activity (Katz et al., 1981). However, in one study, it was demonstrated that, unlike normal animals, rats subjected to chronic stress failed to increase their fluid intake when sucrose or saccharin was added to their drinking water (Katz, 1982). This suggests that chronic stress may depress the activity of brain reward systems. The observation that responding for brain stimulation reward is suppressed by a single session of unavoidable electric shock (see Zacharko and Anisman, Chapter 16, this volume) also suggests that prolonged or uncontrollable stress may cause anhedonia.

In an attempt to create a procedure that models the levels of stress encountered in daily living more realistically than either traumatic electric shock or the severe chronic stress regime used by Katz (1982), we devised a substantially milder chronic stress regime in which each of the elements is, in itself, only mildly stressful. Typical elements included periods of food or water deprivation, overnight illumination, tilting of the cage or changes of cage mates. Rats subjected chronically to this variety of low grade stressors reduce their consumption of, and preference for, highly rewarding weak solutions of sucrose and saccharin. This deficit may model the anhedonia that is a central feature of endogenous depressions. In support of this interpretation, we have recently observed that the rewarding properties of food, as assessed in the place preference paradigm, were markedly attenuated in chronically stressed animals (Figure 1). Subsequent experiments showed a similar insensitivity of stressed animals to the rewarding effects of dilute or concentrated sucrose solutions, amphetamine, and the D2 agonist quinpirole (Papp et al., 1991a, b). These experiments using the place preference paradigm suggest that chronic mild stress causes a generalized decrease in sensitivity to rewards.

The impairment of sucrose consumption in stressed animals is restored to normal after several weeks of treatment with the tricyclic anti-depressants DMI, imipramine or amitriptyline. Induction of the deficit requires anything

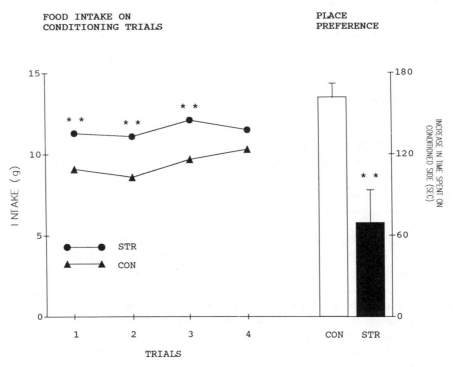

Figure 1. Place preference conditioning following 5 weeks of unpredictable mild stress. 20-hour food-deprived rats (*n*=8/group) were trained in a chamber containing two distinct sides. On each of 4 days, the animals were confined in the non-preferred side of the chamber and allowed free access to food. Stressed animals (STR) showed a small but significant increase in food intake (left). *P<0.05; **P<0.01. When subsequently allowed free access to both sides of the chamber (right), controls (CON) showed a substantial increase in time spent in the initially non-preferred side, but now food-associated, side. The place conditioning was greatly attenuated in stressed animals

between 1 and 4 weeks of stress (in different experiments), and reversal of the deficit by anti-depressants requires between 2 and 5 weeks of treatment; the results of a typical experiment are shown in Figure 2. Following the cessation of stress, behaviour remains abnormal in untreated animals for at least 2 weeks (Willner et al., 1987, 1990a; Muscat et al., 1988; Sampson et al., 1990).

Mechanisms of Anti-Depressant Action

We have carried out a series of experiments to examine the mechanism by which anti-depressants normalize behaviour in the chronic mild stress model. In the first study, rats were exposed to stress for a total of 10 weeks, and once each week, were offered for 1 hour a choice between water and a highly rewarding 1 per cent sucrose solution. After 4 weeks, sucrose intakes in stressed animals were significantly lower than in controls, and half of each group commenced treatment with imipramine (6 mg/kg i.p. each evening). After a further 4 weeks, sucrose intake in the imipramine-treated stressed animals returned to normal. The animals continued to receive stress and/or imipramine, and in the final week, half of each group received a

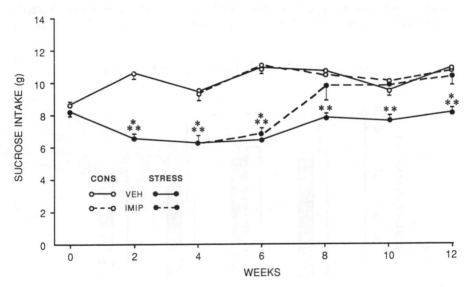

Figure 2. Reduction of sucrose consumption by chronic mild stress and its restoration by imipramine (IMIP). Stress (closed circles) was administered for a total of 12 weeks. Imipramine treatment (5 mg/kg daily) commenced after 4 weeks of stress (dotted lines). Imipramine restored normal behaviour after 4 weeks of treatment in the stressed animals, but had no effect in non-stressed controls. $**P<0.01$; $***P<0.001$

single administration of a low dose (0.15 mg/kg) of the DA receptor antagonist pimozide 4 hours before the fluid intake test. Pimozide selectively abolished the restoration of sucrose consumption in imipramine-treated stressed animals, but was without effect in vehicle-treated stressed animals or in non-stressed animals (Figure 3; Muscat et al., 1990). At higher doses, pimozide also decreased sucrose consumption and preference in non-stressed animals (Towell et al., 1987). The selective effect of a lower dose in imipramine-treated stressed animals strongly suggests that the mechanism of action of imipramine in this model is an increase in the responsiveness of postsynaptic DA receptors.

In a second experiment, we examined the involvement of DA in the action of two other tricyclics, amitriptyline (AMI) and DMI, and also the relative contribution of the DA receptor subtypes. Whereas in the first experiment the effect of pimozide was tested in animals still receiving imipramine, in this study, animals were tested following withdrawal from anti-depressants to exclude the possibility of unwanted pharmacokinetic interactions that might occur in animals receiving acute neuroleptic and chronic anti-depressant treatment concurrently. Stress was administered for a total of 12 weeks, and the anti-depressants were administered daily from week 3 to week 9 (5 mg/kg in weeks 3–6 and 2.5 mg/kg in weeks 7–9). Fluid intake was measured in two-bottle tests, using 1 per cent sucrose versus water during weeks 1–8 and a cocktail of 1 per cent sucrose with 0.1

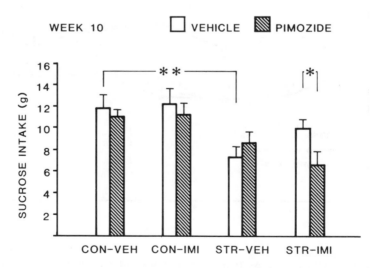

Figure 3. Effect of pimozide (hatched bars) on sucrose consumption in stressed (STR) and non-stressed (CON) animals treated chronically with imipramine (IMI) or vehicle (VEH). Stress was administered for a total of 10 weeks, and imipramine from week 5 onwards. *$P<0.05$; **$P<0.01$. (From Muscat et al., 1990)

per cent saccharin versus water, thereafter. Effects of acute pretreatment with the DA receptor antagonists SCH 23390 (8 μg/kg) and sulpiride (50 mg/kg) were tested on days 7 and 14 of withdrawal, respectively. The results were essentially the same as those of the earlier experiment: consumption of the sweet cocktail was selectively decreased in both groups of anti-depressant-treated stressed animals, but unaffected in any of the other experimental groups (Sampson et al., 1990). These effects were seen with both the specific D1 antagonist SCH 23390 and the specific D2 antagonist sulpiride. This lack of specificity is to be expected, given that, at higher doses, both SCH 23390 and sulpiride also decrease sucrose consumption and preference in non-stressed animals (Muscat and Willner, 1989).

A third experiment examined the potential involvement of 5-HT in the chronic stress model. Rats were subjected to a chronic varied mild stress regime, as in earlier experiments, for a total of 12 weeks; from week 4 onwards, half the animals were administered imipramine (5 mg/kg) daily. Consumption of a 0.7 per cent sucrose solution (measured weekly in a 1-hour single-bottle test) was decreased by stress but restored to normal by imipramine. During week 12, all animals received single doses of the specific D2 antagonist raclopride (100 μg/kg), the 5-HT antagonist metergoline (1 mg/kg), and saline prior to fluid consumption tests, on different days. As with the other DA antagonists, raclopride selectively decreased sucrose intake in imipramine-treated stressed animals without affecting consumption in any other group. However, metergoline increased sucrose consumption in all groups. The results confirm a dopaminergic mechanism of anti-depressant action in this model, but do not provide evidence for serotonergic involvement (Muscat et al., 1990).

Physiological Effects of Chronic Mild Stress

In addition to their decreased sensitivity to sweet rewards, animals subjected to chronic mild stress resemble normal animals treated with neuroleptic drugs in a number of other respects: for example, a decreased rate of food consumption, increased consumption of very sweet foods, and a decreased sensitivity to the anorectic effects of amphetamine or apomorphine and to the orectic effects of 8-hydroxy-DPAT (Muscat et al., 1988, 1989b). As noted earlier, stressed animals are sensitive to the rewarding effects of the D2 agonist quinpirole in the place preference paradigm, and we have recently observed that they are also subsensitive to the locomotor stimulant effect of quinpirole (Papp et al., 1991b). These observations, together with the evidence implicating DA in the therapeutic effects of anti-depressant drugs in this model, suggested that chronic mild stress might lead to a decrease in the level of dopaminergic transmission. In collaboration with Drs K. Golembiowska and V. Klimek we therefore measured various parameters of DA function after 7 weeks' exposure to mild stress and in matched control animals. As stressed animals lose weight, a second control group was included in the study, consisting of animals that were food-deprived and fed one meal a day, but not otherwise stressed.

The results are summarized in Figure 4. Contrary to our expectations, the stressed animals showed a marked increase in the levels of DA and all three of its major metabolites, combined with a substantial decrease in the number of D2 receptors, and a smaller (and non-significant) decrease in D1 receptor numbers. These changes were seen only in samples of limbic forebrain (primarily the nucleus accumbens and olfactory tubercle); they were not present in samples of caudate nucleus.

Although stress did not alter the metabolite:transmitter ratios, the receptor changes are strongly indicative of an increase in the release of DA in limbic forebrain, together with an increase in DA synthesis. Increases in 5-HT and its metabolite 5-HIAA were also observed, and again, were only present in limbic forebrain samples; receptor binding parameters were not measured for 5-HT (Willner et al. 1990a). Subsequent studies, in collaboration with Drs J. Stamford and Z. Kruk, used fast cyclic voltammetry to confirm *in*

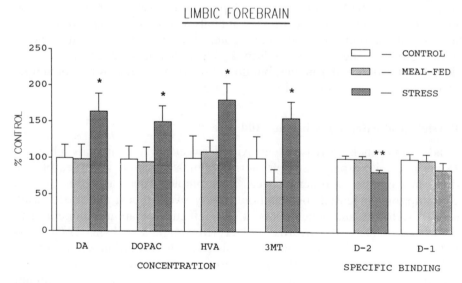

Figure 4. Effects of chronic mild stress (7 weeks) on DA function in the limbic forebrain. Compared to non-stressed and low-weight (meal-fed) controls, stressed animals had higher levels of DA and its metabolites dihydroxyphenylacetic acid (DOPAC), homovanillic acid (HVA) and 3-methoxytyramine (3MT), but a decrease in the specific binding of [³H]spiroperidol to D-2 receptors. *$P<0.05$; **$P<0.01$. (Drawn from data reported in Willner et al, 1990c)

vivo that DA release is increased in the nucleus accumbens of animals subjected to chronic mild stress (Stamford et al., 1991).

These data provide a means of understanding the effect of chronic mild stress on responsiveness to a sweet reward. Stress is known to increase the turnover of DA in the mesolimbic system (Di Chiara et al., Chapter 14; Zacharko and Anisman, Chapter 16, this volume), and tolerance to this effect fails to develop under the chronic mild stress regime, probably owing to its unpredictability (Kant et al., 1983). The observed decrease in D2 receptor sensitivity most likely represents an adaptive response to chronic overstimulation by released DA. As a result of these two countervailing changes, the mesolimbic DA system operates at a new equilibrium, based on increased DA turnover and decreased receptor sensitivity. Because the baseline of presynaptic DA activity is higher, stronger levels of stimulation may be necessary to elicit further increases. Thus, stimuli that would normally activate the system may now be prevented from doing so, and postsynaptic receptors are less responsive to any additional DA that may be released. A tonic increase in 5-HT release would also tend to depress sucrose intake (Garattini et al., 1986), but this effect may be offset by a decrease in 5-HT receptor function, which we have not determined.

CONCLUDING REMARKS

The results obtained using the chronic mild stress model are internally consistent in suggesting that chronic mild stress may disable transmission in the mesolimbic DA system by constraining the response to phasic stimulation. However, the way in these data are reconciled with the clinical evidence of decreased DA turnover in retarded depressions is not immediately apparent. One obvious possibility is that the chronic mild stress model is simply irrelevant to understanding depression. It seems unwise, however, simply to ignore these data, considering how close the model lies to the theoretical mainstream in proposing an important aetiological role for stress in depression (Anisman and Zacharko, 1982; Willner, 1987). A second possibility is that both melancholia and chronic mild stress involve reduced DA function, but the precise mechanisms vary. Another way of looking at this question is to ask whether a relationship between chronic mild stress and melancholia can be demonstrated clinically. We have attempted to address this issue by administering a questionnaire that measures the perceived frequency and severity of minor stresses in melancholic and non-melancholic patients matched for severity, and in non-depressed volunteers. The three groups did not differ in the frequency of stressors they reported, but the perceived severity of stress was substantially higher in the melancholic patients; the non-melancholic patients were indistinguishable from the normal controls (Willner et al., 1990b).

The third possibility, which seems to us the most likely, is that it is the clinical observation of low CSF HVA in retarded patients that is misleading and irrelevant. These data assess DA release from nigrostriatal neurons, and therefore do not address the hypothesis of mesolimbic dysfunction in melancholia. However, it is possible that CSF levels of DA itself do provide an estimate of mesolimbic activity. A correlation has been reported between CSF DA levels and extraversion (King et al., 1986); extraversion has been conceptualized as a tendency to over-react to positive incentives (Gray, 1971), and so may reflect the level of activity in the mesolimbic DA system. In contrast to the HVA data, and consistent with the results of the chronic mild stress model, Gjerris (1988; Gjerris et al., 1987) has reported that CSF levels of DA are elevated in melancholic patients.

The major strengths of the mesolimbic dysfunction hypothesis lie in its collateral support. The behavioural evidence that the mesolimbic system plays a crucial (if not yet fully determined) role in rewarded behaviour is extremely strong, and, as we have demonstrated, can be used to develop realistic and productive animal models of depression (see Zacharko and Anisman, Chapter 16, this volume). The evidence that anti-depressants enhance mesolimbic DA function is also compelling, and these effects can be shown to be of functional relevance. The weakness of the hypothesis is in its clinical base. We have no useful information on the release of DA from mesolimbic terminals in melancholia, or on the state of DA receptors, though both of these issues could now be addressed by brain imaging techniques. Similarly, there is little clinical information to confirm a dopaminergic component to anti-depressant action, though again these studies could readily be carried out using techniques derived from those used routinely in animal models. An important priority in the development of an understanding of the role of DA in depression must now be to attempt to redress the imbalance between the preclinical and the clinical evidence.

ACKNOWLEDGEMENT

The chronic mild stress experiments described in this chapter were partly supported by the Medical Research Council of Great Britain.

REFERENCES

Agren, H. and Terenius, L. (1985) Hallucinations in patients with major depression: interaction between CSF monoaminergic and endorphinergic indices. *Journal of Affective Disorders* **9**, 25–34.

Anizman, H.A. and Zacharo, R.M. (1982) Depression: The predisposing influence of stress. *Behavioral and Brain Sciences* **5**, 89–137.

Asnis, G. (1977) Parkinson's disease, depression and ECT: a review and case study. *American Journal of Psychiatry* **134**, 191–195.

Banki, C.M., Molnar, G. and Vojnik, M. (1981) Cerebrospinal fluid amine metabolites, tryptophan and clinical parameters in depression. *Journal of Affective Disorders* **3**, 91–99.

Borsini, F. and Meli, A. (1990) The forced swimming test: its contribution to the understanding of the mechanism of action of antidepressants. In: Gessa, G.L. and Serra, G. (eds.) *Dopamine and Mental Depression (Advances in the Biosciences)*. New York: Pergamon Press, pp. 63–76.

Borsini, F., Lecci, A., Mancinelli, A., D'Aronno, V. and Meli, A. (1988) Stimulation of dopamine D-2 but not D-1 receptors reduces immobility time of rats in the forced swimming test: implication for antidepressant activity. *European Journal of Pharmacology* **148**, 301–307.

Bunney, W.E. and Davis, J.M. (1965) Norepinephrine in depressive reactions. *Archives of General Psychiatry* **13**, 483–494.

Cervo, L. and Samanin, R. (1987) Evidence that dopamine mechanisms in the nucleus accumbens are selectively involved in the effect of desipramine in the forced swimming test. *Neuropharmacology* **26**, 1469–1472.

Cervo, L. and Samanin, R. (1988) Repeated treatment with imipramine and amitriptyline reduces the immobility of rats in the swimming test by enhancing dopamine mechanisms in the nucleus accumbens. *Journal of Pharmacy and Pharmacology* **40**, 155–156.

Clark, D. and White, F. (1987) D1 dopamine receptor—the search for a function: a critical evaluation of D1/D2 dopamine receptor classification and its functional implications. *Synapse* **1**, 347–388.

Creese, I. and Snyder, S.H. (1978) Behavioral and biochemical properties of the dopamine receptor. In: Lipton, M.A., DiMascio, A. and Killam, K.F. (eds) *Psychopharmacology: A Generation of Progress*. New York: Raven, pp. 377–388.

Csernansky, J.G., Csernansky, C.A. and Hollister, L.E. (1985) ^{3}[H]-Sulpiride labels mesolimbic non-dopaminergic sites that bind antidepressant drugs. *Experientia* **41**, 1419–1421.

Danysz, W., Archer, T. and Fowler, C. (1990) Screening for antidepressant activity. In: Willner, P. (ed.) *Behavioural Models in Psychopharmacology: Theoretical, Industrial and Clinical Perspectives*. Cambridge: Cambridge University Press, pp. 126–156.

del Zompo, M., Boccheta, A., Bernardi, F., Burrai, C. and Corsini, G. U. (1990) Clinical evidence for a role of dopaminergic systems in depressive syndromes. In: Gessa, G.L. and Serra, G. (eds) *Dopamine and Mental Depression (Advances in the Biosciences)*. New York: Pergamon Press, pp. 177–184.

De Montis, M.G., Devoto, P., Gessa, G.L., Porcella, A., Serra, G. and Tagliamonte, A. (1990) Possible role of DA receptors in the mechanism of action of antidepressants. In: Gessa, G.L. and Serra, G. (eds) *Dopamine and Mental Depression (Advances in the Biosciences)*. New York: Pergamon Press, pp. 147–157.

Duterte-Boucher, D., Leclere, J.F., Panissaud, C. and Costentin, J. (1988) Acute effects of direct dopamine agonists in the mouse behavioral despair test. *European Journal of Pharmacology* **154**, 185–189.

Fibiger, H.C. and Phillips, A.G. (1981) Increased intracranial self-stimulation in rats after long-term administration of desipramine. *Science* **214**, 683–684.

Garattini, S., Mennini, T., Bendotti, C., Invernizzi, R. and Samanin, R. (1986) Neurochemical mechanism of action of drugs which modify feeding via the serotonergic system. *Appetite* **7**, 15–38 (suppl).

406 *Willner et al.*

Gessa, G.L., Porceddu, M.L., Collu, M., Mereu, G., Serra, M., Ongini, E. and Biggio, G. (1985) Sedation and sleep induced by high doses of apomorphine after blockade of D1 receptors by SCH-23390. *European Journal of Pharmacology* **109**, 269–274.

Gjerris, A. (1988) Do concentrations of neurotransmitters in lumbar CSF reflect cerebral dysfunction in depression? *Acta Psychiatrica Scandinavica* **345**, 21–24 (suppl).

Gjerris, A., Werdelin, L., Rafaelson, O.J., Alling, C. and Christensen, N.J. (1987) CSF dopamine increased in depression: CSF dopamine, noradrenaline and their metabolites in depressed patients and in controls. *Journal of Affective Disorders* **13**, 279–286.

Goodwin, F.K. (1972) Behavioral effects of L-DOPA in man. In: Shader, R.I. (ed.) *Psychiatric Complications of Medical Drugs*. New York: Raven, pp. 149–174.

Goodwin, F.K. and Sack, R.L. (1974) Central dopamine function in affective illness: evidence from precursors, enzyme inhibitors, and studies of central dopamine turnover. In: Usdin, E. (ed.) *Neuropsychopharmacology of Monoamines and their Regulatory Enzymes*. New York: Raven, pp. 261–279.

Goodwin, F.K., Ebert, M.H. and Bunney, W.E. (1972) Mental effects of reserpine in man: a review. In: Shader, R.I. (ed.) *Psychiatric Complications of Medical Drugs*. New York: Raven, pp. 73–101.

Gray, J.A. (1971) *The Psychology of Fear and Stress*. London: Weidenfeld.

Hartmann, E. and Cravens, J. (1973) The effects of long term administration of psychotropic drugs on human sleep: III. The effects of amitriptyline. *Psychopharmacologia* **33**, 185–202.

Jimerson, D.C. (1987) Role of dopamine mechanisms in affective disorders. In: Meltzer, H.Y. (ed.) *Psychopharmacology: The Third Generation of Progress*. New York: Raven, pp. 505–511.

Kant, G.J., Lenox, R.H., Bunwell, B.N., Margey, E.H., Pennington, L.L. and Meyerhoff, J.L. (1983) Habituation to stress is stressor specific. *Pharmacology Biochemistry and Behavior* **22**, 631–634.

Katz, R.J. (1982) Animal model of depression: pharmacological sensitivity of a hedonic deficit. *Pharmacology Biochemistry and Behavior* **16**, 965–968.

Katz, R.J., Roth, K.A. and Carroll, B.J. (1981) Acute and chronic stress effects on open field activity in the rat: implications for a model of depression. *Neuroscience and Biobehavioral Reviews* **5**, 259–264.

King, R.J., Mefford, I.N., Wang, C., Murchinson, A., Caligari, E.J. and Berger, P.A. (1986) CSF dopamine levels correlate with extraversion in depressed patients. *Psychiatric Research* **19**, 305–310.

Klimek, V. and Maj, J. (1990) The effect of antidepressant drugs given repeatedly on the binding of ^{3}H-SCH 23390 and ^{3}H-spiperone to dopaminergic receptors. In: Gessa, G.L. and Serra, G. (eds) *Dopamine and Mental Depression (Advances in the Biosciences)*. New York: Pergamon Press, pp. 159–166.

Klimek, V. and Nielsen, E.B. (1987) Chronic treatment with antidepressants decreases the number of [^{3}H]SCH 23390 binding sites in the rat striatum and limbic system. *European Journal of Pharmacology* **139**, 163–169.

Maj, J. (1990) Behavioural effects of antidepressant drugs given repeatedly on the dopaminergic system. In: Gessa, G.L. and Serra, G. (eds) *Dopamine and Mental Depression (Advances in the Biosciences)*. New York: Pergamon Press, pp. 139–146.

Maj, J. and Wedzony, K. (1985) Repeated treatment with imipramine or amitriptyline increases the locomotor response of rats to (+)-amphetamine given into the nucleus accumbens. *Journal of Pharmacy and Pharmacology* **37**, 362–364.

Maj, J. and Wedzony, K. (1988) The influence of oxaprotaline enantiomers given repeatedly on the behavioural effects of d-amphetamine and dopamine injected into the nucleus accumbens. *European Journal of Pharmacology* **145**, 97–103.

Maj, J., Wedzony, K. and Klimek, V. (1987) Desipramine given repeatedly enhances behavioural effects of dopamine and d-amphetamine injected into the nucleus accumbens. *European Journal of Pharmacology* **140**, 179–185.

Maj, J., Papp, M., Skuza, G., Bigajska, K. and Zazula, M. (1989) The influence of repeated treatment with imipramine, (+)- and (−)-oxaprotiline on behavioural effects of dopamine D-1 and D-2 agonists. *Journal of Neural Transmission* **76**, 29–38.

Martin-Iverson, M., Leclere, J.F. and Fibiger, H.C. (1983) Cholinergic-dopaminergic interactions and the mechanisms of action of antidepressants. *European Journal of Pharmacology* **94**, 193–201.

Mayeux, R., Stern, Y., Williams, J.B., Cote, L., Frantz, A. and Dyrenfurth, I. (1986) Clinical and biochemical features of depression in Parkinson's disease. *American Journal of Psychiatry* **143**, 756–759.

McCarter, B.D. and Kokkinidis, L. (1988) The effects of long-term administration and antidepressant drugs on intracranial self-stimulation responding in rats. *Pharmacology Biochemistry and Behavior* **31**, 243–247.

McDowell, F., Markham, C., Lee, J., Treciokas, L. and Ansel, R. (1971) The clinical use of levadopa in the treatment of Parkinson's disease. In: McDowell, F. and Markham, C. (eds) *Recent Advances in Parkinson's Disease*. Oxford: Blackwell Scientific Publications, pp. 175–201.

Minter, R.E. and Mandell, M.R. (1979) The treatment of psychotic major depression with drugs and electroconvulsive therapy. *Journal of Nervous and Mental Disorders* **167**, 726–733.

Molander, L. and Randrup, A. (1976) Effects of thymoleptics on behaviour associated with changes in brain dopamine. II. Modification and potentiation of apomorphine-induced stimulation of mice. *Psychopharmacology* **49**, 139–144.

Mouret, J., LeMoine, P. and Minuit, M. (1987) Marqueurs polygraphiques, cliniques et therapeutiques des depressions dopamino-dependantes (DDD). *Comptes Rendus de l'Academie de Science Paris serie III* **305**, 301–306.

Mouret, J., LeMoine, P., Minuit, M. and Robelin, N. (1988) La L-tyrosine guerit, immediatement et a long terme, les depressions dopamino-dependantes (DDD). Étude clinique et polygraphique. *Comptes Rendus de l'Academie de Science Paris serie III* **306**, 93–98.

Murphy, D.L. (1972) L-dopa, behavioral activation and psychopathology. *Research Publications of the Association for Research in Nervous and Mental Disorders* **50**, 472–493.

Muscat, R. and Willner, P. (1989) Effects of selective dopamine receptor antagonists on sucrose consumption and preference. *Psychopharmacology* **99**, 98–102.

Muscat, R., Towell, A. and Willner, P. (1988) Changes in dopamine autoreceptor sensitivity in an animal model of depression. *Psychopharmacology* **94**, 545–550.

Muscat, R., Phillips, G., Nunn, J., Wood, N., Montgomery, A. and Willner, P. (1989a) D1/D2 receptor interactions in the control of feeding and post-prandial satiety. *Behavioural Pharmacology* **1**, 13 (suppl 1).

Muscat, R., Sampson, D., Phillips, G. and Willner, P. (1989b) Animal model of depression: indirect evidence of dopamine dysfunction. *Behavioural Pharmacology* **1**, 55 (suppl 1).

Muscat, R., Sampson, D. and Willner, P. (1990) Dopaminergic mechanism of imipramine action on an animal model of depression. *Biological Psychiatry* **27**, 223–230.

Nelson, J.C. (1987) The use of antipsychotic drugs in the treatment of depression. In: Zohar, J. and Belmaker, R.H. (eds) *Treating Resistant Depression*. New York: PMA Corporation, pp. 131–146.

Nelson, J.C. and Bowers, M.B. (1978) Delusional unipolar depression: description and drug treatment. *Archives of General Psychiatry* **35**, 1321–1328.

Nielsen, E.B. and Andersen, P.H. (1990) GBR 12909: a new potent and selective dopamine uptake inhibitor. In: Gessa, G.L. and Serra, G. (eds) *Dopamine and Mental Depression (Advances in the Biosciences)*. New York: Pergamon Press, pp. 101–108.

Papp, M. (1988) Different effects of short- and long-term treatment with imipramine on the apomorphine- and food-induced place preference conditioning in rats. *Pharmacology Biochemistry and Behavior* **30**, 889–893.

Papp, M. (1989) Differential effects of short- and long-term antidepressant treatments on the food-induced place preference conditioning in rats. *Behavioral Pharmacology* **1**, 69–74.

Papp, M., Willner, P. and Muscat, R. (1991a) An animal model of anhedonia. *Psychopharmacology* (in press).

Papp, M., Muscat, R. and Willner, P. (1991b) Subsensitivity of reward – related dopamine receptors in an animal model of depression. Submitted.

Perry, E.K. (1987) Cortical neurotransmitter chemistry in Alzheimer's disease. In: Meltzer, H.Y. (ed.) *Psychopharmacology: The Third Generation of Progress*. New York: Raven, pp. 887–895.

Phillips, A.C. and Fibiger, H.C. (1987) Anatomical and neurochemical substrates of drug reward determined by the conditioned place preference technique. In: Bozarth, M.A. (ed.) *Methods of Assessing the Reinforcing Properties of Abused Drugs*. New York: Springer, pp. 275–290.

Plaznik, A. and Kostowski, W. (1987) The effects of antidepressant drugs and electroconvulsive shocks on the functioning of the mesolimbic dopaminergic system: a behavioural study. *European Journal of Pharmacology* **135**, 389–396.

Plaznik, A., Danysz, W. and Kostowski, W. (1985) Mesolimbic noradrenaline but not dopamine is responsible for organization of rats behaviour in the forced swim test and anti-immobilizing effect of desipramine. *Polish Journal of Pharmacology and Pharmacy* **37**, 347–357.

Porsolt, R.D. (1981) Behavioural despair. In: Enna, S.J., Malick, J.B. and Richelson, E. (eds) *Antidepressants: Neurochemical Behavioral and Clinical Perspectives*. New York: Raven, pp. 121–140.

Porsolt, R.D., Anton, G., Blavet, M. and Jalfre, M. (1978) Behavioural despair in rats, a new model sensitive to antidepressant treatments. *European Journal of Pharmacology* **47**, 379–391.

Post, R.M., Kotin, J., Goodwin, F.K. and Gordon, E. (1973) Psychomotor activity and cerebrospinal fluid metabolites in affective illness. *American Journal of Psychiatry* **130**, 67–72.

Pulvirenti, L. and Samanin, R. (1986) Antagonism by dopamine, but not noradrenaline receptor blockers of the anti-immobility activity of desipramine after different treatment schedules in the rat. *Pharmacological Research Communications* **18**, 73–80.

Randrup, A., Munkvad, I., Fog, R., Gerlach, J., Molander, L., Kjellberg, B. and Scheel-Kruger, J. (1975) Mania, depression and brain dopamine. In: Essman, W.B. and Valzelli, L. (eds) *Current Developments in Psychopharmacology, Vol. 2*. New York: Spectrum, pp. 206–248.

Raskin, A., Schulterbrandt, J.G., Reatig, N. and McKeon, J.J. (1970) Differential response to chlorpromazine, imipramine and placebo—a study of subgroups of hospitalized patients. *Archives of General Psychiatry* **23**, 164–173.

Robertson, M.M. and Trimble, M.R. (1981) Neuroleptics as antidepressants. *Neuropharmacology* **20**, 1335–1336.

Robertson, M.M. and Trimble, M.R. (1982) Major tranquillizers used as antidepressants: a review. *Journal of Affective Disorders* **4**, 173–193.

Robins, A.H. (1976) Depression in patients with Parkinsonism. *British Journal of Psychiatry* **128**, 141–145.

Roy, A., Pickar, D., Linnoila, M., Doran, A.R., Ninan, P. and Paul, S.M. (1985) Cerebrospinal fluid monoamine and monoamine metabolite concentrations in melancholia. *Psychiatry Research* **15**, 281–292.

Sampson, D., Muscat, R. and Willner, P. (1990) Reversal of antidepressant action by dopamine antagonists in an animal model of depression. *Psychopharmacology* (in press).

Scavone, C., Aizenstein, M.L., De Lucia, R. and Da Silva Planeta, C. (1986) Chronic imipramine administration reduces apomorphine inhibitory effects. *European Journal of Pharmacology* **132**, 263–267.

Schildkraut, J.J. (1965) The catecholamine hypothesis of affective disorders: a review of supporting evidence. *American Journal of Psychiatry* **122**, 509–522.

Serra, G., Argiolas, A., Fadda, F., Melis, M.R. and Gessa, G.L. (1979) Chronic treatment with antidepressants prevents the inhibitory effect of small doses of apomorphine on dopamine synthesis and motor activity. *Life Science* **25**, 415–424.

Sourkes, T.L. (1973) On the origin of homovanillic acid (HVA) in the cerebrospinal fluid. *Journal of Neural Transmission* **34**, 153–157.

Stamford, J.A., Muscat, R., O'Connor, J.J., Patel, J., Trout, S.J., Wieczorek, W.J., Kruk, Z.L. and Willner, P. (1991) Voltammetric evidence that subsensitivity to reward following chronic mild stress is associated with increase release of mesolimbic dopamine. Submitted.

Sulser, F., Owens, M.L. and Dingell, J.V. (1966) On the mechanism of amphetamine potentiation by desipramine. *Life Science* **5**, 2005–2010.

Sweeney, D., Nelson, C., Bowers, M., Maas, J. and Heninger, G. (1978) Delusional versus non-delusional depression: Neurochemical differences. *Lancet* **ii**, 100–101.

Theohar, C., Fischer-Cornellson, K., Akesson, H.O., Ansari, J., Gerlach, G., Ohman, R., Ose, E. and Stegink, A.J. (1981) Bromocriptine as antidepressant: double-blind comparative study with imipramine in psychogenic and endogenous depression. *Current Therapeutic Research* **30**, 830–842.

Towell, A., Muscat, R. and Willner, P. (1986a) Apomorphine anorexia: the role of dopamine cell body autoreceptors. *Psychopharmacology* **89**, 65–68.

Towell, A., Willner, P. and Muscat, R. (1986b) Behavioural evidence for autoreceptor subsensitivity in the mesolimbic dopamine system during withdrawal from antidepressant drugs. *Psychopharmacology* **90**, 64–71.

Towell, A., Muscat, R. and Willner, P. (1987) Effects of pimozide on sucrose consumption and preference. *Psychopharmacology* **92**, 262–264.

Vaccheri, A., Dall'Olio, R., Gaggi, R., Gandolfi, O. and Montanaro, N. (1984) Antidepressant versus neuroleptic activities of sulpiride isomers in four animal models of depression. *Psychopharmacology* **83**, 28–33.

Van Praag, H.M. and Korf, J. (1975) Central monamine deficiency in depression: causative or secondary phenomenon? *Pharmacopsychiatry* **8**, 321–326.

Van Praag, H.M., Korf, J. and Schut, T. (1973) Cerebral monoamines and depression. An investigation with the probenecid technique. *Archives of General Psychiatry* **28**, 827–831.

Van Praag, H.M., Korf, J., Lakke, J.P.W.F. and Schut, T. (1975) Dopamine metabolism in depression, psychoses, and Parkinson's disease: the problem of specificity of biological variables in behavior disorders. *Psychological Medicine* **5**, 138–146.

Waehrens, J. and Gerlach, J. (1981) Bromocriptine and imipramine in endogenous depression: a double-blind controlled trial in out-patients. *Journal of Affective Disorders* **3**, 193–202.

Willner, P. (1983) Dopamine and depression: a review of recent evidence. *Brain Research Reviews* **6**, 211–224.

Willner, P. (1985) *Depression: A Psychobiological Synthesis*. New York: Wiley.

Willner, P. (1987) The anatomy of melancholy: the catecholamine hypothesis of depression revisited. *Reviews in Neuroscience* **1**, 77–99.

Willner, P. (1989) Sensitization to the actions of antidepressant drugs. In: Emmett-Oglesby, M.W. and Goudie, A.J. (eds) *Psychoactive Drugs: Tolerance and Sensitization*. Clifton New Jersey: Humana Press, pp. 407–459.

Willner, P., Towell, A. and Muscat, R. (1985) Apomorphine anorexia: a behavioural and neuropharmacological analysis. *Psychopharmacology* **87**, 351–356.

Willner, P., Towell, A., Sampson, D., Muscat, R. and Sophokleous, S. (1987) Reduction of sucrose preference by chronic mild stress and its restoration by a tricyclic antidepressant. *Psychopharmacology* **93**, 358–364.

Willner, P., Golembiowska, K., Klimek, V. and Muscat, R. (1990a) Changes in mesolimbic dopamine may explain stress-induced anhedonia. *Psychobiology* (in press).

Willner, P., Wilkes, M. and Orwin, O. (1990b) Attributional style and perceived stress in endogenous and reactive depression. *Journal of Affective Disorders* **18**, 281–287.

16

Stressor-Provoked Alterations of Intracranial Self-Stimulation in the Mesocorticolimbic System: an Animal Model of Depression

ROBERT M. ZACHARKO AND HYMIE ANISMAN

Psychology Department, Carleton University, Ottawa, Ontario,
Canada K1S 5B6

INTRODUCTION

It has been suggested that aversive life events may contribute to the expression or exacerbation of a variety of physical and psychological disorders (Akiskal and McKinney, 1973; Sklar and Anisman, 1981; Anisman and Zacharko, 1982). Although the nature of the relationship between stressors and pathology remains to be elucidated, considerable effort has been devoted to the development of animal analogs of human disorders, particularly depression (Willner, 1984). These have included analyses which focused on potential cognitive alterations associated with stressor-induced behavioral deficits (Maier and Seligman, 1976), descriptions of stressor-provoked neurochemical (Anisman, 1984; Zacharko and Anisman, 1989) or hormonal alterations (Makara et al., 1986), as well as the evaluation of pharmacological manipulations which attenuate stressor-induced behavioral disturbances (Zacharko et al., 1984b; Willner, 1987; Shanks and Anisman, 1989).

In developing animal models of human depression it is desirable that the behavior(s) examined be reminiscent of the symptoms of human depression,

The Mesolimbic Dopamine System: From Motivation to Action.
Edited by P. Willner and J. Scheel-Krüger

© 1991 John Wiley & Sons Ltd

and that the treatments effective in ameliorating the clinical syndrome are also effective in eliminating the behavioral disturbances in animals. Additionally, it should be considered that in human depression the symptom profile may vary considerably across individuals, and likewise the effectiveness of treatments in alleviating the symptoms of the illness may vary across subjects. The present review will focus on the effects of stressors on responding for intracranial self-stimulation (ICSS), which may be indicative of the anhedonia which is one of the characteristic symptoms of depression. Moreover, we document some of the fundamental variables which influence the alterations of stressor-induced self-stimulation performance. Finally, we describe strain differences in response to stressors, since such a variable may serve as a rough parallel for the inter-individual differences in the symptom profile seen in human depression.

STRESSOR-INDUCED CENTRAL NEUROCHEMICAL ALTERATIONS

Uncontrollable stressors induce variations in the turnover and concentrations of central catecholamines and serotonin (5-HT), and may influence the sensitivity of presynaptic and postsynaptic receptors (Weiss and Goodman, 1984; Anisman and Zacharko, 1986). Among other things, it appears that the effectiveness of stressors in provoking these amine changes is dependent upon stressor severity, controllability, chronicity and predictability, as well as the brain region being examined. Moreover, it appears that the amine variations may be subject to conditioning or sensitization, such that stressor application may have long-lasting repercussions upon re-exposure to the stressor or to cues previously associated with the stressor. The noradrenaline (NA) and 5-HT alterations, as well as the variations in receptor sensitivity associated with stressor exposure, have been described extensively (Glavin, 1985; Stone, 1987; Zacharko and Anisman, 1989), and thus the present review will focus primarily on the stressor-provoked alterations of dopamine (DA) activity.

The data concerning the NA and 5-HT alterations associated with stressor exposure suggested that activity within the dorsal and ventral noradrenergic bundles (Abercrombie et al., 1986; Stone, 1987; Abercrombie and Jacobs, 1988; Simson and Weiss, 1988), as well as the raphe system (Palkovits et al., 1976), were significantly altered by stressors. Despite the early reports suggesting limited effects of stressors on DA activity (Anisman, 1978), it has become abundantly clear that profound DA alterations may be provoked by stressors, but that such effects are restricted to only a few brain regions. For instance, the stressor-provoked DA changes were limited primarily to the arcuate nucleus of the hypothalamus (Kvetnansky et al., 1976), selective portions of the septum (Saavedra, 1982), and to the mesolimbic/mesocortical system (henceforth referred to as the mesocorticolimbic system) (Herve et al., 1979; Thierry et al., 1979; Blanc et al., 1980; Tassin et al., 1980; Herman et al., 1982; Dantzer et al., 1984). In other DA-rich areas, such as the substantia nigra and caudate (i.e. the nigrostriatal system), stressors were typically without effect (Zacharko and Anisman, 1989). The magnitude of the stressor-induced mesocorticolimbic DA variations appeared to vary with the specific brain region being considered. For instance, it is generally accepted that stressor-induced alterations of DA metabolism, as revealed by increases in the levels of 3,4-dihydroxyphenylacetic acid (DOPAC), are more conspicuous in the mesocortex than in the nucleus accumbens (Anisman and Zacharko, 1986; Antelman et al., 1988).

It has been argued that the stressor-induced increases of mesocorticolimbic DA activity followed from the activation of the ventral tegmental area (VTA) (Bannon et al., 1983). In particular, variations in mesolimbic and mesocortical DA activity were related to the electrophysiological properties of the A10 neurons projecting to these sites, the specific receptor types in the nucleus accumbens and the mesocortex, as well as variations in the sensitivity of feedback inhibition (see ensuing sections, and White, Chapter 3, this volume). However, analyses of stressor-induced DA activity and concentrations with the VTA yielded inconsistent results. For example, while Claustre et al. (1986) failed to detect elevations of the DA metabolite in the A10 region, Deutch et al. (1985) reported that uncontrollable footshock provoked a significant accumulation of DOPAC in the VTA. Interestingly, Deutch et al. (1985) identified distinct populations of DA neurons within the tegmental field which appeared to be differentially affected by stressor presentation. The release of dendritic DA in the A10 region following stressor application would normally function to regulate DA neuronal activity and attenuate the neurochemical response to the aversive stimulus in terminal regions. The failure to detect such an inhibition (mesocortical DA turnover was approximately twice that of the midbrain tegmental area) suggested a subpopulation of A10 neurons which lacked autoreceptors. This subpopulation of DA neurons, which appeared to sustain their neuronal activity in response to stressors, was correlated with the size of the mesocortical projection field (Swanson, 1982). As such, it would appear that DA neurons in the VTA are not homogeneously activated by stressors. Thus, the between-laboratory differences concerning the effects of stressors on DA activity within the A10 region may stem from the precise portions of the tegmentum that were included in the biochemical analyses. Indeed, Mantz et al. (1989) recently reported that tail-pinch provoked a significant increase in mesocortical DA activity, but such an effect was absent in either the nucleus accumbens or the septum. Consistent with the results of Deutch et al. (1985), which suggested that tegmental neurons were differentially activated by stressors, Mantz et al. (1989) observed that the response of mesocortical neurons to tail-pinch stress was not uniform. While the majority of mesocortical neurons responded with increased activation, some neurons were inhibited. Moreover, the effects of such manipulation on mesocortical DA activity appeared to be specific to tail-pinch. Other forms of sensory stimulation, including light touch or pressure, were ineffective in modifying the activity of DA neurons in the mesocortex. It should also be considered that Roth et al. (1988) reported that while uncontrollable footshock augmented DOPAC accumulation in the A10 region, immobilization stress did not elicit such an effect. Taken together, these observations suggest that the responsivity of the mesocorticolimbic system to stressors is dependent upon the nature of the stressor employed and the sensitivity of specific A10 neurons which project to distinct regions of the mesocortex.

The pattern of DA alterations reported from the nucleus accumbens following stressor presentation has not been uniformly consistent. Fadda et al. (1978) reported that footshock provoked a significant elevation of DOPAC in both the mesocortex and the nucleus accumbens. Similar observations have been reported by Thierry et al. (1979), Claustre et al. (1986) and Dantzer et al. (1984). In contrast, Laveille et al. (1978) as well as Deutch et al. (1985), failed to observe such an effect. In the former study, DOPAC:DA ratios were used to estimate the effects of stressors on central DA activity. This approach, however, has been criticized since it fails to indicate whether the change is due to increased DOPAC accumulation, reduced DA levels, or a combination of the two (Bannon and Roth, 1983).

Furthermore, in the report of Deutch et al. (1985), as well as Bowers et al. (1987a), it was observed that stressors affect the levels of homovanillic acid (HVA) or the HVA:DA ratio in the mesolimbic system, but not in the substantia nigra. As depicted in Figure 1, research conducted in this laboratory (Anisman and Zacharko, 1986) has also revealed that footshock provoked relatively small changes of DA activity in the substantia nigra, while in the frontal cortex DOPAC accumulation was markedly increased, even by a relatively small number of shock presentations. Moreover, consistent with the findings of Deutch et al. (1985), DOPAC accumulation in the nucleus accumbens was not appreciably increased by footshock, while HVA was increased by more than 50%. Despite the inconsistencies which have appeared concerning the effects of stressors on DA activity, it appears that stressor-induced DA turnover is most prominent in the mesocortex, followed by the nucleus accumbens, and is minimal in the striatum.

Although DA neuronal activity within the striatum has been shown to be relatively insensitive to the effects of environmental insults, there are some reports that specific stressors may provoke amine alterations. For example, Dunn and File (1983) reported that a combination of cold plus restraint effectively reduced DA levels and increased the DOPAC:DA ratio in the

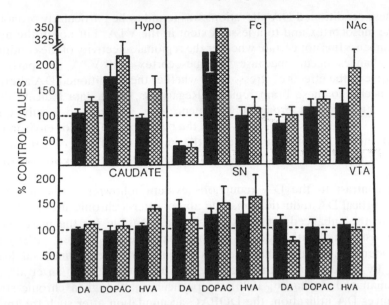

Figure 1. Dopamine (DA), 3,4-dihydroxyphenylacetic acid (DOPAC), and homovanillic acid (HVA) are shown as a percentage of control values (±SEM) in the hypothalamus (Hypo), frontal cortex (Fc), nucleus accumbens (NAc), caudate, substantia nigra (SN) and ventral tegmentum (VTA) of CD-1 mice that received either 30 shocks (black bars) or 360 shocks (hatched bars) of 150 µA of 2-second duration. (From Anisman and Zacharko, 1986)

striatum, mesocortex and nucleus accumbens, with the mesocortical DA alterations being most prominent. A subsequent report by Heyes et al. (1988) indicated that exercise stress (to exhaustion) provoked a significant elevation of DA, DOPAC and HVA levels in the striatum. Thus, under some conditions, particularly those involving a thermoregulatory response or when the stressor imposes stringent motoric requirements (exercise), nigrostriatal DA activity may be affected. Such effects, however, should be differentiated from those induced by a stressor *per se* (Anisman and Zacharko, 1986).

In addition to the immediate effect of a stressor on DA lability within the mesocortical system, such amine alterations may also be subject to conditioning. For example, the stressor-induced increase of DA turnover within the mesocortical system can be reinduced by cues previously associated with uncontrollable footshock (Herman et al., 1982). Such an effect was not apparent in the nucleus accumbens and several other brain regions examined (e.g. amygdala and olfactory tubercle). Similar observations were reported by Deutch et al. (1985) in both the mesocortex and the VTA. The magnitude of these conditioned DA alterations was found to be particularly pronounced in the mesocortex and to a lesser extent in the VTA, but not in the nucleus accumbens. It is not certain whether the regional selectivity of the conditioned DA changes occurs because the mesocortex and VTA are particularly sensitive to the effects of stressors, or whether the conditioned DA alterations are specific to these brain regions. Regardless, these data indicate that an acute stressor may proactively influence the response to a subsequently applied stressor. As such, analysis of the behavioral effects of environmental insults needs to consider not only the immediate effects of stressors, but also the long-term repercussions that may be engendered by stressor-related cues.

In contrast to the DA reductions evident following an acute stressor, mesocortical DA reductions may be absent after a chronic stressor regimen. Unlike the enhanced synthesis which is responsible for the increased NA levels associated with repeated stressor exposure (Irwin et al., 1986), there is evidence suggesting that the DA adaptation is determined, at least in part, by moderation of the excessive DA utilization (Herman et al., 1982; Anisman and Zacharko, 1986). In particular, although a chronic stressor enhances DA utilization, the DOPAC accumulation after such treatment is less pronounced than after an acute stressor. In accordance with the data indicating that DA mesocortical neurons are particularly responsive to stressors, Kramarcy et al. (1984) reported that the enhanced DOPAC accumulation associated with acute footshock was also accompanied by enhanced DA synthesis, as determined from the accumulation of [³H]-DA following incubation with [³H]-tyrosine. Curiously, following repeated stressor application, the enhanced DA synthesis typically associated with acute shock was absent. Unfortunately, the latter effect was exhibited in a separate experiment where the effects of acute shock were not monitored. The absence of the necessary comparison group in this experiment prevents a strong conclusion from being drawn.

STRESSORS AND THE MESOCORTICOLIMBIC SYSTEM: REGIONAL CONSIDERATIONS

The anatomical, electrophysiological and neurochemical organization of the mesocorticolimbic system is provided in several comprehensive reports (Oades and Halliday, 1987; Part 1 of this volume). Accordingly, the following description is provided only to draw attention to a number of points considered relevant to a discussion of stressor-induced alterations in the mesocorticolimbic system.

It is abundantly clear that the midbrain DA neurons are not homogeneous (Oades and Halliday, 1987), and both DA- and non-DA-containing neurons have been identified within the tegmental field (Thierry et al., 1988). As indicated earlier, this heterogeneity may underlie the divergent results reported for the effects of stressor presentation on the responsivity of the tegmentum and its projection sites (Roth et al., 1988). Although the largest tegmental projections appear to be those of the mesolimbic system, and the nucleus accumbens in particular, the mesocortical innervation from the VTA has received increasingly greater attention owing to the decidedly unambiguous behavioral and neurochemical results associated with stressor presentation. The mesocortical projection field has been divided into several subsystems. Perhaps the most significant of these with respect to the effects of stressors on DA neuronal activity is the anteromedial DA system which arises from the medial tegmental area. Amine utilization within this pathway exceeds that of either the mesolimbic or mesostriatal system under basal conditions and also that of adjacent cortical areas to which the tegmentum projects (Bannon and Roth, 1983). It will be recalled, as well, that the anteromedial cortex corresponds to the region in which a significant elevation of DOPAC was observed following stressor presentation, and where cues previously associated with the stressor were effective in eliciting enhanced DA turnover (Deutch et al., 1985).

The cells of origin of the suprarhinal system have been verified along the dorsolateral aspects of the A10 area and project dorsally to the sulcal cortex. There are currently no experimental data available which assess the effects of stressors on DA turnover within the sulcal cortex or compare this region with the anteromedial cortex. Both the piriform and the entorhinal cortices also receive significant DA input. The former system receives its input from both the VTA as well as the medial portions of the substantia nigra, while the latter system is derived from the lateral portions of the VTA. The presentation of mild intermittent footshock, however, is ineffective in altering levels of DA or its metabolite DOPAC in either of these cortical regions in the rat (Roth et al., 1988).

Taken together, there appears to be sufficient evidence to suggest that there is considerable variability in tegmental innervation of the mesocortex, and that these projection sites differ considerably in their responsivity to stressors. The sensitivity of some of these subregions within the mesocortex to stressors and to cues associated with a stressor remains to be determined.

STRESSORS AND BEHAVIOR

Uncontrollable stressors have been shown to induce a wide array of behavioral disturbances, including shuttle escape performance (Maier and Seligman, 1976; Anisman et al., 1979), response perseveration (Anisman et al., 1984), appetitively motivated behaviors (Rosellini et al., 1982), exploratory patterns (Bruto and Anisman, 1983), swim performance (Weiss et al., 1981) and dominance hierarchies (Williams, 1982). Despite the assertion that performance deficits associated with stressors may stem from alterations in motivation, none of these paradigms adequately address this issue. This is particularly surprising given that alterations in motivation or the presence of an anhedonia are fundamental characteristics of depression. In the shuttle escape task, for example, assessment of motivational change may be compromised by the induction of motoric alterations induced by the stressor (Zacharko and Anisman, 1984), while in appetitively motivated paradigms, acquisition of response-outcome associations may be due to associative or non-associative factors (e.g. attentional disturbances: Minor et al., 1984, 1988). Furthermore, in the latter paradigms, the necessity of food deprivation imposes a chronic stressor which can interfere with an adequate assessment of potential reward alterations. Some investigators have attempted to circumvent these problems by investigating the effects of stressors on saccharin consumption (Katz, 1982). While this paradigm appears to be sensitive to the imposition of a stressor, it is difficult to determine whether the alterations of saccharin consumption represent an anhedonia or a component of an anorexic response (Willner et al., Chapter 15, this volume).

Research conducted in this laboratory has focused on the potential effects of stressors on motivational and reward processes by assessing ICSS from various brain regions. Following the initial revision of the catecholamine hypothesis of ICSS by German and Bowden (1974), which postulated a major role for DA, the theory has undergone significant modification (Wise, 1982; Fibiger and Phillips, 1988; Wise and Rompre, 1989; Phillips et al., Chapter 8; Bozarth, Chapter 12, this volume). The basic premise of the theory that areas rich in DA, or sites through which the major DA pathways traverse, are particularly effective in sustaining ICSS remains largely intact. It has been suggested, however, that DA activity and the expression of ICSS may be modulated by several other transmitters, depending on the brain region under consideration (e.g. opiate peptides, acetylcholine, NA, 5-HT) (Koob, 1989).

In an initial series of experiments (Zacharko et al., 1983a), CD-1 mice were trained to respond for ICSS from either the substantia nigra, nucleus accumbens or the medial forebrain bundle (MFB). The latter electrode placements were positioned along the edges of the internal capsule to ensure activation of the rostrally coursing DA pathways (Phillips, 1984). As shown in Figure 2, subsequent exposure to escapable footshock did not influence responding for self-stimulation from any of the areas. However, in mice exposed to an identical amount of footshock (applied in a yoked paradigm), appreciable reductions of responding for brain stimulation were evident when the stimulating electrode was implanted in either the nucleus accumbens or the MFB. These disturbances of ICSS were relatively longlasting, being as marked 1 week after footshock as they were immediately after stressor

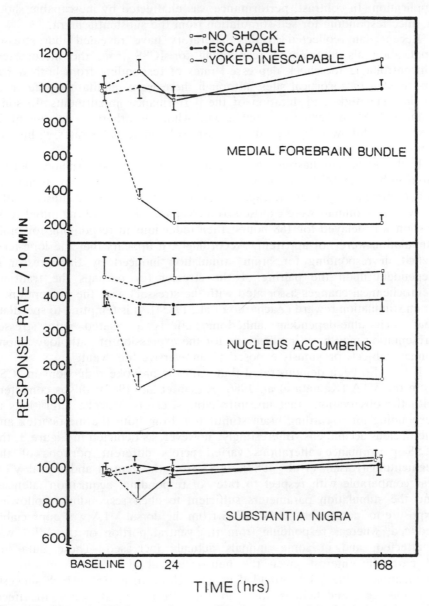

Figure 2. Mean (±SEM) rate of responding for intracranial stimulation over a 10-minute period from the medial forebrain bundle (top), nucleus accumbens (middle), and substantia nigra (bottom) among CD-1 mice that had been exposed to either escapable shock, yoked inescapable shock or no shock. Baseline rates represent responding on the day prior to shock treatment. Mice were tested immediately (0), and again 24 and 168 hours after the shock session. (From Zacharko et al., 1983a)

application. In contrast, performance was unaffected by inescapable shock in mice responding for self-stimulation from the substantia nigra.

Recent data collected in this laboratory have revealed that stressor application also influenced responding for ICSS from the mesocortex. Uncontrollable footshock depressed rates of responding from both dorsal and medial mesocortical sites, although there were qualitative differences in the magnitude and duration of the performance impairments. In some animals ICSS deficits were persistent, while in others a decrement in responding followed by a gradual return to baseline ICSS rates within 168 hours after stressor termination.

It should be emphasized that the long-term ICSS performance deficits from either the MFB or the nucleus accumbens were evident in animals tested immediately after inescapable shock and then re-tested subsequently. However, if animals were exposed to inescapable shock and the initial ICSS session was delayed for 168 hours, then reductions in responding for brain stimulation were not apparent. Accordingly, it appears that the long-term deficit in responding for brain stimulation induced by the stressor is dependent upon the pairing of the stressor (or perhaps the transient neurochemical changes associated with the stressor) with the perception of brain stimulation reward (Zacharko et al., 1983a). It is tempting to speculate that such time-dependent anhedonic effects associated with stressor presentation may have implications for the expression of pathology among human subjects previously exposed to an aversive life event.

It has also been demonstrated that stressors provoke reductions in ICSS from the VTA (Kamata et al. 1986; Kasian et al., 1987); this is consistent with the observations that uncontrollable stressors provoke alterations in responding for rewarding brain stimulation from both the mesocortex and the nucleus accumbens. Interestingly, however, as depicted in Figure 3, the ICSS performance alterations varied across different portions of the tegmentum (Kasian et al., 1987). ICSS from the ventral and dorsal VTA was comparable with respect to rates of responding, acquisition latencies and the stimulation parameters sufficient to elicit responding. Following exposure to inescapable shock, ICSS from the dorsal VTA was appreciably reduced, whereas responding from the ventral portion of the VTA was unaffected, and in some animals actually increased. These data are of particular interest given the neurochemical and electrophysiological delineation of the VTA provided by Deutch et al. (1985), which suggests that the tegmental field is not uniformly affected by stressors. In effect, these data provide a functional differentiation of different portions of the VTA commensurate with earlier biochemical and electrophysiological data suggesting that the midbrain tegmentum is not a homogenous structure.

It is unlikely that the impairments in responding for ICSS from mesolimbic sites were peculiar to the stimulation parameters employed during training.

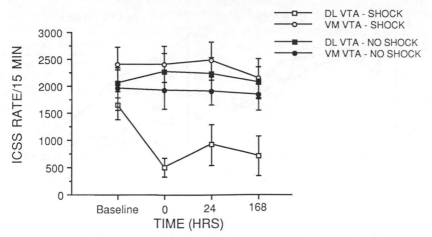

Figure 3. Mean (±SEM) rate of responding for electrical brain stimulation among CD-1 mice implanted with electrodes in either the dorsal (DL) or ventral (VM) portion of the VTA during baseline training, and at several intervals (immediately (0), and again at 24 and 168 hours) after exposure to uncontrollable footshock or no shock. (From Zacharko et al., 1990a)

Bowers et al. (1987b) employed a descending current intensity paradigm in which animals were initially trained to respond for ICSS at currents which were sufficient to elicit moderate rates of responding. Animals were then permitted a single baseline session in the current intensity paradigm wherein the highest current employed was significantly above that used during training. The brain stimulation currents were then automatically reduced in 10 μA decrements at 3-minute intervals over the course of a 30-minute test-session. Following exposure to inescapable shock, ICSS from the nucleus accumbens was reduced at the upper current range, but was unaffected at lower current intensities. Responding for brain stimulation from the substantia nigra was unaffected by the stressor at any of the currents examined. In a subsequent study, Zacharko et al. (1990a) observed that footshock was also effective in reducing responding for brain stimulation in this current intensity paradigm when electrodes were positioned in the dorsal aspects of the tegmental field, but not when the stimulating electrode was verified in the ventral portions of the VTA (Figure 4). Interestingly, the magnitude of the behavioral deficits observed from the tegmentum was considerably more pronounced than that observed from the nucleus accumbens.

Taken together, it would appear that stressors reduce the rewarding value of electrical brain stimulation from the mesocorticolimbic system at both the point of origin of this pathway and at its terminal sites. However, the time course for such an effect was dependent on the brain region in which

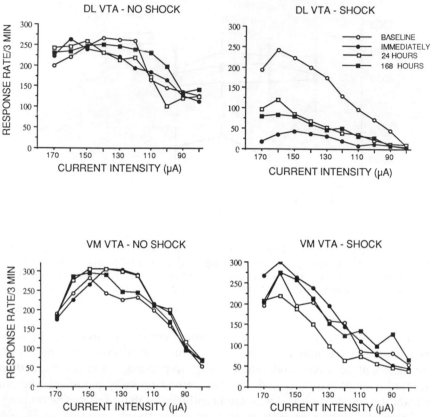

Figure 4. Mean rate of responding for electrical brain stimulation from either the ventral (VM) or dorsal (DL) aspects of the VTA. Baselines rates of responding are provided, as well as performance at each of three intervals (0, 24 and 168 hours) after exposure to either inescapable footshock or no shock. Mice were tested in a descending (170–80 µA) current intensity paradigm, in which animals were permitted to respond for 3 minutes at each current intensity, which decreased in 10 µA steps over the course of the 30-minute test-session. (From Zacharko et al., 1989a)

the stimulating electrode was positioned (e.g. dorsal and medial aspects of the mesocortex; ventral and dorsal portions of the VTA). Moreover, it appeared that the emergence of the ICSS disturbances, at least within the MFB and the nucleus accumbens, was dependent upon stressor controllability. Finally, in contrast to the effects of stressor application on mesolimbic ICSS, exposure to the stressor hardly affected responding for ICSS from the substantia nigra. Inasmuch as a stressor does not readily influence nigrostriatal DA activity, these data provide prima facie evidence in favor of the view that stressor-provoked DA alterations in the mesolimbic system contribute to alterations of self-stimulation performance.

STRESSOR INDUCED BEHAVIORAL IMPAIRMENTS AND ANTI-DEPRESSANTS

Early theories of depression (Schildkraut, 1965; van Praag, 1979) focused on the potential dysfunction of central NA and 5-HT activity, respectively. Accordingly, it is not surprising to find that many current animal models of depression, and particularly those postulating a relationship between stressors and depression, likewise emphasized these particular amines and largely ignored a role for DA. The dearth of attention devoted to DA in subserving depression was, of course, reinforced by the findings that the major anti-depressants were relatively ineffective in altering DA neural transmission (Rothschild, 1988). However, the therapeutic efficacy of second-generation anti-depressants with known DA activity, and reports that desmethylimipramine (DMI) likewise had predictable effects on central reward state (Fibiger and Phillips, 1981; Rothschild, 1988), suggested that central DA dysfunction may be associated with depression.

In a recent series of reports, Mouret et al. (1987, 1988) argued that a DA-dependent depression could be identified on the basis of qualitative differences in sleep patterns, anhedonia and feelings of guilt, and responsivity to pharmacological interventions which augmented central DA activity. Sack et al. (1988) argued that altered DA turnover among endogenously depressed patients was not secondary to nigrostriatal dysfunction, postulating a potential role for the mesocorticolimbic system in depression. Taken together, these data suggest that some of the symptoms of depression and their treatment may be linked to dysfunction of a motivational system (Willner et al., Chapter 15, this volume, for review).

Increasingly greater attention has been devoted to the possibility that, in addition to their effects on central NA and 5-HT activity or on receptor sensitivity, anti-depressant agents may also exert their therapeutic effects by altering central DA activity. Indeed, there are sufficient data to suggest that a variety of anti-depressant agents which are clinically effective appear to potentiate DA activity within the mesolimbic system (see Willner et al., Chapter 15, this volume for review).

In accordance with the view that repeated anti-depressant treatment may influence DA neuronal activity, chronic treatment with DMI lowered the threshold for ICSS among animals implanted with electrodes in the VTA (Fibiger and Phillips, 1981). Such an effect was recently replicated when electrodes were positioned in the MFB in a region described as the site of the rostrally coursing mesolimbic pathway (McCarter and Kokkinidis, 1988). In our laboratory, chronic DMI treatment did not influence the rate of responding for ICSS from the nucleus accumbens, although threshold determinations were not conducted in this particular study. Of particular interest, however, was the finding that administration of DMI for 15 days prior to uncontrollable footshock was effective in attenuating ICSS performance deficits from this region (Zacharko et al., 1984b). The rate of responding for ICSS from the nucleus accumbens was reduced immediately following stressor presentation, but ICSS rates were comparable to those of control animals 24 and 168 hours after initial stressor presentation (Figure 5).

In addition to the prophylactic effects of DMI, chronic DMI treatment also eliminated the disturbance of ICSS from the nucleus accumbens induced by a previously applied stressor (Zacharko et al., 1984a; Zacharko et al. 1989b). However, it was observed that there was considerable variability in the effects of the anti-depressant treatment. In particular, although chronic DMI administration was effective in ameliorating stressor-induced deficits in ICSS in the majority of animals (65%), in some mice performance was unaffected by DMI administration, while other animals showed an initial

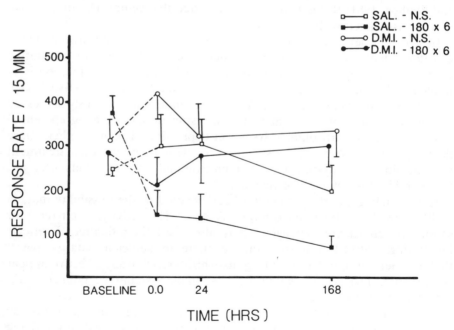

Figure 5. Mean (±SEM) number of responses for electrical stimulation from the nucleus accumbens over a 15-minute period among mice that were exposed to 180 shocks (180 × 6) or no shock (N.S.). Mice had received treatment with either desmethylimipramine (D.M.I.), 5.0 mg/kg twice a day for 15 days, or saline (SAL.) prior to stress treatment. Mice were tested for ICSS immediately (0), and again at 24 and 168 hours after the shock treatment. (From Zacharko, et al., 1984)

recovery followed by a further reduction in responding for ICSS. Moreover, in animals which failed to exhibit response decrements following exposure to inescapable shock, subsequent treatment with DMI actually impaired responding. As yet unpublished data from this laboratory have revealed a similar pattern of responding following chronic DMI treatment in mice with electrodes positioned in the mesocortex. The variations in ICSS from the nucleus accumbens and from the mesocortex could not be accounted for on the basis of variations in electrode placement. Accordingly, it would appear that although DMI is generally effective in reversing stressor-induced reward alterations from the mesolimbic system, the therapeutic efficacy of DMI is subject to considerable inter-individual variability.

It will be recalled that, following chronic stressor application, the reduction of DA and NA concentrations ordinarily associated with acute shock were eliminated. In a similar fashion, we observed that the disturbances of ICSS from the nucleus accumbens evident after a single shock session were absent in mice that received shocks over a period of 15 days (Zacharko et al., 1983b). We suggested that, while adaptive changes ordinarily occur in response to repeated stressor application, depression may ensue when the adaptive changes do not occur either as a result of organismic (e.g. age or strain) or experiential factors (e.g. following a stressor regimen which does not lend itself to adaptation, such as a regimen involving intermittent, unpredictable stressors of various forms: see Willner et al., Chapter 15, this volume). In accordance with this position, we observed that when behavioral adaptation was not evident following a repeated stressor regimen (i.e. the depression of ICSS persisted), chronic treatment with DMI ameliorated the behavioral impairment. However, when the repeated stressor treatment led to amelioration of the behavioral disturbances, then treatment with DMI tended to disrupt responding for ICSS from the nucleus accumbens (Zacharko et al., 1984a).

OPIOIDS AND CENTRAL DA ACTIVITY

Despite growing evidence indicating that DA activity is altered following exposure to aversive environmental events, there are also data implicating neuropeptide modulation of such stressor-induced amine alterations (Kalivas et al., 1988). Such arguments were prompted by immunocytochemical techniques which suggested a potential link between DA and neuropeptides in the VTA (Johansson et al., 1978; Hökfelt et al., 1979; Uhl et al., 1979; Johnson et al., 1980). The observation that the midbrain tegmental area appeared to be a focal point in the mediation of reward associated with maintenance of drug self-administration (Roberts and Koob, 1982), and place conditioning (Phillips and LePiane, 1980), as well as ICSS (Broekkamp et al., 1979), prompted considerable interest in the potential influence of neuropeptides in the mediation of rewarded behavior (see Cooper, Chapter

13, this volume). For example, Phillips and LePiane (1982 and Phillips et al. 1983) reported that intracerebral administration of the enkephalin analog, D-Ala^2-Met^5-enkephalinamide (DALA) into the A10 region produced a dose-dependent enhancement of conditioned place preference. Broekkamp et al. (1979) demonstrated similar effects with respect to brain stimulation reward. Experimental attempts to identify the specific opioid receptor associated with the enhancement of tegmental DA activity were ambiguous owing to the mixed nature of the agonists employed. For example, A10 activation induced by DALA affected both the μ and δ receptors. Recently developed enkephalin analogs, including Try-D-Ala-Gly-NMe-Phe-Gly-ol (DAGO) and [D-Pen^{2,5}]-enkephalin (DPEN), which differ considerably in their relative activation of μ and δ receptors, permitted a more precise description of the mechanisms underlying the activation of the DA substrate in the tegmentum. Latimer et al. (1987) and Vezina et al. (1987) determined that the increased activation of DA neurons, the resultant accumulation of DOPAC concentrations, and the behavioral concomitants associated with such activation followed from stimulation of μ rather than δ receptors in the A10 region. Furthermore, Kalivas and Abhold (1987) reported that stressors promoted the release of enkephalins within the tegmental area. Pharmacological manipulations which prevented such neuropeptide activity attenuated the increase in DA activity within the nucleus accumbens and the mesocortex, and largely eliminated the behavioral concomitants of the stressor. It might be added that enkephalin release within the tegmentum was restricted to the ventral portion of the tegmental field, and that no such alterations were evident in the dorsal A10 region.

The demonstration of an enkephalin–DA link within the A10 region appears to represent only the first stage of a rather complex neuromodulatory interaction. Lisoprawski et al. (1981), for example, reported that substance P was depleted within the VTA in rats exposed to inescapable footshock, while Bannon et al. (1983) reported that monoclonal antibodies directed against substance P prevented activation of mesocortical DA neurons ordinarily induced by a stressor. Subsequent investigations (Kalivas et al., 1985; Takano et al., 1985) revealed that the tachykinins, substance P and substance K, appeared to be equally distributed in the VTA, although substance K was demonstrably more potent in the promotion of locomotor activity. Such findings have prompted some investigators to suggest that the behavioral and neurochemical effects of substance P administration may actually be mediated through the substance K receptor (Kelley et al., 1985, 1989). Finally, the report of DA co-localization of the neuropeptide neurotensin in the tegmentum suggested an additional link in the stressor-induced neurochemical profile (Hökfelt et al., 1984; Studler et al., 1988). For example, Kalivas and Taylor (1985) observed that daily administration of neurotensin into the tegmental area produced a progressive increase in locomotor activity and an associated elevation of DOPAC in the nucleus accumbens. Likewise, Deutch et al. (1987) demonstrated that mild footshock increased neurotensin concentration in the tegmental area, and that this effect was associated with elevated levels of DOPAC in the mesocortex.

It will be recalled that conditioning/sensitization of DA activity has been reported with respect to the mesocorticolimbic system among animals re-exposed to a mild stressor or to cues previously associated with a stressor. That such conditioning of DA activity might conceivably fall under the influence of endogenous opioid activity has been suggested by several lines of evidence. Kalivas (1985) and Kalivas and Duffy (1987) reported that repeated morphine or enkephalin administration induced a progressive increase in behavioral output and DA turnover in the VTA, the nucleus accumbens and the mesocortex following challenge doses of the respective opioids. Behavioral cross-sensitization has also been reported from the tegmentum between cocaine and DAGO (DuMars et al., 1988). Finally, Kalivas et al. (1986) reported behavioral and neurochemical cross-sensitiz-ation between animals subjected to daily footshock or intra-VTA DALA administration. In particular, it was demonstrated that the stressor-provoked increase of DA metabolism within the nucleus accumbens was greatly enhanced in rats that had previously received DALA administration into the VTA over a 5-day period.

We have recently observed that opioid manipulations effectively influenced the disruption of responding for ICSS from the dorsal VTA ordinarily induced by inescapable footshock (Wolfe and Zacharko, 1990). As seen in Figure 6, acute intraventricular administration of 1 µg DALA in a 1 µl volume antagonized the marked (85%) reduction of ICSS from the VTA induced by uncontrollable footshock. The enkephalin was administered during the 'immediate' post-stressor interval, 15 minutes after the introduction of the mice to the self-stimulation chambers (Figure 6). It is particularly noteworthy that the behavioral effect of DALA could be distinguished from that observed following DMI administration. In particular, while the DALA treatment effectively eliminated the disruption of self-stimulation immediately after inescapable shock, when animals were tested 24 and 168 hours later (in the non-drug state), the performance deficits were again evident (see lower panels of Figure 6). Thus, DALA had only a transient effect on the disruption of ICSS induced by inescapable shock. In contrast, the antagonism of the stressor-provoked reductions of self-stimulation from the nucleus accumbens engendered by repeated DMI treatment appeared at more protracted intervals. Whether DMI has transient or longlasting effects on the stressor-induced reduction of ICSS from the VTA remains to be determined. However, this preparation may be ideally suited to distinguish between the effects of DALA and anti-depressant treatments.

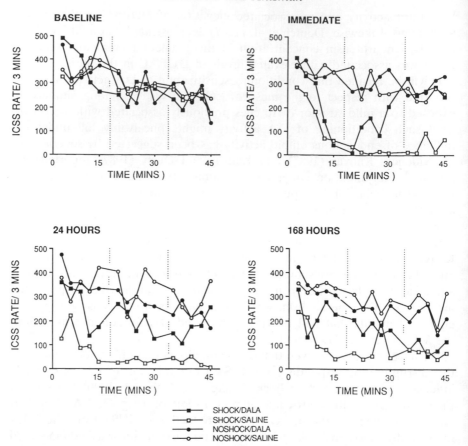

Figure 6. Mean rate of responding for electrical brain stimulation from the dorsal aspects of the VTA among mice exposed to either inescapable footshock or no shock. Self-stimulation rates were assessed during baseline and at three post-stressors intervals (immediate (0), and again at 24 and 168 hours). Mice received a single infusion of either DALA (1.0 μg in a volume of 1.0 μl) or saline 15 minutes after commencement of the 'immediate' test-session. (From Wolfe and Zacharko, 1990)

STRAIN-SPECIFIC EFFECTS OF STRESSORS

The presumed biochemical heterogeneity and the inter-individual variability in the symptom profile of depressed individuals has prompted interest in strain-dependent variations in response to stressors among infrahuman subjects. For example, Shanks and Anisman (1988) reported that the deficits in shuttle escape performance following inescapable shock were pronounced in BALB/cByJ and C3H/HeJ mice, modest in the C57BL/6J strain, and absent in DBA/2J mice unless a relatively severe stressor was employed

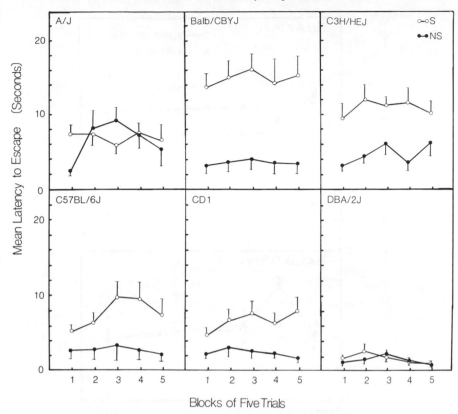

Figure 7. Mean (±SEM) escape latencies over blocks of five trials in each of six strains of mice exposed to either inescapable shock treatment (S) or no shock (NS) 24 hours earlier. (From Shanks and Anisman, 1988)

(Figure 7). However, in a forced swim paradigm, the strain profile was different. For example, inescapable footshock decreased swimming time in C57BL/6J mice, but increased swim time in BALB/cByJ mice and had no effect in DBA/2J mice.

With the use of identical stressor parameters to those described by Shanks and Anisman (1988), it was observed that the effect of uncontrollable footshock on ICSS from the nucleus accumbens was found to vary as a function of the strain of mouse employed (Figure 8). Responding for brain stimulation in the C57BL/6J mice was unaffected by uncontrollable footshock at any of the post-stressor intervals examined. In contrast, BALB/cByJ mice actually increased responding for ICSS immediately following exposure to the stressor, while DBA/2J mice exhibited marked reductions in ICSS (Zacharko et al., 1987). This particular strain profile is markedly different

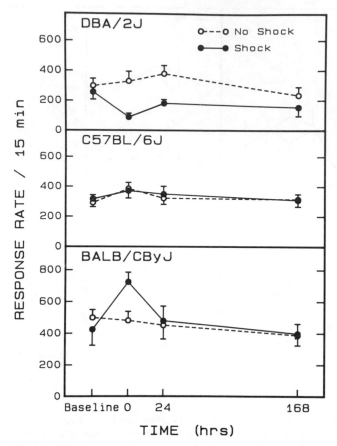

Figure 8. Mean (±SEM) rate of responding for electrical stimulation from the nucleus accumbens in three strains of mice. Animals received a 15-minute test-session prior to treatment (Baseline) and again immediately (0), 24 and 168 hours after exposure to either inescapable footshock (360 shocks of 150 μA of 2-second duration) or no shock. (From Zacharko et al., 1987)

from that observed in the shuttle escape task. Together, these data suggest that the appearance of behavioral deficits in these strains is not simply related to variations in the vulnerability of these animals to the stressors. After all, if a strain was particularly sensitive to a stressor or vulnerable to its effects, then the stressor might have been expected to provoke performance deficits across various tasks in this strain. This was clearly not the case. Rather, the impact of the stressor was dependent upon the specific behavior being considered. In a sense, just as in the case of human depression where individuals may exhibit different symptom profiles, the various strains of mice display different profiles of behavioral disturbances after exposure to inescapable shock.

The stressor-elicited disturbances of self-stimulation vary not only across strains of mice, but also with the brain region supporting ICSS. Recent data collected in this laboratory have revealed that the strain-dependent ICSS response profiles evident in the nucleus accumbens following stressor exposure are fundamentally different when the comparison is extended to the mesocortex and the VTA.

Effects of uncontrollable footshock on ICSS from the mesocortex and accumbens were the same in C57BL/6J mice (no effect) and in DBA/2J mice (persistent decrease). However, in BALB/cByJ mice footshock caused a shortlasting impairment of ICSS from the mesocortex (Figure 9: Zacharko et al. 1990c) as opposed to the increase observed in the nucleus accumbens.

When ICSS from the VTA was assessed, uncontrollable footshock increased self-stimulation rates in both the BALB/cByJ and DBA/2J strains of mice, while ICSS performance was disrupted in the C57BL/6J strain (Kasian and Zacharko, 1989). It should be emphasized that disturbances in reward functioning in the A10 region were confined to the dorsal rather than the ventral portions of the tegmental field; data consistent with the region-specific reward alteration evident from the tegmentum in the non-inbred CD-1 strain of mouse. Evidently interstrain alterations of ICSS provoked by uncontrollable footshock within the mesolimbic and mesocortical systems are not uniform.

Just as in the case of human depression, where the efficacy of anti-depressants may vary appreciably across individuals, the effectiveness of several anti-depressants was dependent upon the strain of mouse being examined, and the specific task in which mice were tested following exposure to inescapable shock. For instance, Shanks and Anisman (1989) observed that the shuttle escape deficits induced by inescapable shock could be antagonized by repeated DMI treatment in A/J mice, but had no effect in either BALB/cByJ, C57BL/6J or CD-1 mice (Figure 10).

Repeated treatment with amitriptyline eliminated the escape disturbance in A/J mice and also reduced (but did not eliminate) the escape deficits in the CD-1 strain. Likewise, in the CD-1 strain, bupropion marginally reduced the escape interference but had no effect in any of the other strains examined (Figure 11). This profile of drug effects could be readily distinguished from that seen when other stressor-induced behavioral responses were examined. It will be recalled that in CD-1 mice chronic DMI treatment eliminated the stressor-provoked ICSS deficits from the nucleus accumbens (Zacharko et al., 1983b) despite the fact that this treatment did not alleviate the stressor-induced escape deficits. In contrast to the CD-1 mice, the stressor-induced disruption of self-stimulation from either the nucleus accumbens or the mesocortex was not affected by repeated treatment with either DMI or

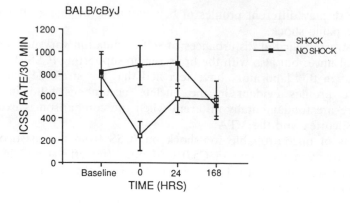

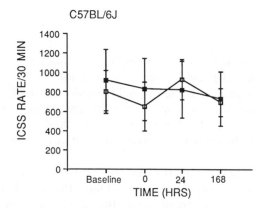

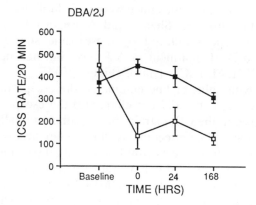

Figure 9. Mean (±SEM) rates of responding for electrical brain stimulation from the mesocortex in each of three strains of mice. Mice received a 30-minute test-session 24 hours prior to treatment, and again immediately (0), 24 and 168 hours after exposure to inescapable shock (360 shocks of 150 μA of 2-second duration) or no shock. (From Zacharko et al., 1990c)

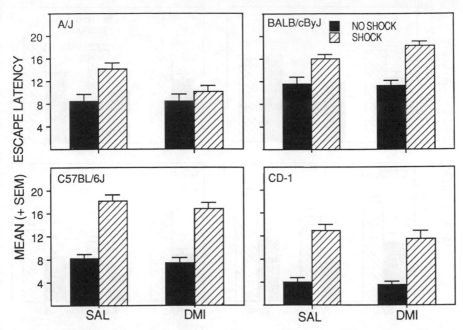

Figure 10. Mean (±SEM) escape latencies (seconds) in four strains of mice that had been exposed to inescapable shock (360 shocks of 300 μA of 2-second duration) or no shock, and tested in a shuttle escape task 15 days later. Mice received either saline (SAL) or desmethylimipramine (DMI: 5.0 mg/kg twice/day) for 14 days and were tested 1 hour after the final drug treatment. (From Shanks and Anisman, 1989)

amitriptyline in DBA/2J mice (Baillie et al., 1988). In effect, these data suggest that the effectiveness of anti-depressants may be specific to some of the effects (symptoms) elicited by inescapable shock, but may not alleviate the entire constellation of disturbances induced by a stressor. Moreover, the specific symptoms affected by the drug treatments appear to be strain-dependent.

Several investigators have reported that the stressor-provoked alterations of catecholamine activity vary across strains of mice (Cabib et al., 1988a, 1988b). In our laboratory the effectiveness of stressors in altering amine activity not only varied with the strain of mouse examined, but also with the brain region under consideration. For instance, inescapable footshock increased DOPAC accumulation in the nucleus accumbens in four of six strains of mice examined, namely the A/J, C57BL/6J, C3H/HeJ and DBA/2J mice, but only in the A/J strain were such alterations associated with significant DA reductions. In contrast, BALB/cByJ mice exhibited significant DA depletion in the nucleus accumbens in the absence of accompanying

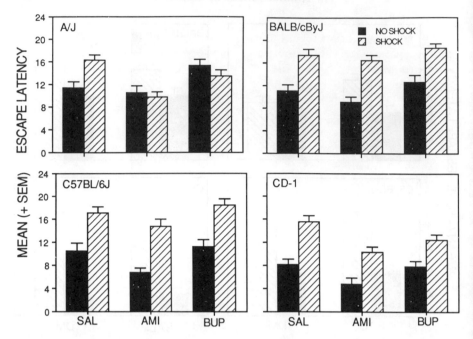

Figure 11. Mean (±SEM) escape latencies (seconds) in four strains of mice that had been exposed to inescapable shock (360 shocks of 300 μA of 2-second duration) or no shock, and tested in a shuttle escape task 15 days later. Mice had received either saline (SAL), amitriptyline hydrochloride (AMI: 5.0 mg/kg twice/day) or bupropion hydrochloride (BUP: 5.0 mg/kg twice/day) for 14 days, and were tested 1 hour after the final drug treatment. Amitriptyline eliminated the escape deficit in A/J mice, and both amitriptyline and bupropion reduced (but did not eliminate) the deficit in CD-1 mice. In A/J mice, bupropion increased escape latencies in control animals, but had no effect in the stressed animals. (From Shanks and Anisman, 1989)

alterations of DOPAC levels. When the mesocortex was considered, a different strain profile emerged. Once again, pronounced DA reductions were evident in A/J and BALB/cByJ mice. Such alterations were associated with significant accumulation of both DOPAC and HVA in the BALB/cByJ mice while only HVA was affected in the A/J strain. In CD-1 mice, only DOPAC levels were found to be enhanced significantly by the stressor. Finally, in the VTA the strain pattern was different from either that of the mesocortex or the nucleus accumbens. The most pronounced reductions of DA were apparent in the CD-1, DBA/2J and BALB/cByJ mice relative to the remaining strains, and only in the CD-1 mice was there an appreciable increase of DOPAC accumulation.

Clearly, while a stressor may induce marked alterations of DA activity in some strains of mice, such an effect may be restricted to only some brain regions. A particular strain may be vulnerable to stressor-provoked DA alterations in one brain region and not another, while in a second strain an opposite pattern of vulnerability may be apparent. If the stressor-induced DA variations were primarily responsible for the alterations of self-stimulation described earlier, then it would have been expected that the pattern of DA alterations induced by stressors would parallel the alterations of ICSS performance across the different strains and brain regions. However, as far as we could determine, there was no apparent congruity between stressor-induced alterations of DA activity and ICSS. However, given that ICSS is a fairly complex behavior which is probably governed by the interaction of several transmitters, the lack of behavioral and neurochemical congruity is not altogether surprising.

CONCLUSIONS

Consistent with the view that stressful events may contribute to the onset of depression in humans, it has been demonstrated that, in animals, exposure to uncontrollable stressors may engender behavioral disturbances reminiscent of the human disorder. Most notably, animals exposed to inescapable footshock exhibit a marked and long lasting anhedonia as gauged by disturbances of responding for electrical brain stimulation from the mesocorticolimbic system. While depression has typically been associated with alterations of NA and 5-HT turnover or receptor activity, it seems clear that stressor-induced DA variations may also contribute to the behavioral profile seen in animals. In addition, there is reason to suspect that the stressor-provoked DA changes may be influenced by neuropeptide activity.

The appearance of the stressor-induced behavioral disturbances may be dependent on a number of experiential and organismic variables, including genetic factors. Thus, the symptom profile exerted by a stressor in one strain of mouse may be very different from that seen in a second strain. Likewise, the neurochemical consequences of a stressor may vary with the brain region being examined, and it seems that the therapeutic efficacy of anti-depressants will be dependent on the specific symptoms elicited by the stressor in particular mouse strains. It is suggested that the symptoms engendered by a stressor may be dependent on the nature of the neurochemical alterations that are provoked and the brain regions in which these occur. Individual (or interstrain) differences exist with respect to the vulnerability to these neurochemical disturbances, and might thus account for the diverse behavioral profiles seen in response to a stressor. Presumably, the effectiveness of anti-depressants is governed by the nature of the neurochemical factors subserving the symptoms of the disorder.

ACKNOWLEDGEMENTS

This work was supported by grants MA-8130 from the Medical Research Council of Canada, and Grant A1087 from the Natural Sciences and Engineering Research Council of Canada.

REFERENCES

Abercrombie, E.D. and Jacobs, B.L. (1988) Systemic naloxone administration potentiates locus coeruleus noradrenergic neuronal activity under stressful but not non-stressful conditions. *Brain Research* **441**, 362–366.

Abercrombie, E.D., Wilkinson, L.O. and Jacobs, B.L. (1986) Environmental stress and activity of locus coeruleus noradrenergic neurons in freely moving cats. *Society for Neuroscience Abstracts* **123**, 1134.

Akiskal, H.S. and McKinney, W.T. (1973) Depressive disorders: towards a unified hypothesis. *Science* **82**, 20–29.

Anisman, H. (1978) Neurochemical changes elicited by stress: behavioral correlates. In: Anisman, H. and Bignami, G. (eds) *Psychopharmacology of Aversively Motivated Behavior* New York: Plenum, pp. 119–172.

Anisman, H. (1984) Vulnerability to depression: contribution of stress. In: Post, R.M. and Ballenger, J.C. (eds) *Neurobiology of Mood Disorders*. Baltimore: Williams and Wilkins, pp. 204–238.

Anisman, H. and Zacharko, R.M. (1982) Depression: the predisposing influence of stress. *Behavioral and Brain Sciences* **5**, 89–137.

Anisman, H. and Zacharko, R.M. (1986) Behavioral and neurochemical consequences associated with stressors. *Annals of the New York Academy of Sciences* **467**, 205–225.

Anisman, H., Remington, G. and Sklar, L.S. (1979) Effects of inescapable shock on subsequent escape performance: catecholaminergic and cholinergic mediation of response initiation and maintenance. *Psychopharmacology* **61**, 107–124.

Anisman, H., Hamilton, M.E. and Zacharko, R.M. (1984) Cue and response choice acquisition and reversal after exposure to uncontrollable shock: induction of response perseveration. *Journal of Experimental Psychology* **10**, 229–243.

Antelman, S.A., Knopf, S., Caggiula, A.R., Kocan, D., Lysle, D.T. and Edwards, D.J. (1988) Stress and enhanced dopamine utilization in the frontal cortex: the myth and the reality. *Annals of the New York Academy of Sciences* **537**, 262–272.

Baillie, P., Wolfe, C., MacNeil, G., Kasian, M. and Zacharko, R.M. (1988) Antidepressant specificity in the reversal of performance deficits in intracranial self-stimulation from mesolimbic and mesocortical sites in the DBA/2J mouse strain. *Society for Neuroscience Abstracts* **14**, 45.

Bannon, M.J. and Roth, R.H. (1983) Pharmacology of mesocortical dopamine neurons. *Pharmacological Reviews* **35**, 53–68.

Bannon, M.J., Elliott, P.J., Alpert, J.E., Goedert, M., Iversen, S.D. and Iversen, L.L. (1983) Role of endogenous substance P in stress-induced activation of mesocortical dopamine neurons. *Nature* **306**, 791–792.

Blanc, G., Herve, D., Simon, H., Lisoprawski, A., Glowinski, J. and Tassin, J.-P. (1980) Response to stress of mesocortico-frontal dopaminergic neurons in rats after long-term isolation. *Nature* **284**, 265–267.

Bowers, M.B., Bannon, M.J. and Hoffman, F.J. (1987a) Activation of forebrain dopamine systems by phencyclidine and footshock stress: evidence for distinct mechanisms. *Psychopharmacology* **93**, 133–135.

Bowers, W.J., Zacharko, R.M. and Anisman, H. (1987b) Evaluation of stressor effects on intracranial self-stimulation from the nucleus accumbens and the substantia nigra in a current intensity paradigm. *Behavioral Brain Research* **23**, 85–93.

Broekkamp, C.L., Phillips, A.G. and Cools, A.R. (1979) Facilitation of self-stimulation behavior following intracerebral microinjections of opioids into the ventral tegmental area. *Pharmacology Biochemistry and Behavior* **11**, 289–295.

Bruto, V. and Anisman, H. (1983) Alterations of exploratory patterns induced by uncontrollable shock. *Behavioral and Neural Biology* **37**, 302–316.

Cabib, S., Kempf, E., Schleef, C., Mele, A. and Puglisi-Allegra, S. (1988a) Different effects of acute and chronic stress on two dopamine mediated behaviors in the mouse. *Physiology and Behavior* **43**, 223–227.

Cabib, S., Kempf, E., Schleef, C., Oliverio, A. and Puglisi-Allegra, S. (1988b) Effects of immobilization stress on dopamine and its metabolites in different brain regions of the mouse: role of genotype and stress duration. *Brain Research* **441**, 153–160.

Claustre, Y., Rivy, J., Dennis, T. and Scatton, B. (1986) Pharmacological studies on stress-induced increase in frontal cortical dopamine metabolism in the rat. *Journal of Pharmacology and Experimental Therapeutics* **238**, 693–700.

Dantzer, R., Guilloneau, D., Mormede, P., Herman, J.P. and LeMoal (1984) Influence of shock-induced fighting and social factors on dopamine turnover in cortical and limbic areas in the rat. *Pharmacology Biochemistry and Behavior* **20**, 331–335.

Deutch, A.Y., Tam, S-Y. and Roth, R.H. (1985) Footshock and conditioned stress increase 3,4-dihydroxyphenylacetic acid (DOPAC) in the ventral tegmental area but not substantia nigra. *Brain Research* **333**, 143–146.

Deutch, A.Y., Bean, A.J., Bissette, G., Nemeroff, C.B., Robbins, R.J. and Roth, R.H. (1987) Stress-induced alterations in neurotensin, somatostatin and corticotropin-releasing factor in mesotelencephalic dopamine brain regions. *Brain Research* **417**, 350–354.

DuMars, L.A., Rodger, L.D. and Kalivas, P.W. (1988) Behavioral cross-sensitization between cocaine and enkephalin in the A10 dopamine region. *Behavioral Brain Research* **27**, 87–91.

Dunn, A.J. and File, S.A. (1983) Cold restraint alters dopamine metabolism in frontal cortex, nucleus accumbens and striatum. *Physiology and Behavior* **31**, 511–513.

Fadda, F., Argiolas, A., Melis, M., Tissari, A., Onali, P. and Gessa, G. (1978) Stress induced increase in 3,4-dihydroxyphenylacetic acid (DOPAC) levels in the cerebral cortex but not in the nucleus accumbens: reversal by diazepam. *Life Sciences* **23**, 2219–2224.

Fibiger, H.C. and Phillips, A.G. (1981) Increased intracranial self-stimulation in rats after long term administration of desipramine. *Science* **124**, 683–684.

Fibiger, H.C. and Phillips, A.G. (1988) Mesocorticolimbic dopamine systems and reward. *Annals of the New York Academy of Sciences* **537**, 206–215.

German, D.C. and Bowden, D.M. (1974) Catecholamine systems as the neural substrate for intra-cranial self-stimulation: an hypothesis. *Brain Research* **73**, 381–419.

Glavin, G.B. (1985) Stress and brain noradrenaline: a review. *Neuroscience and Biobehavioral Reviews* **9**, 233–243.

Herman, J.P., Guillonneau, R., Dantzer, R., Scatton, B., Semerdjian-Rouquier, L. and LeMoal, M. (1982) Differential effects of inescapable footshocks and of stimuli previously paired with inescapable footshocks on dopamine turnover in cortical and limbic areas of the rat. *Life Sciences* 30, 2207–2214.

Herve, D., Tassin, J.-P., Barthelemy, C., Blanc, G., Labveille, S. and Glowinski, J. (1979) Difference in the reactivity of the mesocortical dopaminergic neurons to stress in the BALB/C and C57 BL/6 mice. *Life Sciences* 25, 1659–1664.

Heyes, M.P., Garnett, E.S. and Coates, G. (1988) Nigrostriatal dopaminergic activity is increased during exhaustive exercise stress in rats. *Life Sciences* 42, 1537–1542.

Hökfelt, T., Terenius, L., Kuypers, H.G.J.M. and Dann, O. (1979) Evidence for enkephalin immunoreactive neurons in the medulla oblongata projecting to the spinal cord. *Neuroscience Letters* 14, 55–60.

Hökfelt, T., Everitt, B.J., Theodorsson-Norheim, E. and Goldstein, M. (1984) Occurrence of neurotensin-like immunoreactivity in subpopulations of hypothalamic, mesencephalic, and medullary catecholamine neurons. *Journal of Comparative Neurology* 222, 543–559.

Irwin, J., Ahluwalia, P. and Anisman, H. (1986) Sensitization of norepinephrine activity following acute and chronic footshock. *Brain Research* 379, 98–103.

Johansson, O., Hökfelt, T., Elde, R.P., Schultzberger, T. and Terenius, L. (1978) Immunohistochemical distribution of enkephalin neurons. In: Costa, E. and Trabucchi, M. (eds) *The Endorphins*. New York: Raven, pp. 51–70.

Johnson, R.P., Sar, M. and Stumpf, W. (1980) A topographic localization of enkephalin on the dopamine neurons of the rat substantia nigra and ventral tegmental area demonstrated by combined histofluorescence-immunocytochemistry. *Brain Research* 194, 566–571.

Kalivas, P.W. (1985) Sensitization to repeated enkephalin administration into the ventral tegmental area of the rat. II. Involvement of the mesolimbic dopamine system. *Journal of Pharmacology and Experimental Therapeutics* 235, 544–550.

Kalivas, P.W. and Abhold, R. (1987) Enkephalin release into the ventral tegmental area in response to stress: modulation of mesocorticolimbic dopamine. *Brain Research* 414, 339–348.

Kalivas, P.W. and Duffy, P. (1987) Sensitization to repeated morphine injection in the rat: possible involvment of A10 dopamine neurons. *Journal of Pharmacology and Experimental Therapeutics* 241, 204–212.

Kalivas, P.W. and Taylor, S. (1985) Behavioral and neurochemical effect of daily injection with neurotensin into the ventral tegmental area. *Brain Research* 358, 70–76.

Kalivas, P.W., Deutch, A.Y., Maggio, J.E., Mantyh, P.W. and Roth, R.H. (1985) Substance K and substance P in the ventral tegmental area. *Neuroscience Letters* 57, 241–246.

Kalivas, P.W., Richardson-Carlson, R. and Van Orden, G. (1986) Cross sensitization between foot shock stress and enkephalin-induced motor activity. *Biological Psychiatry* 21, 939–950.

Kalivas, P.W., Duffy, P., Dilts, R. and Abhold, R. (1988) Enkephalin modulation of A10 dopamine neurons: a role in dopamine sensitization. *Annals of the New York Academy of Sciences* 537, 405–414.

Kamata, K., Yoshida, S. and Kameyama, T. (1986) Antagonism of footshock stress-induced inhibition of intracranial self-stimulation by naloxone or methamphetamine. *Brain Research* 371, 197–200.

Kasian, M. and Zacharko, R.M. (1989) Strain differences in responding for self-stimulation from the ventral tegmentum following acute and chronic shock. *Society for Neuroscience Abstracts* **15**, 1135.

Kasian, M., Zacharko, R.M. and Anisman, H. (1987) Regional variations in stressor provoked alterations of intracranial self-stimulation from the ventral tegmental area. *Society for Neuroscience Abstracts* **13**, 1551.

Katz, R.J. (1982) Animal model of depression: pharmacological sensitivity of a hedonic deficit. *Pharmacology Biochemistry and Behavior* **16**, 965–968.

Kelley, A.E., Cador, M. and Stinus, L. (1985) Behavioral analysis of the effect of substance P injected into the ventral mesencephalon on investigatory and spontaneous motor behavior in the rat. *Psychopharmacology* **85**, 37–46.

Kelley, A.E., Cador, M., Stinus, L. and LeMoal, M. (1989) Neurotensin, substance P, neurokinin-α, and enkephalin: injection into ventral tegmental area in the rat produces differential effects on operant responding. *Psychopharmacology* **97**, 243–252.

Koob, G.F. (1989) Anhedonia as an animal model of depression. In: Koob, G.F., Ehlers, C.L. and Kupfer, D.J. (eds) *Animal Models of Depression*. Boston: Birkhauser, pp. 162–183.

Kramarcy, N.R., Delanoy, R.L. and Dunn, A.J. (1984) Footshock treatment activates catecholamine synthesis in slices of mouse brain regions. *Brain Research* **290**, 311–319.

Kvetnansky, R., Mitro, A., Palkovits, M., Brownstein, M., Torda, T., Vigas, M. and Mikulaj, L. (1976) Catecholamines in individual hypothalamic nuclei in stressed rats. In: Usdin, E., Kvetnansky, R. and Kopin, I.J. (eds) *Catecholamines and Stress*. New York: Elsevier, pp. 39–50.

Latimer, L.G., Duffy, P. and Kalivas, P.W. (1987) Mu opioid receptor involvement in enkephalin activation of dopamine neurons in the ventral tegmental areas. *Journal of Pharmacology and Experimental Therapeutics* **241**, 328–337.

Laveille, S., Tassin, J., Thierry, A., Blanc, G., Herve, D., Barthelemy, C. and Glowinski, J. (1978) Blockade by benzodiazepines of the selective high increase in dopamine turnover induced by stress in mesocortical dopaminergic neurons of the rat. *Brain Research* **168**, 585–594.

Lisoprawski, A., Blanc, G. and Glowinski, J. (1981) Activation by stress of the habenulo-interpeduncular substance P neurons in the rat. *Neuroscience Letters* **25**, 47–51.

Maier, S.F. and Seligman, M.E.P. (1976) Learned helplessness: theory and evidence. *Journal of Experimental Psychology: General* **105**, 3–46.

Makara, G.B., Kvetnansky, R., Jezova, D., Jindra, A., Kakucska, I. and Oprsalova, Z. (1986) Plasma catecholamines do not participate in pituitary-adrenal activation by immobilization stress in rats with transection of nerve fibres to the median eminence. *Endocrinology* **119**, 1757–1762.

Mantz, J., Thierry, A.M. and Glowinski, J. (1989) Effect of noxious tail pinch on the discharge rate of mesocortical and mesolimbic dopamine neurons: selective activation of the mesocortical system. *Brain Research* **476**, 377–381.

McCarter, B.D. and Kokkinidis, L. (1988) The effects of long term administration of antidepressant drugs on intracranial self-stimulation responding in rats. *Pharmacology Biochemistry and Behavior* **31**, 243–247.

Minor, T.R., Jackson, R.L. and Maier, S.F. (1984) Effects of task-irrelevant cues and reinforcement delay on choice-escape learning following inescapable shock: evidence for a deficit in selective attention. *Journal of Experimental Psychology: Animal Behavior Processes* **10**, 543–556.

Minor, T.R., Pelleymounter, M.A. and Maier, S.F. (1988) Uncontrollable shock, forebrain norepinephrine, and stimulus selection during choice escape learning. *Psychobiology* **16**, 135–145.

Mouret, J., Lemoine, P. and Minuit, M.-P. (1987) Sleep polygraphic, clinical and therapeutic markers of dopamine dependent depressions (DDD). *Comptes Rendus de L'Academie des Sciences Paris* **306**, 93–98.

Mouret, J., Lemoine, P., Minuit, M.-P. and Robelin, N. (1988) Immediate and long-lasting treatment of dopamine dependent depressions (DDD) by L-tyrosine. A clinical and polygraphic study. *Comptes Rendus de L'Academie des Sciences Paris* **305**, 301–306.

Oades, R.D. and Halliday, G.M. (1987) Ventral tegmental (A10) system: Neurobiology 1. Anatomy and connectivity. *Brain Research Review* **12**, 117–165.

Palkovits, M., Brownstein, M., Kizer, J.S., Saavedra, J.M. and Kopin, I.J. (1976) Effect of stress on serotonin and tryptophan hydroxylase activity of brain nuclei. In: Usdin, E., Kvetnansky, R. and Kopin, I.J. (eds) *Catecholamines and Stress*. New York: Elsevier, pp. 51–59.

Phillips, A.G. (1984) Brain reward circuitry: a case for separate systems. *Brain Research Bulletin* **12**, 195–201.

Phillips, A.G. and LePiane, F. (1980) Reinforcing effects of morphine microinjection into the ventral tegmental area. *Pharmacology Biochemistry and Behavior* **12**, 965–968.

Phillips, A.G. and LePiane, F.G. (1982) Reward produced by microinjection of (D-Ala^2) Met^5-enkephalinamide into the ventral tegmental area. *Behavioral Brain Research* **5**, 225–229.

Phillips, A.G., LePiane, F.G. and Fibiger, H.C. (1983) Dopaminergic mediation of reward produced by direct injection of enkephalin into the ventral tegmental area of the rat. *Life Sciences* **33**, 2505–2511.

Roberts, D.C.S. and Koob, G. (1982) Disruption of cocaine self-administration following 6-hydroxydopamine lesions of the ventral tegmental area in rats. *Pharmacology Biochemistry and Behavior* **17**, 901–904.

Rosellini, R.A., DeCola, J.P. and Shapiro, N.R. (1982) Cross-motivational effects of inescapable shock are associative in nature. *Journal of Experimental Psychology: Animal Behavior Processes* **8**, 376–388.

Roth, R.H., Tam, S-Y., Ida, Y., Yang, J-X. and Deutch, Y. (1988) Stress and mesocorticolimbic dopamine system. *Annals of the New York Academy of Sciences* **537**, 138–147.

Rothschild, A.J. (1988) Biology of depression. *Medical Clinics of North America* **72**, 765–790.

Saavedra, J.M. (1982) Changes in dopamine, noradrenaline and adrenaline in specific septal and preoptic nuclei after immobilization stress. *Neuroendocrinology* **35**, 396–401.

Sack, D.A., James, S.P., Doran, A.R., Sherer, M.A., Linnoila, M. and Wehr, T.A. (1988) The diurnal variation in plasma homovanillic acid level persists but the variation in 3-methoxy-4-hydroxyphenylglycol level is abolished under constant conditions. *Archives of General Psychiatry* **45**, 162–166.

Schildkraut, J.J. (1965) The catecholamine hypothesis of affective disorders: a review of supportive evidence. *American Journal of Psychiatry* **122**, 509–522.

Shanks, N. and Anisman, H. (1988) Stressor-provoked behavioral changes in six strains of mice. *Behavioral Neuroscience* **102**, 894–905.

Shanks, N. and Anisman, H. (1989) Strain-specific effects of antidepressants on escape deficits induced by inescapable shock. *Psychopharmacology* **99**, 122–128.

Simson, P.E. and Weiss, J.M. (1988) Altered activity of the locus coeruleus in an animal model of depression. *Neuropsychopharmacology* **1**, 287–295.

Sklar, L.S. and Anisman, H. (1981) Stress and cancer. *Psychological Bulletin* **89**, 369–406.

Stone, E.A. (1987) Central cyclic-AMP-linked noradrenergic receptors: new findings on properties as related to the actions of stress. *Neuroscience and Biobehavioral Reviews* **11**, 391–398.

Studler, J-M., Kitabgi, P., Tramu, G., Herve, D., Glowinski, J. and Tassin, J-P. (1988) Extensive co-localization of neurotensin with dopamine in rat mesocortico-frontal dopaminergic neurons. *Neuropeptides* **11**, 95–100.

Swanson, L. (1982) The projections of the ventral tegmental area and adjacent regions: a combined fluorescent retrograde tracer and immunofluorescence study in the rat. *Brain Research Bulletin* **9**, 321–353.

Takano, Y., Takeda, Y., Yamada, K. and Kamiya, H. (1985) Substance K, a novel tachykinin injected bilaterally into the ventral tegmental area of rats increases behavioral response. *Life Sciences* **37**, 2507–2514.

Tassin, J.-P., Herve, D., Blanc, G. and Glowinski, J. (1980) Differential effects of a two-minute open-field session on dopamine utilization in the frontal cortices of BALB/C and C57BL/6 mice. *Neuroscience Letters* **17**, 67–71.

Thierry, A., Tassin, J.-P., Blanc, G., and Glowinski, J. (1979) Selective activation of the mesocortical dopamine system by stress. *Nature* **263**, 242–244.

Thierry, A.M., Mantz, J., Milla, C. and Glowinski, J. (1988) Influence of the mesocortical/prefrontal dopamine neurons on their target cells. *Annals of the New York Academy of Sciences* **537**, 101–111.

Uhl, G.R., Goodman, R.R., Kuhar, M.J., Childers, S.R. and Snyder, S.H. (1979) Immunohistochemical mapping of enkephalin containing cell bodies, fibres and nerve terminals in the brain stem of the rat. *Brain Research* **166**, 75–94.

Van Praag, H.M. (1979) Central serotonin. Its relation to depression, vulnerability and depression prophylaxis. In: Objols, E., Ballus, C., Gonzales-Monclus, E. and Pujol, J. (eds) *Biological Psychiatry Today*. New York: Elsevier, pp. 485–496.

Vezina, P., Kalivas, P.W. and Stewart, J. (1987) Sensitization to the locomotor effects of morphine and the specific opioid receptor agonist, DAGO, administered repeatedly to the ventral tegmental area but not to the nucleus accumbens. *Brain Research* **417**, 51–58.

Weiss, J.M. and Goodman, P.A. (1984) Neurochemical mechanisms underlying stress-induced depression. In: Field, T., McCabe, P. and Schneiderman, N. (eds) *Stress and Coping*. Hillsdale, New Jersey: Lawrence Erlbaum, pp. 93–116.

Weiss, J.M., Goodman, P.A., Losito, B.G., Corrigan, S., Charry, J.M. and Bailey, W.H. (1981) Behavioral depression produced by an uncontrollable stressor: relationship to norepinephrine, dopamine and serotonin levels in various regions of rat brain. *Brain Research Reviews* **3**, 157–205.

Williams, J.L. (1982) Influence of shock controllability by dominant rats on subsequent attack and defensive behaviours toward colony intruders. *Animal Learning and Behavior* **10**, 305–315.

Willner, P. (1984) The validity of animal models of depression. *Psychopharmacology* **83**, 1–16.

Willner, P. (1987) The anatomy of melancholy: the catecholamine hypothesis of depression revisited. *Reviews in Neuroscience* **1**, 77–99.

Wise, R.A. (1982) Neuroleptics and operant behavior: the anhedonia hypothesis. *Behavioral and Brain Sciences* **5**, 39–87.

442   *Zacharko and Anisman*

Wise, R.A. and Rompre, P.P. (1989) Brain dopamine and reward. *Annual Review of Psychology* **40**, 191–225.

Wolfe, C. and Zacharko, R.M. D-Ala^2-Met^5-enkephalinamide attenuates stressor induced alterations in intracranial self-stimulation from the dorsal A10 region. *Society for Neuroscience Abstracts* **16**, 444.

Zacharko, R.M. and Anisman, H. (1984) Motor, motivational and anti-nociceptive consequences of stress: contribution of neurochemical change. In: Tricklebank, M.D. and Curzon, G. (eds) *Stress-Induced Analgesia.* New York: Wiley, pp. 33–66.

Zacharko, R.M. and Anisman, H. (1989) Pharmacological, biochemical, and behavioral analyses of depression: animal models. In: Koob, G.F., Ehlers, C.L. and Kupfer, D.J. (eds) *Animal Models of Depression.* Boston: Birkhauser, pp. 204–238.

Zacharko, R.M., Bowers, W.J., Kokkinidis, L. and Anisman, H. (1983a) Region specific reductions of intracranial self-stimulation after uncontrollable stress: possible effects on reward processes. *Behavioral Brain Research* **9**, 129–141.

Zacharko, R.M., Bowers, W.J., Prince, C. and Anisman, H. (1983b) Behavioral alterations following repeated exposure to uncontrollable foot-shock or desmethyli-mipramine. *Society for Neuroscience Abstracts* **9**, 561.

Zacharko, R.M., Bowers, W.J. and Anisman, H. (1984a) Responding for brain stimulation: stress and desmethylimipramine. *Progress in Neuro-Psychopharmacology and Biological Psychiatry* **8**, 601–606.

Zacharko, R.M., Bowers, W.J., Kelley, M.S. and Anisman, H. (1984b) Prevention of stressor-induced disturbances of self-stimulation by desmethylimipramine. *Brain Research* **321**, 175–179.

Zacharko, R.M., Lalonde, G.T., Kasian, M. and Anisman, H. (1987) Strain-specific effects of inescapable shock on intracranial self-stimulation from the nucleus accumbens. *Brain Research* **426**, 164–168.

Zacharko, R.M., Kasian, M., MacNeil, G. and Anisman, H. (1990a) Stressor induced behavioural alterations in intracranial self-stimulation from the ventral tegmental area: evidence for regional variations. *Brain Research Bulletin* **25** (in press).

Zacharko, R.M., Kasian, M., MacNeil, G. and Anisman, H. (1990b) Behavioural alterations in intracranial self-stimulation from the nucleus accumbens following repeated exposure to uncontrollable footshock: therapeutic efficacy of chronic desmethylimipramine (in preparation).

Zacharo, R.M., Gilmore, W., MacNeil, G., Kasian, M. and Anisman, H. (1990c) Stressor induced variations of intracranial self-stimulation from the mesocortex in several strains of mice. *Brain Research* (in press).

17

Animal Models of Mania

ROBERT M. POST, SUSAN R.B. WEISS AND AGU
PERT

Biological Psychiatry Branch, National Institute of Mental Health,
9000 Rockville Pike, Bethesda MD 20892, USA

INTRODUCTION

There are few well accepted animal models of the psychiatric disorders. Controversy abounds regarding what might constitute an adequate animal model for depression, particularly since mood and cognitive changes play such a major role in the syndrome and are difficult to verify in animals (Willner, 1984, 1986; Overmeier and Patterson, 1988; McKinney, 1989; Kornetsky, 1989). Perhaps the situation is a little less problematic when considering animal models of mania, where psychomotor alterations are critical, if not pathognomonic, components of the syndrome. In addition to hyperactivity, Robbins and Sahakian (1981) have proposed that elation (defined as a decrease in threshold for intracranial self-stimulation), irritability and depression should also be present in an adequate model of mania.

While a variety of animal models of mania have been proposed (Robbins and Sahakian, 1981), the major focus of this manuscript will be on the psychomotor stimulants; other models, discussed in detail by Robbins and Sahakian (1981), will be mentioned only briefly. The effects of psychomotor stimulants meet many of the formal criteria for an animal model. There is considerable homology in the behaviors induced to those observed in the manic syndrome. The pharmacology of this model is, at least partially, parallel to that observed clinically in mania, and, most important for the purposes of this volume, mesolimbic dopaminergic substrates appear to be critically involved. In addition, stimulant-induced behaviors have been well characterized in animals and humans, the latter mimicking many aspects of the manic syndrome.

The Mesolimbic Dopamine System: From Motivation to Action.
Edited by P. Willner and J. Scheel-Krüger

© 1991 John Wiley & Sons Ltd

The stimulant model also offers a unique perspective for changes in behavior and biology that develop with repeated or chronic administration. These may be important for the longitudinal course of manic-depressive illness, with its tendency for recurrence and increased rapidity of cycling and manic onsets. Given the potential role of stressors in the induction of mania (Hall et al., 1977; Ambelas, 1979; Silverstone and Romans-Clarkson, 1989), it is not without interest that some stimulant-induced changes show cross-sensitization to at least some types of stressors (Post, 1975; Antelman et al., 1980; Antelman and Chiodo, 1984; Kalivas and Duffy, 1989).

Parenthetically, there is great interest in the biology of stimulant-induced behavioral alterations because of the current pandemic of cocaine use and abuse. Thus, independent of its validity as a model of mania, study of the acute and chronic effects of cocaine is of considerable importance in its own right. While amphetamine and cocaine share many properties and clinical effects, suggesting that their common stimulant properties account for this similarity, most of this chapter will focus on cocaine as a model of mania because of its recent intense research interest.

Other models of mania have been proposed but, in most instances, they have been studied less intensively or have either less face- or cross-validity. The more important of these models will be reviewed briefly. The morphine model has much to recommend it in terms of important defining characteristics of the manic syndrome. Not only does morphine produce biphasic changes in motor activity (i.e. initial motor depression with hyperactivity in a late phase), but administration of this compound to people is associated with mood elevation and euphoria. However, in contrast to the decreased need for sleep in the manic syndrome, administration of morphine in people is associated with a sedative component and periods of hypersomnia (though W.E. Bunney, in a personal communication, has emphasized that many manic patients 'nod' off to sleep periodically in a similar fashion to opiate-intoxicated individuals). The morphine model is of interest given the evidence linking locomotor stimulating effects of opiates to mesolimbic dopaminergic substrates (Broekkamp et al., 1979; Kelley et al., 1980; Joyce et al., 1981; Kalivas et al., 1983; see also Cooper, Chapter 13, this volume).

Robinson and Justice (1986) and Robinson (1989) have presented an interesting model in which right-sided cortical lesions induced by ligation of the middle cerebral artery produce a syndrome of hyperactivity associated with decreases in noradrenaline (NA) in the locus coeruleus and dopamine (DA) in the substantia nigra. The tricyclic anti-depressant desipramine (DMI) prevented the development of hyperactivity. While this has been considered a model of depression, it is of interest that Robinson and associates have found that, while left-sided lesions in people tend to be associated with depression, right-sided lesions are associated with the manic syndrome, although stroke syndromes producing mania appear to be exceedingly rare compared with those productive of depression (Bakchine et al., 1989). In notable contrast to the great predominance of depression over mania associated with stroke syndromes, most endocrinopathies, seizure disorders and a variety of other inducers of secondary affective illness, there appears to be an unusually high incidence of mania associated with multiple sclerosis (Joffe et al., 1987). Thus, the human illness of multiple sclerosis, with the current ability to image brain lesions with MRI, may provide important clues for neuroanatomical substrates involved in mania.

A variety of brain lesions have been associated with hyperactivity in animals and have been proposed as relevant to mania (Robbins and Sahakian, 1981). These include lesions of the hippocampus, septum, frontal cortex, and DA-rich areas including the caudate, nucleus accumbens and ventral mesencephalic tegmentum (VTA). While raphe lesions and serotonergic manipulations may also produce hyperactivity, the lesions involving DA systems are of particular interest in light of evidence linking DA to mania and DA blockade to therapeutic clinical effects (Gerner et al., 1976; Post, 1981a; Jimerson and Post, 1984).

Primate separation models have usually been considered for their resemblance to depressive syndromes (McKinney, 1989). However, the initial phases of reaction to maternal separation or to social separation in the peer paradigm contain a syndrome of agitation, vocalization, hyperactivity, decreased sleep, and a variety of other behaviors and symptoms that appear to mirror those in mania. This 'protest' syndrome lasts only briefly and then gives way to a despair phase. Nonetheless, the biphasic nature of the locomotor activation associated with this syndrome may provide an interesting analogy for biphasic mood changes, i.e. activated behavior followed by depression. In a parallel fashion, study of the mechanisms underlying the biphasic mood changes in the opposite direction achieved by morphine in the rodent (sedation-depression followed by marked motor hyperactivity) may be an interesting focal point for switch mechanisms from depression to mania.

Given the fact that a series of clinical studies document differential anti-manic responsivity as a function of pattern of switch, these animal models may be of particular interest. Kukopulos et al. (1980), Grof et al. (1987) and Haag et al. (1987) have all demonstrated that the pattern of mania followed by depression and then a 'well' interval shows a high responsivity to treatment with lithium carbonate. In contrast, patients presenting with the opposite pattern of depression switching into mania and then a well interval appear to be highly resistant to the acute and prophylactic effects of lithium carbonate. These data also highlight the pharmacological heterogeneity of the manic syndrome and its importance for animal models.

The separation-induced model of protest followed by despair is also a particularly interesting model in terms of the literature on stress and the induction of mania. Thus, it would appear that separation and loss, often thought to be critical precipitating factors in the induction of depression, may also be associated with mania. Recently, a syndrome of funereal mania, where loss and bereavement appear to precipitate manic episodes directly, has been re-documented (Kubacki, 1986). In this fashion, primate separation may be an interesting model in which to focus on the role of psychosocial precipitants to the activated phase of this syndrome. Moreover, adult squirrel monkeys remain hyperactive and agitated, i.e. animals appear to show only a protest phase of reaction and not evidence of the 'despair' reaction typical of adult rhesus monkeys (Suomi et al., 1981; Winslow et al., 1989). Thus, more detailed elucidation of the pathophysiological mechanisms involved in this separation model syndrome may provide particular insights into biochemical and physiological variables underlying activated as opposed to despair-like reactions to appropriate psychosocial stressors.

PSYCHOMOTOR STIMULANT EFFECTS AS A MODEL OF MANIA

Phenomenology

Psychomotor stimulants, when administered acutely to humans, appear to mimic rather faithfully the manic syndrome. Low doses are associated with increases in alertness and arousal often accompanied by a sense of mood elevation, increased vigor and decreased need for sleep. Higher doses administered acutely may be associated with profound euphoria, grandiosity, and delusional proportions in the sense of power and social facility. As in the manic syndrome, there may be total insomnia without a sense of fatigue. Thus, with high doses, a picture of a full-blown manic syndrome can be induced, often attaining psychotic proportions. With high doses and chronic administration, a syndrome of paranoid psychosis can occur that very much resembles that of paranoid schizophrenia (Connell and Akkerhuis, 1958; Ellinwood, 1967; Angrist and Gershon, 1970; Griffith et al., 1970; Bell, 1973). However, Kraepelin (1921), Carlson and Goodwin (1973), and others have emphasized that full-blown stage 3 manic psychosis can very much resemble that of paranoid schizophrenia and be extremely difficult to differentiate. As such, repeated high-dose psychomotor stimulant administration may closely model dysphoric and psychotic mania.

Some of the elements of euphoric and dysphoric mania are outlined in Table 1. The current epidemic of cocaine use provides ample documentation of dysphoric components of the syndrome which progressively emerge with chronic administration. While there has previously been some debate regarding the extent to which cocaine withdrawal has contributed to the dysphoria, recent studies by Sherer and colleagues (1988) indicate that

Table 1. Cocaine as a model for mania in evolution

Acute/low dose models	Chronic/high dose models
Hypomania	*Dysphoric mania*
Euphoria	Irritability and dysphoria
Motor activation	Stereotypy
Enhanced verbal output	Loquacious rambling
Social contacts	Loss of social cues
Productive	Unproductive
Sense of well-being	Grandiosity
Sense of power	Delusions
Heightened sensory awareness	Sensory distortions and hallucinations
Decreased need for sleep	Sleeplessness
Increased sex drive	Decreased sex drive
Alertness and hypervigilance	Paranoia
Demanding and confrontative	Aggressive and violent

dysphoric and psychotic elements can occur in the context of steady-state levels of cocaine maintained by intravenous infusion. Dysphoric components of cocaine have long been widely recognized in the street use of cocaine with various methods being employed in an attempt to decrease cocaine-induced anxiety (opiates (speedballing), marijuana or barbiturates and the like).

Various descriptions in the literature also emphasize the range of cocaine effects from euphoric activation to the marked manic-like and psychotic components. Freud noted the energizing and mood-elevating properties of cocaine.

> After a short time (10–20 minutes), the subject feels as though he had been raised to the full height of intellectual and bodily vigor, in a state of euphoria . . . one can perform mental and physical work with great endurance, and the otherwise urgent needs of rest, food, and sleep are thrust aside, as it were. . . . the individual disposition plays a major role in the effects of cocaine, perhaps a more important role than with other alkaloids. The subjective phenomena after ingestion of coca differ from person to person, and only few persons experience, like myself, a pure euphoria without alteration. Others already experience slight intoxication, hyperkinesia, and talkativeness after the same amount of cocaine, while still others have no subjective symptoms of the effects of coca at all . . .
> Sigmund Freud (1854) (cited in Freud, 1970)

Others have written as follows.

> It was when I got back into that familiar snow feeling that I began to want to talk. Cocaine produces, for those who sniff its powdery white crystals, an illusion of supreme well-being, and a soaring over-confidence in both physical and mental

ability. You think that you could whip the heavyweight champion: and that you are smarter than everybody.

Malcolm X (1945) (cited in Gay et al., 1973)

When you shoot coke in the mainline there is a rush of pure pleasure to the head. Ten minutes later you want another shot. Intravenous C is electricity through the brain, activating cocaine pleasure connections. There is no withdrawal syndrome with C. It is a need of the brain alone.

William Burroughs (1966) (cited in Gay et al., 1973)

Mental weakness, accompanied by irritability, erroneous conclusions, suspicion, bitterness towards his environment, a false interpretation of things, groundless jealousy, etc., bring about in the individual, now suffering from insomnia, illusions of the senses while fully conscious. Hallucinations of vision, hearing, smell and taste, disturbances in the sexual sphere and the general condition master those who are severely affected. In many cocainomaniacs confusional insanity preceded by general mental disorders, vacancy of mind as in delirium tremens, extreme alarm due to false impressions, set in. A cocainist who had snuffed 3.25 gr. cocaine armed himself for protection against imaginary enemies; another in an attack of acute mania jumped overboard into the water; another broke the furniture and crockery into pieces and attacked a friend.

Louis Lewin (1931)

I imagined every one was looking at me and watching me; even when locked in my own room, I could not persuade myself there were not watchers outside, with my eyes glued to imaginary peepholes. If I ventured into the street I thought I was followed and that the passers-by made remarks about me; I thought my vice was known to all, and on all sides I could hear the widespread word 'Cocaine . . .'. It is curious that directly after the effect of cocaine had passed away all the suspicions and delusions vanished instantly. I could see the absurdity and impossibility of the idea that the whole town was watching and talking about one obscure individual. I realized the folly of thinking that spies were in the room above, watching me through holes pierced in the ceiling. Yet, the overpowering desire to repeat the dose would overtake me, and almost instantly after taking it all delusions would return in full force, and no reasoning would banish them.

Wilson (1955) (cited in Woods and Downs 1973)

Abnormal sensations in the peripheral nerves cause the patient to believe there are animals under his skin. The result is frequently self-mutilation, and by a false application of subjective impressions, the mutilation of members of his family, in order to remove the foreign substance from the body. A woman injured herself with needles in order to kill the 'cocaine bugs'. A man who suffered from twinges and pains in the arms and feet thought he was being forcibly electrocuted. He thought he could see electric wires leading to his body.

Louis Lewin (1931)

In these quotes and other descriptions in the literature (Gay et al., 1973; Gawin and Ellinwood, 1988), the potential evolution from euphoric to dysphoric/psychotic effects is highlighted and most of the DSM-III-R criteria for hypomania and mania are recognized and met.

Recurrent Manic Episodes: Behavioral Sensitization as a Model

While most animal models have focused on reproduction of the elements of the acute manic syndrome, the psychomotor stimulant model provides unique abilities to examine the consequences of repeated administration. As such, it may provide an interesting model for the longitudinal course of manic illness, which tends to be characterized by repeated episodes. The median course of manic and depressive episodes in a group of 82 refractory bipolar patients studied at the National Institute of Mental Health shows a pattern of acceleration of episodes much like that reported by Kraepelin in the prepsychopharmacological era (Squillace et al., 1984; Roy-Byrne et al., 1985; Post et al., 1988). Based on the data of Grof and others (1974), in patients not preselected for such refractoriness, there is considerable evidence for an acceleration of the course of illness with repeated episodes, i.e. on average the duration of the well interval between episodes decreases as a function of successive episodes (Squillace et al., 1984). Patients with a first episode of mania appear to run a more malignant course than those with a first episode of depression (Roy-Byrne et al., 1985). Moreover, patients with dysphoric mania, particularly women, tended to have a much more severe course of illness characterized by relative lithium-refractoriness and an increased number of hospitalizations (Post et al., 1989).

In addition to the accelerating course of illness, there is some evidence that, with repetition of manic episodes, the onsets of individual episodes may reach their maximum intensity more rapidly (Post et al., 1981a). In a small group of patients examined for manic onsets during a medication-free interval, those who achieved full intensity of their mania within the first several days had a greater number of prior episodes than those who had more gradual manic onsets. While these data need to be replicated in a larger sample of patients, they are of considerable interest in light of the data on psychomotor stimulant administration reviewed below, indicating that onsets of peak locomotor hyperactivity or the initiation of stereotypy occurs earlier upon repeated administration of the drug.

Acute Pharmacology

An important validating criterion for an animal model is the pharmacological specificity. In this regard, morphine-induced hyperactivity is highly sensitive to suppression with lithium carbonate (Carroll and Sharp, 1971). Lithium appears to have inconsistent effects in suppressing acute amphetamine- or cocaine-induced locomotor activity, and is usually ineffective or may exacerbate stimulant-induced stereotypies (Robbins and Sahakian, 1981). Is it possible that this distinction could reflect not only lithium's general ineffectiveness in schizophrenic-like psychosis (which stereotypy is thought to model), but also in dysphoric mania (Post et al., 1989)?

However, a variety of other agents used in the clinical treatment of mania are effective in suppressing psychomotor stimulant-induced syndromes in experimental animals. The neuroleptic drugs are widely used for their anti-manic properties and are able to inhibit amphetamine- and cocaine-induced locomotor activity. Physostigmine appears uniquely capable of inducing essentially immediate reversibility of the manic syndrome in people (Janowsky et al., 1973). In a parallel fashion, physostigmine is capable of inhibiting amphetamine- and cocaine-induced locomotor hyperactivity (Post et al., unpublished data). Bunney and associates (1971) have reported that the inhibitor of catecholamine biosynthesis, α-methylparatyrosine (AMPT), is also an effective anti-manic agent. AMPT is also capable of inhibiting amphetamine- and cocaine-induced hyperactivity (see Figure 3.3 in Post, 1981b).

The inhibition of these syndromes by neuroleptics and AMPT leaves open the question of the relative dependence on dopaminergic versus neuroadrenergic function. It appears that amphetamine- and cocaine-induced hyperactivity are critically dependent on dopaminergic function, particularly that involving the nucleus accumbens. Lesions of the nucleus accumbens which selectively deplete DA (greater than 90 per cent) inhibit cocaine- and amphetamine-induced locomotor hyperactivity in experimental animals (Kelly et al., 1975; Kelly and Iversen, 1976; Pijnenburg et al., 1976). Moreover, the intravenous self-administration of cocaine and amphetamine is blocked by lesions in this area (Roberts et al., 1980; Pettit et al., 1984), suggesting the importance of the nucleus accumbens in the rewarding properties of these agents. Animals will bar-press for intracranial self-administration of amphetamine into the nucleus accumbens, although the same does not occur for cocaine (Goeders and Smith, 1983, 1984), and it is unclear whether the local anesthetic effects of cocaine or some other factor accounts for this discrepant result. In contrast, animals will work for cocaine-induced intracranial administration into the frontal cortex (Goeders and Smith, 1983, 1984). Thus, to the extent that self-administration reflects the reward value of these agents and may serve as an indirect measure of positive hedonic drive, if not euphoria, mesolimbic and mesocortical substrates appear integrally involved in amphetamine and cocaine reward, respectively.

Recent data using *in vivo* dialysis also indicate the importance of increases in DA release in the stimulant actions of amphetamine and cocaine (Glue et al., 1988; Bunney and Moghaddam, 1988; Hurd and Ungerstedt, 1989a, b; DiChiara and Imperato, 1988; Kaliv s and Duffy, 1989). Dose-related increases in DA levels have been observed in striatum and nucleus accumbens. In contrast to the report of Di Chiara and Imperato (1988), who administered cocaine systematically, Glue et al. (1988) found a greater magnitude of increase in DA levels in striatum than in nucleus accumbens following focal application. Increases in DA were of considerably less magnitude and were not dose-related in the frontal cortex, however (Glue et al., 1988).

COCAINE-INDUCED BEHAVIORAL SENSITIZATION AS A MODEL FOR THE INCREASED VULNERABILITY TO MANIC RECURRENCE

Phenomenology

Repeated administration of psychomotor stimulant produces a syndrome of hyperactivity that is more rapid in onset and increased in magnitude compared with the first administration (Segal, 1975; Post and Rose, 1976; Kilbey and Ellinwood, 1977; Shuster et al., 1977; Stripling and Ellinwood, 1977). This change in responsivity appears to be relatively longlasting (see Table 1 in Post and Contel, 1983). The sensitization effect depends on both dose and number of stimulant administrations (Figure 1). Following a series of cocaine injections, an increased response can be documented up to several months later. While a single dose of cocaine (10 mg/kg i.p.) does not produce behavioral sensitization, repetition of this dose for several days produces a long-lasting sensitization that can be evoked by an injection of saline in the same environment in which cocaine is usually administered (Post et al., 1981b). A single high dose of cocaine (40 mg/kg i.p.) produces a behavioral sensitization to a low dose of cocaine (10 mg/kg) which lasts approximately 5–7 days and is not evident in response to a saline challenge (Weiss et al., 1989a). Repeated administration of this high dose of cocaine (40 mg/kg i.p.) for 3 days produces increases in stereotypic responses. This is of considerable interest from the perspective that stereotypic components are observed in humans following chronic cocaine administration and have also been noted by Kraepelin (1921) and other observers to be a component of the manic syndrome.

An important component of stimulant-induced behavioral sensitization appears to be conditioned (Ellinwood, 1971; Tilson and Rech, 1973; Ellinwood and Kilbey, 1975; Post et al., 1981b; Hinson and Poulos, 1981; Schiff, 1982). That is, animals are more reactive if cocaine is readministered in the same test-cage (Post et al., 1981b; Weiss et al., 1989a). Cocaine-induced behavioral sensitization achieved with a single high dose of cocaine (40 mg/kg i.p.) appears to be entirely context-dependent (Weiss et al., 1989a). That is, animals receiving cocaine in a different cage are no more responsive to challenge than saline-pretreated controls (Figure 2). In contrast, animals receiving cocaine in the test-cage are markedly more reactive to challenge the next day, i.e. they show context-dependent, cocaine-induced behavioral sensitization. It is of interest, to the extent that repeated high doses of cocaine model dysphoric mania, that behavioral sensitization

COCAINE		EFFECT							
Number of Injections	Dose mg/kg i.p.	Behavioral Sensitization Duration	Activity Context Dep.	Activity Indep.	Stereotypy Context Dep.	Stereotypy Indep.	Saline Conditioning	Sensitization Neuroleptic Independent	Seizure Kindling · Death
↑↑↑ (large)	COC$_{65}$								++ · ++
☓10 days	COC$_{160}$ subcut. (K. Gale)	++		++	++			++	
✦✦✦✦✦✦✦✦✦✦	COC$_{10}$	++ months	++	0				++	
↑↑↑	COC$_{40}$	+	0	++	++	++	±		
↑	COC$_{40}$	++ days	++	0	0	0	0	0	
↑ ↑ ↑	COC$_{20}$	0 0	0	0	0	+			
✦ ✦ ✦	COC$_{10}$	0 0	0	0	0	0			
✦	COC$_{10}$	0 0							

Figure 1. Size and number of arrows indicate dose of cocaine and number of administrations. COC, cocaine; subscript, dose in mg/kg administered once daily i.p. except in the study of Gale (1984), when doses were subcutaneous; 0, no effect; ±, equivocal; +, moderate effect; ++, marked or definite effect. Effects of cocaine increase are more persistent with increases in either dose or number of repetitions. The highest doses also become less dependent on environmental context and conditioning, and are associated with seizures, kindling and associated lethality. Thus, effects shift from dopaminergic-mediated behavioral sensitization (motor endpoints) to local anesthetic-mediated kindling (seizure endpoints) as the dose is increased

achieved with cocaine (40 mg/kg i.p.) for 3 consecutive days shows both a context-dependent and a context-independent component, as illustrated in Figure 3.

Pharmacology of Context-Dependent Sensitization

A pharmacological dissection of the single high dose cocaine sensitization paradigm has been conducted in this laboratory, in which cocaine

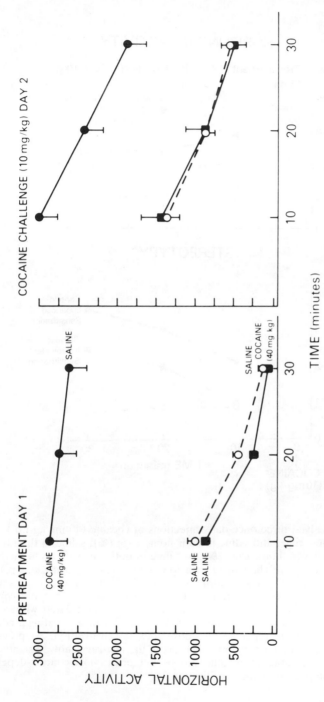

Figure 2. Horizontal locomotor activity is illustrated for three groups of rats ($n=10$/group) receiving the following day-1 pretreatments: cocaine in the test-cage and saline in the home cage (●); saline in the test-cage and cocaine in the home cage (■); saline in both cages (○) (left). Horizontal activity is illustrated for these three groups following a cocaine challenge (10 mg/kg) (right). Only the rats that received cocaine in the test-apparatus on day 1 showed sensitization to cocaine on day 2 (right)

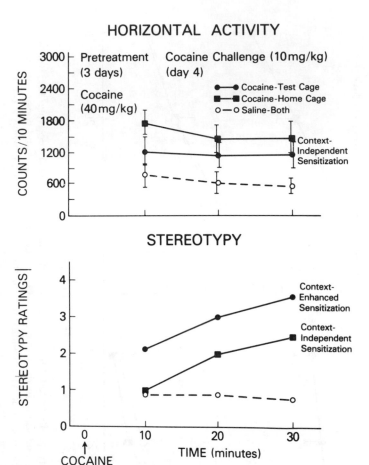

Figure 3. Rats received three once-daily injections of cocaine (40 mg/kg i.p.) in the Plexiglas activity test-cage, and saline in their home cage (●), saline in the test-cage and cocaine in their wire home cage (■), or saline in both cages (○). On the fourth day, all three groups were challenged with low dose cocaine (10 mg/kg i.p.), and locomotor counts were recorded (top), and stereotypy rated every 10 minutes (bottom). Both groups of cocaine pretreated animals showed greater stereotypy than saline controls to the low dose challenge on day 4. Those pretreated with cocaine in the home cage showed more stereotypy than saline controls, revealing a context-independent component to repeated high dose cocaine sensitization. As previously noted, those that received cocaine in the context of the test-cage showed significantly greater stereotypy than either of the other groups, demonstrating a context-dependent or conditioned component of the sensitization

(40 mg/kg i.p.) or saline is administered on day 1 followed by a challenge dose of cocaine (10 mg/kg) on day 2 (Weiss et al., 1989a). Using the neuroleptic haloperidol at doses of either 0.2 or 0.5 mg/kg, a remarkable dissociation has been observed. Haloperidol blocked the development, but not the expression, of cocaine-induced behavioral sensitization. That is, if haloperidol is given prior to the cocaine treatment on day 1, not only is a substantial portion of cocaine-induced locomotor hyperactivity inhibited, but the animals do not show an increased response to the low dose challenge of cocaine the next day (Weiss et al., 1989a). In contrast, once cocaine-induced running activity has been induced on day 1, haloperidol administered prior to the day 2 challenge is unable to block the effect of the prior cocaine sensitization (Figure 4B). In another experiment (Weiss et al., 1989a) these results were extended with the demonstration that prior cocaine administration did not interfere with neuroleptic effects. In this study, both groups of animals were pretreated with cocaine; one group in the home cage and the second group in the test-cage. Neuroleptics again did not block the expression of cocaine-induced sensitization.

Our findings extend previous observations (Beninger and Hahn, 1983; Beninger and Herz, 1986; Tadokoro and Kuribara, 1986) using different stimulants and neuroleptics, different species of animals, and a cocaine, rather than saline, challenge. However, in each study neuroleptics were able to block the development, but not the expression, of stimulant-induced behavioral sensitization. These data suggest that, under a variety of circumstances, doses of neuroleptics that are capable of blocking acute stimulant-induced behaviors are unable to block the sensitized or conditioned component of repeated stimulant administration. Thus, one would predict that dopaminergic lesions induced after cocaine-induced behaviors were manifest would also be ineffective in blocking the sensitization phenomenon.

These data suggest that dopaminergic substrates are critically important for the induction (development) of cocaine-induced behavioral sensitization, but that once cocaine-induced behaviors are manifest, the expression of sensitization is no longer critically dependent on dopaminergic mechanisms. There are ample parallels for this pharmacological dysjunction based on the temporal phase of evolution of a syndrome in other paradigms thought to represent models of learning and memory. For example, agents that block the development of electrophysiological kindling or induction of long-term potentiation (LTP) are often different from those that interfere with the maintenance of these phenomena (Collingridge and Bliss, 1987; Post et al., 1991). Similarly, Cador and associates (Chapter 9, this volume) have implicated DA in the acquisition, but not the maintenance, of conditioned reinforcement (Klimek et al., 1989; Bozarth, Chapter 12, this volume).

To the extent that cocaine-induced behavioral sensitization provides a model for repeated and/or dysphoric manic episodes, these data also provide

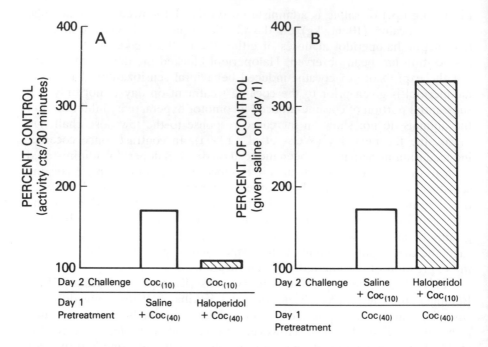

Figure 4. The total horizontal activity (30 minutes) in the experimental groups is expressed as the percentage of activity in the control groups. **A** Effect of haloperidol (0.2 mg/kg i.p.) on the development of cocaine sensitization. The control groups were pretreated with saline alone for the cocaine plus saline group, and haloperidol alone for the cocaine plus haloperidol group. Only the group of rats that received cocaine without haloperidol on day 1 showed sensitization to cocaine on the following day (unshaded column). Haloperidol pretreatment on day 1 blocked the development of cocaine sensitization (shaded column). **B** Effect of haloperidol (0.2 mg/kg i.p.) on the expression of cocaine sensitization. Haloperidol was administered to animals only prior to the cocaine rechallenge on day 2 (shaded column). Both control groups in this study received saline on day 1. As illustrated, the haloperidol-pretreated (day 2) animals showed robust sensitization based on the prior cocaine exposure (shaded column) as did animals tested without neuroleptics (open column). Thus, moderate doses of haloperidol (0.2 mg/kg) or high doses (0.5 mg/kg, not illustrated) did not block the expression of cocaine sensitization (**B**) but did block its development (**A**)

a potential model for neuroleptic refractoriness in these states (Post and Weiss, 1988). Based on our preclinical observations, one would predict that some components of the manic syndrome would be less responsive to neuroleptics after many occurrences of untreated episodes as compared with instances where treatment begins with the initial episode. While, to our knowledge, this proposition has not been systematically studied in recurrent or dysphoric mania, Wyatt and associates (1988) have reviewed the evidence that late treatment of schizophrenic syndromes with neuroleptics is less effective than earlier treatment. Bowers et al. (1988) also found that a history of prior drug abuse, especially involving cocaine, was associated with poor response to neuroleptics. Thus, at least for some psychotic syndromes, the preliminary evidence is consistent with the prediction derived from the behavioral sensitization model that initial early or preventive treatment with neuroleptics might be more effective than later treatment.

When clinical syndromes are neuroleptic-refractory, other pharmacological manipulations may be more effective. In this regard, other pharmacological interventions do not appear to share with neuroleptics the dissociation observed on the sensitization model (Weiss et al., 1989a). The benzodiazepines, for example, appear capable of blocking both the development and the expression of cocaine-induced behavioral sensitization in this paradigm. The same is true for the α_2-adrenergic agonist clonidine. These data are of interest in relation to preliminary evidence indicating the possible anti-manic effects of the benzodiazepine clonazepam (Chouinard et al., 1983; Chouinard, 1988) and of clonidine (Jouvent et al., 1980, 1988; Bakchine et al., 1989), although the most recent data raise doubts about clonazepam (Aronson et al., 1989), and double-blind studies of clonidine in acute mania do not support its efficacy compared with placebo (Janicak et al., 1989).

In contrast to diazepam and clonidine, the anti-convulsant carbamazepine, which has been demonstrated to possess anti-manic activity in 14 double-blind clinical trials (Post et al., 1987a, 1991), is not effective in blocking either the development or the expression of cocaine-induced behavioral sensitization (Post et al., 1984a; Weiss et al., 1990 and unpublished observations). While preliminary data suggest that lithium might be effective in the repeated low dose cocaine-induced behavioral sensitization paradigm (Post et al., 1984b), this anti-manic agent has not been systematically tested in the acute high dose 1-day sensitization paradigm. Thus, with the exception of carbamazepine, preliminary evidence suggests that pharmacoresponsivity in acute and repeated manic syndrome may parallel that observed with behavioral sensitization (Table 2).

Given the partial parallelism of the behavior and pharmacology in cocaine-induced behavioral sensitization to that observed in the full-blown or dysphoric manic syndrome, Pert, Weiss and associates undertook a series of studies to explore systematically the neural substrates involved in cocaine-induced behavioral sensitization. Strategies employed included lesions, local injections, deoxyglucose administration, receptor autoradiography, *in situ* hybridization and *in vivo* dialysis.

Table 2. Pharmacology of manic and cocaine syndromes

	Mania			Cocaine		
					Sensitization	
	Hypomania	Full blown	Dysphoric	Acute	Development	Expression
Lithium	+++	++	+	+	(+)	0
Neuroleptics	+++	+++	(+)	+++	+++	0
Carbamazepine	(+)	+++	(++)	0	0	
Physostigmine	+++	(+++)		++		
AMPT	++	(++)		++		
Benzodiazepines						
Diazepam	++	++		++	++	++
Clonazepam			±			
Clonidine	(+)	(+)		++	0	++

+++ Markedly effective
++ Very effective
+ Mildly effective
± Equivocal
0 Not effective
( ) Few studies or inconsistent results

Mesolimbic DA Lesions and Behavioral Sensitization

A series of lesion studies has implicated mesolimbic dopaminergic substrates as critical to cocaine-induced behavioral sensitization. It was observed in separate studies that selective dopaminergic lesions of the nucleus accumbens or of the amygdala, which themselves were insufficient to inhibit day 1 cocaine-induced hyperactivity (Figure 5a), were associated with an inhibition of cocaine-induced sensitization on day 2 (Figure 5b). In contrast, lesions of the dorsal (Figure 5b) and ventral hippocampus and cerebellum were without effect. While it may be argued that the amygdala lesions increased activity following saline and this accounted for the lack of sensitization, a similar increase after saline occurred with dorsal hippocampal lesions and yet sensitization to cocaine was still evident. Moreover, Deminiere et al. (1988) reported that 6-hydroxydopamine (6-OHDA) lesion of the amygdala increased amphetamine-induced locomotor activity and intravenous self-administration, suggesting that lesioned animals are more sensitive to the reinforcing properties of psychomotor stimulants. Thus, the lack of sensitization in our amygdala-lesioned animals does not appear attributable to either the increase in baseline activity or loss of rewarding effects of the drug.

The degree of depletion of DA in the nucleus accumbens was approximately 65 per cent which probably accounts for the inability of these lesions to block the cocaine-induced hyperactivity (40 mg/kg) on day 1. Nonetheless, this lesion did block sensitization, as revealed by the low dose challenge on day 2. Similar findings with amphetamine have been reported by Gold et al. (1988). The nucleus accumbens has been implicated in the locomotor activating effects of cocaine and reward properties of some psychomotor stimulants. Since many drugs that are self-administered are also associated with increases in locomotor activity, it is possible that these two effects of a drug are linked. Thus, lesions of the nucleus accumbens may interfere with sensitization through interruption of a critical structure for integrating the reward value of a stimulus with behavior.

In another series of studies, we have also found that either electrolytic lesions of the amygdala or selective depletions of DA (approximately 60 per cent) in the amygdala achieved with 6-OHDA and DMI were able to block the behavioral sensitization effect without impairing day 1 cocaine-induced hyperactivity. In the case of amygdala lesions, we surmise that the lesions may be interfering with the environmental-context-dependent component of the behavioral sensitization, as the amygdala receives polysensory information from association areas of cortex (van Hoesen, 1985; Murray and Mishkin, 1985; Aggleton and Mishkin, 1986), and may thus be involved in the formation of associations between different aspects of environmental events (Cador et al., Chapter 9, this volume). In our paradigm

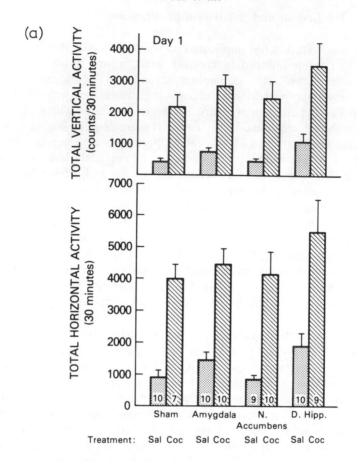

Figure 5a. Total horizontal and vertical (rearing) locomotor activity during the 30-minute test (mean and standard error) is illustrated for groups of rats that received lesions in one of the following areas: sham (surgical control); amygdala; nucleus accumbens (N. Accumbens; 6-OHDA); or dorsal hippocampus (D. Hipp.). The number of subjects in each group is illustrated in the bars in the lower half of the figure. Rats from each of these groups that received cocaine (40 mg/kg) exhibited hyperactivity compared with saline-treated controls, indicating that the lesions did not substantially interfere with the initial induction of cocaine-induced hyperactivity. **b** Horizontal and vertical locomotor activity in response to a cocaine challenge (10 mg/kg) is illustrated for the same animals shown in **a**. Rats with sham lesions or lesions of the dorsal hippocampus showed an enhanced response to cocaine compared with saline-pretreated controls. Rats with lesions of the amygdala or nucleus accumbens failed to show a differential response to the cocaine. Note that while dorsal hippocampal-lesioned animals showed enhanced activity compared to the sham-operated controls (as did animals with lesions of the amygdala and nucleus accumbens), they nevertheless showed a significant differential effect of prior cocaine (day 1) compared to prior saline.

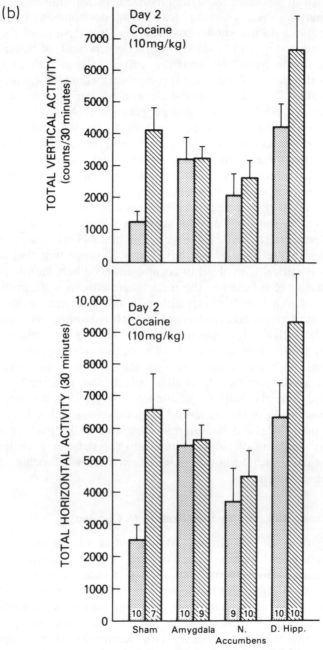

the rats learn to associate the drug environment with the drug effect, since those animals injected with the drug in an environment other than the testing apparatus do not show sensitization. Thus, lesions of the amygdala could be interfering with the associative component of sensitization. A critical test of the hypothesis that the amygdala is selectively involved in the context-dependent (conditioned) component would be whether amygdala lesions would block the context-independent component of behavioral sensitization achieved with a repeated high dose (40 mg/kg × 3) cocaine paradigm (see Figure 3). This experiment has not yet been carried out. If this prediction is confirmed, the data would suggest that two different elements of the mesolimbic dopaminergic system (nucleus accumbens and amygdala) may affect cocaine-induced behavioral sensitization by interfering with different components or inputs.

Rats showed increased responses to local injections of amphetamine into the nucleus accumbens but not the striatum following cocaine-pretreatment (see Figures 5.13a, b and 5.14 in Post et al., 1987b). These data are in agreement with the findings presented above, suggesting that the nucleus accumbens is critically involved in cocaine-induced behavioral sensitization. The rats that were injected in the nucleus accumbens were pretreated with cocaine (10 mg/kg for 10 days), either in the test-cage or in their home cage. A control group received saline in both environments. Amphetamine (10 μg, bilaterally), administered into the nucleus accumbens, increased responsivity in the animals treated with cocaine in the context of the test-cage, but not in those treated with cocaine in the home cage or in the saline-pretreated controls. A similar effect was observed when saline was injected into the nucleus accumbens, suggesting the importance of conditioning factors in the enhanced responsiveness rather than alterations in the sensitivity of the dopaminergic substrates in the nucleus accumbens. In contrast, injections of amphetamine into the striatum revealed no effect of prior cocaine injection in rats that were treated with cocaine for 17 days in either environment.

Local Glucose Utilization in Sensitization to Cocaine

The effects of acute and chronic administration of low and high doses of cocaine on regional metabolic activity of rat brain structures have been evaluated using 2-deoxyglucose methodology. Cocaine (10 mg/kg i.p.) acutely increases glucose utilization in the striatum, lateral septum, frontal parietal cortex, substantia nigra zona reticulata and posterior thalamic nucleus. Metabolic activity decreased in the lateral habenula and parafascicular nucleus of the thalamus. Porrino and Kornetsky (1988) reported that intravenous administration of cocaine (0.5 and 1.0 mg/kg) increased glucose utilization in the medial prefrontal cortex and nucleus accumbens, and decreased it in the lateral habenula (1.0 mg/kg). In their studies, more widespread effects were observed at higher doses (5.0 mg/kg i.v.); changes were prominent in extrapyramidal and limbic structures, including the hippocampus and olfactory tubercle. Following repeated cocaine administration (10 mg/kg i.p.) for 16 days, we found glucose utilization was additionally increased in the cerebellum, suggesting that this neural substrate may conceivably participate in the long-term effects of cocaine-induced behavioral sensitization. Athough lesions of the deep cerebellar nuclei were unable to block cocaine-induced behavioral sensitization achieved in the single high dose paradigm, the effect of many repetitions of cocaine may involve additional structures (i.e. cerebellar hemispheres), and is consistent with observations that behavioral sensitization following multiple injections is both longer lasting than in the single high dose paradigm and is revealed in response to saline administration.

Acute injections of high doses of cocaine (40 mg/kg i.p.) increased glucose utilization in the striatum as well as in the ventrolateral thalamus, globus pallidus, red nucleus, and substantia nigra zona compacta and zona reticulata. Again, with repeated administration of this dose, glucose utilization was increased in the cerebellum, superior colliculus and frontoparietal somatosensory cortex. In addition, when cocaine-kindled seizures were produced in response to the repeated injection of cocaine (40 mg/kg), prominent increases in metabolic activity were observed in the ventral pallidum, olfactory tubercle, nucleus accumbens, anterior olfactory area, subthalamic nucleus, substantia nigra, dorsomedial and ventromedial nucleus of the hypothalamus, ventral hippocampus and several brain stem reticular nuclei, perhaps as part of the motor outflow associated with the seizure.

Thus, while dopaminergic substrates appear to be highly involved in acute psychomotor stimulant administration, the deoxyglucose studies reveal additional structures, such as cerebellum, that appear to be activated with repeated administration of either low or high doses. Cocaine-induced seizures appear additionally to activate intensely a series of DA-rich ventral striatal structures.

Lack of Change in DA Receptors and Tyrosine Hydroxylase in Behavioral Sensitization

In preliminary studies using the DA ligands [³H]SCH 23390 and [³H]raclopride to label D_1 and D_2 receptors, respectively, differences in receptor binding were not observed following repeated administration of cocaine compared with saline. Moreover, no change in the levels of tyrosine hydroxylase was observed, as measured by *in situ* hybridization of its mRNA (Richfield and Pert, unpublished observations). Thus, behavioral sensitization may not involve alterations in DA receptors or tyrosine hydroxylase activity in striatal, mesolimbic or mesocortical areas of the brain. Interestingly, Cools et al. (Chapter 6, this volume) have reported that sensitization to cocaine is blocked by phentolamine administration on either the priming day or the test-day. These data, taken with our clonidine findings, implicate noradrenergic mechanisms in cocaine sensitization.

DA Levels: *In Vivo* Dialysis

Studies with *in vivo* dialysis conducted by Glue et al. (1988) indicate that extracellular DA levels in the striatum are increased following chronic cocaine administration when animals are tested with parenterally administered cocaine, but not when cocaine is introduced focally into dialysis probes in the striatum. These data are consistent with our findings of no effect of direct administration of amphetamine into the striatum of cocaine-sensitized animals compared with controls. They further suggest the possibility that alterations in DA release are mediated by changes in the dopaminergic cell body regions (i.e. VTA), rather than in the terminal fields. These data are convergent with a growing body of data indicating that stimulant-induced behavioral sensitization may be associated with desensitization of DA autoreceptors, leading to a subsequent increase in release in terminal field areas (Robinson and Becker, 1986; Kalivas et al., 1988; White et al., 1989). Further confirmation of this hypothesis is derived from the data of Kalivas et al. (1988) who found increases in extracellular DA in the nucleus accumbens in awake animals following repeated cocaine administration. Repeated cocaine also increased extracellular DA in the nucleus accumbens of chloral hydrate-anesthetized animals in the studies of Pert and Mele (unpublished observation, 1989).

CONCLUSIONS

Clinical observations, systematic studies in volunteers and anecdotal reports all suggest that acute psychomotor stimulant administration models many aspects of acute hypomania or mania, depending on dose and route of administration. Repeated administration of stimulants may model changes that occur with repeated episodes of mania, including increases in severity, dysphoria, rapidity of onset and vulnerability to recurrence. Mesolimbic and mesocortical dopaminergic mechanisms may be critically involved in both the acute and repeated aspects of psychomotor stimulant administration, as revealed by a variety of experimental techniques in the rat. These data are convergent with a substantial body of preclinical and clinical data indicating that dopaminergic mechanisms may be critical to the manic syndrome (Gerner et al., 1976; Post et al., 1980; Jimerson and Post, 1984). Locomotor hyperactivity and the reward value of amphetamine and cocaine (as revealed by i.v. self-administration) may depend in part on dopaminergic mechanisms located in the nucleus accumbens. This area of the brain also appears critical to cocaine-induced behavioral sensitization. In addition, dopaminergic mechanisms in the amygdala may be important to the environmental context component of behavioral sensitization. A variety of other neural substrates are also potentially involved, as revealed by 2-deoxyglucose studies suggesting that the cerebellum may be important in the effects of repeated cocaine administration. *In vivo* dialysis holds great promise for specific documentation of local changes in DA in relationship to on-going behavior in awake animals, and the study of Kalivas et al. (1988) suggests that changes in the nucleus accumbens are involved in cocaine-induced behavioral sensitization.

While animal models obviously have considerable limitations, as outlined in the introduction and elsewhere (Robbins and Sahakian, 1981; Willner, 1986; McKinney, 1989; Kornetsky, 1989), in that they usually cannot fulfil all of the requirements for a model of a given syndrome, the current analysis suggests the heuristic value of the psychomotor stimulant models of acute and repeated episodes of mania. These studies provisionally implicate neuroanatomical and biochemical pathways involved in the acute and chronic phenomena, providing novel hypotheses for preclinical testing as well as areas for focused exploration and direct testing in the clinic. With new imaging techniques currently available, direct tests of the role of mesolimbic DA in manic syndromes are already being performed (Baxter et al., 1988). These regional explorations will greatly extend previous studies of CSF amine metabolites that can only provide global measures of dopaminergic functions (Post et al., 1980). To the extent that autopsy data becomes available in the manic syndrome, perhaps the discrete regions implicated in the stimulant model and in the human PET scan studies can also be directly confirmed or refuted.

Although the various elements of the psychomotor stimulant syndrome may not provide completely valid models for mania, the data accumulated will certainly provide a valid model for the effects of acute and chronic psychomotor stimulants in humans. Given the current pandemic of cocaine use in the US and other countries, such studies of the role of mesolimbic DA substrates in the progressive behavioral and convulsive toxicities of this stimulant should provide important data in their own right, and, hopefully, be productive of suitable treatment interventions. Already, a variety of potential treatments involving dopaminergic mechanisms have been suggested, including bromocriptine, desipramine, carbamazepine, re-uptake blockers, partial DA agonists and flupenthixol (Dackis and Golds, 1985; Gawin and Ellinwood, 1988; Rothman et al., 1989; Giannini et al., 1989; Weiss et al., 1989b; Halikas et al., 1989; Baldessarini, personal communication, 1988). To the extent that these agents are effective in the treatment of different aspects of cocaine syndromes in people (blockade of acute or chronic effects, inhibition of craving, and so on), they may further support a role for DA. To the extent that these emerging treatments of the stimulant syndrome in people converge with effective pharmacological treatments for mania, they will provide added validity for the psychomotor stimulant model of the manic syndrome.

REFERENCES

Aggleton, J.P. and Mishkin, M. (1986) The amygdala: sensory gateway to the emotions. In: Kellerman, H. and Plutchik, R. (eds) *Emotion: Theory, Research, and Experience, Vol. 3.* New York: Academic Press, pp. 281–299.

Ambelas, A. (1979) Psychologically stressful events in the precipitation of manic episodes. *British Journal of Psychiatry* **135**, 15–21.

Angrist, B. and Gershon, S. (1970) The phenomenology of experimentally induced amphetamine psychosis: preliminary observations. *Biological Psychiatry* **2**, 95–107.

Antelman, S.M. and Chiodo, L.A. (1984) Stress: its effect in interactions among biogenic amines and role in the induction and treatment of disease. In: Iversen, L.S., Iversen, S.D. and Snyder, S.H. (eds) *Handbook of Psychopharmacology.* New York: Plenum Press, pp. 279–341.

Antelman, S.M., Eichler, A.J., Black, C.A. and Kocan, D. (1980) Interchangeability of stress and amphetamine in sensitization. *Science* **207**, 329–331.

Aronson, T.A., Shukla, S. and Hirschowitz, J. (1989) Clonazepam treatment of five lithium-refractory patients with bipolar disorder. *American Journal of Psychiatry* **146**, 77–80.

Bakchine, S., Lacomblez, L., Benoit, N., Parisot, D., Chain, F. and Lhermitte, F. (1989) Manic-like state after bilateral orbito-frontal and right temporo-parietal injury: efficacy of clonidine. *Neurology* **39**, 777–781.

Baxter, L.R. Jr, Schwartz, J.M., Phelps, M.E., Mazziotta, J.C., Barrio, J., Rawson, R.A., Engel, J., Guze, B.H., Selin, C. and Sumida, R. (1988) Localization of neurochemical effects of cocaine and other stimulants in the human brain. *Journal of Clinical Psychiatry* **49**, 23–26.

Bell, D.S. (1973) The experimental reproduction of amphetamine psychosis. *Archives of General Psychiatry* **29**, 35–40.

Beninger, R.J. and Hahn, B.L. (1983) Pimozide blocks establishment but not expression of amphetamine-produced environment-specific conditioning. *Science* **220**, 1304–1306.

Beninger, R.J. and Herz, R.S. (1986) Pimozide blocks establishment but not expression of cocaine-produced environment-specific conditioning. *Life Science* **38**, 1425–1431.

Bowers, M.B., Jatlow, P.I. and Mazure, C.M. (1988) Psychogenic drug use and early neuroleptic response. *Abstracts, American College of Neuropsychopharmacology (ACNP).* Vanderbilt University, Nashville, Tennessee, p. 161.

Broekkamp, C.L.E., Phillips, A.G. and Cools, A.S. (1979) Stimulant effects of enkephalin injection into the dopaminergic A10 area. *Nature* **278**, 560–562.

Bunney, B.S. and Moghaddam, B. (1988) Dopamine release in the rat medial prefrontal cortex measured by *in vivo* microdialysis. *Abstracts, American College of Neuropsychopharmacology (ACNP) San Juan, Puerto Rico,* p. 14.

Bunney, W.E. Jr, Brodie, H.K.H., Murphy, D.L. and Goodwin, F.K. (1971) Studies of alpha-methyl-para-tyrosine, L-dopa, and L-tryptophan in depression and mania. *American Journal of Psychiatry* **127**, 872–881.

Carlson, G.A. and Goodwin, F.K. (1973) The stages of mania. A longitudinal analysis of the manic episode. *Archives of General Psychiatry* **28**, 221–228.

Carroll, B.J. and Sharp, P.T. (1971) Rubidium and lithium: opposite effects on amine-mediated excitement. *Science* **172**, 1355–1357.

Chouinard, G. (1988) The use of benzodiazepines in the treatment of manic-depressive illness. *Journal of Clinical Psychiatry* **49**, 15–20.

Chouinard, G., Young, S.N. and Annable, L. (1983) Antimanic effect of clonazapam. *Biological Psychiatry* **18**, 451–466.

Collingridge, G.L. and Bliss, T.V.P. (1987) NMDA receptors—their role in long-term potentiation. *Trends in Neuroscience* **10**, 288–293.

Connell, P.H. and Akkerhuis, G.W. (1958) *Amphetamine Psychosis (Maudsley Monograph No. 5)*. New York: Oxford University Press.

Dackis, C.A. and Gold, M.S. (1985) Pharmacological approaches to cocaine addiction. *Journal of Substance Abuse and Treatment* **2**, 139–145.

Deminiere, J.M., Taghzouti, K., Tassin, J.P., Le Moal, M. and Simon, H. (1988) Increased sensitivity to amphetamine and facilitation of amphetamine self-administration after 6-hydroxydopamine lesions of the amygdala. *Psychopharmacology* **94**, 232–236.

Di Chiara, G. and Imperato, A. (1988) Opposite effects of mu and kappa opiate agonists on dopamine release in the nucleus accumbens and in the dorsal caudate of freely moving rats. *Journal of Pharmacology and Experimental Therapeutics* **244**, 1067–1080.

Ellinwood, E.H. Jr (1967) Amphetamine psychosis I: description of the individuals and process. *Journal of Nervous and Mental Disorders* **144**, 273–283.

Ellinwood, E.H. Jr (1971) 'Accidental conditioning' with chronic methamphetamine intoxication: implications for a theory of drug habituation. *Psychopharmacologia* **21**, 131–138.

Ellinwood, E.H. Jr and Kilbey, M.M. (1975) Amphetamine stereotypy: the influence of environmental factors and prepotent behavioral patterns on its topography and development. *Biological Psychiatry* **10**, 2–16.

Freud, S. (1970) On the general effects of cocaine. *Drug Dependence* **5**, 15.

Gale, K. (1984) Catecholamine-independent behavioral and neurochemical effects of cocaine in rats. In: Sharp, C.W. (ed.) *Mechanisms of Tolerance and Dependence, NIDA Research Monograph Series No. 54*. Washington DC: US Government Printing Office, pp. 323–332.

Gawin, F.H. and Ellinwood, E.H. Jr (1988) Cocaine and other stimulants. Actions, abuse, and treatment. *New England Journal of Medicine* **318**, 1173–1182.

Gay, G.R., Sheppard, C.W., Inaba, D.S. and Newmeyer, J.A. (1973) Cocaine in perspective: 'Gift from the sun god' to 'The rich man's drug'. *Drug Forum* **2**, 409–430.

Gerner, R.H., Post, R.M. and Bunney, W.E. Jr (1976) A dopaminergic mechanism in mania. *American Journal of Psychiatry* **133**, 1177–1180.

Giannini, A.J., Folts, D.J., Feather, J.N. and Sullivan, B.S. (1989) Bromocryptine and amantadine in cocaine detoxification. *Psychiatry Research* **29**, 11–16.

Glue, P., Mele, A., Chiueh, C.C., Nutt, D.J. and Pert, A. (1988) Microdialysis and tissue level studies of presynaptic dopamine function in chronically cocaine-treated rats. *Society for Neuroscience Abstracts* **18**, 740–775.

Goeders, N.E. and Smith, J.E. (1983) Cortical dopaminergic involvement in cocaine reinforcement. *Science* **221**, 773.

Goeders, N.E. and Smith, J.E. (1984) Parameters of intracranial self-administration of cocaine into the medial prefrontal cortex. *National Institute on Drug Abuse Research Monograph, Series 55*, 132–137.

Gold, L.H., Swerdlow, N.R. and Koob, G.F. (1988) The role of mesolimbic dopamine in conditioned locomotion produced by amphetamine. *Behavioral Neuroscience* **102**, 544–552.

Griffith, J.D., Cavanaugh, J.H., Held, J. and Oates, J.A. (1970) Experimental psychosis induced by the administration of d-amphetamine. In: Costa, E. and Garattini, S. (eds) *International Symposium on Amphetamines and Related Compounds*. New York: Raven Press, pp. 897–904.

Grof, E., Haag, M., Grof, P. and Haag, H. (1987) Lithium response and the sequence of episode polarities: preliminary report on a Hamilton sample. *Progress in Neuropsychopharmacology and Biological Psychiatry* **11**, 199–203.

Grof, P., Angst, J. and Haines, T. (1974) The clinical course of depression: practical issues. In: Schattauer, F.K. (ed.) *Symposia Medica Hoest; Classification and Prediction of Outcome of Depression, Vol. 8*. New York: Schattauer, pp. 141–148.

Haag, H., Heidorn, A., Haag, M. and Greil, W. (1987) Sequence of affective polarity and lithium response: preliminary report on Munich sample. *Progress in Neuropsychopharmacology and Biological Psychiatry* **11**, 205–208.

Halikas, J., Kemp, K., Kuhn, K., Carlson, G. and Crea, F. (1989) Carbamazepine for cocaine addiction? *Lancet* **i**, 623–624.

Hall, K.S., Dunner, D.L., Zeller, G. and Fieve, R.R. (1977) Bipolar illness: a prospective study of life events. *Comprehensive Psychiatry* **18**, 497–502.

Hinson, R.E. and Poulos, C.X. (1981) Sensitization to the behavioral effects of cocaine: modification by Pavlovian conditioning. *Pharmacology Biochemistry and Behavior* **15**, 559–562.

Hurd, Y.L. and Ungerstedt, U. (1989a). Cocaine: an *in vivo* microdialysis evaluation of its acute action on dopamine transmission in rat striatum. *Synapse* **3**, 48–54.

Hurd, Y.L. and Ungerstedt, U. (1989b) *In vivo* neurochemical profile of dopamine uptake inhibitors and releasers in rat caudate-putamen. *European Journal of Pharmacology* **166**, 251–260.

Janicak, P.G., Sharma, R.P., Easton, M., Comaty, J.E. and Davis, J.M. (1989) A double-blind, placebo controlled trial of clonidine in the treatment of acute mania. *Psychopharmacology Bulletin* **25**, 243–245.

Janowsky, D.S., El-Yousef, M.K. and Davis, J.M. (1973) Parasympathetic suppression of manic symptoms by physostigmine. *Archives of General Psychiatry* **28**, 542–547.

Jimerson, D.C. and Post, R.M. (1984) Psychomotor stimulants and dopamine agonists in depression. In: Post, R.M. and Ballenger, J.C. (eds) *Neurobiology of Mood Disorders*. Baltimore: Williams and Wilkins, pp. 619–628.

Joffe, R.T., Lippert, G.P., Gray, T.A., Sawa, G. and Horvath, Z. (1987) Mood disorder and multiple sclerosis. *Archives of Neurology* **44**, 376–378.

Jouvent, R., Lecrubier, Y. and Puech, A.J. (1980) Antimanic effect of clonidine. *American Journal of Psychiatry* **137**, 1275–1276.

Jouvent, R., Lecrubier, Y., Hardy, M.C. and Widlocher, D. (1988) Clonidine and neuroleptic-resistant mania. *British Journal of Psychiatry* **152**, 293–294.

Joyce, E.M., Koob, G.F., Strucker, R., Iversen, S.D. and Bloom, F. (1981) The behavioral effects of enkephalin analogues injected into the ventral tegmental area of the globus pallidus. *Brain Research* **221**, 359–370.

Kalivas, P.W. and Duffy, P. (1989) Similar effects of daily cocaine and stress on mesocorticolimbic dopamine neurotransmission in the rat. *Biological Psychiatry* **25**, 913–928.

Kalivas, P.W., Widerlov, E., Stanley, D., Breese, G.R. and Prange, A.J. (1983) Enkephalin action on the mesolimbic system: a dopamine-dependent and a dopamine-independent increase in locomotor activity. *Journal of Pharmacology and Experimental Therapeutics* **227**, 229–237.

Kalivas, P.W., Duffy, P., Dumars, L.A. and Skinner, C. (1988) Behavioral and neurochemical effects of acute and daily cocaine administration in rats. *Journal of Pharmacology and Experimental Therapeutics* **245**, 485–492.

Kelley, A.E., Stinus, L. and Iversen, S.D. (1980) Interaction between D-Ala-Met-enkephalin, A10 dopaminergic neurons, and spontaneous behavior in the rat. *Behavioral Brain Research* **1**, 3–24.

Kelly, P.H. and Iversen, S.D. (1976) Selective 6-OHDA-induced destruction of mesolimbic dopamine neurons: abolition of psychostimulant-induced locomotor activity in rats. *European Journal of Pharmacology* **40**, 45–56.

Kelly, P.H., Sevior, P.W. and Iversen, S.D. (1975) Amphetamine and apomorphine responses in the rat following 6-OHDA lesions of the nucleus accumbens, septi and corpus striatum. *Brain Research* **94**, 507–522.

Kilbey, M.M. and Ellinwood, E.H. Jr (1977) Reversed tolerance to stimulant-induced abnormal behavior. *Life Science* **20**, 1063–1076.

Klimek, V., Krieger, R., Ryan, C.N. and Scheel-Kruger, J. (1989) The role of dopamine and glutamate in the nucleus accumbens and striatum for external and internal cue directed behaviour in the Morris water maze. *Behavioural Pharmacology* **1** (suppl 11).

Kornetsky, C. (1989) Animal models: promises and problems. In: Koob, G.F., Ehlers, C.L. and Kupfer, D.J. (eds) *Animal Models of Depression*. Boston: Birkhauser, pp. 18–29.

Kraepelin, E. (1921) *Manic-Depressive Insanity and Paranoia*. Edinburgh: E. and S. Livingstone.

Kubacki, A. (1986) Male and female mania. *Canadian Journal of Psychiatry* **31**, 70–72.

Kukopulos, A., Reginaldi, D., Laddomada, P., Floris, G., Serra, G. and Tondo, L. (1980) Course of the manic-depressive cycle and changes caused by treatment. *Pharmakopsychiatrica* **13**, 156–167.

Lewin, L. (1931) *Phantastica: Narcotic and Stimulating Drugs*. New York: E.P. Dutton and Company.

McKinney, W.T. (1989) Basis of development of animal models in psychiatry: an overview. In: Koob, G.F., Ehlers, C.L. and Kupfer, D.J. (eds) *Animal Models of Depression*. Boston: Birkhkauser, pp. 3–17.

Murray, E.A. and Mishkin, M. (1985) Amygdalectomy impairs cross-modal association in monkeys. *Science* **228**, 604–606.

Overmier, J.B. and Patterson, J. (1988) Animal models of human psychopathology. *Animal Models of Psychiatric Disorders* **1**, 1–35.

Pettit, H.O., Ettenberg, A., Bloom, F.E. and Koob, G.F. (1984) Destruction of dopamine in the nucleus accumbens selectively attenuates cocaine but not heroin self-administration in rats. *Psychopharmacology* **84**, 167–173.

Pijnenburg, A.J.J., Honig, W.M.M., van der Heyden, J.A.M. and van Rossum, J.M. (1976) Effects of chemical stimulation of the mesolimbic dopamine system upon locomotor activity. *European Journal of Pharmacology* **35**, 45–58.

Porrino, L.J. and Kornetsky, C. (1988) The effects of cocaine on local cerebral metabolic activity. *NIDA Research Monograph* **88**, 92–106.

Post, R.M. (1975) Cocaine psychoses: a continuum model. *American Journal of Psychiatry* **132**, 225–231.

Post, R.M. (1981a) Biochemical theories of mania. In: Belmaker, R.H. and van Praag, H.M. (eds) *Mania: An Evolving Concept*. New York: Spectrum, pp. 217–265.

Post, R.M. (1981b) Psychomotor stimulants as activators of normal and pathological behavior: implications for the excesses of mania. In: Mule, S.J. (ed.) *Behavior in Excess: An Examination of the Volitional Disorders.* New York: Macmillan Publishing Company, pp. 64–94.

Post, R.M. and Contel, N.R. (1983) Human and animal studies of cocaine: implications for development of behavioral pathology. In: Creese, I. (ed.) *Stimulants: Neurochemical, Behavioral, and Clinical Perspective.* New York: Raven Press, pp. 169–203.

Post, R.M. and Rose, H. (1976) Increasing effects of repetitive cocaine administration in the rat. *Nature* **260**, 731–732.

Post, R.M. and Weiss, S.R.B. (1988) Stimulant-induced behavioral sensitization: a model for neuroleptic nonresponsiveness (commentary to the paper by R.J. Beninger). In: Simon, P., Soubrie, P. and Wildlocher, D. (eds) *Animal Models of Psychiatric Disorders.* Basel: S. Karger, pp. 52–60.

Post, R.M., Jimerson, D.C., Bunney, W.E. Jr and Goodwin, F.K. (1980) Dopamine and mania: behavioral and biochemical effects of the dopamine receptor blocker pimozide. *Psychopharmacology* **67**, 297–305.

Post, R.M., Ballenger, J.C., Rey, A.C. and Bunney, W.E. Jr (1981a) Slow and rapid onset of manic episodes: implications for underlying biology. *Psychiatry Research* **4**, 229–237.

Post, R.M., Lockfeld, A., Squillace, K.M. and Contel, N.R. (1981b) Drug–environment interaction: context dependency of cocaine-induced behavioral sensitization. *Life Science* **28**, 755–760.

Post, R.M., Ballenger, J.C., Uhde, T.W. and Bunney, W.E. Jr (1984a) Efficacy of carbamazepine in manic-depressive illness: implications for underlying mechanisms. In: Post, R.M. and Ballenger, J.C. (eds) *Neurobiology of Mood Disorders.* Baltimore: Williams and Wilkins, pp. 777–816.

Post, R.M., Weiss, S.R.B. and Pert, A. (1984b) Differential effects of carbamazepine and lithium on sensitization and kindling. *Progress in Neuropsychopharmacology and Biological Psychiatry* **8**, 425–434.

Post, R.M., Uhde, T.W., Roy-Byrne, P.P. and Joffe, R.T. (1987a) Correlates of antimanic response to carbamazepine. *Psychiatry Research* **21**, 71–83.

Post, R.M., Weiss, S.R.B., Pert, A. and Uhde, T.W. (1987b) Chronic cocaine administration: sensitization and kindling effects. In: Raskin, A. and Fisher, S. (eds) *Cocaine: Clinical and Biobehavioral Aspects.* New York: Oxford University Press, pp. 109–173.

Post, R.M., Roy-Byrne, P.P. and Uhde, T.W. (1988) Graphic representation of the life course of illness in patients with affective disorder. *American Journal of Psychiatry* **145**, 844–848.

Post, R.M., Rubinow, D.R., Uhde, T.W., Roy-Byrne, P.P., Linnoila, M., Rosoff, A. and Cowdry, R.W. (1989) Dysphoric mania: clinical and biological correlates. *Archives of General Psychiatry* **46**, 353–358.

Post, R.M., Altshuler, L.L., Ketter, T., Denicoff, K. and Weiss, S.R.B. (1991) Antiepileptic drugs in affective illness: clinical and theoretical implications. In: Smith, D.B., Treiman, D.M. and Trimble, M.R. (eds) *Advances in Neurology. Vol. 55: Proceedings of the International Symposium on Neurobehavioral Problems in Epilepsy: Scientific Basis, Insights, and Hypotheses.* New York: Raven Press (in press).

Robbins, T.W. and Sahakian, B.J. (1981) Animal models of mania. In: Belmaker, R.H. and van Praag, H.M. (eds) *Mania: An Evolving Concept.* New York: Spectrum, pp. 143–216.

Roberts, D.C.S., Koob, G.F., Klonoff, P. and Fibiger, H.C. (1980) Extinction and recovery of cocaine self-administration following 6-hydroxydopamine lesions of the nucleus accumbens. *Pharmacology Biochemistry and Behavior* **12**, 781–787.

Robinson, R.G. (1989) The use of an animal model to study post-stroke depression. In: Koob, G.F., Ehlers, C.L. and Kupfer, D.J. (eds) *Animal Models of Depression*. Boston: Birkhauser, pp. 74–98.

Robinson, T.E. and Becker, J.B. (1986) Enduring changes in brain and behavior produced by chronic amphetamine administration: a review and evaluation of animal models of amphetamine psychosis. *Brain Research Reviews* **11**, 157–198.

Robinson, R.G. and Justice, A. (1986) Mechanisms of lateralized hyperactivity following focal brain injury in the rat. *Pharmacology Biochemistry and Behavior* **25**, 263–267.

Rothman, R.B., Mele, A., Reid, A.A., Akunne, H., Greig, N., Thurkauf, A., Rice, K.C. and Pert, A. (1989) Tight binding dopamine reuptake inhibitors as cocaine antagonists: a strategy for drug development. *FEBS Letters* **257**, 341–344.

Roy-Byrne, P.P., Post, R.M., Uhde, T.W., Porcu, T. and Davis, D.D. (1985) The longitudinal course of recurrent affective illness: life chart data from research patients at NIMH. *Acta Psychiatrica Scandinavica* **71**, 5–34.

Schiff, S.R. (1982) Conditioned dopaminergic activity. *Biological Psychiatry* **17**, 135–154.

Segal, D.S. (1975) Behavioral and neurochemical correlates of repeated d-amphetamine administration. In: Mandell, A.J. (ed.) *Advances in Biochemical Psychopharmacology XIII: Neurobiological Mechanisms of Adaptation and Behavior*. New York: Raven Press, pp. 247–262.

Sherer, M.A., Kumor, K.M., Cone, E.J. and Jaffe, J.H. (1988) Suspiciousness induced by four-hour intravenous infusions of cocaine. Preliminary findings. *Archives of General Psychiatry* **45**, 673–677.

Shuster, L., Yu, G. and Bates, A. (1977) Sensitization to cocaine stimulation in mice. *Psychopharmacology* **52**, 185–190.

Silverstone, T. and Romans-Clarkson, S. (1989) Bipolar affective disorder: causes and prevention of relapse. *British Journal of Psychiatry* **154**, 321–335.

Squillace, K., Post, R.M., Savard, R. and Erwin, M. (1984) Life charting of the longitudinal course of recurrent affective illness. In: Post, R.M. and Ballenger, J.C. (eds) *Neurobiology of Mood Disorders*. Baltimore: Williams and Wilkins, pp. 38–59.

Stripling, J.S. and Ellinwood, E.H. Jr (1977) Sensitization to cocaine following chronic administration in the rat. In: Ellinwood, E.H. and Kilbey, M.M. (eds) *Cocaine and Other Stimulants*. New York: Plenum Press, pp. 327–351.

Suomi, S.J., Kraemer, G.W., Baysinger, C.M. and De Lizio, R.D. (1981) Inherited and experimental factors associated with individual differences in anxious behavior displayed by rhesus monkeys. In: Klein, D.F. and Rabbin, J. (eds) *Anxiety: New Research and Changing Concepts*. New York: Raven Press, pp. 179–200.

Tadokoro, S. and Kuribara, H. (1986) Reverse tolerance to the ambulation-increasing effect of methamphetamine in mice as an animal model of amphetamine psychosis. *Psychopharmacology Bulletin* **22**, 757–762.

Tilson, H.A. and Rech, R.H. (1973) Conditioned drug effects and absence of tolerance to d-amphetamine induced motor activity. *Pharmacology Biochemistry and Behavior* **1**, 149–153.

Van Hoesen, G.W. (1985) Neural systems of the non-primate forebrain implicated in memory. *Annals of the New York Academy of Science* **444**, 97–112.

Weiss, S.R.B., Post, R.M., Pert, A., Woodward, R. and Murman, D. (1989a) Role of conditioning in cocaine-induced behavioral sensitization: differential effect of haloperidol. *Pharmacology Biochemistry and Behavior* **34**, 655–661.

Weiss, S.R.B., Post, R.M., Szele, F., Woodward, R. and Nierenberg, J. (1989b) Chronic carbamazepine inhibits the development of local-anesthetic seizures kindled by cocaine and lidocaine. *Brain Research* **497**, 72–79.

Weiss, S.R.B., Post, R.M., Costello, M., Nutt, D.J. and Tandeciarz, S. (1990) Carbamazepine retards the development of cocaine-kindled seizures but not sensitization to cocaine-induced hyperactivity. *Neuropsychopharmacology* **3**, 273–281.

White, F.J., Henry, D.J. and Ackerman, J.M. (1989) Electrophysiological effects of repeated cocaine administration on the mesoaccumbens dopamine system. *Behavioural Pharmacology* **1**, 42 (suppl 1).

Willner, P. (1984) The validity of animal models of depression. *Psychopharmacology* **83**, 1–16.

Willner, P. (1986) Validation criteria for animal models of human mental disorders: learned helplessness as a paradigm case. *Progress in Neuropsychopharmacology and Biological Psychiatry* **10**, 677–690.

Winslow, J.T., Newman, J.D. and Insel, T.R. (1989) CRH and alpha-helical-CRH modulate behavioral measures of arousal in monkeys. *Pharmacology Biochemistry and Behavior* **32**, 919–926.

Woods, J.H. and Downs, D.A. (1973) Psychopharmacology of cocaine. In: *Drug Use in America: Problem in Perspective, Technical Papers of the Second Report of the National Commission on Marihuana and Drug Abuse, Appendix 1, Patterns and Consequences of Drug Use*. Washington DC: US Government Printing Office, p. 116.

Wyatt, R.J., Alexander, R.C., Egan, M.S. and Kirsh, D.G. (1988) Schizophrenia: just the facts. What do we know, how well do we know it? *Schizophrenia Research* **1**, 3–18.

18

Individual Vulnerability to Drug Self-Administration: Action of Corticosterone on Dopaminergic Systems as a Possible Pathophysiological Mechanism

PIER VINCENZO PIAZZA, JEAN-MARIE DEMINIÈRE,
STEFANIA MACCARI, MICHEL LE MOAL,
PIERRE MORMÈDE AND HERVÉ SIMON

Psychobiologie des Comportements Adaptatifs, INSERM U. 259, Université de Bordeaux II, Domaine de Carreire, rue Camille Saint-Saëns, 33077 Bordeaux Cedex, France

INTRODUCTION

The Dopaminergic System and Physiological/Pathological Behavior

Current knowledge of the physiological role of dopaminergic (DA) neurons indicates that these cells act primarily as a modulatory network rather than having a specific function (Simon and Le Moal, 1984, 1988; see also Cador et al., Chapter 9, this volume). Thus, modification of the activity of these neurons affects a wide range of animal behaviors (Ungerstedt, 1971; Le Moal et al., 1975; Marshal et al., 1980; Robbins and Everitt, 1982; Piazza et al., 1987, 1988). Three lines of evidence support a modulatory role. First, the behavioral deficit induced by lesion of the DA afferents to a given structure resembles the result of deregulation of the whole structure (Simon and Le Moal, 1984, 1988). Second, lesion of the DA projection in a structure

The Mesolimbic Dopamine System: From Motivation to Action.
Edited by P. Willner and J. Scheel-Krüger

© 1991 John Wiley & Sons Ltd

does not suppress the function of that structure. Thus, it is possible to reverse the deficit induced by a DA lesion by administration of DA agonists, intracerebral graft of embryonic DA neurons (Dunnett et al., 1983, Herman et al., 1985, 1988), and environmental conditions increasing DA liberation (Taghzouti et al., 1986). Third, there are interactive relationships between different components of the DA system. For example, an increase in DA activity in the frontal cortex or in the amygdala can induce a corresponding decrease in the nucleus accumbens (Louilot et al., 1986, 1989), and the activation of A10 DA neurons may inhibit behaviors mediated by A9 DA neurons, such as circling (Piazza et al., 1989a).

The modulatory role that DA neurons exercise on different nervous system functions may explain the efficacy of DA replacement therapy in a variety of human pathological conditions involving sensorimotor (Hornykiewicz, 1963), emotional (Pert et al., 1978; Major et al., 1979) and cognitive functions (Creese et al., 1976; Seeman, 1980). Surprisingly, given the wide-ranging relationships between DA and psychopathology, there is little experimental evidence on how a change in DA activity induces a psychopathological state. Part of the difficulty in the search for psychopathological mechanisms involving DA cells may relate to the difficulty of devising suitable experimental models of human psychopathology and/or to our incomplete understanding of the role of DA neurons in behavior.

Life Experiences, Dopaminergic Neurons and Corticosterone

The DA system is implicated in the physiological response to 'stressful' environmental conditions. In animals, DA neurons participate in three different ways in the response to intense and painful environmental stimulation, which is considered as a model of stress. First, stress activates these neurons. A number of studies have shown that experiences such as electric footshock, restraint and tail-pinch increase DA release (Thierry et al., 1976; Blanc et al., 1980; D'Angio et al., 1987; Dunn, 1988; Roth et al., 1988). Second, certain behaviors, often described as adjunctive behaviors (Falk, 1977; Wetherington, 1982), exhibited by animals in response to particular environmental influences depend on the integrity of DA systems. Thus, the polydipsia displayed by food-deprived rats on a fixed-interval food reinforcement schedule (Falk, 1969), or the compulsive eating induced by a mild pinching of the tail (Antelman et al., 1976) are disrupted by DA lesions (Antelman et al., 1975; Robbins and Koob, 1980). Third, repeated environmental, as well as pharmacological, activation of DA cells augments (sensitizes) the behavioral (Antelman and Eichler, 1979; Antelman et al., 1980; Herman et al., 1984; Robinson, 1984; Robinson and Becker, 1986; Antelman, 1988) and biochemical (Robinson and Becker, 1982; Robinson et al., 1985, 1987) responses of DA neurons to subsequent activation.

Interestingly, this change in DA activity also seems to influence the propensity of individual animals to perform displacement activities such as schedule-induced polydipsia (Mittelman et al., 1986) and tail-pinch-induced eating (Antelman et al., 1980). The intensity of such behaviors is enhanced by repeated exposure to psychostimulants. Thus, DA neurons not only participate in the responses to acute environmental activations, but may also be a substrate for the influence of past experiences on the subject's current response to the environment.

Although certain environmental and pharmacological stimuli appear to be able to modify permanently the influence of DA activity on behavior, it is still not clear how this is mediated. Steroid hormones, and particularly corticosterone, may be the link. Three different lines of evidence support this idea. First, plasma and brain levels of corticosterone are modified by the environmental and pharmacological stimulations that alter DA activity. For example, corticosterone levels are increased by a wide variety of experiences such as a novel environment, immobilization, electric footshocks and rearing conditions (Bohus et al., 1982; Dantzer and Mormède, 1983; Sachser, 1986), as well as by administration of amphetamine (Knych and Eisenberg, 1979). Second, DA cells have glucocorticoid receptors (Härfstrand et al., 1986). Third, the activity of DA neurons is modified by injection of corticosterone (Imperato et al., 1989). An interaction between corticosterone and DA neurons could thus serve as a biological substrate, mediating the effects of stressful experiences on behavior.

Vulnerability to Acquisition of Amphetamine Self-Administration: an Experimental Model for the Study of Pathological Behavior

To make progress in the analysis of a possible role of the interaction between environmental stimulations, steroids and DA in behavioral pathology, an animal model that enables the independent manipulation of each factor is essential. Furthermore, such a model must also be relevant to human pathology. Fortunately, such a model is available, and it has its origin in human deviant behavior. Self-administration of psychoactive drugs can be viewed as a response to unfavorable environmental conditions or to certain psychopathological states (Khantzian, 1985; Marlatt et al., 1988). Animals will also self-administer psychoactive drugs (Weeks, 1962), and this behavior involves DA transmission (Koob and Bloom, 1988). Therefore, self-administration provides a good model for the study of the mechanisms involving interactions between life events, steroids and DA function.

The clinical study of addiction has indicated that a main factor influencing drug intake in humans is an individual's vulnerability to the reinforcing effects of the drug. As stated by O'Brien et al. (1986): '... Some addicts go for months or years using heroin or cocaine only on week-ends before becoming a daily (addicted) user. Others report that they had such an intense positive response that they became addicted with the first dose...'. We thus focused our attention on the problem of drug vulnerability.

The dopaminergic mesolimbic system is considered to be the main cerebral site mediating the acquisition (Deminière et al., 1988a) and maintenance (Koob and Bloom, 1988) of amphetamine self-administration. An increase in vulnerability to acquire amphetamine self-administration is associated with an increased reactivity of DA neurons to psychostimulants. For example, a lesion of A10 neurons that induces an enhanced psychomotor response to amphetamine also increases the vulnerability to self-administer this drug (Le Moal et al., 1979; Deminière et al., 1984). Opposite changes of DA activity in the nucleus accumbens (increase) and in the frontal cortex (decrease) are also thought to mediate the increases in psychomotor reactivity to psychostimulants and vulnerability to self-administer such drugs (Deminière et al., 1988a, 1989). Lesion of the amygdala with 6-hydroxydopamine (6-OHDA) (Deminière et al., 1988b) or an electrolytic lesion of the ventral raphe nuclei (Simon et al., 1980), both of which induce this biochemical pattern, also increase both the vulnerability to self-administer amphetamine and the psychomotor effects of this drug.

In this chapter, the interactions between life events, corticosterone and DA are examined as a possible biological substrate of vulnerability to self-administer amphetamine. Three working hypotheses have underpinned our approach: (1) Certain experiences may increase the vulnerability to acquire amphetamine self-administration by modifying the reactivity of mesencephalic DA neurons; (2) vulnerability may not only be experimentally induced, but may also be predicted in individual animals by assessing their reactivity to environmental and pharmacological stimulations; and (3) steroid hormones may influence the psychomotor and reinforcing effects of amphetamine.

METHODOLOGICAL APPROACHES

Drug Self-Administration as an Experimental Model of Drug Addiction

Animals self-administer a large number of compounds, including all drugs that induce addiction in man. For this reason, self-administration has been proposed as a tool for the investigation of the potential addictive properties of new psychoactive compounds as well as for the experimental study of addiction (Weeks, 1962; Pickens and Harris, 1968; Schuster and Thompson, 1969).

In this model, a chronic intracardiac catheter, exiting in the mild scapular region, connects the blood system of a freely moving animal to a syringe-driven pump. During self-administration sessions, the subject, by switching on the pump, self-infuses the contents of the syringe. The pump may be switched on by pressing a lever or by the introduction of the animal's nose in a hole in the wall of the cage (the latter device was employed in our experiments). The self-administration cage also contains an identical device that does not activate the pump (defined as inactive), which is utilized to record exploration of the environment and locomotor activity. An animal is considered to perform an active self-administration only when the number of responses on the active device is significantly higher than that on the inactive device (95 per cent confidence limits).

Two different paradigms of self-administration are commonly used, retention and acquisition. The two paradigms differ in their experimental procedure, and address different questions. In the retention paradigm, higher doses of drug are delivered at each injection, the session is of relatively long duration, and the behavior is studied after stabilization. The retention paradigm has been employed to investigate the neural basis maintaining self-administration behavior, especially the phenomenon of dependence. In the acquisition paradigm, attention is focused on the first days of contact with the drug. Lower doses are used, and the sessions last only 30 minutes. The acquisition paradigm has been used to study the propensity of the individual to develop self-administration (Deminière et al., 1989), and individual differences in vulnerability to drug reinforcing effects are readily observed using this paradigm (Piazza et al., 1989b). The acquisition paradigm was therefore used in all our experiments on individual vulnerability to drug self-administration.

Locomotor Response to Amphetamine as a Behavioral Index of DA Activity in the Mesolimbic System

The relationship between the reinforcing properties of amphetamine and DA activity in the mesolimbic system is an interesting aspect of the influence of experience or steroids on DA systems. Although amphetamine acts on other aminergic systems of the brain, the locomotor response to this drug seems specifically dependent on DA. Furthermore, amphetamine-induced locomotion seems to be mediated specifically by activation of mesolimbic DA projections (Creese and Iversen, 1975). In the following experiments, amphetamine-induced self-administration was correlated with the psycho-motor effects of this drug. Locomotor activity was measured automatically in a circular corridor (10 cm wide and 70 cm in diameter) by four photoelectric cells placed at the perpendicular axes of the apparatus.

LIFE EVENTS, THE DA SYSTEM AND AMPHETAMINE SELF-ADMINISTRATION

It has been found that various environmental stimulations modify the reactivity of animals to psychostimulants. For example, after repeated exposure to tail-pinch (Antelman et al., 1980) or electric footshock (Herman et al., 1984), rats exhibit an enhanced response to amphetamine. It has been suggested that the repeated activation of DA neurons by environmental stimuli may sensitize the response of these cells to a new challenge (Antelman et al., 1980; Robinson and Becker, 1986). The main evidence that certain experiences enhance the response to amphetamine by stimulating DA neurons is that repeated pharmacological activation of these cells (by intracerebral injections) increases the response to this drug in a similar way to the environmental stimulation (Kalivas and Weber, 1988). Comparison of the effects of repeated environmental stimulation and amphetamine injections may thus represent a useful model for investigation of the influence of experience-induced change in DA systems on the vulnerability to develop drug-taking behavior.

A repeated light pinching of the rat's tail was selected as the environmental stimulus. This procedure induces an increase in DA release in the nucleus accumbens (D'Angio et al., 1987) that is thought to be implicated in self-administration behavior (Koob and Bloom, 1988). Repeated treatment with tail-pinch (four 1-minute daily sessions for 15 days) induced an increase of both the locomotor response to amphetamine (1 mg/kg i.p.) and self-administration of amphetamine (Figure 1A).

Repeated treatment with amphetamine (four injections, 1.5 mg/kg i.p. 4-day intervals) had very similar effects on both responses (Figure 1B), and when the effects of the two treatments, expressed as a percentage increase over controls, were compared, no difference was found for either amphetamine-induced self-administration or locomotor activity (Figure 2).

The effects of other life experiences on the psychomotor and reinforcing effects of amphetamine have also been studied in our laboratory. Among these, social competition appears to have a strong influence on the acquisition of amphetamine self-administration. Colonies of male rats housed with female rats (colonies with a higher level of competition) have a higher level of acquisition of amphetamine self-administration ($F(1,40)=16.33$, $P<0.0001$) than colonies of male rats without females (colonies considered to be at a low level of competition). Early experience also seems to influence amphetamine self-administration. Thus, a significant increase in the acquisition of self-administration of this drug ($F(5,140)=3.9$, $P<0.001$) has been found in adult rats (4-month-old) whose mothers had been submitted to a restraint procedure (half an hour twice a day) during the third and fourth weeks of gestation. In both models, an increase in the reinforcing properties

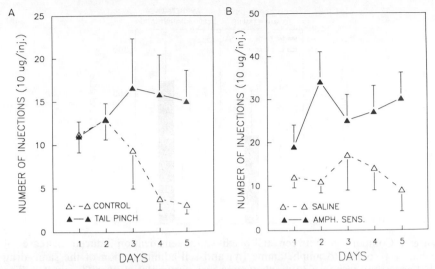

Figure 1. A, Self-administration of amphetamine (10 μg/injection) after repeated (15 days, four trials of 1-minute per day) tail-pinch and in control subjects. The two groups differed over the 5 days (F(1,21)=2.85, *P*<0.05). Locomotor responses to amphetamine (1 mg/kg i.p.) were also increased by tail-pinch (results not shown: control, 580±40; tail-pinch, 830±60; F(1,21)=3.42, *P*<0.05). **B**, Self-administration of amphetamine (10 μg/injection) after repeated injections (four injections 3 days apart) of amphetamine (1.5 mg/kg i.p.) or saline (0.9 per cent NaCl). The two groups differed over the 5 days (F(1,28)=4.25, *P*=0.02). Locomotor responses to amphetamine were also increased by repeated administration (results not shown: first injection, 1512±30; fourth injection, 2245±80; F(1,15)=16.8, *P*<0.001)

of amphetamine accompanied an increase in the psychomotor effect of the drug.

In conclusion, these results indicate that experience can increase the vulnerability to acquire amphetamine self-administration. Furthermore, self-administration was always studied at least 1 week after the end of the stressful condition. This lends support to the notion that the lasting effect of experiences may be 'stored' in DA neurons.

FACTORS PREDICTIVE OF INDIVIDUAL VULNERABILITY TO ACQUIRE AMPHETAMINE SELF-ADMINISTRATION

The previous results suggested that animals with a higher locomotor response to amphetamine should also exhibit a higher vulnerability to self-administer this drug. Given the interchangeable effects of environmental and pharmacological stimulation on amphetamine response, a behavioral parameter expressing the reactivity to environmental stimulation might predict an

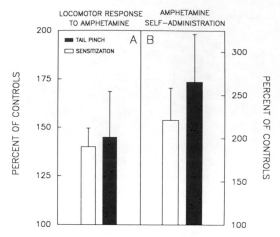

Figure 2. Comparison between tail-pinch- and sensitization-induced increase of locomotor response to amphetamine (**A**) and self-administration of the same drug (**B**). Locomotor response to amphetamine was accumulated over 90 minutes. The two treatments were compared on the last day of self-administration. No differences were found between the increase (expressed as percentage of controls) induced by tail-pinch and amphetamine sensitization on either variable

individual's vulnerability to amphetamine self-administration. The reactivity to a novel environment was chosen for these experiments since: (**1**) animals that have received strong environmental stimulation have higher locomotor activity in a novel environment (West and Michael, 1988); (**2**) the experience of a novel environment is employed as an animal model of psychological stress (Mormède, 1983), as it induces a similar release of corticosterone to that induced by electric footshock (Dantzer and Mormède, 1983); and (**3**) DA activity is involved in the behavioral response to a novel environment (Robbins and Everitt, 1982).

The novel environment consisted of a circular corridor (10 cm wide and 70 cm diameter). The locomotor response was recorded for 2 hours and the number of photocell counts cumulated over this period was used as an index of the individual's reactivity to the novel environment. The activity scores of individual animals ranged from 120 to 1200 photocell counts. The locomotor response to an acute amphetamine injection was studied in two different groups of animals (doses of 0.3 mg/kg i.v. or 1.5 mg/kg i.p.). Two variables were used to characterize the psychomotor effects of amphetamine: first, the reactivity to the drug, expressed by the locomotor response accumulated over the interval required for the drug to express its maximum effect (10 minutes for the 0.3 mg/kg i.v. dose, 30 minutes for the 1.5 mg/kg i.p. dose); and second, the total effect of the drug, expressed by the locomotor response cumulated over the whole period in which amphetamine induced an increase in locomotor activity (90 minutes and, 180 minutes, respectively). Locomotor activity in the novel environment was positively correlated with the reactivity to amphetamine at both doses of the drug (for 0.3 mg/kg i.v., $r=0.75$, $P<0.001$; for 1.5 mg/kg i.p., $r=0.47$, $P=0.02$), but the total response to the drug was positively correlated with novelty-induced locomotion only when the 0.3 mg/kg i.v. dose was used ($r=0.84$, $P<0.01$). The reinforcing effect of amphetamine was evaluated from the intake of the drug accumulated over 5 days of testing for self-administration. Locomotor activity in the novel environment and the drug intake during self-administration were also positively correlated ($r=0.62$, $P<0.01$).

Differences for all the variables studied were found between two groups of animals singled out on the basis of their locomotor activity in the novel environment. The first group (high responders, HR) contained all the animals with an activity score above the median, and the second (low responders, LR) contained all other animals. Thus, HR rats which showed a higher locomotor response in the novel environment (Figure 3A) also showed a greater psychomotor reactivity to 0.3 mg/kg i.v. (Figure 3B) and 1.5 mg/kg i.p. (Figure 3C) of amphetamine, as well as a greater vulnerability to acquire amphetamine self-administration (Figure 4).

This division in HR and LR animals may be of value for investigation of the biological basis of vulnerability to acquire amphetamine self-administration. One insight provided by this model concerns the relevance of a sensitized state of DA neurons to the etiology of vulnerability to self-administration. Repeated exposure to amphetamine may augment the vulnerability to self-administration of resistant subjects, or may simply increase intake in already vulnerable animals. To answer this question, a group of animals was first categorized according to their locomotor response to novelty, and then repeatedly injected with amphetamine (four injections, 1.5 mg/kg i.p. 3-day intervals) or saline.

The two groups of animals responded differently to repeated exposure to amphetamine. Amphetamine sensitization increased the locomotor response of LR groups to amphetamine, whereas it did not change the response of the HR animals (Figure 5) which behaved as if they were already sensitized. In addition, amphetamine sensitization also increased the vulnerability to acquire amphetamine self-administration in the LR group (Figure 6).

In conclusion, these results indicate that novelty-induced locomotor activity may represent a non-invasive factor predictive of individual reactivity to the psychomotor and reinforcing effect of amphetamine. Furthermore, a sensitized state of DA neuronal transmission may be an important determinant of individual vulnerability to acquire amphetamine self-administration.

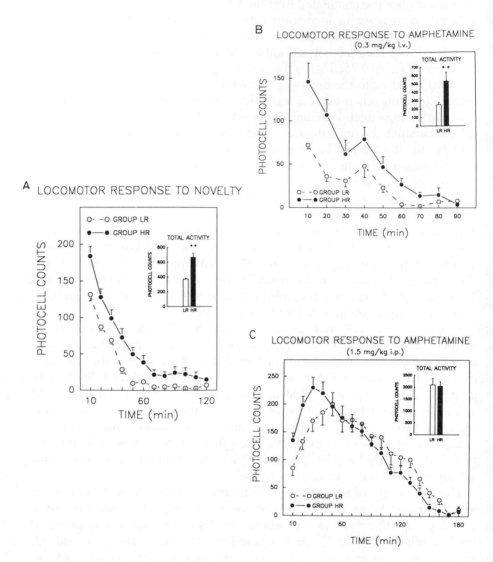

Figure 3. A, Locomotor activity in a novel environment of LR (low responders) and HR (high responders) groups of rats. The two groups differed in total locomotor activity (F(1,28)=17.3; P=0.0003). **B**, Locomotor activity after amphetamine (0.3 mg/kg IV) of the LR (low responders in the novel environment) and HR (high responders in the novel environment) groups. HR rats exhibited a stronger response to the drug (F(1,14)=7.91, P<0.01). **C**, Locomotor activity after amphetamine (1.5 mg/kg i.p.) of the LR (low responders in the novel environment) and HR (high responders in the novel environment) groups. HR rats had a faster locomotor response to the drug (ANOVA Group × Time interaction, F(7,476)=2.23; P=0.003)

AMPHETAMINE SELF—ADMINISTRATION

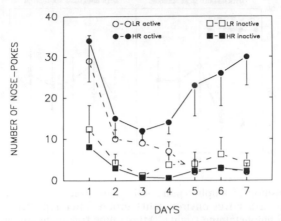

Figure 4. Amphetamine self-administration (10 µg/injection) of LR (low responders in the novel environment) and HR (high responders in the novel environment) groups. The two groups differed in their acquisition of amphetamine self-administration. While both groups discriminated between the active and inactive holes in the first 2 days of testing, only HR animals acquired and maintained self-administration of amphetamine (ANOVA Group × Hole interaction, F(1,18)=11.94, P=0.002)

AMPHETAMINE SENSITIZATION

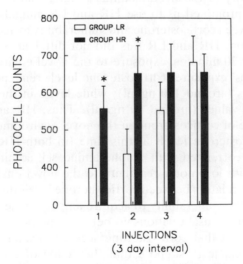

Figure 5. Effect of amphetamine sensitization on amphetamine-induced locomotor activity in groups of animals defined by their locomotor activity in a novel environment (LR, low responders; HR, high responders). The difference in locomotor activity between the two groups (accumulated over 30 minutes) was abolished over the four injections. *P<0.05(ANOVA)

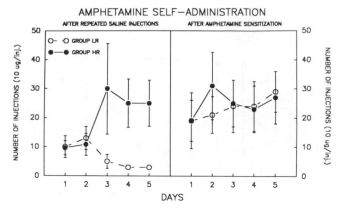

Figure 6. Acquisition of amphetamine self-administration of LR and HR (low and high responders in a novel environment) groups after repeated administration of saline (left) and amphetamine (right). After saline treatment, the groups differed in their acquisition of self-administration, both in terms of total amphetamine administered over 5 days ($F(1,18)=7.21$; $P=0.01$), and in terms of the number of injections over the different days ($F(4,48)=3.81$; $P=0.01$). After amphetamine sensitization, there was no difference between the two groups.

CORTICOSTERONE AND AMPHETAMINE-INDUCED BEHAVIORS

The high reactivity of the hypothalamus–pituitary–adrenal axis to environmental changes prompted us to use HR and LR animals to investigate the relationship between corticosterone and vulnerability to acquire amphetamine self-administration. HR and LR rats did not differ in corticosterone levels before and after 30 minutes' exposure to the novel environment. However, after 120 minutes' exposure, corticosterone levels remained high in the HR group of animals (around 180 ng/ml), while levels in the LR rats returned to pre-exposure values (around 40 ng/ml). Thus, HR animals displayed a sustained release of corticosterone in the novel environment ($F(1,14)=4.93$, $P<0.05$). Corticosterone levels at this time (in both HR and LR animals) were positively correlated with amphetamine self-administration ($r=0.63$, $P<0.01$), and with locomotor reactivity to the novel environment ($r=0.62$, $P<0.01$). The correlation between corticosterone levels during environmental stimulation and the vulnerability to acquire amphetamine self-administration does not imply any causal relationship between the two. Nevertheless, given the activating effect that corticosterone seems to exercise on DA neurons, it is not unreasonable to suppose that the action of this hormone on DA cells may influence the psychomotor and reinforcing effect of amphetamine. The difference between HR and LR animals may provide a clue to the role of corticosterone on the intensity of an individual's response to amphetamine.

Although HR animals have higher levels of corticosterone than LR rats after 120 minutes' exposure to novelty, there was no difference in corticosterone liberation between the two groups in the first 30 minutes of exposure to novelty. Thus, if the locomotor response to amphetamine is dependent on corticosterone levels, the differences between the two groups in amphetamine-induced locomotion should be greater if the drug is injected after 120 minutes of exposure to novelty than when it is injected after 30 minutes. Although the HR animals always had a higher response to amphetamine, the extent of the difference between the two groups did depend on the time of injection. When amphetamine was injected after 30 minutes of exposure to novelty there was a 42.8 per cent difference between the HR and LR animals, which increased to 138.5 per cent when the drug was injected after 120 minutes (Figure 7).

A second component of the influence of corticosterone on the locomotor response to amphetamine can be investigated by administration of corticosterone after a period of habituation in the test-apparatus to allow endogenous corticosterone levels to return to normal. For this experiment, rats were implanted with intracardiac catheters, and, after a recovery period of 5 days, were tested for their locomotor response to amphetamine in the

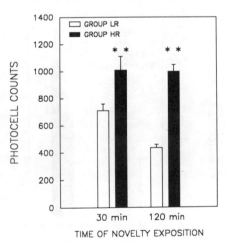

Figure 7. Locomotor effects of intravenous amphetamine injection (0.3 mg/kg) at different durations of exposure to the novel environment. When amphetamine was administered after 120 minutes of exposure to novelty the difference in response between LR and HR animals (low and high responders in the novel environment) was significantly increased (Group: $F(1,58)=47.9$, **$P<0.001$; Group $\times$ Time interaction: $F(2,58)=3.52$, $P<0.05$)

circular corridor. On day 1, after a habituation period to the apparatus of 2 hours, animals were infused through the intracardiac catheter with 0.9 per cent NaCl saline solution (1 ml/kg), and their activity recorded for 1.5 hours. After this period, they were infused with 3 mg/kg of corticosterone-21-hemisuccinate dissolved in saline solution. On days 2 and 3, using the same schedule and following a Latin square design, animals received corticosterone-21-hemisuccinate-BSA (3 mg/kg i.v.) or saline solution, followed after 10 minutes by an amphetamine injection (0.3 mg/kg i.v.). Injection of corticosterone had no effect on locomotor activity *per se*, but it significantly increased the locomotor response to amphetamine (Figure 8).

In a different experiment, the influence of corticosterone levels on the vulnerability to acquire amphetamine self-administration was tested. Corticosterone was injected through the cardiac catheter 10 minutes before the start of the self-administration session. This pretreatment increased the vulnerability to acquire amphetamine self-administration in the resistant animals (LR group). Corticosterone induced amphetamine self-administration in LR rats even if they had not acquired this behavior after 8 days of testing (Figure 9).

Thus, corticosterone seems to increase not only the psychomotor, but

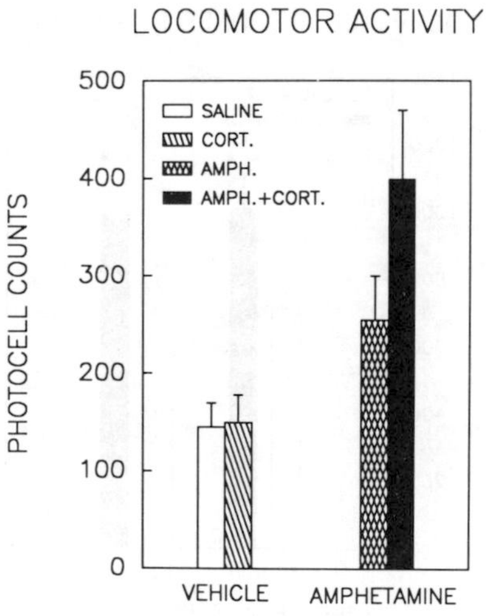

Figure 8. Effect of intravenous infusion of corticosterone-21-hemisuccinate-BSA-Sigma (CORT., 3 mg/kg IV) on amphetamine-induced (0.3 mg/kg IV) locomotor activity. Corticosterone did not increase locomotor activity when compared to the effect of a vehicle injection (0.9 per cent NaCl saline solution). However, a pretreatment with this hormone significantly increased the locomotor response to amphetamine (AMPH) (ANOVA $F(3,15)=5.75$; $P=0.007$)

AMPHETAMINE SELF–ADMINISTRATION

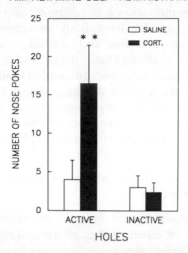

Figure 9. Effect of intravenous infusion of corticosterone-21-hemisuccinate-BSA-Sigma (CORT., 3 mg/kg IV) on amphetamine self-administration behavior of LR ($n=7$) (low responders rats which had previously failed to acquire self-administration). LR animals, which did not develop self-administration after a saline injection (i.e. no difference between nose-pokes in active and passive holes), vigorously self-administered the drug after the infusion of corticosterone, as shown by increase in the number of nose-pokes in the active hole. **$P<0.01$(ANOVA)

also the reinforcing properties of amphetamine. This is in line with the effect of pretreatment with corticosterone on the acquired self-administration of the HR animals. After corticosterone, the HR rats reduced their intake of the drug. A similar phenomenon during the maintenance of well established amphetamine self-administration is typically observed when the amount of drug delivered for each injection is increased (Koob, 1984), or when the animals are injected with amphetamine before the self-administration session (Risner and Jones, 1976). This reduction in drug intake has been interpreted as an attempt by the animal to maintain a constant reinforcing effect of the drug (Koob, 1984).

In conclusion, the corticosterone response appears to predict vulnerability of an individual to amphetamine self-administration. Corticosterone also seems to influence both the psychomotor and reinforcing effects of amphetamine.

CONCLUSIONS

Our results tend to confirm our working hypotheses. First, animal models of stress, as well as repeated administration of amphetamine, increase the psychomotor and reinforcing effects of amphetamine. Second, individual vulnerability to self-administration is predictable, and animals with a higher locomotor response to novelty have both an enhanced response to the psychomotor effect of amphetamine and increased vulnerability to develop amphetamine self-administration. Third, the steroid hormone corticosterone seems to influence individual responses to amphetamine. Thus, animals with an enhanced corticosterone response during exposure to a novel environment are also more sensitive to the psychomotor and reinforcing effects of amphetamine. Furthermore, administration of this hormone augments both the locomotor and the reinforcing effects of amphetamine.

Increase of Amphetamine Self-Administration by Life Events: the DA System as a Possible Substrate

The increase in self-administration induced by amphetamine sensitization could be attributed to an effect of this pharmacological procedure on the DA system. Although amphetamine acts on other monoaminergic systems, both sensitization (Robinson and Becker, 1986) and self-administration (Koob and Bloom, 1988) are thought to be mediated essentially via DA systems. Although experience considered as stressful for the animal induces a variety of biochemical changes, a marked increase in DA release in the mesolimbic system is a salient finding. Thus, a sensitization-like effect on mesolimbic DA projections by repeated environmental stimulation might be responsible for the enhanced reinforcing action of amphetamine. This idea is supported by the comparable effects of tail-pinch and amphetamine sensitization on the acquisition of self-administration. In fact, as both tail-pinch and repeated amphetamine administration affect the DA neural system as well as the propensity to self-administer stimulants, it is plausible that the effects of environmental experiences on the development of this pathological behavior are mediated by the DA system.

Individual Reactivity to Environmental Challenges Predicts both the Psychomotor and the Reinforcing Effects of Amphetamine

The higher novelty-induced locomotor activity of vulnerable animals is open to various interpretations. Locomotor reactivity to novelty may be an expression of both exploratory behavior (Robbins, 1977) and of reactivity to stress. Indeed, exposure to novelty is considered to be a model of psychological stress (Mormède, 1983), and it raises plasma corticosterone to levels comparable to those induced by electric shocks (Dantzer and Mormède, 1983). Furthermore, novelty-induced locomotion is increased by previous experience that is regarded as stressful (West and Michael, 1988), is decreased by adrenalectomy, and is increased by a corticosterone injection

(Veldhuis et al., 1982). Three main findings throw more light on this behavioral parameter. First, HR animals release more corticosterone during exposure to novelty. Second, when rats are allowed to choose between two familiar arms of a Y maze and a novel arm, rats with a higher reactivity to amphetamine display neophobia (lower preference for the novel environment) (unpublished results). Third, repeated amphetamine injections reduce the propensity to investigate novelty (unpublished results). Animals which are more vulnerable to psychostimulants may thus be more reactive to stressful environments.

A rapid increase in locomotor activity seems to be the most consistent feature differentiating the psychomotor response of HR and LR rats to amphetamine. This difference is observed for different doses of amphetamine, whereas the difference in the total response to the drug disappears at high doses (1.5 mg/kg i.p.). A fast psychomotor response to amphetamine may be an important index of a change in the activity of the DA mesolimbic system (Creese and Iversen, 1975), which may underlie the greater vulnerability to drug addiction. In humans, the rate of development of dependence is related to the speed with which the effects of a drug are experienced after administration. The faster response of the HR group may be akin to the 'rush' experienced by the drug abuser a few seconds after inhalation or intravenous injection of a psychostimulant. Two additional results lend support to this idea. First, a similar relationship between locomotor reactivity to amphetamine and self-administration vulnerability has been observed after electrolytic lesions of the ventral tegmental area (Le Moal et al., 1979). The lesioned rats showed an initial enhanced reactivity to amphetamine, and also exhibited a dramatic increase in acquisition of self-administration. Second, if the reactivity of the psychomotor effect of amphetamine of LR rats is increased by repeated injection of the drug, vulnerability of these rats to acquire amphetamine self-administration is also increased.

Vulnerable animals (HR group or stressed subjects) are always more reactive to the psychomotor effect of amphetamine, and/or display a higher locomotor activity in the novel environment. This result raises the question of whether the differences in the acquisition of self-administration observed in our experiments were due to differences in the reinforcing effect of amphetamine or whether they were due to differences in novelty- or amphetamine-induced locomotor activity? Indeed, more activity in the self-administration cage may lead to greater hole exploration, thereby increasing the probability of learning the association between the hole and the administration of amphetamine. However, in all experiments the animals that showed a higher vulnerability to acquire self-administration displayed no more nose pokes in the inactive hole than controls. Thus, the differences observed in the acquisition of self-administration cannot be attributed to differences in exploratory behavior or in the locomotor effect of amphetamine. Likewise, during the first days of testing, animals did not differ in number of nose-pokes in the active hole, and so they had an equal probability of learning the association between the active hole and amphetamine administration. Furthermore, it has recently been reported (Lett, 1989) that repeated amphetamine injections increase the reinforcing properties of the drug in a place preference test which is independent of the psychomotor effects of the drug.

Corticosterone Action on DA as a Possible Physiopathological Mechanism of Vulnerability to Amphetamine Self-Administration

The mesolimbic DA system and especially its projection in the nucleus accumbens may be the neural substrate of corticosterone action on amphetamine responses. Thus, corticosterone administration stimulates DA release in the accumbens (Imperato et al., 1989), possibly via glucocorticoid receptors located on DA cells (Härfstrand et al., 1986). Corticosterone may also mediate the influence of life experiences on amphetamine self-administration. Thus, animal models of stress lead to an increase in the release of corticosterone. The stimulatory effect of this hormone on DA neurons may also be responsible for the lasting effect of environmental stimulation on reactivity to amphetamine. It has been shown that animals which have experienced strong stimuli, such as electric shocks, release more corticosterone than controls in response to new environmental stimulation (Hashimoto et al., 1988; Caggiula et al., 1989). Since normal activities of laboratory animals, such as the cleaning of the home cage (Maccari et al., unpublished results), lead to corticosterone release, rats with an enhanced hormone response may maintain DA neurons in a sensitized state. This change in DA activity may be responsible for an enhanced vulnerability to self-administration. This is in line with the fact that HR animals, which release more corticosterone after exposure to a novel environment, also show a higher locomotor response to amphetamine and a greater vulnerability to acquire amphetamine self-administration.

The hypothesis that corticosterone may play a role in the induction and maintenance of a sensitized state of DA neurons is further supported by the permissive role played by the hypothalamus–pituitary–adrenal axis on sensitization to amphetamine. For example, adrenalectomy (Rivet et al., 1989) or corticotropin-releasing factor (CRF) antagonists (Cole et al., 1989) block the behavioral sensitization that follows repeated amphetamine injections or restraint. Intraventricular injection of CRF increases the psychomotor effect of amphetamine (Cole and Koob, 1989), while repeated injection of this peptide induces a behavioral sensitization to amphetamine (Cador et al., 1989). An understanding of the mechanisms by which certain experiences de-regulate the activity of the hypothalamus–pituitary–adrenal axis may thus throw more light on the physiological mechanisms sustaining some types of pathological behavior.

In conclusion, our findings suggest that interactions between environmental stimulation, corticosterone and DA may constitute a pathophysiological mechanism underlying vulnerability to self-administer amphetamine. Given the relevance for human pathology of the self-administration model, our results provide an experimental contribution to the hypothesis that certain pathological behaviors may stem from alterations in DA system activity. Environmental experiences and corticosterone may impinge on DA neuronal activity, forming a pathophysiological chain whose end result is an abnormality in behavioral adaptation.

REFERENCES

Antelman, S.M. (1988) Stressor-induced sensitization to subsequent stress: implications for the development and treatment of clinical disorders. In: Kalivas, P.W. (ed.) *Sensitization in the Central Nervous System*. New York: Academic Press, pp. 227–259.

Antelman, S.M. and Eichler, A.J. (1979) Persistent effects of stress on dopamine-related behaviors: clinical implications. In: Usdin, E., Kopin, I.J. and Barchas, J. (eds) *Catecholamines: Basic and Clinical Frontiers*. New York: Pergamon, pp. 1759–1761.

Antelman, S.M., Szechtman, H., Chin, P. and Fisher, A.E. (1975) Tail pinch-induced eating, gnawing and licking behavior in rats: dependence on the nigrostriatal dopamine system. *Brain Research* **99**, 319–337.

Antelman, S.M., Rowland, N.E. and Fisher, A.E. (1976) Stimulation bound ingestive behavior: a view from the tail. *Physiology and Behavior* **17**, 743–748.

Antelman, S.M., Eichler, A.J., Black, C.A. and Kocan, D. (1980) Interchangeability of stress and amphetamine in sensitization. *Science* **20**, 7329–7331.

Blanc, G., Hervé, D., Simon, H., Lisoprawski, A., Glowinski, J. and Tassin, J.-P. (1980) Response to stress of mesocortico-frontal dopaminergic neurones in rats after long-term isolation. *Nature* **284**, 265–267.

Bohus, B., De Kloet, E.R. and Veldhuis, H.D. (1982) Adrenal steroids and behavioral adaptation: relationship to brain corticoid receptors. In: Ganten, D. and Pfaff, D. (eds) *Adrenal Actions on Brain*. New York: Springer-Verlag, pp. 108–148.

Cador, M., Cole, B.J., Koob, G.F., Stinus, L. and Le Moal, M. (1989) Central administration of CRF produces sensitization of amphetamine-induced behaviour. *Society for Neuroscience Abstracts* **15**, 252.

Caggiula, A.R., Antelman, S.M., Aul, E., Knopf, S. and Edwards, D.J. (1989) Prior stress attenuates the analgesic response but sensitizes the corticosterone and cortical dopamine responses to stress 10 days later. *Psychopharmacology* **99**, 233–237.

Cole, B.J. and Koob, G.F. (1989) Low doses of corticotropin-releasing factor potentiate amphetamine-induced stereotyped behavior. *Psychopharmacology* **99**, 27–33.

Cole, B.J., Cador, M., Stinus, L., Koob, G.F. and Le Moal, M. (1989) Endogenous

CRF: Role in stress- and amphetamine-induced sensitization of forebrain dopamine systems. *Society for Neuroscience Abstracts* **15**, 252.

Creese, I. and Iversen, S.D. (1975) The pharmacological and anatomical substrates of the amphetamine responses in the rat. *Brain Research* **83**, 419–436.

Creese, I., Burt, D.R. and Snyder, S.H. (1976) Dopamine receptor binding predicts clinical and pharmacological potencies of antischizophrenic drugs. *Science* **192**, 481–482.

D'Angio, M., Serrano, A., Rivy, J.P. and Scatton, B. (1987) Tail-pinch stress increase extracellular DOPAC levels (as measured by *in vivo* voltammetry) in the rat nucleus accumbens but not frontal cortex: antagonism by diazepam and zolpidem. *Brain Research* **409**, 169–174.

Dantzer, R. and Mormède, P. (1983) Stress in farm animals: a need for reevaluation. *Journal of Animal Science* **56**, 6–18.

Deminiere, J.M., Simon, H., Herman, J.P. and Le Moal, M. (1984) 6-Hydroxydopamine lesion of the dopamine mesocorticolimbic cell bodies increases (+)-amphetamine self-administration. *Psychopharmacology* **83**, 281–284.

Deminiere, J.M., Le Moal, M. and Simon, H. (1988a) Catecholamine neuronal systems and (+)-amphetamine administration in the rat. In: Sandler, M. (ed.) *Progress in Catecholamine Research, Part A*. New York: Alan R. Liss, Inc., pp. 489–494.

Deminiere, J.M., Taghzouti, K., Tassin, J.-P., Le Moal, M., and Simon, H. (1988b) Increased sensitivity to amphetamine and facilitation of amphetamine self-administration after 6-hydroxydopamine lesions of the amygdala. *Psychopharmacology* **94**, 229–236.

Deminiere, J.M., Piazza, P.V., Le Moal, M., and Simon, H. (1989) Experimental approach to individual vulnerability to psychostimulant addiction. *Neuroscience and Biobehavioral Reviews* **13**, 141–147.

Dunn, A.J. (1988) Stress related activation of cerebral dopaminergic systems. *Annals of the New York Academy of Sciences* 188–205.

Dunnet, S.B., Björklund, A., Schmidt, R.H., Stenevi, U. and Iversen, S.D. (1983) Intracerebral grafting of neuronal cell suspensions: IV. Behavioural recovery in rats with unilateral 6-OHDA lesions following implantation of nigral cell suspensions in different forebrain sites. *Acta Physiologica Scandinavica* **522**, 29–36 (suppl).

Falk, J.L. (1969) Conditions producing psychogenic polydipsia in animals. *Annals of the New York Academy of Sciences* **157**, 569–593.

Falk, J.L. (1977) The origins and functions of adjunctive behavior. *Animal Learning and Behavior* **5**, 325–335.

Härfstrand, A., Fuxe, K., Cintra, A., Agnati, L.F., Zini, I., Wilkström, A.C., Okret, S., Zhao-Ying, Yu, Goldstein, M., Steinbusch, H., Verhofstad, A. and Gustafsson, J.A. (1986) Glucocorticoid receptor immunoreactivity in monoaminergic neurons in the rat brain. *Proceedings of the National Academy of Science USA* **83**, 9779–9783.

Hashimoto, K., Suemaru, S., Takao, T., Sugawara, M. Makino, S. and Ota, Z. (1988) Corticotropin-releasing hormone and pituitary-adrenocortical responses in chronically stressed rats. *Regulatory Peptides* **23**, 117–126.

Herman, J.P., Stinus, L. and Le Moal, M. (1984) Repeated stress increases locomotor response to amphetamine. *Psychopharmacology* **84**, 431–435.

Herman, J.P., Nadaud, D., Chouli, K., Taghzouti, K., Simon, H. and Le Moal, M. (1985) Pharmacological and behavioral analysis of dopaminergic grafts placed into the nucleus accumbens. In: Björklund, A. and Stenevi, U. (eds) *Neural Grafting in the Mammalian CNS*. Amsterdam: Elsevier, pp. 519–528.

Herman, J.P., Chouli, K., Abrous, N., Dulluc, J. and Le Moal, M. (1988) Effects of intra-accumbens dopaminergic grafts on behavioral deficits induced by 6-OHDA lesions of the nucleus accumbens or A10 dopaminergic neurons: a comparison. *Behavioral Brain Research* **29**, 73–83.

Hornykiewicz, O. (1963) Die topische Localisation das Verhalten von Noradrenalin und Dopamin (3-Hydroxytyramin) in der Substantia Nigra des normalen und Parkinson-kranken Menschen. *Wiener Klinische Wochenschrift* **57**, 309–312.

Imperato, A., Puglisi-Allegra, S., Casolini, P., Zocchi, A. and Angelucci, L. (1989) Stress-induced enhancement of dopamine and acetylcholine release in limbic structure, role of corticosterone. *European Journal of Pharmacology* **165**, 337–339.

Kalivas, P.W. and Weber, B. (1988) Amphetamine injection into the ventral mesencephalon sensitized rats to peripheral amphetamine and cocaine. *Journal of Pharmacology and Experimental Therapeutics* **254**, 1095–1102.

Khantzian, E.J. (1985) The self-medication hypothesis of addictive disorders: focus on heroin and cocaine dependence. *American Journal of Psychiatry* **142**, 1259–1264.

Koob, G.F. (1984) Separate neurochemical substrate for cocaine and heroin reinforcement. In: Church, R.M., Commons, M.L., Stellar, J. and Wagner, A.R. (eds) *Quantitative Analysis of Behavior: Biological Determinants of Behavior, Vol. 7.* Hillsdale New Jersey: Lawrence Erlbaum Associates Inc., pp. 45–56.

Koob, G.F. and Bloom, F.E. (1988) Cellular and molecular basis of drug dependence. *Science* **242**, 715–723.

Knych E.T. and Eisenberg, R.M. (1979) Effect of amphetamine on plasma corticosterone in the conscious rat. *Neuroendocrinology* **29**, 110–118.

Le Moal, M., Galey, D. and Cardo, B. (1975) Behavioral effects of local injections of 6-hydroxydopamine in the medial ventral tegmentum in the rat. Possible role of the mesolimbic dopaminergic system. *Brain Research* **88**, 190–194.

Le Moal, M., Stinus, L. and Simon, H. (1979) Increased sensitivity to (+)-amphetamine self-administered by rats following mesocorticolimbic dopamine neurones destruction. *Nature* **280**, 156–158.

Lett, B.T. (1989) Repeated exposures intensify rather than diminish the rewarding effects of amphetamine, morphine and cocaine. *Psychopharmacology* **98**, 357–362.

Louilot, A., Le Moal, M. and Simon, H. (1986) Functional interdependence between the dopaminergic neurons innervating the amygdala and the nucleus accumbens: *in vivo* voltammetry as a tool for functional anatomy. *Annals of the New York Academy of Science* **473**, 496–498.

Louilot, A., Le Moal, M. and Simon, H. (1989) Opposite influences of dopaminergic pathways to the prefrontal cortex or the septum on the dopaminergic transmission in the nucleus accumbens. An *in vivo* voltammetric study. *Neuroscience* **29**, 45–56.

Major, L., Murphy, D.L. and Lipper, S. (1979) Effects of clorgyline and pargyline on deaminated metabolites of norepinephrine, dopamine and serotonin in human cerebrospinal fluid. *Journal of Neurochemistry* **32**, 229–231.

Marlatt, G.A., Baer, J.S., Donovan, D.M. and Kivlahan, D.R. (1988) Addictive behaviors: etiology and treatment. *Annual Review of Psychology* **39**, 223–252.

Marshall, J.F., Berrios, N. and Sawyer, S. (1980) Neostriatal dopamine and sensory inattention. *Journal of Comparative and Physiological Psychology* **94**, 833–845.

Mittleman, G.M., Castaneda, E., Robinson, T.E. and Valenstein, E.S. (1986) The propensity for non-regulatory ingestive behavior is related to differences in dopamine systems: behavioral and biochemical evidence. *Behavioral Neuroscience* **100**, 213–220.

Mormède, P. (1983) The vasopressin receptor antagonist dPTyr(Me)AVP does not prevent stress-induced ACTH and corticosterone release. *Nature* **302**, 345–346.

O'Brien, C.P., Ehrman, R.N. and Terns, J.N. (1986) Classical conditioning in human opioid dependence. In: Goldberg, S.R. and Stolerman, I.P. (eds) *Behavioral Analysis of Drug Dependence*. London: Academic Press, pp. 329–338.

Pert, A., Rosenblatt, J.E., Sivit, C., Pert, C.B. and Bunney, W.E. (1978) Long term treatment with lithium prevents the development of dopamine receptor supersensitivity. *Science* **201**, 171–173.

Piazza, P.V., Ferdico, M., Benigno, A., Crescimanno G. and Amato, G. (1987) Inhibitory effect of the ventral tegmental A10 region on the hypothalamic defense reaction: evidence for a possible dopaminergic mediation. *Brain Research* **413**, 356–359.

Piazza, P.V., Ferdico, M., Russo, D., Crescimanno, G., Benigno, A. and Amato, G. (1988) Facilitatory effect of ventral tegmental area A10 region on the attack behavior in the cat: possible dopaminergic role on selective attention. *Experimental Brain Research* **72**, 109–116.

Piazza, P.V., Russo, D., Ferdico, M., Crescimanno, G., Benigno, A. and Amato, G. (1989a) The influence of dopaminergic A10 neurons on the motor pattern evoked by substantia nigra (pars compacta) stimulation. *Behavioral Brain Research* **31**, 273–278.

Piazza, P.V., Deminiere, J.M., Le Moal, M. and Simon, H. (1989b) Factors that predict individual vulnerability to amphetamine self-administration. *Science* **245**, 1511–1513.

Pickens, R. and Harris, W.C. (1968) Self-administration of d-amphetamine by rats. *Psychopharmacologia* (Berlin) **12**, 158–163.

Risner, M.E. and Jones, B.E. (1976) Role of noradrenergic and dopaminergic processes in amphetamine self-administration. *Pharmacology Biochemistry and Behavior* **5**, 477–482.

Rivet, J.M., Stinus, L., Le Moal, M. and Mormède, P. (1989) Behavioral sensitization to amphetamine is dependent on corticosteroid receptors activation. *Brain Research* **498**, 149–153.

Robbins, T.W. (1977) A critique of the methods available for the measurement of spontaneous motor activity. In: Iversen, L.L., Iversen, S.D. and Snyder, S.H. (eds) *Handbook of Psychopharmacology, Vol. 7*. New York: Plenum Press, pp. 37–80.

Robbins, T.W. and Everitt, B.J. (1982) Functional studies of the central catecholamines. *International Review of Neurobiology* **23**, 303–365.

Robbins, T.W. and Koob, G.F. (1980) Selective disruption of displacement behavior by lesion of the mesolimbic DA system. *Nature* **285**, 409–412.

Robinson, T.E. (1984) Behavioral sensitization: characterization of enduring changes in rotational behavior produced by intermittent injections of amphetamine in male and female rats. *Psychopharmacology* **84**, 466–475.

Robinson, T.E. and Becker, J.B. (1982) Behavioral sensitization is accompanied by an enhancement in amphetamine-stimulated dopamine release from striatal tissue *in vitro*. *European Journal of Pharmacology* **85**, 253–254.

Robinson, T.E. and Becker, J.B. (1986) Enduring changes in brain and behavior produced by chronic amphetamine administration: a review and evaluation of animal models of amphetamine psychosis. *Brain Research Reviews* **11**, 157–198.

Robinson, T.E., Becker, J.B., Moore, C.J., Castaneda, E. and Mittleman, G. (1985) Enduring enhancement in frontal cortex dopamine utilization in an animal model of amphetamine psychosis. *Brain Research* **343**, 374–377.

Robinson, T.E., Becker, J.B., Young, E.A., Akil, H. and Castaneda, E. (1987) The effects of footshock stress on regional brain dopamine metabolism and pituitary B-endorphin release in rats previously sensitized to amphetamine. *Neuropharmacology* **26**, 679–691.

Roth, R.H., Tam, S.-Y., Ida, Y., Yang, J.-X. and Deutsch, A. (1988) Stress and the mesocorticolimbic dopamine system. *Annals of the New York Academy of Sciences* 138–147.

Sachser, N. (1986) Short-term responses of plasma norepinephrine, epinephrine, glucocorticoid and testosterone titers to social and non-social stressors in male guinea pigs of different social status. *Physiology and Behavior* **39**, 11–20.

Schuster, C.R. and Thompson, T. (1969) Self-administration and behavioral dependence on drugs. *Annual Review of Pharmacology* **9**, 483–502.

Seeman, P. (1980) Dopamine receptors. *Pharmacological Reviews* **32**, 229–313.

Simon, H. and Le Moal, M. (1984) Mesencephalic dopaminergic neurons: functional role. In: Usdin, E., Carlson, A., Dahlström, A. and Engel, S. (eds) *Catecholamines: Neuropharmacology and Central Nervous System. Theoretical Aspects.* New York: Alan R. Liss, pp. 293–307.

Simon, H. and Le Moal, M. (1988) Mesencephalic dopaminergic neurons: role in the general economy of the brain. *Annals of the New York Academy of Science* **537**, 235–253.

Simon, H., Stinus, L. and Le Moal, M. (1980) Effets de la lésion des noyaux du raphé sur l'auto-administration de d-amphetamine chez le rat: augmentation considerable de l'appétence aux toxiques. *Comptes Rendues de l'Academie de Science (III)* **290**, 225–258.

Taghzouti, K., Simon, H. and Le Moal, M. (1986) Disturbances in exploratory behavior and functional recovery in the Y and radial maze following dopamine depletion of the lateral septum. *Behavioral and Neural Biology* **45**, 48–56.

Thierry, A.M., Tassin, J.-P., Blanc, G. and Glowinski, J. (1976) Selective activation of the mesocortical dopaminergic system by stress. *Nature* **263**, 242–244.

Ungerstedt, U. (1971) Adipsia and aphagia after 6-hydroxydopamine induced degeneration of the nigro-striatal dopamine system. *Acta Physiologica Scandinavica* **83** (suppl), 95–122 (suppl 367).

Veldhuis, H.D., De Kloet, E.R., Van Zosten, I. and Bohus, B. (1982) Adrenalectomy reduces exploratory activity in the rat: a specific role for corticosterone. *Hormones and Behavior* **16**, 191–198.

Weeks, J.R. (1962) Experimental morphine addiction: method for automatic intravenous injections in unrestrained rats. *Science* **138**, 143–144.

West, C.H.K. and Michael, R.P. (1988) Mild stress influence sex differences in exploratory and amphetamine-enhanced activity in rats. *Behavioral Brain Research* **30**, 95–97.

Wetherington, C.L. (1982) Is adjunctive behavior a third class of behavior? *Neuroscience and Biobehavioral Reviews* **6**, 329–350.

19

Cognitive Deficits in Schizophrenia and Parkinson's Disease: Neural Basis and the Role of Dopamine

T.W. ROBBINS

Department of Experimental Psychology, University of Cambridge, Downing Street, Cambridge CB2 3EB, UK

INTRODUCTION

Parkinson's disease (PD) and schizophrenia are, of course, very different clinical disorders, and yet they have some aspects in common. Both have been associated with the dysfunctioning of the central dopaminergic systems and both lead to cognitive disorders, some of which resemble those produced by frontal lobe damage. In both cases, too, the cognitive deficits have to some extent been overshadowed by the importance of the core symptoms, which are mainly motoric in the former case and psychotic in the latter. The relationships between, respectively, the psychotic and cognitive symptoms in schizophrenia and the motor and cognitive deficits in PD are unclear. To what extent are the symptoms of schizophrenia, for example, determined by a fundamental cognitive impairment? Are these two types of symptom perhaps relatively independent? The psychotic and motor symptoms may also at least partly determine the cognitive failures and at the very least greatly complicate their assessment. For example, it has been suggested that many of the cognitive symptoms of PD may be due secondarily to motor dysfunction (Marsden, 1982). Poor performance of patients with PD or schizophrenia on neuropsychological tests could also potentially result

The Mesolimbic Dopamine System: From Motivation to Action.
Edited by P. Willner and J. Scheel-Krüger

© 1991 John Wiley & Sons Ltd

from motivational factors such as possible depression in PD (Mayeux et al., 1981; Starkstein et al., 1989) and apathy in schizophrenia. Probably for these reasons, until recently little emphasis has been placed on the intellectual deterioration that can occur in either condition. This is perhaps surprising in view of the long history of study of cognitive impairment in both schizophrenia and PD. For example, Kraepelin (1919) documented extensively cognitive deficits in psychotic patients and introduced the term 'dementia praecox', whereas an increased incidence of dementia has been known for some time to occur in the parkinsonian population (see Quinn et al., 1986).

Crow (1980) revived interest in the cognitive deficit in schizophrenia by defining two distinct subtypes of schizophrenia: a Type I syndrome which he associated with positive psychotic symptoms, no cognitive deficit and with elevated striatal D2 receptors; and a Type II syndrome which he associated with negative symptoms (such as social withdrawal), a cognitive 'defect state', and evidence of neuropathology provided by evidence of enlarged ventricles. Useful as this distinction has been at a heuristic level, there are several problems associated with it. For example, some patients apparently exhibit at the same time both Type I and Type II symptoms. Second, 'thought disorder', perhaps the cardinal symptom of schizophrenia, is difficult to categorize as either a Type I or Type II symptom; in addition to positive instances of thought derailment, such as neologisms, thought disorder can also manifest itself as a poverty in the contents of the thinking. Third, some symptoms, such as 'response stereotypy', are difficult to characterize as negative symptoms, and yet are most clearly associated with the Type II rather than the Type I syndrome (Frith and Done, 1983). Fourth, stereotypy in experimental animals has also been most closely associated with elevated striatal dopamine (DA) function (Robbins et al., 1990), which would also lead one to expect an increased incidence of stereotypy in Type I rather than Type II schizophrenia. Finally, it would appear that cognitive dysfunction can occur in Type I schizophrenia. For these reasons, it is unclear that the Type I/Type II distinction is of great utility in the analysis of the cognitive dysfunction in schizophrenia.

There is accumulating evidence that cognitive dysfunction can occur even in early-in-the-course, unmedicated subjects with PD (Brown and Marsden, 1988a). This may be quite distinct from the state of parkinsonian dementia, which could result from a combination of the pathological and biochemical changes of PD, and subclinical degrees of Alzheimer's disease, to produce a wide spectrum of clinical presentations of apparent 'parkinsonian dementia' (Quinn et al., 1986). The neuropathology of the cognitive deficit in PD is also difficult to define. As well as the striatal DA loss, there is evidence of noradrenergic, serotoninergic, dopaminergic and cholinergic deafferentation of the cortex in PD (Agid et al., 1987). Any of these changes, alone or in various combinations, could be responsible for cognitive dysfunction. There is the further possibility of cognitive deficit due to the L-DOPA medication itself, which has been suggested to contribute to some of the 'frontal lobe'-like impairments of PD (Gotham et al., 1988), although this would not account for deficits in the unmedicated state.

DIMENSIONS OF ANALYSIS

To understand the nature and significance of the cognitive deficits in schizophrenia and PD, it is useful to consider them along several dimensions. The first of these is the heterogeneity of deficits in both conditions. The symptomatic heterogeneity of schizophrenia has, of course, been recognized for a long time, and previous authors have already considered possible implications for the cognitive dysfunctioning that occurs in schizophrenia (Robertson and Taylor, 1985). This heterogeneity to some extent transcends the subcategories used earlier this century (such as hebephrenia and paranoia), as well as the Type I/Type II distinction made above. The important point is that, like the psychotic symptoms, different combinations of cognitive disturbance are likely to coexist in the same individual. Therefore, in any study of the cognitive impairment in schizophrenia, it is essential that the clinical characteristics of the population are made explicit. Heterogeneity of cognitive deficits in PD has been less clearly documented, but seems plausible, based, for example, on the huge variety of deficits reviewed by Brown and Marsden (1988a), and our own experience that individual variability is high, particularly in the early-in-the-course PD patients (Morris et al., 1988; Sahakian et al., 1988).

The other main dimensions to be considered are neuropathological and neuropsychological in nature. Thus, the second dimension to be considered is that of laterality of symptoms. Both PD and schizophrenia may present with lateralized symptoms. The major symptoms of hemi-parkinsonism may be apparent in the early-in-the-course PD patients, although there is no evidence of bias to a particular side. Psychotic symptoms, such as visual hallucinations, have also been described as lateralized to the right visual hemifield (Bracha et al., 1985). Perhaps surprisingly, there is also considerable evidence for a consistent motor turning bias in schizophrenics (towards the left side of space) (Bracha, 1987). More controversial is the evidence implicating specific left hemispheric dysfunction in schizophrenia, which hypothetically results from lateralized brain damage or from callosal abnormality, or both (Flor-Henry, 1983; Doty, 1989). This evidence of functional lateralization is intriguing in view of some evidence of lateralized signs of neuropathology in schizophrenia, particularly in the temporal lobe (Reynolds, 1988). By contrast, there has been much less evidence of lateralization of cognitive deficit in PD, although the possibility should certainly not be discounted (see Taylor et al., 1986; Direnfeld et al., 1984, for positive evidence, and Boller et al., 1984; Huber et al., 1989, for negative evidence).

Another useful dimension is that of cortical and subcortical dementia. This distinction was originally introduced by Albert et al. (1974) to distinguish those deficits in dementia, such as apraxia, agnosia and aphasia, that seemed to be primarily of neocortical origin, and those such as forgetfulness, slowness of thought and motivational impairment, that could apparently arise from largely subcortical damage in disorders such as progressive supranuclear palsy. Neuropsychological analysis of the deficits of PD show that it can be considered as another example of subcortical dementia (Agid et al., 1987; Brown and Marsden, 1988a). The apparent slowness of thought in schizophrenia also suggests that it may provide another example of subcortical dementia (Nelson et al., 1990; Pantelis et al., 1990). However, the subcortical/cortical dichotomy is perhaps most useful as an heuristic for describing different clusters of symptoms rather than having important neuroanatomical implications. It is obvious, for example, that the monoaminergic deafferentation of the cortex that occurs in PD may result from subcortical pathology, but would nevertheless influence the functioning of projections that innervate the cerebral cortex and thus presumably alter cortical functioning. Similarly, damage restricted to elements of the basal ganglia, such as the pallidum, would also affect the expression of cortical functioning, via, for example, defined corticostriatal feedback loops (Alexander et al., 1986), particularly those involving interactions between the frontal cortex and the striatum. Indeed, Albert et al. (1974), and others, have noted the similarity of symptoms in 'subcortical dementia' to those seen following frontal lobe damage; as we shall see, 'frontostriatal dementia' may be an even more apt description. However, the dichotomy implied in subcortical/cortical divisions of dementia is useful to bear in mind when trying to understand the reason that patients may perform accurately, but excessively slowly, or, alternatively, patients who perform perhaps at the normal speed, but inaccurately. In neural terms, this difference in performance may correspond to an output from a neural network which is intact, but lacks some modulatory factor that determines its rate of output, versus output from a network severely distorted by structural damage. These may be good analogies for understanding the contributions of the ascending monoaminergic systems to neural networks of their terminal domains in normal and aberrant cognitive processing.

Definition of the exact role of the monoaminergic, particularly dopaminergic, systems in the cognitive symptoms of schizophrenia and PD is of considerable importance. The earliest, but perhaps by now, naive view would be that dopaminergic hypoactivity could potentially account for the PD cognitive impairment, whereas dopaminergic hyperactivity might be relevant to the schizophrenic counterpart. However, there are several problems with this simple hypothesis. First, it fails to take into account the importance of possible regional differences in DA activity. This is important in two respects. First, PD is generally considered to result primarily from degeneration of the DA-containing cells projecting to the caudate putamen or dorsal striatum whereas (on the basis of rather flimsy evidence) it is generally believed that psychosis is a manifestation of DA hyperactivity in structures such as the nucleus accumbens, which forms part of the ventral striatum. Second, there is now considerable, though controversial, evidence that frontal cortical DA activity is reciprocally related to subcortical DA activity. Thus, underactivity of the frontal cortical DA system may result paradoxically in overactivity of the subcortical DA projections (Bannon and Roth, 1983; Blanc et al., 1980). The other major problem is the possibility that schizophrenia can be associated with hypoactivity of the DA systems as well as hyperactivity. Indeed, some of the post-mortem neurochemical evidence favours the former possibility (Mackay, 1980).

This chapter will concentrate on the hypothesis that schizophrenic and PD cognitive abnormality arises primarily from frontostriatal dysfunction, although other possibilities will be considered. The major burden of explanation for this hypothesis is how dopaminergic abnormalities could potentially interact with other forms of pathology to produce the cognitive deficits in schizophrenia. In PD, the question of subcortical/cortical interaction may be less acute, but the modulatory role in cognition of the major monoaminergic and cholinergic projections to the cortex and striatum must be specified. Other major problems lie in explanation of the heterogeneity of deficits in PD and schizophrenia, and their possibly lateralized nature. It will be argued that the comparison between these disorders is useful for understanding the cognitive disorders associated with each condition. It will also be argued that it is useful to take into account the relevant evidence from animal experiments, whether in the domains of neurobiology or behavioural neuroscience. While it would be naive to suggest that it is possible to model the cognitive abnormalities of schizophrenia and even PD in animal experiments, it will be argued that considerable progress can be made in understanding the organization and functions of the systems implicated in these clinical disorders. Moreover, progress can be made in understanding the causal role of perturbations in particular neurochemical or neural systems using experimental tests with animals. The degree to which such information can be extrapolated to the clinic is facilitated when comparable tests are used for both animal and human subjects; several examples of this strategy will also be reviewed in this chapter.

THEORIES OF COGNITIVE DYSFUNCTION IN PD AND SCHIZOPHRENIA

If the cognitive deficits of PD and schizophrenia do indeed result from a similar neural substrate, then it is important to know in what way the deficits differ in these disorders, and to have a viable theory which can explain both the common and different aspects of the deficits. Frith (1987) has recently proposed such a theory and this will be a convenient starting point for the discussion. He acknowledges that theories of the cognitive dysfunction in schizophrenia based on the concept of a 'defective filter' (Frith, 1979) are probably incorrect; rather, the core deficit in schizophrenia is an impairment in the selection and control of actions. This, of course, is far more readily compatible with neuropsychological theories based on the premise of frontostriatal dysfunction in schizophrenia (Robbins and Sahakian, 1983; Evenden and Ryan, 1988; Joyce, 1988). According to Frith (1987), the main deficit in PD is the inability to translate willed intentions into action (Figure 1). Willed intentions refer to the class of actions that are not elicited directly by environmental stimuli, but are 'spontaneous' and are controlled mainly by interoceptive stimuli. The problem in schizophrenia, as described by Frith, is not in the translation of volition into action, but in the control and generation of volitions. In acute (Type 1) schizophrenia, the patient is hypothesized to have lost the central monitoring mechanism by which actions are matched with plans. The mismatch that occurs in schizophrenia leads to a subjective state conducive to paranoia and delusional thought disorder.

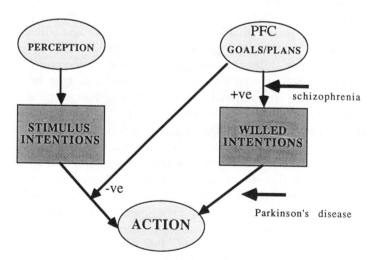

Figure 1. Diagrammatic representation of Frith's (1987) hypothesis. PFC, prefrontal cortex; +ve, positive symptoms; −ve, negative symptoms

A similar hypothesis has been proposed by Robbins and Sahakian (1983) who, however, emphasize the possible importance of the induction of spontaneous hyperactive response tendencies over which the patient feels he or she has no control. According to Frith (1987), in chronic (Type II) schizophrenia, the problem is the lack of planning *per se*, which results in a poverty of thought and action.

These hypothetical deficits are mapped by Frith (1987) onto hypothetical neural substrates. In PD, the lesion is at the level of the basal ganglia; in schizophrenia the deficit is located in the frontal cortex and results in impaired control of action by the basal ganglia. In fact, the significance of frontostriatal interactions in the psychopathology of psychosis had also been noted by Robbins and Sahakian (1983), who elaborated the Norman and Shallice model of action control (Shallice, 1982) at the neural level.

According to the Norman and Shallice model (Figure 2), it is necessary to postulate a 'supervisory' process to account for efficient response selection in certain situations. This supervisory process provides attentional resources which bias the decision towards one response (for example, an action) or another. Normally, 'schemas' that represent the performance of particular responses (such as actions) are triggered by such agents as external stimuli.

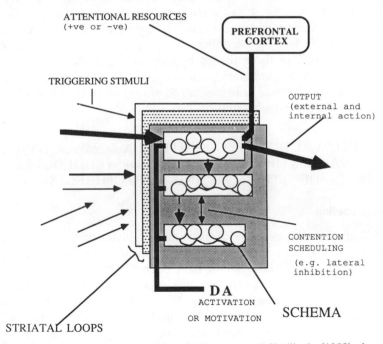

Figure 2. Diagrammatic representation of Norman and Shallice's (1980) theory of 'attention to action', as elaborated by Robbins and Sahakian (1983) in neural terms

Choice between responses is hypothetically mediated by a relatively automatic and autonomous process called contention scheduling. However, supervisory processes are required when there is no automatic response to be selected, as in new learning situations, or when there is a conflict between two or more dominant responses, as occurs, for example, during distraction. The model proposed by Norman and Shallice has the great advantage of being able to predict both increased distraction and increased perseveration, depending on the precise situation, when the supervisory process (which they attribute to the frontal cortex) is disrupted. Without a supervisory influence during distraction, responses to the irrelevant triggering stimulus cannot be suppressed. Without a supervisory influence in extinction, when a response is no longer rewarded, the previously dominant, but now ineffective, response continues unabated because of the removal of the supervisory function. Robbins and Sahakian (1983) suggested that the interaction between the supervisory process and response selection occurred at the level of the basal ganglia, and was also modulated by an activational (subsuming motivational) influence of the ascending striatal DA innervation. The relationships between these ideas and those of Frith (1987; see Figure 1) seem quite clear.

These theories all predict that a cardinal feature of the cognitive deficit produced by frontostriatal dysfunction lies in the production of deficits in initiative and planning which can result in apparently aimless, perseverative behaviour in the face of changing environmental circumstances. We will now consider some of the evidence to support this prediction in PD and in schizophrenia, by a comparative analysis of the impairments in PD and schizophrenia at all levels of organization of output, from the level of simple motor function to that of cognition.

FROM ACTION TO COGNITION: A COMPARATIVE ANALYSIS OF SELECTED NEUROPSYCHOLOGICAL DEFICITS IN PD AND SCHIZOPHRENIA

Motor Function

Consistent with the possibility of basal ganglia involvement in schizophrenia is the late occurrence of abnormal spontaneous movements termed orofacial or limb dyskinesias. Although these have been linked with chronic neuroleptic treatment and consequent DA receptor supersensitivity, there are grounds for believing that the movements may also depend upon other factors such as age. In addition, in experimental animals, frontal lobe damage has been observed to promote the occurrence of such movements after chronic neuroleptic treatment (Gunne et al., 1982), and several studies have shown that the stereotyped oral movements induced by d-amphetamine that are known to depend upon striatal DA activity are also exacerbated by frontal lobe damage (Iversen, 1971). Recent clinical analyses have come to the conclusion that the incidence of some of the tardive dyskinesias (particularly of the orofacial variety) may be more prevalent in schizophrenics with predominantly negative symptoms, including intellectual deterioration (Barnes, 1988). This association, which appears to run against the hypothesis that chronic neuroleptic treatment is responsible, is substantiated by the findings of systematic relationships between tardive movements and indices of brain (particularly frontal) damage and basal ganglia hypometabolism (Waddington and Youssef, 1986).

As in PD (Bloxham et al., 1984; Robbins and Brown, 1990), there is also evidence for dysfunction in schizophrenics in those processes by which actions are initiated. One of the most striking of the deficits in schizophrenia is the slowing of reaction time, which is exacerbated under certain test conditions, suggestive of changes in response set (Shakow, 1971). Given the strong evidence that implicates changes in reaction time performance to the operation of fronto-striatal circuitry (Goldberg, 1985; Alivisados and Milner, 1989) it is a plausible hypothesis that both the PD and schizophrenic deficits arise from malfunction of these regions. It is of interest for Frith's model that cognitive and reaction time deficits have both been attributed to impairments in the mechanisms by which stimuli of internal origin activate behaviour (Brown and Marsden, 1988b; Brown and Robbins, 1990; Robbins and Brown, 1990). This is consistent with Frith's model which, similarly, proposes specific deficits in PD patients in the initiation of actions in response to interoceptive cues ('willed intentions') rather than exteroceptive cues ('stimulus intentions'). Unfortunately, as we will find with virtually all of the evidence to be reviewed, there have been no systematic comparisons of reaction time deficits in the same conditions between these two patient groups; these are urgently required, so that the nature of the impairment in action control can be clarified in each case.

Response Stereotypy

Since Bleuler's descriptions of schizophrenia (Bleuler, 1950), it has been recognized that a considerable portion of schizophrenic behaviour is stereotyped in nature, and this has been highlighted by amphetamine-like drugs which induce stereotyped behaviour in experimental animals, as well as evidence of psychotic effects in man (Iversen, 1986; Evenden and Ryan, 1988). Although schizophrenic stereotypies were linked to the adverse effects of institutionalization, there is now considerable evidence that their quite high occurrence in the schizophrenic population is attributable to the condition itself (Jones, 1965).

Until recently, there has been little experimental analysis of stereotyped behaviour in schizophrenics. However, striking stereotyped sequences of behaviour have now been shown to occur in both Type I and Type II schizophrenics in a two-choice guessing paradigm where the sequence of presentation of stimuli is in fact random (Frith and Done, 1983; Lyon et al., 1986). In the Frith and Done study, acute Type I schizophrenics tended to show stereotyped alternation sequences (of the form left–right–left–right), whereas chronic patients (especially when in a cognitive defect state) sometimes adopted marked position biases, responding almost exclusively on one side. These effects did not occur to anywhere near the same extent in patient groups with affective disorder or dementia, and so presumably did not arise from generalized intellectual or motivational impairment; nor were they non-specific products of psychosis, as they did not occur in patients with depression.

The neural substrates for the deficits are unclear, as patients with specific damage of the frontal cortex or striatum have not been assessed in this task. However, there are strong parallels to the stereotyped sequences seen in the schizophrenic groups in the behaviour seen in animals treated with the indirect DA agonist d-amphetamine, performing what is a very similar task to that used by Frith and Done (1983). In this experiment, rats essentially had to 'guess' which of two levers was next to provide food. (Evenden and Robbins, 1983 a, b). The effects depended on the baseline level of switching; when high, the drug tended to reduce the switching tendency. However, when at an intermediate level (as in the case of the Frith and Done experiment), d-amphetamine produced dose-related increases in switching between the two levers at low doses and in perseverating responses (failing to collect earned food pellets) at higher doses (Evenden and Robbins, 1983b). In a direct comparison of the Frith and Done task in normal human subjects receiving amphetamine and marmosets receiving one dose of the drug, amphetamine tended to increase alternation in the human subjects and to induce perseveration in the marmosets (Ridley et al., 1988). It is possible that this discrepancy represents a species difference, but also could plausibly arise from dose-response or baseline differences in the two species. The important conclusion is that d-amphetamine, perhaps through a release of striatal DA, mimics some of the effects seen in both types of schizophrenic subject. By contrast, DA receptor blockade (produced by systemic α-flupenthixol) had no significant effects on switching, even at doses that significantly reduced response rate (Evenden and Robbins, 1983a).

The problem with this extrapolation is that the amphetamine model of psychosis only works well for the positive signs of schizophrenia; thus the significant stereotypy of the Type II state would not be expected. Two possible explanations of this increased stereotypy suggest themselves. First, it could result from striatal DA underactivity as the obverse of the increased switching produced by DA release; it would be interesting to test this hypothesis in normal subjects receiving DA receptor blocking drugs or in PD patients who have striatal DA depletion. In the study of Evenden and Robbins (1983a), the DA receptor blocker α-flupenthixol had no significant effect on switching even at doses that reduced response rate. A second possibility is that the stereotypy results from frontal lobe dysfunction which releases the stereotyped tendencies mediated by the striatum. Frontal lobe damage is well known to increase both spontaneous and amphetamine-induced stereotypies in experimental animals (Iversen, 1971). In both of these cases, then, some forms of behavioural inflexibility can be expected to result from the effects of striatal dopaminergic hyperactivity. The difficulty lies in attempting to distinguish these possibilities from observations of the behavioural output alone. For example, it might be possible to distinguish 'active' and 'passive' forms of stereotyped behaviour by their overall rate or intensity.

Perseveration

Stereotypy is generally considered as a behavioural phenomenon, as in the stereotyped choice of actions described above. However, to the extent that thought itself can be considered as internalized action, it is possible to consider stereotypy in cognitive terms, either in parallel with behavioural stereotypy or even underlying it. One example of cognitive stereotypy is in perseveration during reversal learning, where a previously incorrect response now becomes correct and vice versa. Both frontal and striatal lesions induce impairments in certain forms of reversal learning, largely due to perseverative modes of responding, with the orbitofrontal cortex and its projections to the caudate nucleus being particularly implicated (Jones and Mishkin, 1972; Divac 1984). Frith (1987) suggested that reversal learning is a good example of a task in which the outcome of responses requires a central monitor, and where, in the absence of such monitoring in Type I schizophrenia, perseverative responding would be highly likely. However, simple reversal learning has been relatively little studied in either PD or schizophrenia, doubtless because the task is easy for human subjects. Thus, Downes et al., (1989) found no significant effects of PD on simple or compound visual stimulus discrimination, and Freedman and Oscar-Berman (1989) found significant effects only in PD patients with dementia. Other forms of cognitive flexibility are required in tasks requiring the shifting of attention from one locus to another, and these are considered in further detail below.

Planning

The occurrence of such phenomena as stereotypy and perseveration is often linked with the absence of a plan or 'supervisory attentional mechanism'

(Shallice, 1982). In the absence of such a mechanism, the relatively automatic routines or 'schemata' are controlled solely by a 'contention scheduling system' (Shallice, 1982). Thus, when contingencies change, for example, when goals are altered, as in reversal learning, the system continues to generate the formerly most dominant response, or, when more than one dominant response is available, the system switches uncontrollably between the responses. The operation of these systems for action control has been linked to the relationships between the frontal lobes and the basal ganglia (Robbins and Sahakian, 1983), and is clearly compatible both with the data of Frith and Done (1983, see above) and the theory advanced by Frith (1987).

To test the hypothesis that the frontal lobes are involved in planning, Shallice and McCarthy modified and simplified the well-known Tower of Hanoi problems in which arrangements of discs are moved to specified positions on rods in the shortest possible sequence (Shallice, 1982). The subject is required to study the problem and then make the correct series of moves. The number of moves required is specified and varies from two to five. Using this task, Shallice (1982) was able to demonstrate marked impairments in the accuracy of move sequences in patients with anterior (including frontal), but not posterior, cortical damage. We have modified the Shallice task to be suitable for presentation on a computer VDU, using a touch-sensitive screen to measure the accuracy and latency of the responses (Morris et al., 1988; Owen et al., 1990). We have also included a yoked motor control test in which the subject's motor or reaction times can be subtracted from the overall latency to solve the problems, thus providing a true estimate of 'thinking time'. A group of idiopathic PD patients under medication with L-DOPA was shown to be no less accurate than normal age- and IQ-matched controls. However, the PD patients took longer to think about the problems, particularly prior to the first move (Morris et al., 1988; Figure 3). This is of especial importance for the hypothesis that PD represents a form of subcortical dementia, as the lengthened thinking times could be taken as evidence for the clinical concept of slowed thinking or 'bradyphrenia' (Rogers 1986). A slightly different version of the task and calculation of corrected thinking time has been used to test a group of patients receiving neurosurgery for tumours or epilepsy of the frontal lobes. (Owen et al., 1990). In contrast to the results with PD patients, this study showed that frontal patients were less accurate than controls but were not significantly slower to think about the first move. Therefore, although PD patients are impaired on this 'frontal' task, their deficit is qualitatively different from that of frontal patients. It seems possible that the PD impairment is linked either to specific neurochemical or regional damage of the frontal cortex, or to a disruption of striatal functions. Unfortunately, schizophrenic subjects have not yet been tested in this Tower of London

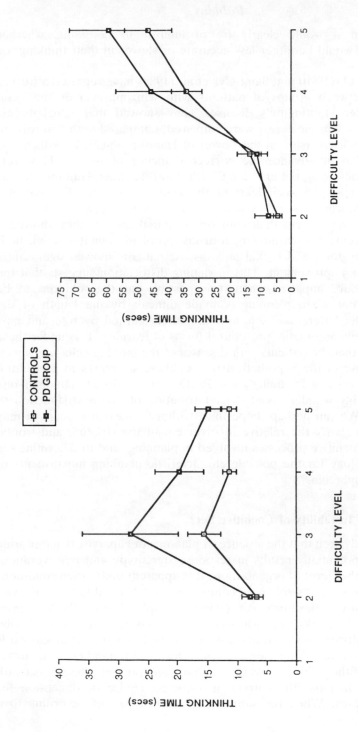

Figure 3. Slowing of thinking time in PD patients for the Tower of London planning problems for two-, three-, four- and five-move problems (level of difficulty). The effects were significant for thinking prior to (left), but not following (right), the first move of each problem. The thinking times were corrected for motor slowing, using a yoked control procedure. The slowing was evident when calculated both for correct solutions only and for all problems attempted. (Reproduced from Morris et al., 1988 with permission)

procedure, but it would clearly be of interest to determine whether schizophrenics would be either less accurate or slower in their thinking, or both.

Goldberg et al. (1990) and Saint-Cyr et al. (1988) have reported a further dissociation between groups of patients with schizophrenia or the basal ganglia disorder Huntington's disease. They showed that schizophrenic patients (mainly chronic cases) were impaired, compared with controls, in solving a three-disc version in the Tower of Hanoi problem, for which it is possible to plan in advance the correct sequence of moves. However, they were significantly better, along with controls, than Huntington's or Parkinson's disease patients in learning the solutions to a four-disc problem, which is too difficult to solve by planning a solution in advance. Although schizophrenics were worse than controls on initial testing, they showed a parallel improvement in learning the four-disc problem when it was repeated, whereas Huntington's and Parkinson's disease patients showed significantly less progressive improvement. This intriguing dissociation suggests that the schizophrenics are impaired when it is possible for the solutions to be planned, but not when planning is made difficult by the length of the problem. In the latter case, solutions are often learned by rote and may involve relatively automatic, procedural forms of learning. It is under these circumstances that the patients with diseases of the basal ganglia are worse, perhaps because of the hypothetical role of these structures in procedural learning (or 'learning by doing', see Butters et al., 1987), although one might reasonably wonder about the contribution of motor dysfunction to such deficits. We can perhaps hope that, within the next few years, it may be possible to clarify the relative involvement of the striatum and frontal cortex in the cognitive processes involved in planning, and to determine the locus of pathology for the possible characteristic planning impairments of PD and schizophrenia.

Inflexibility or Instability of Cognitive Set?

We have already seen that the absence of planning or supervisory monitoring of behaviour potentially results in response stereotypy and perseveration. At an even higher level of organization, it is apparent under such conditions that attentional set gains enhanced control over intellectual functioning with resultant cognitive inflexibility. An obvious example of this is the Wisconsin Card Sorting Test (WCST), which is often used to assess frontal lobe dysfunction (Milner, 1964). In this task, the subject is required to sort cards which vary in three dimensions, colour, form and number. The tester chooses one of these dimensions (e.g. colour) and provides the subject with verbal feedback about the correct or incorrect choice of dimension for sorting each card. When the subject has learned to sort according to a particular dimension, the tester changes the correct dimension to one which was irrelevant (e.g. form). Frontal lobe patients have particular difficulty in switching their choice of dimension, so that they may perseverate in sorting according to the formerly correct dimension. They also achieve fewer correct categories of sorting. According to Milner (1964), patients with dorsolateral prefrontal cortex lesions are particularly susceptible, although impairments have been seen following damage to other frontal regions and, indeed, to other areas of the neocortex, such as the right temporal lobe (Canavan et al., 1988). The importance of this task is that both schizophrenic (Weinberger, 1988) and PD patients (Canavan et al., 1989; Brown and Marsden, 1988a), including early-in-the-course, unmedicated cases (Lees and Smith, 1983), show impaired performance, implicating frontal lobe dysfunction in each condition.

Aberrant WCST performance in PD and schizophrenia poses questions about both the nature of the cognitive deficits and their underlying neural basis. The WCST can be seen both as a test of the ability to abstract, and of the ability to attend selectively to certain stimulus dimensions. In turn, this selective attention may operate at the input stage (filtering out the irrelevant stimulus dimensions) or as a response set (a bias to respond to a particular dimension). Based on the theoretical perspective described above (Frith, 1987), and from other considerations (Robbins and Brown, 1990), we favour the latter possibility. The perseverative responding that can occur in frontal subjects is clearly at a higher level of organization than either the response stereotypy or the perseveration that may occur to a particular reinforced stimulus in reversal learning. In the case of the perseverative errors made in the WCST, the perseveration is not limited to a particular stimulus but to an entire class of stimuli which individually might themselves be novel to the subject. Thus, it is possible that these various forms of perseveration (Sandson and Albert, 1984) reflect the hierarchical organization of response tendencies, ranging from simple motor elements to complex cognitive structures.

Although the WCST is an excellent clinical instrument, its design and complexity make it less suitable for experimental analysis. Downes et al. (1989) have pointed out that the test encompasses principles of matching to sample, conditional and reversal learning, as well as intra- and extra-dimensional shifting. An intra-dimensional (ID) shift occurs when a subject is trained to attend to a particular dimension and is then required to transfer this rule to a novel set of exemplars of that dimension. By contrast, an extra-dimensional (ED) shift occurs when the subject is required to shift to an alternative, usually previously irrelevant, dimension (Mackintosh, 1983). The latter capacity is the core requirement of the WCST, but the requirement of other principles makes it possible for subjects to fail the task for a variety of reasons. Moreover, whereas the WCST is not suitable as an animal learning test, the capacity for ED shifting has been studied intensively in several species (Mackintosh, 1983), and the effects of selective lesions can be studied (Passingham, 1972; Roberts, Everitt and Robbins, unpublished observations).

In a recent study (Downes et al., 1989), ED and ID shifting were assessed directly in groups of unmedicated and medicated PD patients. First, simple discrimination and reversal learning were tested using stimuli varying only in one dimension (shapes or lines). The alternative dimension was then introduced (i.e. shapes or lines) as irrelevant distractors in tests of compound stimulus and reversal learning. Finally, ID and ED non-reversal shifts were introduced, using new examplars of the shape and line stimuli (to avoid perseveration to specific stimuli). The results (Figure 4) showed that both PD groups were impaired at ED, but not ID shifts. There was also some evidence that the unmedicated group was impaired when a distracting dimension was introduced. Thus, the PD patients may suffer not so much from a deficit in 'shifting attitude' (Cools et al., 1984) as from a general impairment in the control exerted by stimuli over behaviour, or what we term an instability of response set. Evidence for this form of impairment comes from studies showing that PD patients commit many non-perseverative errors (sometimes at least as many as in the perseverative error category) as well as achieving significantly fewer categories than normal subjects (Brown and Marsden, 1988a), which may reflect problems in tuning into the appropriate stimulus dimension rather than in perseverative responding. In fact, the situation may be similar in the studies examining WCST performance in schizophrenia (Weinberger, 1988), although the question of non-perseverative errors has not received close attention. Thus, as in the case of subjects receiving neurosurgery of the frontal lobes, both PD and schizophrenia may be associated with the combination of perseveration and distractibility which we argue is most consistent with the hypothesis of an instability of response set resulting from a diminished supervisory frontal lobe influence (Robbins and Sahakian, 1983; Shallice, 1982).

Analysis of the presence of both types of deficit in the same population of schizophrenic subjects is complicated by the nature of the schizophrenic condition. Thus, distractibility may be relatively more common in acute than chronic schizophrenics, just as stereotyped response switching is more prevalent than response perseveration, as described above (Frith and Done, 1983). Recently, acute, but not chronic, medicated schizophrenics have been shown to exhibit impaired latent inhibition (Baruch et al., 1988).

Latent inhibition can be construed as a form of habituation in which non-reinforced pre-exposure to certain stimuli usually results in the subject being less able to learn about those stimuli when they later become associated with reinforcement and hence more salient (Mackintosh, 1983). Thus, for example, if a conditioned stimulus (CS) is pre-exposed without any

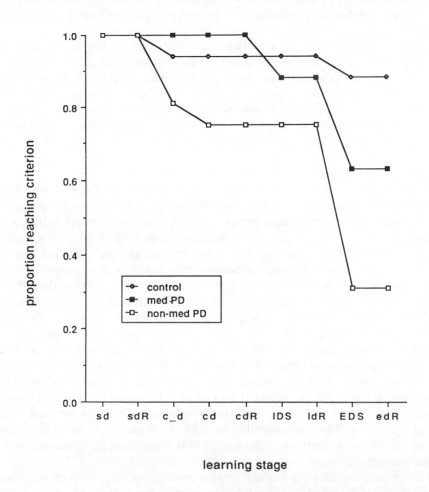

Figure 4. Poor performance of PD patients, both medicated (med) and non-medicated (non-med) when compared with age- and IQ- matched controls on an intra-/extra- dimensional (ID/ED) shift paradigm of attentional set shifting. Patients were tested on a sequence of simple discrimination (sd), reversal (sdR), compound stimulus discrimination (c_d) (i.e. with an added stimulus dimension but not superimposed on the original dimension), then superimposed (cd), then reversal (cdR), before two transfer tests; an ID shift and reversal (IDS, idR), and an ED shift and reversal (EDS, edR). The ordinate shows the proportion of total subjects successful at each stage. Note the steep decline in performance in the ED shift by the PD patients. (From Downes et al., 1989 with permission)

consequence before it becomes an aversive CS through conditioning with shock, then it will be less capable of suppressing responding as a result of the latent inhibition produced by its prior, non-reinforced exposure. Therefore, an impairment in latent inhibition manifests itself as superior learning about pre-exposed cues. The acute schizophrenics of the Baruch et al. study actually performed this phase of the test better than controls, and so it is difficult to claim that their performance resulted from reduced motivation. The deficit in latent inhibition can be understood as one of selective attention, presumably due to heightened distractibility in the pre-exposure stage. Therefore, the intriguing results of Baruch et al. (1988) may indicate that acute schizophrenics tend to be more distractible than the chronic subgroups. Unfortunately, the effects of the neuroleptic medication of the patients have not yet been assessed, neither have there yet been parallel studies in patients with PD, so it is difficult to assess a possible dopaminergic substrate for the latent inhibition deficit from these data alone. Moreover, it is unclear to what extent these changes in latent inhibition are specific to core features of schizophrenia, rather than to non-specific excessive arousal shown in this, and other, clinical groups. The fact that it does not occur in the chronic, medicated state suggests this interpretation. However, it is of interest that in the study of ID/ED shifting described above, the PD subjects generally failed the ED shift task by adopting very sophisticated hypotheses about sequences of correct and incorrect choices, rather than exhibiting gross perseveration. Similar observations have been noted by Flowers and Robertson (1985). Therefore, it appears that the PD patients may have been impaired in shifting to the previously non-reinforced dimension rather than in shifting away from the previously reinforced dimension (Downes et al., 1989). This can be interpreted as an exaggerated response to learned irrelevance, a process related to (but not the same as) latent inhibition. Thus, it is possible that PD patients would show superior latent inhibition or learned irrelevance to controls, hence contrasting with acute schizophrenics.

The potentially exciting feature of the application of paradigms such as learned irrelevance and latent inhibition to patients is that information on the neural and neurochemical substrates for these phenomena is now emerging from psychopharmacological and neuropsychological studies with experimental animals.

NEURAL AND NEUROCHEMICAL BASIS OF COGNITIVE SET INSTABILITY IN PD AND SCHIZOPHRENIA

It is particularly important to determine the neural substrates of the mediation of intact and impaired performance on the WCST in normal controls and patients with PD or schizophrenia. Whether the PD or schizophrenic impairment is at the level of the frontal lobes or basal ganglia is unclear at present. Weinberger (1988) has argued strongly that the impaired WCST performance in schizophrenia is due to hypometabolism of the dorsolateral prefrontal cortex, but the neural substrates of the deficit in PD are less clear.

Weinberger's evidence hinges on the use of cerebral regional blood flow studies conducted in a functional imaging context, where the subject is either resting or performing various cognitive tasks, including the WCST. According to the evidence summarized by Weinberger, chronic schizophrenics exhibit frontal hypometabolism particularly when performing the WCST but not when performing (equally badly) at other tasks, such as Continuous Performance, which involve vigilance and 'effortful processing'. Moreover, this selective hypometabolism is still observed when the patients are unmedicated, which is an important consideration in view of the fact that drugs such as haloperidol appear to produce impairments in 'cognitive shifting' (Berger et al., 1989). Finally, the hypometabolism is hypothesized to depend at least in part upon reduced frontal cortex DA activity. Some evidence for this possibility is derived from two observations: first, measures of the DA metabolite homovanillic acid (HVA) are reduced in CSF samples from the schizophrenic sample participating in the functional imaging studies (Weinberger et al., 1988a). Second, there is some rather surprising evidence that CSF HVA actually provides a reasonably accurate indirect index of frontal cortex DA turnover in experimental primates, perhaps because of the intrinsically higher turnover rate of this DA projection pathway (Elsworth et al., 1987).

Overall, the evidence for frontal hypometabolism in schizophrenia using more sensitive imaging techniques such as PET and NMR seems strong (Buchsbaum and Haier, 1987). However, the evidence from these sources at present provides only limited support for Weinberger's claim of a specific dorsolateral involvement, or that the hypometabolism is especially evident in the functional imaging context of WCST performance. There is also excellent evidence that schizophrenia is associated with hypometabolism of certain structures of the basal ganglia. Some studies have indicated that the largest differences from controls occur in the caudate nucleus whereas others have highlighted the lentiform nucleus (Buchsbaum and Haier, 1987). A contribution of these changes to the impaired WCST performance is plausible, given the relationships between frontostriatal structures and the evidence linking impaired WCST performance in Huntington's disease with atrophy of the caudate nucleus (Weinberger et al., 1988b).

The neural substrates of the parkinsonian deficit on the WCST are less clear, particularly as hypofrontality has been reported for this group during WCST performance (Weinberger et al., 1988b). Another source of clues about the possible neural or neurochemical basis of the WCST deficit comes from the evaluation of the effects of L-DOPA medication in 'on–off' studies with PD patients. In fact, there is not much evidence that L-DOPA has any consistent effect. In a study by Bowen et al. (1975) L-DOPA increased the number of correct responses (mainly by reducing non-perseverative errors), but did not improve the number of categories attained. A more recent study by Gotham et al. (1988) even seemed to indicate that L-DOPA medication impaired performance, particularly on the WCST and other 'frontal' tasks, such as subject-ordered pointing. This impairment may be related to that seen in hyperactive children treated with Ritalin (methylphenidate) on the same task (Dyme et al., 1982) and remind us that hyperactivity, as well as hypoactivity, of the central DA systems may impair WCST performance. However, direct comparisons of performance by PD patients on and off medication for the WCST were not significant in the Gotham et al. study. Furthermore, Pillon et al. (1989) have shown that there is no correlation with the motor response to L-DOPA (a presumed index of striatal dopaminergic activity) and performance on the WCST. They stress instead the possible non-dopaminergic contributions to the intellectual deterioration in PD. Hence, there is no convincing evidence that L-DOPA therapy exerts any specific effect on the WCST, and by implication, that its performance does not depend on dopaminergic mechanisms.

In summary, although it is commonly believed that impairments on the WCST are related to dysfunction of the frontostriatal system, there is no convincing evidence to implicate a particular part of this circuitry or its modulation by ascending dopaminergic activity. From the evidence surveyed, it would appear likely that WCST performance is susceptible to perturbations of distinct portions of the circuitry, although there is a paucity of evidence showing that its performance breaks down in different ways related to these different influences. These considerations strengthen the arguments made above that it is vital that animal analogues of the WCST are developed so that the effects of selective neuropharmacological manipulations, and hence the causal role of particular forms of neuropathology in PD and schizophrenia, can be assessed.

THE CONTRIBUTION OF ANIMAL MODELS TO UNDERSTANDING THE COGNITIVE DEFICITS OF PD AND SCHIZOPHRENIA

Now that clear patterns of cognitive deficits are becoming established in both PD and schizophrenia, it is becoming possible to use information gleaned from animal experiments to test specific hypotheses about the neural and neurochemical bases of the disorders. However, there are problems for this approach because some of the deficits, such as in planning, are not easily modelled in animals and, for those that can be modelled, there is the question of how central those cognitive deficits are to the clinical conditions. Moreover, it is generally necessary to test the effects of many manipulations before the specificity of the behavioural changes in animals can be confidently defined at either the psychological or neural level.

Prefrontal Cortex

In general terms, although the effects of frontal lobe and basal ganglia lesions in animals have been well documented, impairments in tasks such as delayed response and delayed alternation have not been shown to be particularly sensitive to non-demented PD (Freedman and Oscar-Berman, 1989) or schizophrenia. However, it has been important to show that selective DA depletion from the prefrontal cortex, or infusions of DA receptor antagonists, in monkeys produces impairments in delayed alternation (Brozoski et al., 1979). It is also important to be aware that errors made in this task in intact rats are related to indices of DA turnover in prefrontal cortex, but not in subcortical, DA systems (Sahakian et al., 1985). Therefore, it appears that either DA hyperactivity or hypoactivity may be detrimental to the performance of this task, and this provides us with an important general model for how DA dysfunction in the prefrontal cortex may lead to cognitive deficit. What is lacking is an understanding of the types of psychological and physiological conditions that normally produce fluctuations in the activity of the ascending DA systems. For example, both stress and reward-related processes have been implicated and it is not clear how these two hypotheses could be compatible. Of particular importance to the present discussion, isolation has been shown to produce reductions in prefrontal cortex DA turnover in the rat (Blanc et al., 1980; Jones, Robbins and Marsden, unpublished observations), and this may be related to reciprocal increases in DA release in the subcortical DA systems (Blanc et al., 1980; Jones, et al., 1988). Rats reared in isolation have a variety of cognitive deficits including impairments in the radial eight-arm maze (Einon, 1980) and in reversal learning (Jones, Robbins and Marsden, unpublished results), which might be correlates of these neurochemical effects.

Ventral and Dorsal Striatum

From the above discussions, it is apparent that it is difficult to consider the subcortical DA systems independently of the cortical DA projections because of the inverse relationship that often governs interactions between the two (Tassin et al., Chapter 7, this volume). Nevertheless, at least three groups of investigators have considered DA hyperactivity in the nucleus accumbens as a model for the cognitive changes in schizophrenia. Solomon and Staton (1982) have found that systemic chronic or intra-accumbens (but not intracaudate) d-amphetamine can disrupt latent inhibition in an active avoidance procedure in the rat, and Baruch et al. (1988) have mentioned this ventral striatal mechanism as a possible mediator of the disrupted latent inhibition in their acute schizophrenic group.

There is little doubt that d-amphetamine does disrupt latent inhibition in the rat, supporting a role for dopaminergic processes in this phenomenon, but the nature and significance of this effect has to be carefully considered. Whereas Solomon and Staton needed chronic doses of the drug to produce an effect using an active avoidance procedure (where strong latent inhibition is reflected by reduced motor output), Weiner et al. (1984), using an aversive conditioned suppression procedure (where strong latent inhibition is reflected by increased motor output), have shown that low systemic, acute doses of d-amphetamine were sufficient. On the other hand they found in another study that a higher dose (that induces stereotyped behaviour) did not impede latent inhibition. Moreover, they also found that the drug was ineffective when given only in the pre-exposure stage, suggesting that the drug mainly affected the expression rather than the acquisition of latent inhibition. These findings also suggest that there is a correlation between disruption of latent inhibition and the effects of the drug on locomotor activity rather than stereotypy. This would explain the apparent sensitivity of the nucleus accumbens to the disruption of latent inhibition (Solomon and Staton, 1982) as it mediates the locomotor, but not the stereotyped, activities produced by amphetamine (Kelly et al., 1975). An obvious possibility is that the effects on latent inhibition arise indirectly from the locomotor hyperactivity produced by the drug.

A similar question can be raised about the disruptive effects of systemic d-amphetamine or apomorphine in two other models of reported attentional deficits in human schizophrenic subjects; an attentional switching paradigm (Robbins et al., 1986), and a paradigm measuring attention to 'prepulse' stimuli which inhibit the effects of an acoustic startle stimulus (Swerdlow et al., 1988). In these cases, enhanced dopaminergic activity produced by systemic doses of either d-amphetamine or apomorphine disrupted attentional function. In the study by Robbins et al. (1986), disruption by systemic d-amphetamine was completely blocked by mesolimbic DA depletion. In the study by Swerdlow et al. (1988), the disruptive effect of systemic apomorphine was seen in rats with mesolimbic DA depletion and presumed supersensitive DA receptors in the nucleus accumbens, but not in rats with mesofrontal DA depletion. However, the pattern of results from the Robbins et al. study suggested that the mesolimbic DA depletion antagonized the global disruption of behaviour by the drug, rather than having a specific effect on attentional switching. The effects of the drug, both on latent inhibition and prepulse inhibition procedures, might arise from similar disruption. A possible argument against this in the case of latent inhibition, as studied by Weiner and colleagues, is that the disruptive effects of d-amphetamine on latent inhibition are manifested by an enhanced conditioned suppression of responding. An argument against this for the prepulse inhibition task would point to the temporal specificity of the effect.

Another critique of the role of the ventral striatum in attentional processes would refer to the considerable evidence linking this system to reward-related processes (Fibiger and Phillips, 1986; Robbins et al., 1989; Fibiger, Chapter 24; Cador et al., Chapter 9, this volume). It is possible that the effect of amphetamine on latent inhibition could be ascribed in some way to an enhancement of the reinforcing or incentive properties of the pre-exposed stimulus (e.g. because of its novelty). Perhaps this account also represents the best way of interpreting the effects of neuroleptic drugs on latent inhibition; the effects of stimulus pre-exposure would then be exaggerated by the neuroleptic-induced blockade of whatever reinforcing properties the pre-exposed stimulus might possess. There are impressive reports of exaggerated latent inhibition, produced by DA receptor antagonists such as haloperidol (Weiner and Feldon, 1987; Christison et al., 1988), which indicate a specific role for DA receptors in these attentional phenomena. These demonstrations are also consistent with the hypothesis mentioned above, that PD patients might exhibit exaggerations in learned irrelevance or latent inhibition (Downes et al., 1989).

The latent inhibition and other models of attentional dysfunction following ventral striatal DA manipulations are interesting in the context of schizophrenic attentional disorder, but more work is required to establish the anatomical and behavioural specificity of the effects. It remains possible that changes in ventral striatal DA are important in both PD and schizophrenia, but not necessarily for their cognitive changes. For example, the DA-dependent exaggeration of conditioned reinforcing effects of stimuli formerly paired with reward following intra-accumbens amphetamine infusions (Robbins et al., 1989), could conceivably provide a substrate for the formation of delusional (including paranoid) systems if the effects of negative conditioned reinforcers are exaggerated in the same way. It is also of interest that PD patients report less experience of euphoria than do normal or clinically depressed subjects following methylphenidate administration (Cantello et al., 1989) which, in view of the animal evidence (Fibiger and Phillips, 1986), might reflect DA depletion in the ventral, as distinct from the dorsal, striatum. Overall, it seems reasonable to conclude that mesolimbic DA dysfunction would be associated, at least in part, with affective disturbance.

EVALUATION OF THE FRONTOSTRIATAL HYPOTHESIS IN SCHIZOPHRENIA AND PD

On the basis of the evidence reviewed above, it seems reasonable to suppose that frontostriatal dysfunction might be implicated in the cognitive deficits in both schizophrenia and PD. What is far less clear is which precise regions or neurochemical systems are impaired. For example, we still do not know the precise role of DA hypoactivity or hyperactivity in either the frontal cortex or striatum. We do not know which of the frontostriatal 'loops' (Alexander et al., 1986) are implicated. We do not even know whether the primary changes are to be found in the striatum or frontal cortex. There is much the frontostriatal hypothesis fails to explain at present. For example, the range of cognitive deficits in schizophrenia (Liddle, 1987b; Doty, 1989) and PD (Brown and Marsden, 1988a) is broader than we have chosen to survey. In particular, there have been reported problems in perception visuospatial function, verbal and non-verbal memory and learning, which may not implicate frontostriatal systems. Some of these deficits may be specifically frontal in nature, but there exists evidence suggesting that there might also be other neural substrates for them. For example, both PD patients (Canavan et al., 1989; Sahakian et al., 1988) and unmedicated, chronic schizophrenics (Kermali et al., 1987) can exhibit deficits in conditional learning, which could be related to frontal lobe damage, but which could also depend on the dysfunction of other regions such as the temporal lobe (Petrides, 1985). We have also not attempted to account for some of the more specialized deficits in schizophrenia, such as comprehension, which may indicate the existence of lateralized deficits (Flor-Henry, 1983). Finally, we have not attempted to account for heterogeneity, particularly in schizophrenia, either between individuals or within individuals with this disorder.

One of the more promising approaches for dealing with these immense problems has been that of Liddle (1987a, b), analysing the relationships between schizophrenic syndromes, cognitive performance and neurological dysfunction. In earlier work, Liddle (1987a) analysed the correlation between different symptoms in schizophrenia, finding little evidence for a Type I/Type II dichotomy, but a strong segregation of symptoms into three clusters, labelled 'reality distortion' (primarily delusions and hallucinating voices), 'disorganization' (inappropriate affect, poverty of speech content and formal thought disorder), and 'psychomotor poverty' (poverty of speech, decreased spontaneous movement and blunting of affect). In the subsequent study (Liddle, 1987b), he correlated these syndromes with neurological dysfunction and cognitive deficit. The main findings were that: (*1*) the psychomotor poverty syndrome was associated with neurological signs, and poor performance in tests of long-term memory object naming and conceptual thinking; (*2*) the disorganization syndrome was associated with neurological signs, and poor performance in tests of orientation, concentration, immediate recall and word learning; and (*3*) the reality distortion syndrome showed little correlation with either neurological or cognitive dysfunction, except for perhaps a figure-ground perceptual test. Liddle (1987a,b) attempts to relate these patterns to different cortical foci on the basis of other clinical and experimental data. He links the psychomotor poverty and disorganization syndromes hypothetically to damage to the dorsolateral prefrontal cortex and orbitofrontal cortex, respectively. He links the reality distortion syndrome to temporal lobe damage. He attempts to explain the heterogeneity of schizophrenia by suggesting that patients may have different combinations of these forms of damage, consistent with different patterns of cortical damage which may interact further with subcortical changes (e.g. in the ascending DA systems) to produce a spectrum of cognitive and psychotic symptoms in schizophrenia. This is an imaginative hypothesis which has the merit of being testable using the modern imaging techniques. The main problem with the scheme is that it does not readily fit the pattern of neuropsychological deficits that Liddle (1987b) obtained; it is a pity, for example, that few sensitive tests of frontal lobe dysfunction were included in the battery he used.

Liddle's hypothesis could also be conceived within the wider ambit of cortical-striatal loops (Figure 5). It is important to realize, from the scheme of Alexander et al. (1986), that most regions of cortex project onto the striatum and also that, whereas frontal projections serve both the dorsal striatum (especially the caudate nucleus) and the ventral striatum, by contrast, the entorhinal cortex, basolateral amygdala and hippocampus (subiculum) project strongly to structures of the ventral striatum, such as the nucleus accumbens (Groenewegen et al., Chapter 2, this volume). Thus, the cognitive and perhaps psychotic symptoms of schizophrenia may yet be understood within the context of impaired corticostriatal interaction. As these loops presumably interact to produce normal performance, it is possible that the fragmentary nature of schizophrenic behaviour and cognition arises from an impairment in those mechanisms controlling this interactive integration.

In reassessing the possible role of changes in DA systems in schizophrenia, the sheer heterogeneity of the cognitive dysfunction in schizophrenia argues against a single factor, such as DA overactivity, being sufficient to account for them. The DA overactivity hypothesis is also compromised because it fails to account for most of the negative symptoms of schizophrenia, including especially formal thought disorder, a core deficit of the syndrome, as it can occur in both the acute and chronic phases of the disorder. However, the nature of the interaction of striatal DA activity and the functioning of the cortical-striatal loops is a key residual issue. For example, dopaminergic activity could serve to amplify the output of whatever processing occurs in the malfunctioning networks projecting to the striatum, or alternatively

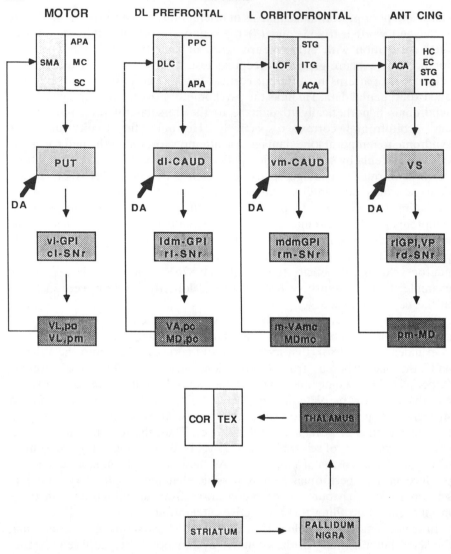

Figure 5. Corticostriatal loops according to the scheme of Alexander et al., 1986. Four of the five loops they depicted are shown here; the motor loop, the dorsolateral (DL) prefrontal cortex (pfc) loop, the lateral (L) orbitofrontal loop and the anterior cingulate (ANT CING) loop. An 'oculomotor' loop is omitted. Note the dopaminergic (DA) inputs to the striatum indicated by thick black arrows. Those cortical structures innervating the striatum are shown in the top of the figure. The 'loop' only projects back to a subset of these cortical regions. ACA, anterior cingulate area; APA, arcuate premotor area; CAUD, caudate; DLC, dorsolateral prefrontal cortex; EC, entorhinal cortex; GPi, internal segment of the globus pallidus; HC, hippocampal

more effectively oppose such output. It is easy to identify possible pathological functional correlates of each type of interaction from the examples provided in this chapter.

By comparison, while the motor symptoms of PD arise, at least in part, from a DA-dependent disruption of the 'motor' cortical-striatal loop, as defined by Alexander et al. (1986) (see Figure 5), there is considerably less evidence that parkinsonian cognitive deficits depend either upon striatal DA loss or upon structural damage in the cortex, as seen for example in MRI studies (Huber et al., 1989). The available evidence suggests that it may be more fruitful to understand the cognitive deficits in PD as resulting from impairments of telencephalic processing produced by variable damage to ascending monoaminergic and cholinergic elements of the reticular core.

ACKNOWLEDGEMENTS

I would like to thank Drs Goldberg and Weinberger for allowing me to cite their unpublished data, and the Wellcome Trust for supporting our experimental research described here.

REFERENCES

Agid, Y., Ruberg, M., Dubois, B. and Pillon, B. (1987) Anatomoclinical and biochemical concepts of subcortical dementia. In: Stahl, S.M., Iversen, S.D. and Goodman, E.C. (eds) *Cognitive Neurochemistry*. Oxford: Oxford University Press, pp. 248–271.

Albert, M.S., Feldman, R.G. and Willis, A.L. (1974) The subcortical dementia of progressive supranuclear palsy. *Journal of Neurology, Neurosurgery and Psychiatry* **37**, 121–130.

Alexander, G.E., DeLong, M. and Strick, P.E. (1986) Parallel organization of functionally segregated circuits linking basal ganglia and cortex. *Annual Review of Neuroscience* **9**, 357–381.

Alivisados, B. and Milner, B. (1989) Effect of temporal or frontal leucotomy on the use of advance information in a choice of reaction time task. *Neuropsychologia* **27**, 495–503.

---

cortex; ITG, inferior temporal gyrus; LOF, lateral orbitofrontal cortex; MC, motor cortex; MDmc, medialis dorsalis pars magnocellularis; MD, medialis dorsalis; MDpc, medialis dorsalis pars parvocellularis; PPC, posterior parietal cortex; PUT, putamen; SC, somatosensory cortex; SMA, supplementary motor cortex; SNr, substantia nigra pars reticulata; STG, superior temporal gyrus; VAmc, ventralis anterior pars magnocellularis; VApc, ventralis anterior pars parvocellularis; VLpm, ventralis lateralis pars medialis; VLpo, ventralis lateralis pars oralis; VP, ventral pallidum; VS, ventral striatum; cl-, caudolateral; dl-, dorsolateral; l-, lateral; ldm-, lateral dorsomedial; m-, medial; mdm-, medial dorsomedial; pm-, posteromedial; rd-, rostrodorsal; rl-, rostrolateral; rm-, rostromedial; vm-, ventromedial; vl-, ventrolateral. The bottom figure indicates the general cortical–striatal–pallidal–thalamic loop

Bannon, M.J. and Roth, R.H. (1983) Pharmacology of mesocortical dopamine neurons. *Pharmacological Reviews* **35**, 53–68.

Barnes, T.R.E. (1988) Tardive dyskinesia: risk factors, pathophysiology and treatment. In: Granville-Grossman, K. (ed.) *Recent Advances in Clinical Psychiatry, Number 6*. London: Churchill Livingstone, pp. 185–205.

Baruch, I., Hemsley, D.R. and Gray, J. (1988) Differential performance of acute and chronic schizophrenics in a latent inhibition task. *Journal of Nervous and Mental Disorders* **176**, 598–606.

Berger, H.J.C., van Hoof, J.J.M., Spaendonck, K.P.M., Horstink, M.W.I., van den Berken, J.H.L., Jaspers, R. and Cools, A.R. (1989) Haloperidol and cognitive shifting. *Neuropsychologia* **27**, 629–639.

Blanc, G., Herve, D., Simon, H., Lisoprawski, A., Glowinski, J. and Tassin, J.-P. (1980) Response to stress of mesocortical frontal depletion in rats after long term isolation. *Nature* **284**, 265–267.

Bleuler, E. (1950) *Dementia Praecox or the Group of Schizophrenias*. New York: Universities Press.

Bloxham, C.A., Mindel, T.A. and Frith, C.D. (1984) Initiation and execution of predictable and unpredictable movements in Parkinson's disease. *Brain* **107**, 371–384.

Boller, F., Passafiume, D., Keefe, N.C., Rogers, K. and Kim, Y. (1984) Visuospatial impairment in Parkinson's disease. *Archives of Neurology* **41**, 485–490.

Bowen, F., Kamienny, R.S., Burns, M.M. and Yahr, M.D. (1975) Parkinsonism: effects of levodopa on concept formation. *Neurology* **25**, 701–704.

Bracha, H.S. (1987) Asymmetric rotation (circling) behavior, a dopamine related asymmetry: preliminary findings in unmedicated and never-medicated schizophrenic patients. *Biological Psychiatry* **22**, 995–1003.

Bracha, H.S., Cabrera, F.J., Karson, C.N. and Bigelow, L.B. (1985) Laterality of visual hallucinations in chronic schizophrenia. *Biological Psychiatry* **20**, 1132–1136.

Brown, R.G. and Marsden, C.D. (1988a) Subcortical dementia; the neuropsychological evidence. *Neuroscience* **25**, 363–387.

Brown, R.G. and Marsden, C.D. (1988b) Internal versus external cues and the control of attention in Parkinson's disease. *Brain* **111**, 323–345.

Brown, V.J. and Robbins, T.W. (1990) Simple and choice reaction time performance following unilateral striatal dopamine depletion in the rat: impaired motor readiness but preserved response preparation. *Brain* (in press).

Brozoski, T.J., Brown, R.M., Rosvold, H.E. and Goldman, P.S. (1979) Cognitive deficits caused by regional depletion of dopamine in the prefrontal cortex of rhesus monkey. *Science* **205**, 929–932.

Buchsbaum, M.S. and Haier, R.J. (1987) Functional and anatomical brain imaging impact on schizophrenia research. *Schizophrenia Bulletin* **13**, 115–132.

Butters, N., Salmon, D.P., Granholm, E., Heindel, W. and Lyon, L. (1987) Neuropsychological differentiation of amnesic and dementing states. In: Stahl, S.M., Iversen, S.D. and Goodman, E. (eds) *Cognitive Neurochemistry*. Oxford: Oxford University Press, pp. 3–20.

Canavan, A.G.M., Passingham, R.E., Marsden, C.D., Quinn, N., Wyke, M. and Polkey, C.E. (1989) The performance on learning tasks of patients in the early stages of Parkinson's disease. *Neuropsychologia* **27**, 141–156.

Cantello, R., Aguggia, M., Gilli, M., Delsedime, M., Chiardo Cutin, I., Riccio, A. and Mutani, R. (1989) Major depression in Parkinson's disease and the mood response to intravenous methylphenidate: possible role of the 'hedonic' dopamine synapse. *Journal of Neurology, Neurosurgery and Psychiatry* **52**, 724–731.

Christison, G.W., Atwater, G.E., Dunn, L.A. and Kilts, C. (1988) Haloperidol enhancement of latent inhibition. Relation to therapeutic action? *Biological Psychiatry* **23**, 746–749.

Cools, A.R., van der Berken, J.H.L., Horstink, M.W.I., van Spaendonck, K.P.M. and Berger, H.J.C. (1984) Cognitive and motor shifting aptitude in Parkinson's disease. *Journal of Neurology, Neurosurgery and Psychiatry* **47**, 443–453.

Crow, T.J. (1980) Molecular pathology of schizophrenia: more than one disease process? *British Medical Journal* **280**, 66–68.

Direnfeld, L.K., Albert, M.L., Volicer, L., Langlais, P.J., Marrquis, J. and Kaplan, E. (1984) Parkinson's disease: the possible relationship of laterality to dementia and neurochemical findings. *Archives of Neurology* **41**, 935–941.

Divac, I. (1984) The neostriatrum viewed orthogonally. *CIBA Foundation Symposium on Functions of the Basal Ganglia* **107**, 201–221.

Doty, R.W. (1989) Schizophrenia: a disease of interhemispheric processes at forebrain and brainstem levels? *Behavioural Brain Research* **34**, 1–33.

Downes, J.J., Roberts, A.C., Sahakian, B.J., Evenden, J.L., Morris, R.G. and Robbins, T.W. (1989) Impaired extradimensional shift performance in medicated and unmedicated Parkinson's disease: evidence for a specific attentional dysfunction. *Neuropsychologia* **27**, 1329–1343.

Dyme, I.Z., Sahakian, B.J., Golinko, B. and Rabe, E.F. (1982) Perseveration induced by methylphenidate in children: preliminary findings. *Progress in Neuropsychopharmacology and Biological Psychiatry* **6**, 269–273.

Einon, D. (1980) Spatial memory and response strategies in rats: age, sex and rearing differences in performance. *Quarterly Journal of Experimental Psychology* **32**, 473–489.

Elsworth, D., Leahy, D.J., Roth, R.J. Jr and Redmond, D.E. Jr (1987) Homovanilic acid concentrations in brain, CSF and plasma as indicators of central dopamine function in primates. *Journal of Neural Transmission* **68**, 51–62.

Evenden, J.L. and Robbins, T.W. (1983a) Increased response switching, perseveration and perseverative switching following d-amphetamine in the rat. *Psychopharmacology* **80**, 67–73.

Evenden, J.L. and Robbins, T.W. (1983b) The effects of d-amphetamine, chlordiazepoxide and alpha flupenthixol on choice and rate measures of reinforcement in the rat. *Psychopharmacology* **79**, 180–186.

Evenden, J.L. and Ryan, C. (1988) Order and disorder of behaviour: the dopamine connection In: Simon, P., Soubrié, P. and Widlocher, D. (eds) *An Inquiry into Schizophrenia and Depression*. Basel: Karger, pp. 49–88.

Fibiger, H.C. and Phillips, A.G. (1986) Reward, motivation and cognition: psychobiology of the mesotelencephalic dopamine systems. In: Bloom, F.E. and Geiger, S.R. (eds) *Handbook of Physiology. The Nervous System, Vol. 4. Intrinsic Regulatory Systems of the Brain*. Bethesda: American Physiological Society, pp. 647–675.

Flor-Henry, P. (1983) Neuropsychological symptoms in patients with psychiatric disorders. In: Heilman, K.M. and Satz, P. (eds) *Neuropsychology of Human Emotion*. New York: Guilford Press, pp. 193–220.

Flowers, K.A. and Robertson, C. (1985) The effect of Parkinson's disease on the ability to maintain cognitive set. *Journal of Neurology, Neurosurgery and Psychiatry* **48**, 517–529.

Freedman, M. and Oscar-Berman, M. (1989) Spatial and visual learning deficits in Alzheimer's and Parkinson's diseases. *Brain and Cognition* **11**, 114–126.

Frith, C.D. (1979) Consciousness, information processing and schizophrenia. *British Journal of Psychiatry* **134**, 225–235.

Frith, C.D. (1987) The positive and negative symptoms of schizophrenia reflect impairments in the perception and initiation of action. *Psychological Medicine* **17**, 631–648.

Frith, C.D. and Done, J. (1983) Stereotyped responding by schizophrenic patients on a two-choice guessing task. *Psychological Medicine* **13**, 779–786.

Goldberg, G. (1985) Supplementary motor area structure and function: review and hypotheses. *Behavioral and Brain Sciences* **8**, 567–616.

Goldberg, T.E., Saint-Cyr, J.A. and Weinberger, D.R. (1990) Assessment of procedural learning and problem solving in schizophrenic patients by Tower of Hanoi type tasks. *Journal of Neuropsychiatry and Clinical Neuroscience* (in press).

Gotham, A.-M., Brown, R.G. and Marsden, C.D. (1988) 'Frontal' cognitive functions in patients with Parkinson's disease 'on': and 'off' levodopa. *Brain* **111**, 299–321.

Gunne, L.M., Graudon, J. and Glaeser, B. (1982) Oral dyskinesia in rats following brain lesions and neuroleptic drug administration. *Psychopharmacology* **77**, 134–139.

Huber, S.J., Shuttleworth, E.C., Christy, J.A., Chakeres, D.W., Curtin, A. and Paulson, G.W. (1989) Magnetic resonance imaging and Parkinson's disease. *Journal of Neurology, Neurosurgery and Psychiatry* **52**, 1221–1235.

Iversen, S.D. (1971) The effect of surgical lesions to frontal cortex and substantia nigra on amphetamine response in rats. *Brain Research* **31**, 295–311.

Iversen, S.D. (1986) Animal models of schizophrenia. In: Bradley, P.B. and Hirsch, S.R. (eds) *The Psychopharmacology of Schizophrenia*. Oxford: Oxford University Press, pp. 71–102.

Jones, B. and Mishkin, M. (1972) Limbic lesions and the problem of stimulus-reinforcement associations. *Experimental Neurology* **36**, 362–377.

Jones, G.H., Hernandez, T.D., Marsden, C.A. and Robbins, T.W. (1988) Enhanced striatal response to d-amphetamine as revealed by intracerebral dialysis following social isolation in rats. *British Journal of Pharmacology* **94**, 349 P.

Jones, I.H. (1965) Observations on schizophrenic stereotypies. *Comprehensive Psychiatry* **6**, 323–335.

Joyce, E.M. (1988) The amphetamine model of schizophrenia: a critique. In: Simon, P., Soubrié, P. and Widlocher, D. (eds) *An Inquiry into Schizophrenia and Depression*. Basel: Karger, pp. 89–100.

Kelly, P.H., Seviour, P. and Iversen, S.D. (1975) Amphetamine and apomorphine responses in the rat following 6-OHDA lesions of the nucleus accumbens septi and corpus striatum. *Brain Research* **94**, 507–522.

Kermali, D., Maj, M., Galderisi, S., Monteleone, P. and Mucci, A. (1987) Conditional associative learning in drug free schizophrenic patients. *Neuropsychobiology* **17**, 30–34.

Kraepelin, E. (1919) *Dementia Praecox and Paraphrenia*. Edinburgh: Churchill Livingstone.

Lees, A.J. and Smith, E. (1983) Cognitive deficits in the early stages of Parkinson's disease. *Brain* **106**, 257–270.

Liddle, P.F. (1987a) The symptoms of chronic schizophrenia: a re-examination of the positive-negative dichotomy. *British Journal of Psychiatry* **151**, 145–151.

Liddle, P.F. (1987b) Schizophrenic syndromes, cognitive performance and neurological dysfunction. *Psychological Medicine* **17**, 49–57.

Lyon, N., Mejsholm, B. and Lyon, M. (1986) Stereotyped responding by schizophrenic outpatient: cross-cultural confirmation of perseverative switching on a two-choice task. *Journal of Psychiatric Research* **20**, 137–150.

Mackay, A.V.P. (1980) Positive and negative schizophrenic symptoms and the role of dopamine. *British Journal of Psychiatry* **137**, 379–386.

Mackintosh, N.J. (1983) *Conditioning and Associative Learning*. Oxford: The Clarendon Press.

Marsden, C.D. (1982) The mysterious motor function of the basal ganglia: the Robert Wartenburg lecture. *Neurology* 32, 514–539.

Mayeux, R., Stern, Y., Rosen, J. and Levanthal, J. (1981) Depression, intellectual impairment, and Parkinson's disease. *Neurology* 31, 645–650.

Milner, B. (1964) Some effects of frontal lobe lesions in man. In: Warren, J.M. and Akert, K. (eds) *The Frontal Granular Cortex and Behaviour*. New York: McGraw-Hill, pp. 313–331.

Morris, R.G., Downes, J.J., Sahakian, B.J., Evenden, J.L., Heald, A. and Robbins, T.W. (1988) Planning and spatial working memory in Parkinson's disease. *Journal of Neurology, Neurosurgery and Psychiatry* 51, 757–766.

Nelson, H.E., Pantelis, C., Carruthers, K., Speller, J., Baxendale, S. and Barnes, T.R.E. (1990) Cognitive functioning and symptomatology in chronic schizophrenia. *Psychological Medicine* 20, 357–365.

Norman, D.A. and Shallice, T. (1980) *Attention to Action: Willed and Automatic Control of Behavior*. University of California: San Diego, Centre for Human Information Processing, Technical Report No. 99.

Owen, A., Downes, J.J., Sahakian, B.J., Polkey, C.E. and Robbins, T.W. (1990) Planning and spatial working memory following frontal lobe damage. *Neuropsychologia* (in press).

Pantelis, C., Barnes, T.R.E. and Nelson, H.E. (1990) Is the concept of subcortical dementia relevant to schizophrenia? (Submitted).

Passingham, R. (1972) Non-reversal shifts after selective prefrontal ablation in monkeys (*Macaca mulatta*). *Neuropsychologia* 10, 41–46.

Petrides, M. (1985) Deficits on conditional associative learning tasks after frontal and temporal lobe lesions in man. *Neuropsychologia* 23, 601–614.

Pillon, B., Dubois, B., Cuismano, G., Bonnet, A.-M. and Lhermitte, A.Y. (1989) Does cognitive impairment in Parkinson's disease result from non-dopaminergic lesions. *Journal of Neurology, Neurosurgery and Psychiatry* 52, 201–206.

Quinn, N., Rossor, M.N. and Marsden, C.D. (1986) Dementia and Parkinson's disease. *British Medical Bulletin* 42, 86–90.

Reynolds, G.P. (1988) Post mortem neurochemistry of schizophrenia. *Psychological Medicine* 18, 793–797.

Ridley, R.M., Baker, H.F., Frith, C.D., Dowdy, J. and Crow, T.J. (1988) Stereotyped responding on a two-choice guessing task by marmosets and humans treated with amphetamine. *Psychopharmacology* 95, 560–564.

Robbins, T.W. and Brown, V.J. (1990) The role of the striatum in the mental chronometry of action: A theoretical review. *Reviews in the Neurosciences* (in press).

Robbins, T.W. and Sahakian, B.J. (1983) Behavioral effects of psychomotor stimulant drugs: clinical and neuropsychological implications. In: Creese, I. (ed.) *Stimulants: Neurochemical, Behavioral and Clinical Perspectives*. New York: Raven Press, pp. 301–338.

Robbins, T.W., Evenden, J.L., Ksir, C., Reading, P., Wood, S. and Carli, M. (1986) The effect of d-amphetamine, alpha flupenthixol and mesolimbic dopamine depletion on a test of attentional switching in the rat. *Psychopharmacology* 90, 72–78.

Robbins, T.W., Cador, M., Taylor, J.R. and Everitt, B.J. (1989) Limbic-striatal interactions in reward-related processes. *Neuroscience and Biobehavioral Reviews* 13, 155–162.

Robbins, T.W., Mittleman, G., O'Brien, J. and Winn, P. (1990) The neuropsychological significance of stereotypy induced by stimulant drugs. In: Cooper, S. and Dourish, C. (eds) *The Neurobiology of Stereotyped Behaviour* Oxford: Clarendon Press, pp. 25–63.

Robertson, G. and Taylor, P.J. (1985) Some cognitive correlates of schizophrenic illness. *Psychological Medicine* **15**, 81–98.

Rogers, D. (1986) Bradyphrenia in Parkinson's disease: a historical review. *Psychological Medicine* **16**, 257–265.

Sahakian, B.J., Sarna, G., Kantamaneni, B.D., Jackson, A., Hutson, P.H. and Curzon, G. (1985) Association between learning and cortical catecholamines in non-drug treated rats. *Psychopharmacology* **86**, 339–343.

Sahakian, B.J., Morris, R.G., Evenden, J.L., Heald, A., Levy, R., Philpot, M. and Robbins, T.W. (1988) A comparative study of visuospatial learning and memory in Alzheimer-type dementia and Parkinson's disease. *Brain* **111**, 695–718.

Saint-Cyr, J.A., Taylor, A.E. and Lang, A.E. (1988) Procedural learning and neostriatal dysfunction in man. *Brain* **111**, 941–959.

Sandson, J. and Albert, M.L. (1984) Varieties of perseveration. *Neuropsychologia* **22**, 715–732.

Shakow, D.J. (1971) Some observations on the psychology (and some fewer, on the biology) of schizophrenia. *Journal of Nervous and Mental Disease* **153**, 300–316.

Shallice, T. (1982) Specific impairments in planning. *Philosophical Transactions of the Royal Society (London)B*, **298**, 199–209.

Solomon, P. and Staton, D. (1982) Differential effects of microinjections of d-amphetamine into the nucleus accumbens or the caudate nucleus on the rat's ability to ignore an irrelevant stimulus. *Biological Psychiatry* **17**, 743–756.

Starkstein, S.E., Preziosi, T.J., Berthier, M.L., Bolduc, P.L., Mayberg, H.S. and Robinson, R.G. (1989) Depression and cognitive impairment in Parkinson's disease. *Brain* **112**, 1141–1154.

Swerdlow, N.R., Koob, G.F., Geyer, M., Mansbach, R. and Braff, D. (1988) A cross-species model of psychosis. In: Simon, P., Soubrié, P. and Widlocher, D. (eds) *An Inquiry into Schizophrenia and Depression* Basel: Karger, pp. 1–18.

Taylor, A.E., Saint-Cyr, J.A. and Lang, A.E. (1986) Frontal lobe dysfunction in Parkinson's disease. *Brain* **109**, 845–883.

Waddington, J.L. and Youssef, H.A. (1986) Late onset involuntary movements in chronic schizophrenia: relationship of 'tardive' dyskinesis to intellectual impairment and negative symptoms. *British Journal of Psychiatry* **149**, 616–620.

Weinberger, D.R. (1988) Schizophrenia and the frontal lobe. *Trends in Neuroscience* **11**, 367–370.

Weinberger, D.R., Berman, K.F. and Illowsky, B.P. (1988a) Physiologic dysfunction of dorsolateral prefrontal cortex in schizophrenia. III. A new cohort and evidence or a monoaminergic mechanism. *Archives of General Psychiatry* **45**, 609–615.

Weinberger, D.R., Berman, K.F., Iadarola, M.K., Driesen, N. and Zec, R.F. (1988b) Prefrontal blood flow and cognitive function in Huntington's disease. *Journal of Neurology, Neurosurgery and Psychiatry* **51**, 94–104.

Weiner, I. and Feldon, J. (1987) Facilitation of latent inhibition by haloperidol in rats. *Psychopharmacology* **91**, 248–253.

Weiner, I., Lubow, R.E. and Feldon, J. (1984) Abolition of the expression but not the acquisition of latent inhibition by chronic amphetamine in rats. *Psychopharmacology* **83**, 194–199.

20

Drug Effects on Brain Lateralization in the Basal Ganglia of Schizophrenics

MONTE S. BUCHSBAUM, RICHARD J. TAFALLA, CHANDRA REYNOLDS, MIGNONE TRENARY, LORI BURGWALD, STEVEN POTKIN AND WILLIAM E. BUNNEY JR

Department of Psychiatry, Brain Imaging Center, UC Irvine, Irvine CA 92717, USA

HEMISPHERIC ASYMMETRY AND PHARMACOLOGICAL RESPONSE IN SCHIZOPHRENIA

Clues to the neuroanatomy of schizophrenia come from both the behavioral deficits and the psychopharmacological response to medication. Psychologists have focused on bizarre verbal productions, disturbed cognitive and attentional function, and defective communication to implicate a left hemisphere site. Psychophysical tasks and scalp EEG recordings have also supported left hemisphere dysfunction (Flor-Henry, 1979). Psychiatrists have been impressed by the dramatic improvements some patients show when treated with neuroleptic drugs, which block the dopamine (DA) receptors. This has suggested that schizophrenia is related to an overactivity of the mesolimbic or other DA neurons. This hypothesis is also partly supported by evidence that DA agonists may increase psychosis, by the relationship between levels of the DA metabolite homovanillic acid and neuroleptic response, and by the findings of increases in receptor binding in autopsy studies of patients with schizophrenia (Losonczy et al., 1987).

Until recently, evidence for these two hypotheses has been largely indirect and obtained in such different experimental settings with such different methods that the two approaches have remained separate. It has been widely

The Mesolimbic Dopamine System: From Motivation to Action.
Edited by P. Willner and J. Scheel-Krüger

© 1991 John Wiley & Sons Ltd

assumed that neurochemical systems (and therefore drug response) are symmetrical, and many autopsy studies have analysed the corpus striatum in only one hemisphere. The laterality studies have often not been linked to controlled drug trials, and have used medicated patients and examined cognitive functions thought to be localized in the cortex of the left or right hemisphere rather than in the basal ganglia. Most theories have relied largely on relatively indirect evidence for either laterality or basal ganglia deficits. Circling behavior in schizophrenics is one such indirect measure with evidence for right subcortical overactivity relative to controls (Bracha, 1987). Other indirect measures of asymmetrical motor activity, suggesting possible basal ganglia asymmetry, include clockwise drawing of circles (Marder and Woods, 1987) and Hoffman reflex asymmetry (Goode and Manning, 1988). Asymmetries in the effects of neuroleptics also provide evidence that asymmetries in motor behavior may be important. However, in such diverse phenomena as neuroleptic-induced dyskinesia (Waziri, 1980), lateralized neuroleptic-induced side-effects (Tomer et al., 1987), and lateralization of emotional expression after neuroleptic treatment (Hartley et al., 1989), the direction of dopaminergic hyperactivity may be difficult to infer.

POSITRON EMISSION TOMOGRAPHY

With positron emission tomography (PET) scanning, direct measurement of regional brain activity has become possible. The earliest PET studies evaluated frontal lobe function since reduced cerebral blood flow in schizophrenics had been observed earlier with the Xenon technique (Ingvar and Franzen, 1974). Widespread support is seen in the literature for low frontal:occipital ratio of glucose metabolism, measured with PET and for cerebral blood flow, measured with ^{133}xenon, in the brain of both medicated and non-medicated schizophrenics (Buchsbaum and Haier, 1987; Williamson, 1987; Weinberger et al., 1988).

EEG δ-activity, often associated clinically with low blood flow or cerebral dysfunction, may also be increased in the frontal lobes of patients with schizophrenia (Buchsbaum et al., 1982; Morihisa et al., 1983; Morstyn et al., 1983; Guenther and Breitling, 1985; Williamson and Mamelak, 1987; Karson et al., 1987; Guich et al., 1989). These studies did not systematically analyse asymmetries. While all found δ-increases in the frontal lobes of schizophrenics, they differed widely in statistical criteria for replication of the initial studies (Guich et al., 1989).

Not all PET studies have presented data on the frontal lobes separately for each hemisphere; in three studies, the reduction in relative metabolic rate in the frontal lobes in schizophrenics has been stronger on the right than on the left, but a significant difference in the hemispheric asymmetry for the frontal:occipital ratio has not been confirmed (Buchsbaum et al., 1984, 1990; Volkow et al., 1987). However, higher frontal lobe left:right ratios were found in normal than in schizophrenic patients by Wolkin et al. (1985).

Glucose metabolism asymmetry in the cortex has not been well demonstrated for the hemispheres as a whole. No significant difference between the metabolic rates of the whole cortex of the right and left hemispheres in resting subjects was found in a number of studies (Buchsbaum et al., 1982; Resnick et al., 1988; Szechtman et al., 1988; Cleghorn et al., 1989). Similarly, Gur et al. (1987) found no overall hemispheric asymmetry difference between normals and schizophrenics, but did observe more severely disturbed patients to have higher left hemisphere values (Gur et al., 1989).

Differences in asymmetry between normals and schizophrenics 'off' medication have not been consistent for the basal ganglia. Most studies (Buchsbaum et al., 1987; Resnick et al., 1988; Szechtman et al., 1988) have failed to find significant asymmetry, although Wolkin et al. (1985) found a higher metabolic rate in the left lentiform nucleus than in the right in normal subjects, and this left elevation was lost in schizophrenics, suggesting a left dysfunction. Early et al. (1987) found a high left globus pallidus:whole brain ratio in patients with schizophrenia, but have not reported right-sided values or statistical evaluation of the asymmetry.

Most PET studies of cerebral metabolism have shown greater effects of dopaminergic drugs on the basal ganglia than on the frontal lobe: this is consistent with the distribution of DA receptors in the brain. In animal studies, manipulation of the dopaminergic system with 6-hydroxydopamine (6-OHDA) injections produced changes in subcortical structures but not in the frontal lobes (Kozlowski and Marshall, 1980), a finding similar to later human studies (DeLisi et al., 1985). We have found a significant increase in metabolic rate in the putamen, greatest on the right, but no statistically significant change in the frontal:occipital ratio in eight schizophrenics scanned both on and off neuroleptics (1.06 on medication, 1.04 off medication (Buchsbaum et al. 1987)). No cortical area showed a statistically significant increase, although a trend ($P<0.10$) appeared toward increased metabolic rates. Further, significant correlations were found between basal ganglia metabolic change with medication and improvement as assessed by the Brief Psychiatric Rating Scale (BPRS). Cohen et al. (1988) found increases in basal ganglia metabolic rate with neuroleptics, as we did, with little effect in the frontal lobes. Increased metabolism in the lentiform nucleus with sulpiride was also found by Wik et al. (1989). This effect was greatest in the right, just as we had observed (Buchsbaum et al., 1987). Gur et al. (1987) found no effect of neuroleptics on the frontal lobe; neither did this group show basal ganglia effects (Resnick et al., 1988). The frontal lobe was one of the few areas that failed to show a significant neuroleptic effect in the study of Wolkin et al. (1985), but the increase in occipital metabolic rate produced a statistically significant decrease in the hypofrontality ratio. Wiesel et al. (1985) and Wik et al. (1989) also reported no significant effect of sulpiride treatment on the frontal lobe. Volkow et al. (1986) found no effects of neuroleptics anywhere in the brain but had only four patients (Type II error estimated at 91 per cent).

It should be noted that no study administered a fixed dose of neuroleptics for a fixed interval in a placebo-controlled random assignment trial; all followed drug-withdrawn patients subsequently treated, confounding order and drug treatment. Analysis of data from a controlled design, with patients performing a task sensitive to the effects of neuroleptics, is clearly needed to resolve this issue.

ASYMMETRY OF RESPONSE TO CLOZAPINE AND THIOTHIXENE

In a follow up of previous studies showing greater effects of neuroleptics in the right putamen, we examined the asymmetries of the response to two medications. In our current studies, twelve patients with schizophrenia served as subjects. Patients (11 men and one woman, average age 28.8 years) met DSM-III criteria for schizophrenia and were off all psychoactive medication for 2 weeks or more before beginning testing. All subjects were right-handed. Subjects with major medical illness, head injury and epilepsy were excluded.

Thiothixene-treated patients were part of a larger double-blind, placebo-controlled, random assignment, 6-week study. These five patients were scanned before treatment with a minimum of 2 weeks off treatment and 1 month or more after treatment when receiving open thiothixene. Brief psychiatric rating scale (BPRS) ratings were obtained during the blind phase of the trial, however. The mean dose was 35.8 mg. Clozapine-treated patients were part of a larger blind trial and received an average dose of 510 mg for 8 weeks.

During the uptake of [^{18}F]deoxyglucose, subjects viewed a screen that presented blurred numbers and were asked to press a button when a zero was presented, as described elsewhere (Buchsbaum et al., 1987). Metabolic rate was assessed in 6×6 mm regions placed stereotaxically in the slices according to a photographic atlas (Matsui and Hirano, 1978), as described elsewhere (Buchsbaum et al., 1987; Buchsbaum et al., 1989). We entered metabolic rate values into a five-way analysis of variance (ANOVA) with independent groups (clozapine, thiothixene), and repeated measures for treatment (before and after), structure (caudate, medial anterior putamen and posterior lateral putamen), level (dorsal, middle and ventral slices through the basal ganglia corresponding to 41 per cent, 34 per cent and 28 per cent of head height) and hemisphere (right and left). This was done to provide a single test of the hypothesis that clozapine and thiothixene would differ in their effect on glucose metabolic rate along a medial–lateral basal ganglia dimension, possibly stronger on the right than on the left. Follow-up *t*-tests would be provided on each region. We also analysed data using relative metabolic rate (the region of interest divided by the whole slice metabolic rate).

Patients treated with clozapine increased their metabolic rates in the basal ganglia, especially the right putamen; patients treated with thiothixene decreased their metabolic rates, especially in the right caudate but least in the right putamen. The effect of clozapine was more uniform across caudate and putamen (changes were in the 3–4 μmol range) in comparison to the effect of thiothixene, which showed the smallest decrease in the right putamen. Similar results were seen for the analysis of relative metabolic rate (Tables 1–3). Exploratory *t*-tests confirmed thiothixene but not clozapine effects in the dorsal caudate and clozapine but not thiothixene effects in the ventral putamen.

CONCLUSION

PET studies on medication effects in schizophrenics undertaken in this laboratory support basal ganglia lateralization only after use of neuroleptics

Table 1. Effects of clozapine and thiothixene on glucose metabolic rate

	Left				Right			
	Before		After		Before		After	
	Mean	s.d.	Mean	s.d.	Mean	s.d.	Mean	s.d.
Clozapine								
Caudate	25.2	3.5	29.7	7.5	27.5	6.7	32.1	7.1
Anterior putamen	27.6	6.4	32.1	8.1	28.1	6.0	34.1	8.1
Posterior putamen	28.0	8.8	32.4	8.7	26.4	8.4	29.5	9.3
Thiothixene								
Caudate	22.5	6.3	19.6	4.9	24.4	6.9	18.7	4.7
Anterior putamen	24.8	4.5	21.7	6.9	27.1	7.3	22.4	5.9
Posterior putamen	23.9	7.1	20.4	7.9	22.0	7.9	20.4	8.8

This difference in pattern was confirmed with the four-way ANOVA interaction (scan day by drug by structure by hemisphere, $F=8.13$; d.f.$=2,20$; $P<0.005$; multivariate TSQ$=27.04$; $F=12.2$; d.f.$=2,9$; $P<0.005$)

Table 2. Effects of clozapine and thiothixene on relative glucose metabolic rate

	Left				Right			
	Before		After		Before		After	
	Mean	s.d.	Mean	s.d.	Mean	s.d.	Mean	s.d.
Clozapine								
Caudate	1.12	0.13	1.16	0.20	1.19	0.15	1.26	0.20
Anterior putamen	1.20	0.16	1.26	0.24	1.22	0.14	1.33	0.20
Posterior putamen	1.21	0.25	1.26	0.25	1.14	0.28	1.14	0.28
Thiothixene								
Caudate	1.11	0.23	1.08	0.23	1.21	0.28	1.04	0.26
Anterior putamen	1.22	0.15	1.15	0.16	1.32	0.14	1.21	0.19
Posterior putamen	1.16	0.21	1.06	0.23	1.06	0.23	1.07	0.28

Scan day by drug by structure by hemisphere interaction, $F=7.58$; d.f.$=2,20$; $P<0.005$; multivariate $T2=24.2$; $F=10.92$; d.f.$=2,9$; $P<0.005$. Scan day by drug interaction, $F=6.93$; d.f.$=1,10$; $P=0.025$

Table 3. Left minus right difference scores before and after drug treatment

	Before	After	Change
Clozapine			
Caudate	−0.07	−0.10	−0.03
Anterior putamen	−0.02	−0.07	−0.05
Posterior putamen	0.07	0.12	0.05
Thiothixene			
Caudate	−0.10	0.04	0.14
Anterior putamen	−0.10	0.06	0.16
Posterior putamen	−0.10	0.01	0.11

in patients engaged in a visual vigilance task. As previously reported, changes are greatest on the right side. Interestingly, a difference in dorsal/ventral metabolic change is seen with the dorsal area showing more thiothixene response and the ventral basal ganglia showing more clozapine response. This is consistent with the differential effects of clozapine and a classical neuroleptic in the paw test, as reported by Ellenbroek and Cools

(1989). The dorsal/ventral striatum difference is prominent in work on stimulus–reward associations (Cador et al., 1989), but is little reported in earlier PET work. PET resolution in our studies is 10 mm in the axial plane; with the typical basal ganglia height of 3 cm, dorsal and ventral striatum can be separated. Matching MRI templates for more precise anatomical localization will add accuracy, and we are currently in the process of collecting such data.

Other sources of information on human asymmetry in the basal ganglia come from autopsy data. Unfortunately, most studies have not analysed samples from both the left and right hemispheres. Reynolds (1983) found DA asymmetries only in the amygdala and not in the caudate, but did not report on the putamen or separate dorsal and ventral regions. However, a study of D2 receptors in the rat revealed significantly higher right than left spiroperidol binding in the striatum (Schneider et al., 1982). This would be consistent with the reported asymmetrical responsivity of the right striatum in man, although cross-species analogies in function are highly questionable. It would, however, certainly seem useful to collect human brain data from both hemispheres in future clinical studies.

Magnetic resonance imaging has also revealed hemispheric asymmetries, including decreased right prefrontal white matter signal intensity in schizophrenics (Rossi et al., 1988), and more marked right than left temporal atrophy (Rossi et al., 1989). Other studies have related ventricular size to lateralization in psychomotor performance (Classen and Fritze, 1989). Detailed studies of the size, shape and anatomic asymmetries of the basal ganglia are yet to be reported, however.

The lateral semiduplication of the brain is still incompletely understood. For the clearly lateralized functions of motor control, the right and left hemisphere activity is more easily understood than for abstract cognitive activity or intense emotions which have no obvious relationship to physical space. The principle of redundancy with a spare hemisphere operates only to a limited extent, but must be considered in relationship to schizophrenia and the relationship between basal ganglia activity, and the possibly asymmetrical emotional and cognitive input into motor action. New direct indices of basal ganglia metabolism and receptor density, available with PET, should prove useful in this effort.

ACKNOWLEDGEMENTS

The authors thank the National Institute of Mental Health (Grant MH40071) and the Center for Neuroscience and Schizophrenia (Grant MH44188) for support of this research. Erin Hazlett, Steve Guich, Cheuk Tang, Brian Regardie, Michelle Solano and Lisa Auslander provided technical support, and Justine Sarashid administrative and secretarial services.

REFERENCES

Bracha, H.S. (1987) Asymmetric rotational (circling) behavior, a dopamine-related asymmetry: preliminary findings in unmedicated and never-medicated schizophrenic patients. *Biological Psychiatry* **22**, 995–1103.

Buchsbaum, M.S. and Haier, R.J. (1987) Functional and anatomical brain imaging: impact on schizophrenia research. *Schizophrenia Bulletin* **13**, 115–132.

Buchsbaum, M.S., Ingvar, D.H., Kessler, R., Waters, R.N., Cappelletti, J., van Kammen, D.P., King, A.C., Johnson, J.L., Manning, R.G., Flynn, R.W., Mann, L.S., Bunney, W.E., Jr and Sokoloff, L. (1982) Cerebral glucography with positron emission tomography. *Archives of General Psychiatry* **39**, 251–259.

Buchsbaum, M.S., Wu, J.C., DeLisi, L.E., Holcomb, H.H., Hazlett, E., Cooper-Langston, K. and Kessler, R. (1987) Positron emission tomography studies of basal ganglia and somatosensory cortex neuroleptic drug effects: differences between normal controls and schizophrenic patients. *Biological Psychiatry* **22**, 479–494.

Buchsbaum, M.S., DeLisi, L.E., Holcomb, H.H., Cappelletti, J., King, A.C., Johnson, J., Hazlett, E., Dowling-Zimmerman, S., Post, R.M., Morihisa, J., Carpenter, W., Cohen, R., Pickar, D., Weinberger, D.R., Margolin, R. and Kessler, R.M. (1984) Antero-posterior gradients in cerebral glucose use in schizophrenia and affective disorders. *Archives of General Psychiatry* **41**, 1159–1166.

Buchsbaum, M.S., Gillin, J.C., Wu, J., Hazlett, E., Sicotte, N., Dupont, R.M. and Bunney, W.E. (1989) Regional cerebral glucose metabolic rate in human sleep assessed by positron emission tomography. *Life Sciences* **45**, 1349–1356.

Buchsbaum, M.S., Nuechterlein, K.H., Haier, R.J., Wu, J., Sicotte, N., Hazlett, E., Asarnow, R., Potkin, S. and Guich, S. (1990) Glucose metabolic rate in normals and schizophrenics during the continuous performance test assessed by positron emission tomography. *British Journal of Psychiatry* **156**, 216–227.

Cador, M., Robbins, T.W. and Everitt, B.J. (1989) Involvement of the amygdala in stimulus-reward associations: interaction with the ventral striatum. *Neuroscience* **30**, 77–86.

Classen, W. and Fritze, J. (1989) Ventricular size, cognitive and psychomotor performance, and laterality in schizophrenia. *Psychiatry Research* **29**, 267–269.

Cleghorn, J.M., Garnett, E.S., Nahmias, C., Firnau, G., Brown, G.M., Kaplan, R., Szechtman, H. and Szechtman, B. (1989) Increased frontal and reduced parietal glucose metabolism in acute untreated schizophrenia. *Psychiatry Research* **28**, 119–133.

Cohen, R.M., Semple, W.E., Gross, M., Nordahl, T.E., Holcomb, H.H., Dowling, M.S. and Pickar, D. (1988) The effect of neuroleptics on dysfunction in a prefrontal substrate of sustained attention in schizophrenia. *Life Sciences* **43**, 1141–1150.

DeLisi, L.E., Holcomb, H.H., Cohen, R.M., Pickar, D., Carpenter, W., Morihisa, J.M., King, A.C., Kessler, R. and Buchsbaum, M.S. (1985) Positron emission tomography in schizophrenic patients with and without neuroleptic medication. *Journal of Cerebral Blood Flow and Metabolism* **5**, 201–206.

Early, T.S., Reiman, E.M., Raichle, M.E. and Spitznagel, E.L. (1987) Left globus pallidus abnormality in never-medicated patients with schizophrenia. *Proceedings of the National Academy of Sciences USA* **84**, 561–563.

Ellenbroek, B.A. and Cools, A.R. (1989) The dorsal and ventral striatum: their differential role in the paw test. *Behavioural Pharmacology* **1**, 49 (suppl 1).

Flor-Henry, P. (1979) On certain aspects of the localization of the cerebral systems regulating and determining emotion. *Biological Psychiatry* **14**, 677–698.

Goode, D.J. and Manning, A.A. (1988) Specific imbalance of right and left sided motor neuron excitability in schizophrenia. *Journal of Neurology, Neurosurgery, and Psychiatry* **51**, 626–629.

Guenther, W. and Breitling, D. (1985) Predominant sensorimotor area left hemisphere dysfunction in schizophrenia measured by brain electrical activity mapping. *Biological Psychiatry* **20**, 515–532.

Guich, S., Buchsbaum, M.S., Burgwald, L., Wu, J., Haier, R., Asarnow, R., Nuecherlein, K. and Potkin, S. (1989) Effect of attention on frontal distribution of delta activity and cerebral metabolic rate in schizophrenia. *Schizophrenia Research* **2**, 439–448.

Gur, R.E., Resnick, S.M., Alavi, A., Gur, R.C., Caroff, S., Dann, R., Silver, F.L., Saykin, A.J., Chawluk, J.B., Kushner, M. and Reivich, M. (1987) Regional brain function in schizophrenia. A positron emission tomography study. *Archives of General Psychiatry* **44**, 119–125.

Gur, R.E., Resnick, S.M. and Gur, R.C. (1989) Laterality and frontality of cerebral blood flow and metabolism in schizophrenia: relationship to symptom specificity. *Psychiatry Research* **27**, 325–334.

Hartley, L.R., Strother, N., Arnold, P.K. and Mulligan, B. (1989) Lateralization of emotional expression under a neuroleptic drug. *Physiology and Behavior* **45**, 917–921.

Ingvar, D.H. and Franzen, G. (1974) Abnormalities of cerebral blood flow distribution in patients with chronic schizophrenia. *Acta Psychiatrica Scandinavica* **50**, 425–462.

Karson, C.N., Coppola, R., Morihisa, J.M. and Weinberger, D.R. (1987) Computed electroencephalographic activity mapping in schizophrenia. *Archives of General Psychiatry* **44**, 514–517.

Kozlowski, M.R. and Marshall, J.F. (1980) Plasticity of [14C]2-deoxy-D-glucose incorporation into neostriatum and related structures in response to dopamine neuron damage and apomorphine replacement. *Brain Research* **197**, 167–183.

Losonczy, M.F., Davidson, M. and Davis, K.L. (1987) The dopamine hypothesis of schizophrenia. In: Meltzer, H.Y. (ed.) *Psychopharmacology: The Third Generation of Progress*. New York: Raven, pp. 715–726.

Marder, L.R. and Woods, D.J. (1987) Left hemispheric overactivation in schizophrenia: relationship to clockwise circling. *Psychiatry Research* **20**, 215–220.

Matsui, T. and Hirano, A. (1978) *An Atlas of the Human Brain for Computerized Tomography*. Tokyo: Igaku-Shoin.

Morihisa, J.M., Duffy, F.H. and Wyatt, R.J. (1983) Brain electrical activity mapping (BEAM) in schizophrenic patients. *Archives of General Psychiatry* **40**, 719–728.

Morstyn, R., Duffy, F.H. and McCarley, R.W. (1983) Altered topography of EEG spectral content in schizophrenia. *Electroencephalography and Clinical Neurophysiology* **56**, 263–271.

Resnick, S.M., Gur, R.E., Alavi, A., Gur, R.C. and Reivich, M. (1988) Positron emission tomography and subcortical glucose metabolism in schizophrenia. *Psychiatry Research* **24**, 1–11.

Reynolds, G.P. (1983) Increased concentrations and lateral asymmetry of amygdala dopamine in schizophrenia. *Nature* **305**, 527–529.

Rossi, A., Stratta, P., Gallucci, M., Amicarelli, I., Passariello, R. and Casacchia, M. (1988) Standardized magnetic resonance image intensity study in schizophrenia. *Psychiatry Research* **25**, 223–231.

Rossi, A., Stratta, P., D'Albenzio, L., Tartaro, A., Schiazza, G., Di Michele, V., Ceccoli, S. and Casacchia, M. (1989) Reduced temporal lobe area in schizophrenia

538   *Buchsbaum et al.*

by magnetic resonance imaging: preliminary evidence. *Psychiatry Research* **29**, 261–263.

Schneider, L.H., Murphy, R.B. and Coons, E.E. (1982) Lateralization of striatal dopamine (D2) receptors in normal rats. *Neuroscience Letters* **33**, 281–284.

Szechtman, H., Nahmias, C., Garnett, S., Firnau, G., Brown, G.M., Kaplan, R.D. and Cleghorn, J.M. (1988) Effect of neuroleptics on altered cerebral glucose metabolism in schizophrenia. *Archives of General Psychiatry* **45**, 523–532.

Tomer, R., Mintz, M., Kempler, S. and Sigal, M. (1987) Lateralized neuroleptic-induced side effects are associated with asymmetric visual evoked potentials. *Psychiatry Research* **22**, 311–318.

Volkow, N.D., Brodie, J.D., Wolf, A.P., Angrist, B., Russell, J. and Cancro, R. (1986) Brain metabolism in patients with schizophrenia before and after acute neuroleptic administration. *Journal of Neurology, Neurosurgery and Psychiatry* **49**, 1190–1202.

Volkow, N.D., Wolf, A.P., Van Gelder, P., Brodie, J.D., Overall, J.E., Cancro, R. and Gomez-Mont, F. (1987) Phenomenological correlates of metabolic activity in 18 patients with chronic schizophrenia. *American Journal of Psychiatry* **144**, 151–158.

Waziri, R. (1980) Lateralization of neuroleptic-induced dyskinesia indicates pharmacologic asymmetry in the brain. *Psychopharmacology* **68**, 51–53.

Weinberger, D.R., Berman, K.F. and Illowsky, B.P. (1988) Physiological dysfunction of dorsolateral prefrontal cortex in schizophrenia. *Archives of General Psychiatry* **45**, 609–615.

Wiesel, F.A., Blomqvist, G., Grietz, T., Nyman, H., Schalling, D., Stone-Elander, S., Widen, L. and Wik, G. (1985) Regional brain glucose metabolism in neuroleptic-free schizophrenic patients in an acute phase of the disease. *Proceedings of the 4th World Congress of Biological Psychiatry*. New York: Elsevier Science Publishing Co., pp. 392–394.

Wik, G., Wiesel, F.A., Sjogren, I., Blomqvist, G., Greitz, T. and Stone-Elander, S. (1989) Effects of sulpiride and chlorpromazine on regional cerebral glucose metabolism in schizophrenic patients as determined by positron emission tomography. *Psychopharmacology* **97**, 309–318.

Williamson, P. (1987) Hypofrontality in schizophrenia: a review of the evidence. *Canadian Journal of Psychiatry* **32**, 399–404.

Williamson, P. and Mamelak, M. (1987) Frontal spectral EEG findings in acutely ill schizophrenics. *Biological Psychiatry* **22**, 1021–1024.

Wolkin, A., Jaeger, J., Brodie, J.D., Wolf, A.P., Fowler, J., Rotrosen, J., Gomez-Mont, F. and Cancro, R. (1985) Persistence of cerebral metabolic abnormalities in chronic schizophrenia as determined by positron emission tomography. *American Journal of Psychiatry* **142**, 564–571.

21

Neuroleptics of the Future

ERIK B. NIELSEN AND PETER H. ANDERSEN

Departments of Behavioral Pharmacology and Biochemical Pharmacology,
CNS division, Novo Nordisk A/S, DK-2880 Bagsvaerd, Denmark

INTRODUCTION

Since the fortuitous discovery of the anti-psychotic properties of chlorpromazine in 1952 by the French physicians Delay and Deniker (Delay and Deniker, 1952), a large number of anti-psychotic drugs have been developed. However, not until recently was it convincingly demonstrated that therapeutic doses of these drugs block dopaminergic receptors in the living human brain, observations which confirmed pharmacological data which had been generated in a variety of situations in animals (Farde et al., 1986, 1988a,b). The association between dopamine (DA) and psychosis is most convincingly apparent when the concentration of drug needed to block DA receptors *in vitro* is plotted against the daily dose necessary to control psychosis, and a very high correlation is obtained (Creese et al., 1976; Seeman, 1980).

In recent years, a distinction has been made between 'classical' and 'atypical' neuroleptics (White and Wang, 1983; Vinick and Kozlowski, 1986; Lowe et al., 1988; Jain et al., 1988; New and Takaki, 1988). Classical neuroleptics (e.g. haloperidol, trifluoperazine and chlorpromazine) induce a variety of common side-effects, i.e. acute extrapyramidal side-effects (extrapyramidal symptoms (EPS); pseudoparkinsonism (rigidity, bradykinesia, tremor), akathisia and dystonias), increased levels of plasma prolactin and orthostatic hypotension (Davis et al., 1983). During long-term treatment, serious, irreversible 'tardive dyskinesias' (TD) may develop in 10–15 per cent of patients (Klawans et al., 1980; Gerlach, 1988a). Many patients also complain of psychological side-effects such as sedation, lack of initiative, depression, somnolence, decreased libido, and a feeling of 'being placed in a box' (Davis et al., 1983). Atypical neuroleptic drugs retain anti-psychotic action in the relative absence of EPS or reduced effect on plasma prolactin,

The Mesolimbic Dopamine System: From Motivation to Action.
Edited by P. Willner and J. Scheel-Krüger

© 1991 John Wiley & Sons Ltd

though the substituted benzamides do have the latter effect. Further, atypical neuroleptics are also antagonists of D2 receptors, although they are relatively weak in this respect. However, in addition to the D2 blocking effect, the compounds act at several other neurotransmitter systems in the brain (Creese, 1983; Andersen, 1988); this indicates that some of these actions may underlie the reduced EPS liability.

The relationship between anti-psychotic drug action and D2 receptor antagonism created a situation whereby, until recently, new anti-psychotic drugs were developed exclusively on the basis of their ability to block DA receptors. However, in the last few years, several new principles for obtaining anti-psychotic drug action have emerged. Some of them are based on indirect ways to modulate dopaminergic neurotransmission for the achievement of anti-psychotic effect, potentially in the relative absence of EPS. Other approaches are based on entirely new principles. The present paper is a brief review of these new approaches.

DA ANTAGONISTS WITH ATYPICAL PROFILE

DA D1 Antagonists

All clinically effective anti-psychotic drugs block DA D2 receptors. A small number of compounds also block non-selectively DA D1 receptors (Andersen et al., 1986). It was not until 1983 that it was discovered that the benzazepine SCH 23390 is a specific and selective antagonist of D1 receptors (Hyttel, 1983). Subsequent characterization revealed that the functional anti-dopaminergic effects of SCH 23390 were similar to those of D2 antagonists (Iorio et al., 1983; Christensen et al., 1984).

However, SCH 23390 lacks effects in tissues containing only D2 receptors, e.g. the mammotrophic cells of the pituitary which are tonically inhibited by DA and thus release prolactin in response to D2 receptor antagonism (Cocchi et al., 1987). Further research showed that D1 receptors exert an enabling role for the expression of DA D2 receptor stimulation (Clark and White, 1987; White, Chapter 3, this volume); therefore, the D1 receptor may exert a crucially important controlling influence on DA function (Clark and White, 1987; White, 1987). When coupled with the fact that there are many D1 receptors in limbic areas (Boyson et al., 1986) and that SCH 23390 is very efficacious in blocking amphetamine-discrimination (Nielsen and Jepsen, 1985), a mesolimbic, behavioral DA assay (Nielsen and Scheel-Kruger, 1986), this may suggest high anti-psychotic potential for D1 antagonists. A number of additional features also make D1 antagonists attractive as anti-psychotic drug candidates. These include the observation that clozapine and structurally similar compounds, which are non-selective for D1/D2 receptors, have high D1 blocking potency *in vivo* (Chipkin and

Latranyi, 1987; Andersen, 1988). Furthermore, D1 receptor function may be enhanced in schizophrenia (Memo et al., 1983). Finally, the mesolimbic DA antagonistic effect of D1 blockers may occur at relatively low occupancy level, indicating, perhaps, a reduced side-effect potential of this class of drugs (Fink-Jensen et al., 1989). The observation that a D1 antagonist (SCH 23390) produces fewer effects on DA metabolism than D2 antagonists also suggests that fewer side-effects may arise from D1 antagonism (Boyar and Altar, 1987).

At present, there are several selective DA D1 antagonists described in the literature. These include: (*1*) SCH 23390 and related 7-hydroxybenzazepines (Barnett et al., 1988); (*2*) benzazepines with fused 5-substituent ring systems (e.g. NO-756 and NO-112; Andersen et al., 1988); (*3*) isoquinolines (e.g. A-69024; Kerkman et al., 1989); and (*4*) benzonaphthazepines (Chipkin et al., 1988). These compounds are at various stages of development; unfortunately, no clinical data are available as yet. Primate data with SCH 23390 suggest that D1 antagonists may be devoid of EPS at doses which exert anti-dopaminergic (anti-conditioned avoidance) effects (Coffin et al., 1989). It remains to be established whether this is due to the poor oral bioavailability of the compound, since it was found that SCH 23390 did elicit EPS similar to those of raclopride in Cebus monkeys (Kistrup and Gerlach, 1987; Gerlach et al., 1986), or if it is due to a difference in the history of the animals in the two studies (naïve versus prior treatment with D2 antagonists).

Substituted Benzamides

The first compound from this class to be extensively characterized was sulpiride (O'Conner and Brown, 1982). It exists in two isomeric forms, the (−)-form being the pharmacologically active isomer. Sulpiride has a limited penetration into the central nervous system, but under *in vitro* conditions is a very potent D2 antagonist (O'Conner and Brown, 1982). It can be speculated that sufficient amounts of sulpiride may penetrate into relevant areas of the central nervous system where dopaminergic functions are pathologically enhanced, whereas the relative occupation of D2 receptors involved in EPS is lower. In particular, the septohippocampal system, as well as other limbic structures, may be a target for the substituted benzamides (Köhler et al., 1981, Bischoff et al., 1982). When given in 'clinically relevant' doses to rats, sulpiride selectively down-regulated the number of spontaneously active DA cells only in the ventral tegmental (A10) area (VTA), but not in the substantia nigra (A9 area) (White and Wang, 1983; Chiodo and Bunney, 1983).

This selective 'depolarization inactivation' was also obtained with other 'atypical', 'mesolimbic-specific' neuroleptics (e.g. sulpiride, clozapine, thioridazine). Metoclopramide appears to be an 'inverse' atypical DA antagonist since it selectively down-regulates A9, rather than A10, DA neurons (White and Wang, 1983), a fact which may parallel the observation that the drug preferentially causes EPS at low doses, while higher doses are needed to obtain anti-psychotic efficacy (Harrington et al., 1983; Stanley et al., 1980).

Numerous substituted benzamides have emerged since sulpiride. Some of the most recent and potent compounds include piquindone (Nakajima and Iwata, 1984), remoxipride (Ogren et al., 1984; Chouinard, 1987) and raclopride (Hall et al., 1988). These newer compounds have a much better ability to penetrate the central nervous system; nevertheless, it appears that they retain a reduced propensity to produce EPS. However, the drugs increase prolactin, as expected from their D2 blocking ability (Memo et al., 1986; Farde et al., 1988a).

It appears that many substituted benzamides bind to the D2 receptor in a sodium-sensitive manner, in contrast to other chemical classes of D2 neuroleptics which are insensitive to sodium (Creese, 1983; see however Nakajima and Iwata, 1984). The significance of this phenomenon is presently unknown.

Clozapine-Like Compounds

Clozapine is an unique anti-psychotic drug. It is a weak, non-selective D1/D2 antagonist (Andersen, 1988) which also binds to a multitude of other receptors including muscarinic, α-adrenergic, 5-HT_2 and histamine receptors (Peroutka and Snyder, 1980; Eichenberger, 1984; Hyttel et al., 1985; Altar et al., 1986; Cohen and Lipinski, 1986; Richelson, 1988). Clozapine has many side-effects, notably sedation, cardiovascular effects and, in some patients, a potentially lethal agranulocytosis (Gerlach, 1988b). Nevertheless, the anti-psychotic potential of clozapine appears to be unprecedented, particularly in otherwise 'treatment refractory' patients (Gerlach, 1988b). Clozapine selectively produces depolarization inactivation of A10 DA cells, similar to sulpiride (White and Wang, 1983; Chiodo and Bunney, 1983). The strong anti-cholinergic effects of clozapine undoubtedly reduce its propensity to cause EPS, but this apparently may not be the sole property which explains its mesolimbic specificity, since, at least in electrophysiological experiments, the α-adrenergic effect of the drug is also of importance (Chiodo and Bunney, 1985). Attempts to develop clozapine-analogs (e.g. fluperlapine) have been hampered by the problem of agranulocytosis.

Recent research has focused on the role of the D1 receptor in the action of clozapine. Thus, Andersen and Braestrup (1986) found that clozapine preferentially binds to an adenylate cyclase-sensitive conformation of the D1 receptor. However, although there are some other D1 antagonists which share this property with clozapine (e.g. NO-756; Andersen et al., 1988), clinical data are not yet available to shed light on the potential role of this effect. It can be expected that future research may lead to an understanding of the unique properties of clozapine, and hence to compounds with fewer side-effects.

Other 'Regionally-Specific' DA Antagonists

Drugs from this class include compounds which, like clozapine, appear to be 'regionally-specific' for mesolimbic DA systems (White and Wang, 1983; Chiodo and Bunney, 1983). Examples are thioridazine and molindone. Although thioridazine has strong anti-cholinergic properties (Snyder et al., 1974), which, to some extent, may explain its relative lack of EPS, it should be noted that thioridazine is largely metabolized into sulforidazine and mesoridazine (Kilts et al., 1984), and that studies on the atypical nature of thioridazine should focus on these substances.

It is also less apparent why molindone is relatively devoid of EPS liability. The drug, or possibly one of its metabolites, has relatively strong monoamine oxidase inhibitory properties (Balsara et al., 1983), a situation which may counteract the D2 blocking effects of molindone. Relatively limited research has been conducted in this potentially fruitful area (Meller, 1982; White and Wang, 1983). It could be envisioned that if the atypical nature of these compounds were explored to a greater extent, drugs with an improved profile may be identified.

Recently, CIBA-Geigy has described tetracyclic D2 antagonists which appear to be selective *in vivo* for hippocampal DA receptors (in comparison to striatal DA receptors) (Bischoff et al., 1988). The clinical data indicate that at least one such compound (savoxepine) may have a reduced propensity to cause EPS (Butler and Bech, 1987). Interestingly, substituted benzamides also appear to be hippocampus-selective in this manner (Bischoff et al., 1982). The basis for this selectivity is unknown, but may involve α-adrenergic mechanisms or a subclass of D2 receptors which, at present, are only poorly characterized (Waldmeier et al., 1982).

D2 Autoreceptor Agonists

By virtue of their lower level of occupancy by endogenous DA, so-called terminal (synthesis-modulating) autoreceptors are more sensitive to DA and other DA agonists when compared with postsynaptic DA receptors (Gariano et al., 1989a,b; White and Wang, 1984). This situation allows for certain partial DA D2 agonists to retain full agonist action at autoreceptors while having little or no agonistic efficacy at postsynaptic receptors. Autoreceptor agonists decrease the synthesis of DA, and may thus functionally mimic the action of postsynaptic antagonists. Furthermore, because of their partial agonist nature, the drugs (ideally) may exert net postsynaptic efficacy no higher than induced by endogenous DA (i.e. such drugs fail to induce strong DA agonistic effects even at high receptor occupancy); thus the potential for postsynaptic receptor–regulatory feedback effects is reduced. Interestingly, autoreceptor agonists produce the same 2-deoxyglucose utilization picture as neuroleptics, e.g. increased utilization of 2-deoxyglucose in the lateral habenula (Palacios and Wiederhold, 1984). Thus, such compounds (e.g. BHT-920, 3-PPP and CGS 15855A) produce sedation when administered to animals, but fail to produce strong classical DA antagonist effects, e.g. catalepsy, postsynaptic DA receptor proliferation or raised levels of plasma prolactin (Arnt, 1987; Clark et al., 1985). However, as agonists often produce desensitization, it can be speculated that such compounds may lose their efficacy over time. This problem has not been studied to any significant extent (Altar et al., 1987). At present, no clinical data are available, except for open clinical trials in which it was found that low (autoreceptor-selective?) doses of *N*-propylnorapomorphine and apomorphine (Tamminga et al., 1978, 1986) were anti-psychotic. Unresolved questions relate to the relative lack of DA autoreceptors in mesocortical areas (White and Wang, 1984), and what role this may play (Meltzer, 1982). However, as many selective (patented) compounds have been described in the literature, clinical data in controlled studies should soon emerge.

Mixed D2/5-HT$_2$ Antagonists

Classical D2 antagonists are endowed with EPS potential. However, it appears that the severity of EPS is reduced with drugs which are also potent 5-HT$_2$ antagonists (Altar et al., 1986; Meltzer, 1988; Nash et al., 1988; see also Svendsen et al., 1986; Janssen et al., 1988; Ugedo et al., 1989). Clozapine, for example, is a quite potent 5-HT$_2$ antagonist, but a weak D2 antagonist. This situation is somewhat in contrast to animal data, which have indicated that side-effects induced in primates with, for example, haloperidol are resistant to simultaneous 5-HT$_2$ blockade (Liebman et al., 1989; Korsgaard et al., 1985). Perhaps simultaneous 5-HT$_2$ blockade renders D2 antagonism a more efficacious anti-psychotic treatment such that lower levels of D2 receptor occupation are necessary; this in turn may lessen EPS severity. Nevertheless, several pharmaceutical companies are developing mixed D2/5-HT$_2$ antagonists. Some examples are risperidone (Janssen: Janssen et al., 1988), tefludazine (Lundbeck: Svendsen et al., 1986) and tiospirone (previously called BMY 13859, MJ 13859 or tiaspirone; Bristol-Myers/SQUIBB: Yevich et al., 1986). The clinical data so far look promising.

DA MODULATORY APPROACHES

Selective 5-HT$_2$ Antagonists

Although it might be expected that mixed DA/5-HT$_2$ antagonists will be, at least as efficacious as selective D2 antagonists, selective 5-HT$_2$ antagonists are also being developed which are claimed to exert anxiolytic and anti-psychotic effects (Ugedo et al., 1989). It was recently shown that a 5-HT$_2$ receptor antagonist ritanserin exerts an activating effect on mesolimbic DA neurons (Ugedo et al., 1989). It was speculated that such an action may be beneficial for treating Type II schizophrenia (with 'negative' symptomatology), since, in such cases, there is evidence of dopaminergic hypofunction.

Glutamate Antagonists

Cortical glutamatergic neurons project to presynaptic DA terminals and thereby exert a modulatory effect on DA release (Maura et al., 1988). This situation may allow for glutamate antagonism as a new anti-psychotic treatment principle. Glutamate receptors exist in several subtypes; thus, N-methyl-D-aspartate (NMDA), quisqualate and kainate receptor subtypes have been described (Honoré, 1989), as well as a modulatory site to NMDA sensitive to glycine (White et al., 1989). In this respect, intracerebral microdialysis work has shown that antagonism of quisqualate receptors by the quisqualate antagonist CNQX can block DA release induced by amphetamine while having no effect on basal DA release (Imperato, personal communication; Honoré, 1989).

There is also the intriguing possibility that glutamate antagonists may provide protection against a putative ischemic process in schizophrenia (Deakin, 1988). Recent evidence demonstrated by Deakin et al. (1989) showed abnormal levels of glutamatergic binding sites in the orbital frontal cortex of schizophrenics. Since glutamatergic neurons project to dopaminergic neurons in the amygdala, this may provide a mechanism which underlies the increased levels of DA in that area (Reynolds, 1983). This provides further evidence for a DA–glutamate link involved in neurotoxicity. Conversely, following ischemia, large amounts of DA are released.

Reports in which dementia, cerebral atrophy and other signs of neurodegeneration are present in schizophrenia (Boronow et al., 1985; Brown et al., 1986) are consistent with a role for glutamate in the disease. The field of glutamate antagonism is very promising for the treatment of ischemia. For example, it was shown recently that the toxicity of the dopaminergic neurotoxin methamphetamine could be prevented by MK-801, a non-competitive antagonist at the NMDA receptor subtype of the glutamate receptor complex (Sonsalla et al., 1989). At present, it appears that the only drugs being developed are NMDA antagonists (competitive, e.g. AP-7, or non-competitive, e.g. MK-801; Iversen et al., 1988) or quisqualate receptor antagonists (Honoré et al., 1988; Honoré, 1989). However, recently glycine receptor antagonists have also been described (Drejer et al., 1989).

5-HT₃ Receptor Antagonists

Antagonists at 5-HT$_3$ receptors were originally developed as drugs for treatment of cancer therapy-induced emesis (Andrews et al., 1988). Subsequent work indicated that the drugs were able to modulate dopaminergic function in the nucleus accumbens. For example, intracerebral dialysis studies showed that 5-HT$_3$ antagonists inhibit DA release in this area (Imperato and Angelucci, 1989; Carboni et al., 1989a). Conversely, a 5-HT$_3$ agonist stimulates DA release (Blandina et al., 1988). Further, 5-HT$_3$ antagonists block nicotine- or morphine-induced place preference, a learned behavior which has been shown to depend on mesolimbic DA systems (Carboni et al., 1989b). Since these systems may be involved in psychosis, it can be anticipated that 5-HT$_3$ antagonists may have anti-psychotic potential. It should be noted that the compounds are not effective in classical models for DA antagonism (e.g. antagonism of stereotyped behavior; Nielsen, unpublished data). However, a recent report showed that chronic treatment with the 5-HT$_3$ antagonist MDL 73147EF decreased the number of spontaneously active DA cells in both the A9 and A10 area; this may be a depolarization inactivation effect similar to that of haloperidol (Sorensen et al., 1989). MDL 73147EF was without effect when given acutely (in contrast to haloperidol). Sorensen et al. (1989) suggested that 5-HT$_3$ antagonists exert anti-psychotic effects when given chronically, but may be devoid of acute EPS liability. Several drugs of this type are under development, although clinical data regarding anti-psychotic potential are not yet available.

Adenosine Compounds

Adenosine is a widely distributed neuromodulator which participates in a multitude of metabolic and regulatory processes (Prémont et al., 1977; Snyder, 1985; Clark et al., 1985; Williams, 1987). There appear to be at least two adenosine receptor subtypes (A1, inhibitory; A2, stimulatory). There is a link between adenosine A2 receptors and DA (Jarvis and Williams, 1987; Abbracchio et al., 1987). For example, the adenosine antagonist caffeine produces dopaminergic-like agonist effects in 6-hydroxy-dopamine (6-OHDA)-lesioned animals, an effect which can be blocked by DA antagonists and A2 agonists (Fredholm et al., 1983). Some A2 agonists have also been shown to exert DA antagonist-like effects in a variety of animal models (Heffner et al., 1985; Jarvis and Williams, 1987; Abbracchio et al., 1987).

Few compounds seem to be in development. Warner-Lambert has described $N^6-(2,2$-diphenyl-ethyl)adenosine (compound 27) as an antipsychotic candidate (Bridges et al., 1987).

NON-DOPAMINERGIC NEUROLEPTICS

Sigma Antagonists

Most drugs today are developed using 'rational' *in vitro* screening for specific, well defined, pharmacological effects, e.g. blockade of a specific receptor. BW 234U (rimcazole), a carbazole compound, however, was found as an antagonist of apomorphine-induced fighting in rats (Davidson et al., 1985; Ferris et al., 1989). It was later discovered that the compound was an antagonist of 'sigma' receptors in the brain. The benzomorphan *N*-allylnormethazocine, or SKF 10047, and related opioids share similar psychotomimetic effects with phencyclidine (PCP) and related analogs (Deutsch et al., 1988; McCann et al., 1989). Ligand-binding studies indicated the existence of distinct 'PCP' and SKF 10047 (or sigma) binding sites (McCann et al., 1989). In pharmacological experiments, it has been difficult to demonstrate clear pharmacological effects arising from putative drug action at sigma receptors (Contreras et al., 1988; Tam et al., 1988; Iwamoto, 1989). Rather, it appears that the PCP-like effect of SKF 10047 is due to its interaction with PCP receptors since it has a high affinity for both PCP and sigma receptors. For example, sigma antagonists such as haloperidol are unable to block the discriminative effects of SKF 10047 (Deutsch et al., 1988; McCann et al., 1989) and, further, in autoradiographic 2-deoxyglucose studies, haloperidol is unable to block the effects of PCP (Piercey and Ray, 1988). It has been claimed, however, that some effects of PCP (stereotyped behavior and ataxia) may result from its actions on sigma receptors (Contreras et al., 1988). It should be noted that recent evidence points to the possibility that sigma 'receptors' in fact constitute a membrane-bound enzyme (because of the non-specific pharmacology, microsomal localization and high density in the liver; McCann et al., 1989).

Other drugs to follow rimcazole include BMY 14802 which was recently characterized electrophysiologically (Matthews et al., 1986; Wachtel and White, 1988), HR 375 (Hock et al., 1985) and tiospirone (Largent et al., 1988). BMY 14802 was found specifically to reverse apomorphine-induced decreases in DA cell firing when given acutely. Chronic BMY 14802 selectively decreased the number of spontaneously active A10 DA cells by a mechanism different from that of anti-psychotic drugs (depolarization inactivation). The interaction between DA systems and sigma receptors is complex, and it is difficult to evaluate to what extent sigma antagonism is a valid therapeutic principle. Clinical experience with BMY 14802 and rimcazole is limited (Deutsch et al., 1988) and is not yet conclusive.

Calcium Channel Antagonists

Some neuroleptics (e.g. trifluoperazine) are potent antagonists of calcium (Ca^{2+}) channels (Deutsch et al., 1988). It has been speculated that this effect may contribute to their anti-psychotic potential particularly to the effect of such drugs on Type II symptomatology (Meltzer et al., 1986). At present, there are few studies on the anti-psychotic potential of Ca^{2+} channel blockers. Recent reports (Pileblad and Carlsson, 1987; Fadda et al., 1989) indicate that Ca^{2+} blockade may lead to decreased DA synthesis in the brain. The clinical utility of this principle has not yet been explored.

CONCLUSIONS

Several interesting new pharmacological approaches are now being developed for the treatment of psychosis. These approaches are largely based on discoveries made in animal models. It is readily apparent, however, that almost all of these approaches center around DA, i.e. the anti-psychotic potential of these new principles evolves from the DA theory of psychosis. This situation is probably related to the fact that the cost of drug development has risen to very high levels; consequently, the pharmaceutical industry is faced with a decreased ability to test entirely new (non-dopaminergic) principles. It can be anticipated that DA-related therapies may not show an efficacy which is substantially superior to that of neuroleptics; however, the potential for side-effects may be reduced. Truly new therapeutic principles may appear only out of serendipity (as with many other pharmaceutical discoveries), or when the biological basis for psychosis is discovered.

ACKNOWLEDGEMENTS

Mrs E. Darmer is thanked for skilful assistance in the preparation of this manuscript.

REFERENCES

Abbracchio, M.P., Colombo, F., DiLuca, M., Zaratin, P. and Cattabeni, F. (1987) Adenosine modulates the dopaminergic function in the nigrostriatal system by interacting with striatal dopamine dependent adenylate cyclase. *Pharmacological Research Communications* **19**, 275–286.
Altar, C.A., Wasley, A.M., Neale, R.F. and Stone, G.A. (1986) Typical and atypical

antipsychotic occupancy of D2 and S2 receptors: an autoradiographic analysis in rat brain. *Brain Research Bulletin* **16**, 517–525.

Altar, C.A., Boyar, W.C. and Wood, P.L. (1987) Dopamine autoreceptor agonists including CGS 15855A decrease dopamine release and metabolism in mouse brain. *European Journal of Pharmacology* **134**, 303–311.

Andersen, P.H. (1988) Comparison of the pharmacological characteristics of [^{3}H] raclopride and [^{3}H]SCH 23390 binding to dopamine receptors in vivo in mouse brain. *European Journal of Pharmacology* **146**, 113–120.

Andersen, P.H. and Braestrup, C. (1986) Evidence for different states of the dopamine D1 receptor: clozapine and fluperlapine may preferentially label an adenylate cyclase-coupled state of the D1 receptor. *Journal of Neurochemistry* **47**, 1822–1831.

Andersen, P.H., Nielsen, E.B., Groenvald, F.C. and Braestrup, C. (1986) Some atypical neuroleptics inhibit [^{3}H]SCH 23390 binding in vivo. *European Journal of Pharmacology* **120**, 143–144.

Andersen, P.H., Groenvald, F.C., Hohlweg, R., Hansen, L.B., Guddal, E. and Braestrup, C. (1988) NO-112, NO-756—new dopamine D1 selective antagonists. *Society for Neuroscience Abstracts* **14**, 935.

Andrews, P.L.R., Rapeport, W.G. and Sanger, G.J. (1988) Neuropharmacology of emesis induced by anti-cancer therapy. *Trends in Pharmacological Science* **9**, 334–341.

Arnt, J. (1987) Behavioral studies of dopamine receptors: evidence for regional selectivity and receptor multiplicity. In: Creese, I. and Fraser, C. (eds) *Structure and Function of Dopamine Receptors*. New York: Alan R. Liss, pp. 199–231.

Balsara, J.J., Gada, V.P., Nandal, N.V. and Chandorkar, A.G. (1983) Psychopharmacological investigation of the monoamine oxidase inhibitory activity of molindone, a dihydroindolone neuroleptic. *Journal of Pharmacy and Pharmacology* **36**, 608–613.

Barnett, A., McQuade, R., Chipkin, R., Vemulapalli, S. and Chiu, P. (1988) The effects of SCH 23390 and related benzazepines on other CNS and peripheral receptor systems. In: Spano, P.F., Biggio, G., Toffano, G. and Gessa G.L. (eds) *Central and Peripheral Dopamine Receptors: Biochemistry and Pharmacology*. Padova, Italy: Liviana Press, pp. 69–79.

Bischoff, S., Bittiger, H., Deleni-Stula, A. and Ortmann, R. (1982) Septo-hippocampal system: target for substituted benzamides. *European Journal of Pharmacology* **79**, 225–232.

Bischoff, S., Christen, P. and Vassout, A. (1988) Blockade of hippocampal dopamine (DA) receptors: a tool for antipsychotics with low extrapyramidal side effects. *Progress in Neuropsychopharmacology and Biological Psychiatry* **12**, 455–467.

Blandina, P., Goldfarb, J. and Green, J.P. (1988) Activation of a 5-HT3 receptor releases dopamine from rat striatal slice. *European Journal of Pharmacology* **155**, 349–350.

Boronow, J., Pickar, D., Ninan, P.T., Roy, A., Hommer, D., Linnoila, M. and Paul, S.M. (1985) Atrophy limited to the third ventricle in chronic schizophrenic patients. *Archives of General Psychiatry* **42**, 266–271.

Boyar, W.C. and Altar, C.A. (1987) Modulation of in vivo dopamine release by D2 but not D1 receptor agonists and antagonists. *Journal of Neurochemistry* **48**, 824–831.

Boyson, S.J., McGonigle, P. and Molinoff, P.B. (1986) Quantitative autoradiographic localization of the D1 and D2 subtypes of dopamine receptors in rat brain. *Journal of Neuroscience* **6**, 3177–3188.

Bridges, A.J., Moos, W.H., Szotek, D.L., Trivedi, B.K., Bristol, J.A., Heffner, T.G., Bruns, R.F. and Downs, D.A. (1987) N6-(2,2-diphenylethyl)adenosine, a novel adenosine receptor agonist with antipsychotic-like activity. *Journal of Medicinal Chemistry* **30**, 1709–1711.

Brown, R., Colter, N., Corsellis, A.N., Crow, T.J., Frith, C.D., Jagoe, R., Johnstone, E.C. and Marsh, L. (1986) Postmortem evidence of structural brain changes in schizophrenia. *Archives of General Psychiatry* **43**, 36–42.

Butler, B. and Bech, P. (1987) Neuroleptic profile of cipazoxapine (Savoxepine), a new tetracyclic dopamine antagonist: clinical validation of the hippocampus versus striatum ratio model of dopamine receptors in animals. A preliminary report. *Pharmacopsychiatry* **20**, 122–126.

Carboni, E., Acquas, E., Frau, R. and Di Chiara, G. (1989a) Differential inhibitory effects of a 5-HT$_3$ antagonist on drug-induced stimulation of dopamine release. *European Journal of Pharmacology* **164**, 515–519.

Carboni, E., Acquas, E., Leone, P. and Di Chiara, G. (1989b) 5-HT3 receptor antagonists block morphine- and nicotine- but not amphetamine-induced reward. *Psychopharmacology* **97**, 175–178.

Chiodo, L.A. and Bunney, B.S. (1983) Typical and atypical neuroleptics: differential effects of chronic administration on the activity of A9 and A10 midbrain dopaminergic neurons. *Journal of Neuroscience* **3**, 1607–1619.

Chiodo, L.A. and Bunney, B.S. (1985) Possible mechanisms by which repeated clozapine administration differentially affects the activity of two subpopulations of midbrain dopamine neurons. *Journal of Neuroscience* **5**, 2539–2544.

Chipkin, R.E. and Latranyi, M.B. (1987) Similarity of clozapine and SCH 23390 in reserpinized rats suggests a common mechanism of action. *European Journal of Pharmacology* **136**, 371–375.

Chipkin, R.E., Iorio, L.C., Coffin, V.L., McQuade, R.D., Berger, J.G. and Barnett, A. (1988) Pharmacological profile of SCH 39166: a dopamine D1 selective benzonaphthazepine with potential antipsychotic activity. *Journal of Pharmacology and Experimental Therapeutics* **247**, 1093–1102.

Chouinard, G. (1987) Early phase II clinical trial of remoxipride in treatment of schizophrenia with measurements of prolactin and neuroleptic activity. *Journal of Clinical Psychopharmacology* **7**, 159–164.

Christensen, A.V., Arnt, J., Hyttel, J., Larsen, J.J. and Svendsen, O. (1984) Pharmacological effects of a specific dopamine D1 antagonist SCH 23390 in comparison with neuroleptics. *Life Science* **34**, 1529–1540.

Clark, D. and White, F.J. (1987) D1 dopamine receptor—the search for a function: a critical evaluation of the D1/D2 dopamine receptor classification and its functional implications. *Synapse* **1**, 347–388.

Clark, D., Hjorth, S. and Carlsson, A. (1985) Dopamine-receptor agonists: mechanisms underlying autoreceptor selectivity. *Journal of Neural Transmission* **62**, 1–52.

Cocchi, D., Ingrassia, S., Rusconi, L., Villa, I. and Muller, E.E. (1987) Absence of D1 dopamine receptors that stimulate prolactin release in the rat pituitary. *European Journal of Pharmacology* **142**, 425–429.

Coffin, V.L., Latranyi, M.B. and Chipkin, R.E. (1989) Acute extrapyramidal syndrome in cebus monkeys: development mediated by dopamine D$_2$ but not D$_1$ receptors. *Journal of Pharmacology and Experimental Therapeutics* **249**, 769–774.

Cohen, B.M. and Lipinski, J.F. (1986) In vivo potencies of antipsychotic drugs in blocking alpha 1 noradrenergic and dopamine D2 receptors: implications for drug mechanisms of action. *Life Science* **39**, 2571–2580.

Contreras, P.C., Contreras, M.L., Compton, R.P. and O'Donohue, T.L. (1988) Biochemical and behavioral characterization of PCP and sigma receptors. In:

Domino, E.F. and Kamenka, J.-M. (eds) *Sigma and Phencyclidine-Like Compounds as Molecular Probes in Biology.* Ann Arbor, MI: NPP Books, pp. 327–334.

Creese, I. (1983) Receptor interactions of neuroleptics. In: Coyle, J.T. and Enna, S.J. (eds) *Neuroleptics: Neurochemical, Behavioral and Clinical Perspectives.* New York: Raven Press, pp. 183–222.

Creese, I., Burt, D.R. and Snyder, S.H. (1976) Dopamine receptor binding predicts clinical and pharmacological potencies of antischizophrenic drugs. *Science* **192**, 481–483.

Davidson, J., Dren, A., Miller, R., Manberg, P., Kilts, C. and Wingfield, M. (1985) BW234: a nondopamine receptor-blocking antipsychotic drug without extrapyramidal side effects? *Drug Development Research* **6**, 13–17.

Davis, J., Janicak, P., Linden, R., Moloney, J. and Pavkovic, I. (1983) Neuroleptics and psychotic disorders. In: Coyle, J.T. and Enna, S.J. (eds) *Neuroleptics: Neurochemical, Behavioral and Clinical Perspectives.* New York: Raven Press, pp. 15–64.

Deakin, J.F.W. (1988) The neurochemistry of schizophrenia. In: Bebbington, P. and McGuffin, P. (eds) *Schizophrenia: the Major Issues.* London: Butterworth Publications, pp. 56–72.

Deakin, J.F.W., Slater, P., Simpson, M.D.C., Gischrist, A.C., Skan, W.J., Royston, M.C., Reynolds, G.P. and Cross, A.J. (1989) Frontal cortical and left temporal glutaminergic dysfunction in schizophrenia. *Journal of Neurochemistry* **52**, 1781–1786.

Delay, J. and Deniker, P. (1952) Le traitement des psychoses par une methode neurolytique derivee de l'hibernotherapie. In J. Boudouresques and J. Bonnal (eds) *Congres des Medicins Aliensites et Neurologistes de France, Vol. 50,* Paris: Masson & Cie Libraires de l'Academie de Medicine, p. 497.

Deutsch, S.I., Weizman, A., Goldman, M.E. and Morihisa, J.M. (1988) The sigma receptor: a novel site implicated in psychosis and antipsychotic drug efficacy. *Clinical Neuropharmacology* **11**, 105–119.

Drejer, J., Sheardown, M., Nielsen, E.O. and Honoré, T. (1989) Glycine reverses the effect of HA-966 on NMDA responses in cultured rat cortical neurons and in chick retina. *Neuroscience Letters* **98**, 333–338.

Eichenberger, E. (1984) Pharmacology of fluperlapine compared with clozapine. *Arzneimittelforschung, Drug Research* **34**, 110–113.

Fadda, F., Gessa, G.L., Mosca, E. and Stefanini, E. (1989) Different effects of the calcium antagonists nimodipine and flunarizine on dopamine metaboism in the rat brain. *Journal of Neural Transmission* **75**, 195–200.

Farde, L., Hall, H., Ehrin, E. and Sedvall, G. (1986) Quantitative analysis of D2 dopamine receptor binding in the living human brain by PET. *Science* **231**, 258–261.

Farde, L., Wiesel, F.-A., Hall, H., Halldin, C. and Sedvall, G. (1988a) Central D2-dopamine receptor occupancy in schizophrenic patients treated with antipsychotic drugs. *Archives of General Psychiatry* **145**, 71–76.

Farde, L., Wiesel, F.A., Jansson, P., Uppfeldt, G., Wahlen, A. and Sedvall, G. (1988b) An open label trial of raclopride in acute schizophrenia. Confirmation of D2-dopamine receptor occupancy by PET. *Psychopharmacology (Berlin)* **94**, 1–7.

Ferris, R.M., Harfenist, M., McKenzie, G.M., Cooper, B., Soroko, F.E. and Maxwell, R.A. (1989) BW 234U (cis-9-[3-(3,5,-dimethyl-1-piperazinyl)-propyl]carbazole dihydrochloride): a novel antipsychotic agent. *Journal of Pharmacy and Pharmacology* **34**, 388–390.

Fink-Jensen, A., Nielsen, E.B. and Andersen, P.H. (1989) Dopamine receptor occupancy in vivo: functional correlates. *Behavioural Pharmacology* **1**, 50 (suppl 1).

Fredholm, B.B., Herrera-Marschitz, M., Jonzon, B., Lindström, K. and Ungerstedt, U. (1983) On the mechanism by which methylxanthenes enhance apomorphine-induced rotation behavior in the rat. *Pharmacology Biochemistry and Behavior* **19**, 535–541.

Gariano, R.F., Sawyer, S.F., Tepper, J.M., Young, S.J. and Groves, P.M. (1989a) Mesocortical dopaminergic neurons. 2. Electrophysiological consequences of terminal autoreceptor activation. *Brain Research Bulletin* **22**, 517–523.

Gariano, R.F., Tepper, J.M., Sawyer, S.F., Young, S.J. and Groves, P.M. (1989b) Mesocortical dopaminergic neurons. 1. Electrophysiological properties and evidence for soma-dendritic autoreceptors. *Brain Research Bulletin* **22**, 511–516.

Gerlach, J. (1988a) Tardive dyskinesia. Pathophysiological mechanisms and clinical trials. *Encephale* **14**, 227–232.

Gerlach, J. (1988b) Future treatment of schizophrenia. In: Casey, D.E. and Christensen, A.V. (eds) *Psychopharmacology: Current Trends* Berlin: Springer-Verlag, pp. 94–104.

Gerlach, J., Casey, D. and Kistrup, K. (1986) D-1 and D-2 receptor manipulation in Cebus monkeys: implication for extrapyramidal syndromes in humans. *Clinical Neuropharmacology* **9**, 131–133 (suppl 4).

Hall, H., Kohler, C., Gawell, L., Farde, L. and Sedvall, G. (1988) Raclopride, a new selective ligand for the dopamine-D2 receptors. *Progress in Neuropsychopharmacology and Biological Psychiatry* **12**, 559–568.

Harrington, R.A., Hamilton, C.W., Brogden, R.N., Linkewich, J.A., Romankiewicz, J.A. and Heel, R.C. (1983) Metoclopramide. An updated review of its pharmacological properties and clinical use. *Drugs* **25**, 451–494.

Heffner, T.G., Downs, D.A., Bristol, J.A. and Bruns, R.F. (1985) Antipsychotic-like effects of adenosine receptor agonists. *Pharmacologist* **27**, 293.

Hock, F.J., Kruse, H., Gerhards, H.J. and Konz, E. (1985) Pharmacological effects of HR 375: a new potential antipsychotic agent. *Drug Development Research* **6**, 301–311.

Honoré, T. (1989) Excitatory amino acid receptor subtypes and specific antagonists. *Medicinal Research Reviews* **9**, 1–23.

Honoré, T., Davies, S.N., Drejer, J., Fletcher, E.J., Jacobsen, P., Lodge, D. and Nielsen, F.E. (1988) Quinoxalinediones: potent competitive non-NMDA glutamate receptor antagonists. *Science* **241**, 701–703.

Hyttel, J. (1983) SCH 23390—the first selective dopamine D-1 antagonist. *European Journal of Pharmacology* **91**, 153–154.

Hyttel, J., Larsen, J.J., Christensen, A.V. and Arnt, J. (1985) Receptor-binding profiles of neuroleptics. *Psychopharmacology Supplement* **2**, 9–18.

Imperato, A. and Angelucci, L. (1989) 5-HT$_3$ receptors control dopamine release in the nucleus accumbens of freely moving rats. *Neuroscience Letters* **101**, 214–217.

Iorio, L.C., Barnett, A., Leitz, F.H., Houser, V.P. and Korduba, C.A. (1983) SCH 23390: a potential benzazepine antipsychotic with unique interactions on dopamine systems. *Journal of Pharmacology and Experimental Therapeutics* **226**, 462–468.

Iversen, L.L., Woodruff, G.N., Kemp, J.A., Foster, A.C., Gill, R. and Wong, E.H.F. (1988) Pharmacology and neuroprotective effects of the NMDA antagonist MK-801. In: Domino, E.F. and Kamenka, J.-M. (eds) *Sigma and Phencyclidine-Like Compounds as Molecular Probes in Biology*. Ann Arbor, MI: NPP Books, pp. 757–766.

Iwamoto, E.T. (1989) Evidence for a model of activation of central sigma systems. *Life Science* **44**, 1547–1555.

Jain, A.K., Kelwala, S. and Gershon, S. (1988) Antipsychotic drugs in schizophrenia: current issues. *International Clinical Psychopharmacology* **3**, 1–30.

Janssen, P.A.J., Niemegeers, C.J.E., Awouters, F., Schellekens, K.H.L., Megens, A.A.H.P. and Meert, T.F. (1988) Pharmacology of risperidone (R 64 766), a new antipsychotic with serotonin-S2 and dopamine-D2 antagonistic properties. *Journal of Pharmacology and Experimental Therapeutics* **244**, 685–693.

Jarvis, M.F. and Williams, M. (1987) Adenosine and dopamine function in the CNS. *Trends in Pharmacological Sciences* **8**, 330–332.

Kerkman, D.J., Ackerman, M., Artman, L.D., MacKenzie, R.G., Johnson, M.C., Bednarz, L., Montana, W., Asin, K.E., Stampfli, H. and Kebabian, J.W. (1989) A-69024: a non-benzazepine antagonist with selectivity for the D-1 dopamine receptor. *European Journal of Pharmacology* **166**, 481–491.

Kilts, C.D., Knight, D.L., Mailman, R.B., Widerlöv, E. and Breese, G.R. (1984) Effects of thioridazine and its metabolites on dopaminergic function: drug metabolism as a determinant of the antidopaminergic actions of thioridazine. *Journal of Pharmacology and Experimental Therapeutics* **231**, 334–342.

Kistrup, K. and Gerlach, J. (1987) Selective D1 and D2 receptor manipulation in Cebus monkeys: relevance for dystonia and dyskinesia in humans. *Pharmacology and Toxicology* **61**, 157–161.

Klawans, H.L., Christopher, G.G. and Perlik, S. (1980) Tardive dyskinesia: review and update. *American Journal of Psychiatry* **137**, 900–908.

Köhler, C., Haglund, L., Ögren, S.-O. and Ängeby, T. (1981) Regional blockade by neuroleptic drugs of in vivo ³H-spiperone binding in the rat brain. Relation to blockade of apomorphine induced hyperactivity and stereotypies. *Journal of Neural Transmission* **52**, 163–173.

Korsgaard, S., Gerlach, J. and Christensson, E. (1985) Behavioral aspects of serotonin-dopamine interaction in the monkey. *Psychopharmacology* **118**, 245–252.

Largent, B.L., Wikström, H., Snowman, A.M. and Snyder, S.H. (1988) Novel antipsychotic drugs share high affinity for sigma receptors. *European Journal of Pharmacology* **155**, 345–347.

Liebman, J.M., Gerhardt, S.C. and Gerber, R. (1989) Effects of 5-HT1A agonists and 5-HT2 antagonists on haloperidol-induced dyskinesias in squirrel monkeys: no evidence for reciprocal 5-HT-dopamine interaction. *Psychopharmacology* **97**, 456–461.

Lowe, J.A., Seeger, T.F. and Vinick, F.J. (1988) Atypical antipsychotics—recent findings and new perspectives. *Medicinal Research Reviews* **8**, 475–497.

Matthews, R.T., McMillen, B.A., Sallis, R. and Blair, D. (1986) Effects of BMY 14802, a potential antipsychotic drug, on rat brain dopaminergic function. *Journal of Pharmacology and Experimental Therapeutics* **239**, 124–131.

Maura, G., Giardi, A. and Raiteri, M. (1988) Release-regulating D-2 dopamine receptors are located on striatal glutamatergic nerve terminals. *Journal of Pharmacology and Experimental Therapeutics* **247**, 680–684.

McCann, D.J., Rabin, R.A., Rens-Domiano, S. and Winter, J.C. (1989) Phency-clidine/SKF-10,047 binding sites: evaluation of function. *Pharmacology Biochemistry and Behavior* **32**, 87–94.

Meller, E. (1982) Chronic molindone treatment: relative inability to elicit dopamine receptor supersensitivity in rats. *Psychopharmacology* **76**, 222–227.

Meltzer, H.Y. (1982) Dopamine autoreceptor stimulation: clinical significance. *Pharmacology Biochemistry and Behavior* **17**, 1–10 (suppl 1).

Meltzer, H.Y. (1988) New insights into schizophrenia through atypical antipsychotic drugs. *Neuropsychopharmacology* **1**, 193–196.

Meltzer, H.Y., Sommers, A.A. and Luchins, D.J. (1986) The effect of neuroleptics and other psychotropic drugs on negative symptoms in schizophrenia. *Journal of Clinical Psychopharmacology* **6**, 329–338.

Memo, M., Kleinman, J.E. and Hanbauer, I. (1983) Coupling of dopamine D-1 recognition sites with adenylate cyclase in nuclei accumbens and caudatus of schizophrenics. *Science* **221**, 1304–1307.

Memo, M., Missale, C., Carruba, M.O. and Spano, P.F. (1986) Pharmacology and biochemistry of dopamine receptors in the central nervous system and peripheral tissue. *Journal of Neural Transmission* **22**, 19–32 (suppl).

Nakajima, T. and Iwata, K. (1984) [3H]Ro 22-1319 (piquindone) binds to the D2 dopaminergic receptor subtype in a sodium-dependent manner. *Molecular Pharmacology* **26**, 430–438.

Nash, J.F., Meltzer, H.Y. and Gudelsky, G.A. (1988) Antagonism of serotonin receptor mediated neuroendocrine and temperature responses by atypical neuroleptics in the rat. *European Journal of Pharmacology* **151**, 463–469.

New, J.W. and Takaki, K.W. (1988) Antipsychotic agents. *Annual Reports in Medicinal Chemistry* **23**, 1–10.

Nielsen, E.B. and Jepsen, S.A. (1985) Antagonism of the amphetamine cue by both classical and atypical antipsychotic drugs. *European Journal of Pharmacology* **111**, 167–176.

Nielsen, E.B. and Scheel-Kruger, J. (1986) Cueing effects of amphetamine and LSD: elicitation by direct microinjection of the drugs into the nucleus accumbens. *European Journal of Pharmacology* **125**, 85–92.

O'Conner, S.E. and Brown, R.A. (1982) The pharmacology of sulpiride—a dopamine receptor antagonist. *General Pharmacology* **13**, 185–193.

Ogren, S.O., Hall, H., Kohler, C., Magnusson, O., Lindbom, L.O. and Angeby, K. (1984) Remoxipride, a new potential antipsychotic compound with selective antidopaminergic actions in the rat brain. *European Journal of Pharmacology* **102**, 459–474.

Palacios, J.M. and Wiederhold, K.H. (1984) Presynaptic dopaminergic agonists modify brain glucose metabolism in a way similar to the neuroleptics. *Neuroscience Letters* **50**, 223–229.

Peroutka, S.J. and Snyder, S.H. (1980) Relationship of neuroleptic drug effects at brain dopamine, serotonin, alpha-adrenergic, and histamine receptors to clinical potency. *American Journal of Psychiatry* **137**, 1518–1522.

Piercey, M.F. and Ray, C.A. (1988) Evidence from 2-DG autoradiography that phencyclidine's functional effects are mediated by specific PCP rather than sigma receptors. In: Domino, E.F. and Kamenka, J.-M. (eds) *Sigma and Phencyclidine-Like Compounds as Molecular Probes in Biology*. Ann Arbor, MI: NPP Books, pp. 285–295.

Pileblad, E. and Carlsson, A. (1987) The Ca^{++}-antagonist nimodipine decreases and the Ca^{++}-agonist BAY K 8644 increases catecholamine synthesis in mouse brain. *Neuropharmacology* **26**, 101–105.

Prémont, J., Perez, M. and Bockaert, J. (1977) Adenosine-sensitive adenylate cyclase in rat striatal homogenates and its relationship to dopamine- and Ca^{2+}-sensitive adenylate cyclases. *Molecular Pharmacology* **13**, 662–670.

Reynolds, G.P. (1983) Increased concentrations and lateral asymmetry of amygdala dopamine in schizophrenia. *Nature* **305**, 527–529.

Richelson, E. (1988) Neuroleptic binding to human brain receptors: relation to clinical effects. *Annals of the New York Academy of Science* **537**, 435–442.

Seeman, P. (1980) Brain dopamine receptors. *Pharmacological Reviews* **32**, 229–313.

Snyder, S.H. (1985) Adenosine as a neuromodulator. *Annual Review of Neuroscience* **8**, 103–124.

Snyder, S.H., Greenberg, D. and Yamamura, H.I. (1974) Antischizophrenic drugs and brain cholinergic receptors. *Archives of General Psychiatry* **31**, 58–61.

Sonsalla, P.K., Nicklas, W.J. and Heikkila, R.E. (1989) Role for excitatory amino acids in methamphetamine-induced nigrostriatal dopaminergic toxicity. *Science* **243**, 398–400.

Sorensen, S.M., Humphreys, T.M. and Palfreyman, M.G. (1989) Effect of acute and chronic MDL 73,147EF, a 5-HT$_3$ receptor antagonist, on A9 and A10 dopamine neurons. *European Journal of Pharmacology* **163**, 115–118.

Stanley, M., Lautin, A., Rotrosen, J., Gershon, S. and Kleinberg, D. (1980) Metoclopramide: antipsychotic efficacy of a drug lacking potency in receptor models. *Psychopharmacology* **71**, 219–225.

Svendsen, O., Arnt, J., Boeck, V., Bögesö, K.P., Christensen, A.V., Hyttel, J. and Larsen, J.-J. (1986) The neuropharmacological profile of tefludazine, a potential antipsychotic drug with dopamine and serotonin receptor antagonistic effects. *Drug Development Research* **7**, 35–47.

Tam, S.W., Steinfels, G.F. and Cook, L. (1988) Biochemical and behavioral aspects of sigma and phencyclidine receptors: similarities and differences. In: Domino, E.F. and Kamenka, J.-M. (eds) *Sigma and Phencyclidine-Like Compounds as Molecular Probes in Biology*. Ann Arbor, MI: NPP Books, pp. 383–396.

Tamminga, C.A., Schaffer, M.H., Smith, R.C. and Davis, J.M. (1978) Apomorphine improves schizophrenic symptoms. *Science* **200**, 567–568.

Tamminga, C.A., Gotts, M.D., Thaker, G.K., Alphs, L.D. and Foster, N.L. (1986) Dopamine agonist treatment of schizophrenia with N-propylnorapomorphine. *Archives of General Psychiatry* **43**, 398–402 (erratum on p. 899).

Ugedo, L., Grenhoff, J. and Svensson, T.H. (1989) Ritanserin, a 5-HT2 receptor antagonist, activates midbrain dopamine neurons by blocking serotonergic inhibition. *Psychopharmacology* **98**, 45–50.

Vinick, F.J. and Kozlowski, M.R. (1986) Atypical antipsychotic agents. *Annual Reports in Medicinal Chemistry* **21**, 1–8.

Wachtel, S.R. and White, F.J. (1988) Electrophysiological effects of BMY 14802, a new potential antipsychotic drug, on midbrain dopamine neurons in the rat: acute and chronic studies. *Journal of Pharmacology and Experimental Therapeutics* **244**, 410–416.

Waldmeier, P.C., Ortmann, R. and Bischoff, S. (1982) Modulation of dopaminergic transmission by alpha-noradrenergic agonists and antagonists: evidence for antidopaminergic properties of some alpha antagonists. *Experientia* **38**, 1168–1176.

White, F.J. (1987) D-1 dopamine receptor stimulation enables the inhibition of nucleus accumbens neurons by a D-2 receptor agonist. *European Journal of Pharmacology* **135**, 101–105.

White, F.J. and Wang, R.Y. (1983) Differential effects of classical and atypical antipsychotic drugs on A9 and A10 dopamine neurons. *Science* **221**, 1054–1057.

White, F.J. and Wang, R.Y. (1984) A10 dopamine neurons: role of autoreceptors in determining firing rate and sensitivity to dopamine agonists. *Life Science* **34**, 1161–1170.

White, W.F., Brown, K.L. and Frank, D.M. (1989) Glycine binding to rat cortex and spinal cord: binding characteristics and pharmacology reveal distinct populations of sites. *Journal of Neurochemistry* **53**, 503–512.

Williams, M. (1987) Purine receptors in mammalian tissues: pharmacology and functional significance. *Annual Review of Pharmacology and Toxicology* **27**, 315–345.

Yevich, J.P., New, J.S., Smith, D.W., Lobeck, W.G., Catt, J.D., Minielli, J.L., Eison, M.S., Taylor, D.P., Riblet, L.A. and Temple, D.L. Jr (1986) Synthesis and biological evaluation of 1-(1,2-benzisothiazol-3-yl)- and (1,2-benzisoxazol-3-yl) piperazine derivatives as potential antipsychotic agents. *Journal of Medicinal Chemistry* **29**, 359–369.

Part 4
FROM MOTIVATION TO ACTION

22

The Mesolimbic System: Principles of Operation

JØRGEN SCHEEL-KRÜGER[1] AND PAUL WILLNER[2]

[1]Psychopharmacological Research Laboratory, St Hans Hospital, DK-4000 Roskilde, Denmark; [2]Department of Psychology, City of London Polytechnic, Old Castle Street, London E1 7NT, UK

INTRODUCTION

The construct of motivation provides a powerful heuristic framework within which to conceptualize the ways in which behaviour is organized, directed and energized in response to bodily needs and salient external stimuli. Early research into the physiological substrates of motivated behaviour focused primarily on the hypothalamus, driven largely by observations of changes in consummatory behaviour following damage to the lateral or ventromedial hypothalamic nuclei (Anand and Brobeck, 1951), and the discovery of intracranial self-stimulation (Margules and Olds, 1962). However, it subsequently became clear that many of the functions originally attributed to the lateral hypothalamus should in fact be attributed to fibre systems traversing this area, and striking similarities were demonstrated between the effects of lateral hypothalamic damage and those of 6-hydroxydopamine (6-OHDA) lesions of the ascending dopamine (DA) projections (Ungerstedt, 1971).

Another most significant development was the identification of the ventral striatum as a 'limbic–motor interface' (Stevens, 1973; Nauta et al., 1978; Mogenson et al., 1980; Heimer et al., 1982). The 'limbic system' has been implicated in emotion and motivation since the very beginnings of physiological psychology (Papez, 1937): the ventral striatum was now seen to be an area in which information from 'limbic' structures, particularly the amygdala and hippocampus, gains access to the motor system (Mogenson et al., 1980; Mogenson, 1987; Cools, 1988). The innervation from the

The Mesolimbic Dopamine System: From Motivation to Action.
Edited by P. Willner and J. Scheel-Krüger

© 1991 John Wiley & Sons Ltd

mesolimbic DA system controls the flow of information through the ventral striatum and thereby fulfils the energizing functions traditionally ascribed to the lateral hypothalamus: the translation of motivation into action. This chapter summarizes our current understanding of its mode of action.

INPUTS TO THE MESOLIMBIC DA SYSTEM

Conditions for Activation

The mesolimbic DA system is powerfully activated by stimuli that predict the imminent delivery of rewards (Phillips et al., Chapter 8, this volume). Stimuli predictive of reward acquire incentive properties: in addition to simply providing information, they also function as motivators to activate and direct behaviour towards the goal (Bindra, 1969; Bozarth, Chapter 12, this volume). However, in contrast to the strong evidence that activity in the mesolimbic system increases in the preparatory phase of appetitive instrumental behaviour, and contrary to earlier reports, the most recent evidence, from studies using *in vivo* electrochemical detection, suggests that the mesolimbic system is not activated further by the delivery of a reward (or that if such activation does occur, its size is small relative to the changes observed during the preparatory phase) (Phillips et al., Chapter 8, this volume).

From a functional perspective it makes very good sense to switch on a system that facilitates active behaviour during the approach to a goal, but to take a more relaxed approach once the goal has been attained. This common-sense notion is supported by the observation that a period of consummatory behaviour, such as feeding (Antin et al., 1975) or even more strikingly, copulation, is typically followed by a period of rest or sleep (which would not be predicted simply from the energy expended in attaining the goal), rather than by the frantic activity that would be expected if rewards stimulated further DA release.

The difficulty in accepting this eminently sensible position is that certain kinds of rewards, namely brain stimulation (at certain sites) and drugs, do activate the mesolimbic system, and furthermore, that this is the basis of their rewarding effects (Bozarth, Chapter 12; Cooper, Chapter 13; Di Chiara et al., Chapter 14; Pulvirenti et al., Chapter 5, this volume). The simple resolution is to accept that there are at least two distinct types of reward. Drug (particularly psychomotor stimulant) reward, brain stimulation reward, and the conditioned reward provided by appetitive incentive stimuli are mediated by activation of the mesolimbic DA system; primary rewards, such as sex or the consumption of food, operate through other non-dopaminergic mechanisms. The concept of a class of rewards defined by psychomotor activation and approach behaviour, and mediated by the mesolimbic DA system, has recently been lucidly expounded by Wise (1989) (see also Bozarth, Chapter 12, this volume). It should be noted that the question of whether rewards activate the mesolimbic system is logically and conceptually distinct from the question of whether DA antagonists blunt the hedonic impact of rewards. DA antagonists would be expected to interfere not only with the effects of activating the mesolimbic system, but also with any permissive effects attributable to the basal release of DA in the unactivated state.

A second condition for activation of the mesolimbic system, less prominent in this book, but equally significant and well established, is stress (Zacharko and Anisman, Chapter 16, this volume). There is some difficulty in reconciling these data with the concept that arousal is rewarding, and there is as yet no fully satisfactory resolution to this paradox. What is clear, however, but frequently overlooked, is that in the presence of a primary or a secondary aversive stimulus, the appropriate action, resulting in avoidance or escape, leads to a more desirable outcome (D'Angio et al., 1988).

In general terms, both stressors and signals predicting reward are stimuli to action. Activation of the mesolimbic DA system serves to facilitate the generation of appropriate behaviour, and to increase its vigour until the goal is attained.

Afferent Pathways

How does information about stress or incentive stimuli reach the ventral tegmental area (VTA), where the A10 DA cells are located? A clue to this question may be obtained by considering the gross anatomy of the afferents to the VTA (see Figure 1).

Afferents from the brainstem and pons, which include serotonergic projections from the dorsal and median raphe nuclei, and noradrenergic projections from the locus coeruleus, may provide non-specific, arousing, sensory stimulation. The VTA receives more specific, processed information via numerous afferents from the forebrain. The most important areas include the medial and lateral (sulcal) prefrontal cortex, nucleus accumbens, septum, bed nucleus of the stria terminalis, ventral pallidum, medial and lateral preoptic areas, lateral and ventromedial nuclei of the hypothalamus, lateral habenula and the central nucleus of the amygdala (Nauta et al., 1978; Swanson, 1982; Björklund and Lindvall, 1986; Oades and Halliday, 1987; Swanson et al., 1987; Alheid and Heimer, 1988; Zahm, 1989).

Based on the substantial number and extent of major afferents to the VTA, it seems reasonable to assume that the A10 DA system may play an important integrative role in the control of behaviour by internal and external events. Unfortunately, our current knowledge still remains incomplete with regard to the specific role of all these afferents to the VTA and the precise

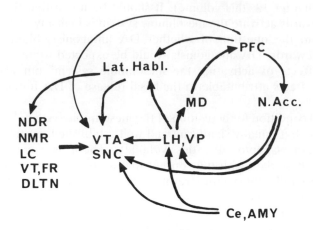

Figure 1. The 'feedback loops' of the mesolimbic dopamine neurons in the ventral tegmental area (VTA) and the medial part of substantia nigra, zona compacta (SNC) include afferents from the central amygdaloid nucleus (Ce, AMY), the lateral hypothalamus (LH), the ventral pallidum (VP), the nucleus accumbens (N. Acc.), the lateral habenular nucleus (Lat. Habl.), nucleus dorsalis raphe (NDR), nucleus medialis raphe (NMR), locus coeruleus (LC), ventral tegmental area (VTA), formatio reticularis (FR) and the dorsolateral tegmental nucleus (DLTN). It must be stressed that it is currently not known whether the loops shown on this figure represent feed-back or feed-forward loops. The prefrontal (PFC) innervation of the VTA seems thus to represent a feed-forward loop

ways in which different inputs, and different neurotransmitters, control distinct groups of mesolimbic DA cells projecting to specific terminal regions (Swanson, 1982; Simon and Le Moal, 1984; Zahm, 1989). Nevertheless, a general picture is beginning to emerge, particularly in relation to afferents from the prefrontal cortex and locus coeruleus on the one hand, and from the amygdala and lateral hypothalamus on the other.

Neurotransmitter Regulation of A10 DA Cells

There is strong pharmacological evidence that the A10 DA cells are tonically regulated by inhibitory somatodendritic DA autoreceptors (White, Chapter 3, this volume). In addition, a number of the afferent projections are reasonably well characterized in terms of neurotransmitter actions in the VTA.

Experiments using electrolytic lesions of the raphe nuclei suggested that serotonin (5-HT) projections from the dorsal and median raphe nuclei inhibit the firing of some A10 DA cells, but that 5-HT afferents from the median raphe nucleus stimulate the DA projection from the VTA to the prefrontal cortex. Thus, there is functional heterogeneity with the VTA (Herve et al., 1981). More recent studies have demonstrated that the inhibitory control of VTA–accumbens cells is mediated by 5-HT$_2$ receptors (Ugedo et al., 1989). Paradoxically, however, local injection of 5-HT into the VTA increases the release of DA in the accumbens (Guan and McBride, 1989). This effect appears to be mediated by 5-HT$_3$ receptors, since 5-HT$_3$ antagonists reduce the release of DA in the accumbens (Costall et al., 1987) or striatum (Blandina et al., 1989), as well as antagonizing the stimulation of DA release in the accumbens by morphine or nicotine (Carboni et al., 1989; Imperato and Angelucci, 1989). Chronic treatment with a 5-HT$_3$ antagonist also decreases the firing rate of both A9 and A10 DA neurons (Sorensen et al., 1989).

The nucleus accumbens, ventral pallidum and lateral habenula all provide an inhibitory GABAergic innervation to both DA and non-DA neurons in the VTA (Arnt and Scheel-Kruger, 1979; Christoph et al., 1986; Nishikawa et al., 1986). Indeed, the locomotor and behavioural stimulation seen after amphetamine administration seems most strongly correlated with the inhibition of non-DA neurons within the VTA and zona reticulata of the substantia nigra (Scheel-Kruger, 1986; Olds 1988). The non-DA VTA neurons actually represent part of the output of the mesolimbic system, providing descending projections towards the brainstem premotor neurons localized, *inter alia*, in the central grey, pontine reticular formation, lateral parabrachial nucleus, pedunculopontine nucleus and locus coeruleus (Beckstead et al., 1979; Phillipson, 1979; Simon et al., 1979; Swanson, 1982; Bjorklund and Lindvall, 1986).

Local injection of GABA agonists in the caudal part of the VTA induces compulsive locomotor stimulation, aggressive attack behaviour and increased food intake in satiated rats. By contrast, in the anterior part of the VTA, GABA agonists induce sedation, whereas GABA antagonists increase locomotor activity (Arnt and Scheel-Kruger, 1979; Tanner, 1979). These data again point to important topographical distinctions within the VTA. The inhibition of locomotion by GABA agonists in the VTA appears to involve both DA and non-DA neurons (Stinus et al., 1982).

The A10 DA cells projecting to the nucleus accumbens are activated by stimulation of nicotinic cholinergic receptors (Carboni et al., 1989; Museo and Wise, 1990; Di Chiara et al., Chapter 14, this volume). The origin of the cholinergic innervation of the VTA may be the ventral parabrachial nucleus (Niijima and Yoshida, 1988; Gould et al., 1989) and the laterodorsal tegmental nucleus, which represents an important integrating nucleus in the limbic circuitry (Groenewegen and Van Dijk, 1984; and personal communication) (see Figure 1).

Peptides and the A10 DA System

The VTA receives a substantial innervation from various peptidergic systems, including enkephalin, dynorphin, substance P, neurokinin-A (NKA) and neurotensin. The origins of these systems are still largely unknown, but may include the nucleus accumbens, basal forebrain, hypothalamus and amygdala. The substance P innervation of the VTA may be involved in stress-induced activation of the mesocortical DA system (Kalivas et al., 1983; Elliott et al., 1986); there is also evidence implicating enkephalin in this effect (Kalivas and Abhold, 1987). It must also be emphasized that the behavioural effects observed after microinjection of enkephalin in the VTA show remarkable similarities to the effects induced by low systemic doses of amphetamine, and include rewarding effects, as assessed in self-administration and place preference paradigms (Kalivas et al., 1983; Cador et al., 1988; Kelley et al., 1989; Cooper, Chapter 13, this volume).

The opioid system stimulates the VTA DA neurons indirectly, by disinhibition, through both μ and δ receptors, whereas dynorphin and other agents acting at κ receptors are inhibitory on the VTA DA cells (Kalivas and Abhold, 1987; Reid et al., 1988; Cooper, Chapter 13, this volume). Interestingly, all of the peptidergic systems produce a differential degree of activation of the VTA–nucleus accumbens, –septal and –cortical DA systems. Substance P preferentially activates the mesocortical projection, whereas NKA preferentially activates DA neurons projecting to the accumbens. Neurotensin activates the VTA–amygdala DA system, in addition to the VTA–accumbens projection (Cador et al., 1989a). The most important conclusion is: '...that each of these peptides has a distinct profile of activation of the dopamine-innervated structures. These results suggest that much attention must be given to the potential heterogeneity within the VTA' (Cador et al., 1989b; see also Sugimoto and Mizuno, 1987; Haber and Groenewegen, 1989; Zahm, 1989). This conclusion receives direct support from studies demonstrating that each peptide has a distinct behavioural profile after local microinjection into the VTA. For example, stimulation of DA receptors by d-ala-met-enkephalin (DALA) facilitates feeding behaviour, while stimulation by neurotensin inhibits feeding, and substance P has no effect. Major differences were also seen in a fixed interval schedule of food reinforcement, whereas all three peptides enhanced locomotor activity (Cador et al., 1986, 1988; Kelley et al., 1989).

Each peptide may act on different subpopulations of DA and non-DA neurons, topographically organized within the VTA and projecting to distinct regions, including the prefrontal cortex, septum, nucleus accumbens, amygdala and entorhinal cortex (Swanson, 1982; Zahm, 1989). As similar findings have already been noted in respect of 5-HT and GABA, anatomical and functional heterogeneity may be a general principle underlying the afferent innervation of the VTA.

Inputs to the VTA from the Prefrontal Cortex and Locus Coeruleus

The DA neurons in the VTA and substantia nigra show two distinct patterns of activity: the monotonic 'pacemaker' pattern and a burst-firing mode. These findings are of considerable interest because this may represent a means by which DA neurons may modulate the activity of a selected mesolimbic region by a focused pattern of synchronized bursting in a subgroup of DA neurons, within distinct parallel output channels.

Bursting activity may be induced within the VTA by two inputs. One is a glutamate/aspartate pathway from the prefrontal cortex. It is well established that the deep layers of prefrontal cortex contain not only the DA terminals but also neurons that project directly to the VTA (Christie et al., 1985; Hardy, 1986; Sesack et al., 1989). Electrical stimulation of the deep layers of the prefrontal cortex has been shown to cause an orthodromic excitation, leading to burst firing in DA neurons within the VTA and medial substantia nigra (Gariano and Groves, 1988). A second input that can induce burst firing in the mesocortical DA system is the noradrenaline (NA) projection from the locus coeruleus (Hervé et al., 1982; Grenhoff and Svensson, 1989). It seems obvious that there may be several alternatives for both feedback and feedforward loops between the NA and DA-innervated prefrontal cortex, the locus coeruleus and the VTA regions innervated by the prefrontal cortex (Oades and Halliday, 1987; Sesack et al., 1989).

Robbins (1988) has proposed that the locus coeruleus NA system becomes active under conditions in which DA activity increases; the effect of stimulating NA release would be to preserve attentional selectivity (Oades, 1985) during episodes of increased arousal and stress. An equally important role for NA, and for the glutamatergic pathway from the prefrontal cortex, may be to stimulate the VTA DA system into burst firing to activate the cognitive processes involved in coping with stressors (D'Angio et al., 1988). The prefrontal cortex may be activated for this purpose by specific patterns of internal and external stimuli, while the locus coeruleus is activated nonspecifically by novel stimuli.

Inputs to the VTA from the Amygdala and Lateral Hypothalamus

The basolateral nucleus of the amygdala receives highly integrated information from all cortical association areas, including prefrontal, parietal, temporal and insular cortex (Papez, 1937; Price et al., 1987; Alheid and Heimer, 1988; Turner et al., 1980). It is firmly established that the amygdala is part of a stimulus-analysing system in the brain (Jones and Mishkin, 1972;

Gaffan et al., 1988; Ono et al., 1989); the processing of information from sensory areas in the occipital lobe of the cerebral cortex, via temporal cortex, to the lateral and basolateral amygdaloid complex has been described in great detail (Aggleton and Mishkin, 1986; Fukuda et al., 1987; Price et al., 1987). Signals from these nuclei pass via the central nucleus of the amygdala to the lateral hypothalamus and basal forebrain, and from there to the VTA (Arbuthnott, 1980; Alheid and Heimer, 1988; Wilson and Rolls, 1990). The VTA also receives information directly from the central nucleus of the amygdala and from the insular cortex (Hardy, 1986; Price et al., 1987; Wallace et al., 1989). The amygdala–VTA projection may utilize somatostatin and/or neurotensin (Cador et al., 1989a; Deutch et al., 1988).

Following the decoding, recognition and cross-modal integration of stimuli by the cortex (Kesner and Di Mattia, 1987; Krushel and Van der Kooy, 1988; Dunn and Everitt, 1988), a major function of the amygdala, as the next processing station, is to provide the appropriate affective associations. Thus, lesions or chemical inactivation of the amygdala cause an inability to integrate environmental stimuli into normal adaptive behaviour. The amygdala plays an essential role in the learning of conditioned reinforcement, and the development of incentive motivation (Aggleton and Mishkin, 1986; Cador et al., Chapter 9, this volume). As discussed below, the effects of lesion to the amygdala are in many respects strikingly similar to those of DA antagonists or lesions of the mesolimbic DA system.

The hierarchical organization of the transmission of information from the amygdala, via the lateral hypothalamus and basal forebrain, to the VTA has been examined most extensively in electrophysiological studies of feeding behaviour (Rolls et al., 1986; Ono et al., 1986, 1989; Nishino et al., 1987; Yamamoto et al., 1989). A particularly noteworthy finding is that a substantial proportion of neurons in the lateral hypothalamus and VTA increase their activity during the anticipatory, searching phase prior to the onset of feeding, and decrease their activity during and after the consummatory phase (Nishino et al., 1987; Yamamoto et al., 1989). Cells have been described, in the lateral hypothalamus and substantia innominata of monkeys and rats, which respond to visual or auditory stimuli that have previously been associated with reward (for example, a drinking tube). Significantly, these responses were seen only following conditioning, and were only obtained when the animal was food- or water-deprived. Thus, activity in these hypothalamic cells closely reflects the incentive value of the conditioned stimulus (Rolls et al., 1986; Wilson and Rolls, 1990). These data indicate that information concerning salient environmental stimuli is transmitted from the amygdala through a gate in the lateral hypothalamus, and is only able to activate the VTA DA cells if the gate is open.

The signals responsible for the gating of neuronal activity in the hypothalamus–VTA system by the degree of motivation (food or water deprivation) may arise from the nucleus of the solitary tract (Figure 2). The posterior part of this nucleus, which receives endogenous visceral inputs, projects directly to the hypothalamus (including the paraventricular and lateral nuclei), the bed nucleus of the stria terminalis, the septum, and the central and medial amygdaloid nuclei (Ter Horst et al., 1989). Thus, all of

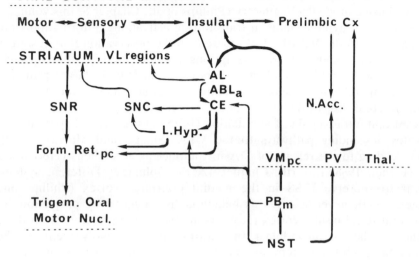

Figure 2. The nucleus of the solitary tract (NST) is one of the primary sensory sites for visceral and taste sensory input, which reach the posterior and anterior areas of NST, respectively. The NST has widespread ascending projections including the parabrachial medial region (PBm), the hypothalamus including the lateral hypothalamus (L. Hyp.), the central amygdaloid nucleus (CE), and the thalamic paraventricuar nucleus (PV, Thal). The anterior–lateral oral–gustatory NST projects via the PB to the posterior ventromedial, parvocellular thalamic nucleus (VMpc). The PB projects also to the CE and the hypothalamus. The efferents from the thalamic taste nucleus (VMpc) reach the insular cortex and the lateral and anterior basolateral amygdaloid nuclei (AL, ABLa). The motor, sensory and insular cortical regions and the ABLa innervate the ventrolateral striatum, VL. The prelimbic cortex and the PV innervate the nucleus accumbens (N. Acc.). The output systems directed towards the trigeminal oral motor nuclei include the formatio reticularis, parvocellular region (Form. Ret. pc) substantia nigra, zona reticularis (SNR), L. Hyp. and CE. The mesolimbic dopamine system from the VTA and medial substantia nigra, zona compacta innervates essential regions of the total feeding system including the prelimbic and insular cortical areas, the N. Acc., ventral striatum, PV, CE and hypothalamus

these nuclei are in a position to relay the current status of interoceptive stimuli towards the VTA DA cell region, where they are integrated with signals arriving from exteroceptive stimuli via the thalamic–visceral cortex–amygdaloid–hypothalamic axis (Price et al., 1987; Krushel and Van der Kooy, 1988).

The electrophysiological data showing activation of the hypothalamus–VTA system in the preparatory phase of instrumental behaviour are highly compatible with the time course of DA release in the nucleus accumbens observed using *in vivo* voltammetry (Phillips et al., Chapter 8, this volume). The role of the hypothalamus in transmitting activational information from the amygdala to the VTA is also apparent in the observation that gustatory preference thresholds for sweet solutions are increased by ibotenic acid lesions of the lateral hypothalamus (Ferssiwi et al., 1987); these results are exactly comparable to those observed after the reduction of DA transmission by neuroleptic drugs (Willner et al., Chapter 10, this volume). It is also relevant that intracranial self-stimulation (ICSS) in the lateral hypothalamus activates descending pathways to the VTA (Shizgal and Murray, 1989), again, leading to the release of DA in the nucleus accumbens (Hernandez and Hoebel, 1988; Bozarth, Chapter 12, this volume). (Different systems appear to subserve ICSS in the medial prefrontal cortex (Phillips and Fibiger, 1989); nevertheless, this behaviour is mediated by projections to the lateral sulcal insular cortex (Robertson, 1989), and probably from there to the basolateral amygdala.) In addition to this involvement of the hypothalamus–VTA system in appetitive behaviours, activation of the VTA DA system has also been found to facilitate attack behaviour in the cat, and to inhibit defensive behaviour following electrical stimulation of the lateral or ventromedial hypothalamus (Piazza et al., 1987, 1988).

THE LIMBIC–MOTOR INTERFACE

Inputs to the Ventral Striatum

In addition to DA and the afferents from the subiculum of the hippocampus, basolateral amygdaloid nucleus and medial prefrontal cortex, other projections to the nucleus accumbens include afferents from the entorhinal cortex and specific midline thalamic nuclei, including the paraventricular nucleus, as well as projections from the brainstem and midbrain, containing the neuromodulators 5-HT, NA, CCK and neurotensin (Groenewegen et al., Chapter 2, this volume).

As in the dorsal striatum (Gimenez-Amaya and Graybiel, 1990), the different afferents to the ventral striatum appear to follow a basic principle of topographical and parallel organization. Thus, afferents from the ventral subiculum, the posterior part of the basal amygdaloid nucleus, the posterior prelimbic and infralimbic cortex, and the paraventricular thalamic nucleus, project to caudal and medial regions of the nucleus accumbens, which is enriched with CCK, whereas afferents from the dorsal subiculum, the anterior part of the basolateral amygdaloid nucleus, the anterior prelimbic cortex, and the parataenial and central thalamic nuclei reach more lateral and rostral areas of the nucleus accumbens (Groenewegen et al., Chapter 2, this volume). From a functional perspective, it is important to add that a topographical organization is also apparent in the inputs to the subiculum and basolateral amygdala. Thus, information from the visceral-related paralimbic and infralimbic cortex projects, via the medial entorhinal cortex, to the ventral subiculum and posterior parts of the basal amygdaloid complex, whereas polysensory and parasensory areas of parietal and temporal cortex project, via the lateral entorhinal cortex, to the dorsal subiculum and anterior parts of the basal amygdaloid complex (Groenewegen et al., 1987; Groenewegen, 1988). These anatomical findings strongly suggest that the nucleus accumbens represents a functionally heterogeneous structure which receives distinct and specific afferent information to be processed within parallel loops.

The exact manner in which the terminal projections of the subiculum, basolateral amygdala and prelimbic cortex relate to one another and to the medium spiny output neurons of the nucleus accumbens remains to be clarified. It is known that hippocampal and mesolimbic DA afferents converge on dendrites or spines of the same GABAergic (Meredith et al., 1990) medium spiny neurons within the nucleus accumbens (Totterdell and Smith, 1989; Groenewegen et al., Chapter 2, this volume). Within the medial nucleus accumbens, interdigitating and complementary patterns of terminals are seen in the afferents from the ventral subiculum and prelimbic cortex (Groenewegen et al., Chapter 2, this volume); similar findings have been reported in dorsal striatum (Selemon and Goldman-Rakic, 1985). It is not currently known whether afferents from the subiculum and amygdala terminate on the same or distinct populations of neurons within the nucleus accumbens. However, within the internal patch and matrix organization of the rostral and caudal regions, the amygdalar and subicular afferents show a complex and, to some extent, distinct pattern of termination (Groenewegen et al., Chapter 2, this volume).

Gating Actions of Mesolimbic DA

There is a striking overlap within the nucleus accumbens, at least at an overall global level, between the areas of termination of the mesolimbic DA afferents, and the afferents from the amygdala, hippocampus and medial frontal cortex (Figure 2, Cador et al., Chapter 9; Groenewegen et al., Chapter 2, this volume). This fact alone would indicate that the mesolimbic

DA system modulates the transmission of information reaching the ventral striatum from these structures, and this deduction is amply confirmed by electrophysiological studies (White, Chapter 3; Mogenson and Yim, Chapter 4, this volume).

The distinction between active and passive behaviour represents a useful, if simplistic, starting point for conceptualizing the distinction between the respective roles of the amygdalar and hippocampal inputs to the ventral striatum. Thus, locomotion is increased by administration of *N*-methyl-D-aspartate (NMDA), or carbachol, to the ventral subiculum, but decreased by administration of NMDA to the basolateral nucleus of the amygdala (Mogenson and Yim, Chapter 4, this volume).

Glutamatergic projections to the nucleus accumbens are responsible for both of these responses, since both were antagonized by the local injection of a glutamate antagonist into the accumbens. The neuromodulatory effect of DA is evident, since both the electrophysiological effects of stimulating the hippocampus or amygdala, and the associated changes in locomotor activity, were also reversed by stimulation of the VTA, or following intra-accumbens injection of DA or the D2 agonist LY 171555 (Mogenson and Yim, Chapter 4, this volume). CCK, which co-exists with DA in afferent terminals, also acts in a neuromodulatory manner as a functional DA antagonist (Wang and Hu, 1986; Mogenson and Yim, Chapter 4, this volume). It is conceivable that changes in the balance of DA and CCK, co-released from mesolimbic neurons, could be involved in the changes that follow prolonged activation of the mesolimbic system (Fibiger, Chapter 24, this volume).

Cools et al. (Chapter 6, this volume) have presented evidence that these gating functions involve NA–DA interactions within the ventral striatum. Thus, activation of β-adrenergic and/or D2 DA receptors within the accumbens is suggested to close the 'hippocampal gate', while their inhibition opens this gate. Conversely, inhibition of α-adrenergic receptors and/or activation of the so-called DA$_i$ receptors in the accumbens are suggested to close the 'amygdaloid gate'. It will be important to establish whether these interactions take place on nucleus accumbens neurons that receive convergent inputs, or whether the gating of open and closed channels represents a switching between distinct types and clusters of output neurons, perhaps containing different neurotransmitters, and producing different output signals. Differences between anatomically distinct regions of the accumbens, as well as the co-existence of various neurotransmitter combinations (CCK–DA, neurotensin–DA, GABA–enkephalin, GABA–substance P, and so on), could also contribute to the generation of distinct outputs. Anatomical differences are known to exist in relation to the behavioural effects of intra-accumbens injections of CCK (Dauge et al., 1989).

The interaction between NA and the mesolimbic DA afferents may not be unique to the nucleus accumbens: it is also seen in the central nucleus of the amygdala (Dunn and Everitt, 1988; Jiang and Oomura, 1988), the extended amygdaloid complex (Alheid and Heimer, 1988), the lateral septum (Durkin et al., 1986; Marighetto et al., 1989), and the medial prefrontal cortex (Tassin et al., Chapter 7, this volume), as well as at the level of the VTA (Grenhoff and Svensson, 1989). For example, stimulation of the VTA has been found to antagonize the excitatory responses of prefrontal neurons to stimulation of the mediodorsal nucleus of the thalamus or to noxious tail-pinch, whereas stimulation of the locus coeruleus has essentially the opposite effect (Mantz et al., 1988). Furthermore, NA receptor blockade can influence the balance of DA turnover between the dorsal striatum and nucleus accumbens (Lane et al., 1988).

The respective roles of NA and DA in information transmission have been studied in greatest detail in the context of feeding-related neuronal activity in the central nucleus of the monkey amygdala, during a visually-guided bar-press task. Many neurons showed activity during the appetitive and consummatory phases. DA inputs appeared to be involved both in responding to conditioned signals (cue lights that trigger a response) and in motor initiation during the feeding phase. By contrast, NA-sensitive (β-adrenergic) cells decreased firing during the feeding phase and in extinction (Nakano et al., 1987; Jiang and Oomura, 1988), which may be relevant to the well established observation that stimulation of β-adrenergic receptors within the central nucleus of the amygdala facilitates memory formation (McGaugh et al., 1988). Interestingly, activity in cholinergic cells in the nucleus basalis innervated from the central nucleus of the amygdala was not correlated with any particular event, but the cholinergic system intensified and enhanced the effectiveness of sensory inputs to both the amygdala and the cortex (Lenard et al., 1989; Alheid and Heimer, 1988; Wilson and Rolls, 1990). These findings demonstrate distinct roles and interactions, within the amygdala, of NA and DA (Cools et al., Chapter 6, this volume) and acetylcholine (ACh). Thus, in addition to their actions in the ventral striatum, DA and NA may also have important neuromodulatory functions at the level of the major output system of the amygdala, the central nucleus. These may involve the whole of the amygdaloid output, directed both 'upstream' towards the bed nucleus of the stria terminalis, the nucleus accumbens, and the magnocellular corticopetal cholinergic cells of the nucleus basalis (the 'cognitive loop') (Alheid and Heimer, 1988; Wilson and Rolls, 1990), and 'downstream' towards the lateral hypothalamus, the VTA, the substantia nigra zona compacta and brainstem autonomic centres (Wallace et al., 1989).

Behavioural Functions of the Amygdala and Hippocampus

The overall function of the limbic system is to a considerable degree determined by the interaction between the two major limbic structures, the amygdala and the hippocampal formation. The amygdala is implicated in emotional and motivational aspects of behaviour, including the formation of stimulus-reinforcement associations; the hippocampus is concerned with the rules that guide performance (Eichenbaum et al., 1986; Ridley et al., 1989). Thus, the amygdala is concerned with the distinct individual attributes of a single stimulus, and also, in the primate, with the integration of stimulus attributes across sensory modalities (Aggleton and Mishkin, 1986; Gaffan et al., 1988): for example, monkeys with amygdalar lesions were unable to recognize visually objects previously learned by touch; by contrast, hippocampal-lesioned animals performed nearly normally on this task (Murray and Mishkin, 1985). While the lateral amygdala encodes and computes the distinct individual elements of each stimulus, the hippocampus is concerned with the overall significance of the relationships among multiple stimuli. In consequence, the hippocampus is able to mediate the storage and retrieval of contextual information (Hirsh, 1974). The whole hippocampal formation (parahippocampal–entorhinal cortex and the hippocampus proper) thus represents a supramodal or 'post-associational' cortex which generates a combined representation of all incoming information (Eichenbaum et al, 1988; Witter et al., 1989), that enables the organism to create and switch to new and arbitrary patterns of behaviour; this function is carried out in collaboration with the prefrontal cortex (Eichenbaum et al., 1986, 1988; Kesner and Di Mattia, 1987; Goldman-Rakic, 1987a, b; Ridley et al., 1989; Rudy and Sutherland, 1989).

The hippocampus and amygdala receive the same set of multimodal inputs. However, the hippocampus receives the information only after supramodal processing within the parahippocampal–entorhinal cortex (Witter et al., 1989), whereas the amygdala may receive direct sensory inputs via the brainstem and hypothalamic visceral and autonomic relays, and also via unisensory and polysensory cortical association areas (Price et al., 1987). Furthermore, the basolateral amygdala is potentially able, via the subiculum–entorhinal path, to gate an important stream of multimodal sensory information entering the parahippocampal–hippocampal system. The entorhinal cortex, which integrates limbic and associative cortical inputs, is potentially able to control activity in all of the relevant output channels directed to other multimodal association cortical areas, in addition to the subiculum, hippocampus, basolateral amygdaloid nucleus and the nucleus accumbens (Witter et al., 1989).

The Septal Area

In an early review, Cormier (1981) proposed the septum as the structure coordinating the interaction between the amygdala and hippocampus. This role is now largely attributed to the nucleus accumbens, since the major efferent projections of the amygdala are directed towards the accumbens rather than the septum. However, some aspects of Cormier's review are still of interest in the light of our current knowledge. Cormier noted that lesions of the lateral septum disrupt the output of the hippocampus (considered as a habituation system), and consequently release the amygdala (the reinforcement system) from inhibition; this explains why lateral septal lesions increase the appetitive value of a secondary reinforcer associated with food (Cormier, 1981). In contrast to this reciprocal relationship between the lateral septum and amygdala in the control of behavioural responses to motivationally significant stimuli, the medial septum was suggested to act as a relay through which the amygdala is able to activate the hippocampal habituation system. These concepts of septal function should now be integrated with our current knowledge that the essential afferent and efferent sensory inputs to the hippocampal formation pass through the entorhinal cortex, and that the nucleus accumbens undoubtedly represents the major output station.

It is also necessary to recognize the neuromodulatory role of DA within the septum. DA afferents to the lateral septum exercise a tonic inhibitory control via GABAergic interneurons on the cholinergic neurons of the septohippocampal formation (Galey et al., 1985, 1989; Durkin et al., 1986). ACh is crucial for learning and memory processes within the hippocampus, probably by acting as a gain amplification system for afferent sensory stimuli (Lenard et al., 1989; Ridley et al., 1989). DA may thus inhibit hippocampal information processing at the input stage, via the lateral septum, as well as at the output stage, via the nucleus accumbens. It is of interest in this context that NA terminals in the septum exert an α-receptor-mediated excitatory influence on the cholinergic cells of the septohippocampal pathway (Marighetto et al., 1989). The functional activity of the hippocampus may thus be determined by the NA:DA balance, not only within the nucleus accumbens and prefrontal cortex (Cools et al., Chapter 6; Tassin et al., Chapter 7, this volume), but also within the septum.

Interaction of DA with the Amygdala–Accumbens Pathway

The amygdala influences and regulates the autonomic system, visceral functions, reactions to stressors and novelty, reproduction, ingestive behaviour, social behaviour, attention, learning, memory and goal-directed behaviour. In addition to receiving highly processed information from the external environment, transmitted via polysensory associational cortical areas to the basolateral nucleus, the amygdala also receives a substantial volume of information from the internal environment (Figure 2). Thus, the central nucleus receives a direct innervation from the visceral and autonomic relay stations in the pons and mesencephalon: the dorsal motor nucleus of the tenth nerve, the nucleus of the solitary tract, the parabrachial nucleus and the central gray, as well as heavy reciprocal connections from the whole of the ventromedial and lateral hypothalamus. The amygdaloid complex therefore plays a central integrative role in the normal functioning of the limbic system (Ono et al., 1985; Price et al., 1987). Alheid and Heimer (1988) have recently advanced the concept of the 'extended amygdala', which includes the DA-innervated centromedial amygdala, the substantia innominata and ventral pallidum (including the corticopetal cholinergic neurons), the bed nucleus of the stria terminalis and the medial part of the nucleus accumbens. This complex is considered to control and gate the ascending (cortical and accumbens) and descending (hypothalamus, VTA and brainstem) output of the entire limbic system.

The effects of damage to the amygdala, together with a consideration of its afferent and efferent connections, suggest that this structure may be essential in the creation of incentive motivation (Bindra, 1969). Thus, the amygdala seems to be essential in the formation and maintenance of associations between motivationally significant stimuli, both within and between sensory modalities (Aggleton and Mishkin, 1986; Price et al., 1987; Gaffan et al., 1988). Indeed, Cormier (1981) has argued that only stimuli processed through the amygdala can become conditioned reinforcers.

The mesolimbic DA system is also critically involved in the activation of behaviour by motivationally significant stimuli (Beninger, 1983; Cador et al., 1989b; Everitt et al., 1989; Cador et al., Chapter 9, this volume). It is therefore not surprising that the literature contains numerous instances of almost identical behavioural effects following lesions of the amygdala and following DA receptor blockade or DA lesions within the nucleus accumbens. For example, amygdala-lesioned animals show a marked inflexibility of behaviour in response to the omission of expected rewards in a variety of different behavioural paradigms (Kemble and Beckham, 1970; Henke, 1977; Goomas et al., 1980; Riolobos, 1986; Siegel et al., 1988; Dunn and Everitt, 1988; Cador et al., 1989b; Everitt et al., 1989; Cador et al., Chapter 9, this volume); very similar effects are seen following DA receptor blockade, or 6-OHDA or ibotenic acid lesions, of the nucleus accumbens (Simon and Le Moal, 1984; Taghzouti et al., 1985; Salamone 1986, 1988; Willner et al., 1988; Annett et al., 1989; Salamone, Chapter 23, this volume).

The projection from the amygdala to the nucleus accumbens is the crucial output in the establishment of previously neutral stimuli as conditioned reinforcers (Cador et al., 1989b; Everitt et al., 1989). NMDA lesions of the basolateral amygdaloid nucleus decreased the ability of conditioned reinforcers (stimuli associated with food or sex) to support new learning, but this impairment was ameliorated by intra-accumbens injection of amphetamine. Lesion of the amygdala diminished considerably (but did not totally abolish) the response to the conditioned reinforcer. There may thus be an additional contribution of other limbic afferents to the nucleus accumbens (Cador et al., Chapter 9, this volume).

These results indicate that response-specific information about conditioned reinforcers originating from the amygdala is 'gain-amplified' in its effect on motor output by DA in the ventral striatum. The interpretation of a non-specific behavioural amplification by DA with regard to the quantitative activational aspects of motivated behaviour has received considerable support in several behavioural paradigms related to appetitive or aversive conditioned behaviour (Cador et al., Chapter 9; Salamone, Chapter 23, this volume). Such findings strongly support the concept that the ventral striatum functions as an interface to translate limbic 'motivational–emotional' determinants of behaviour into motor actions (Stevens, 1973; Mogenson et al., 1980; Mogenson, 1987; Cools, 1988).

Information controlling the directional aspects of behaviour may be determined by inputs to the ventral striatum from limbic structures and the cortex. There is evidence that cortical projections to the dorsal striatum may be involved in the establishment of memory for stimulus attributes (Kesner and DiMattia, 1987; Goldman-Rakic, 1987a), and DA also functions in the dorsal striatum to modulate and improve the retention of conditioned reinforcement (Packard and White, 1989; Packard et al., 1989; Robbins et al., 1989).

In addition to its role in conditioned reinforcement, the amygdala can also specify and determine the unconditioned stereotyped behavioural response to DA receptor stimulation in the ventrolateral striatum in drug-naive rats. In recent experiments, local injection of the GABA agonist muscimol (5–25 ng) into the anterior basolateral amygdala completely antagonized apomorphine (1–2.5 mg/kg)-induced stereotyped licking/gnawing activity without antagonism of stereotyped sniffing/head movement. In contrast, disinhibition of the output from the basolateral amygdala after local injection of the GABA antagonists picrotoxin or bicuculline (100 ng) enhanced the licking/gnawing activity following low doses (0.25–0.5 mg/kg) of apomorphine (Scheel-Kruger et al., in preparation). The licking/gnawing syndrome is observed after the combined local injection of D1 and D2 agonists into the ventrolateral region of the striatum (Kelley et al., 1988; Scheel-Kruger et al., in preparation). This striatal region is directly innervated by the anterior part of the basolateral amygdala, and also by the cortical oral motor area and the insular cortical taste area (Krushel and Van der Kooy, 1988) (see Figure 2). Stereotyped licking/gnawing behaviour induced by direct DA agonists may thus be related to information concerning salient exteroceptive stimuli (in this case, wire netting or food), controlled and transmitted via the amygdala.

As noted earlier, in addition to these interactions in the ventral striatum, DA also directly modulates the amygdala output. The functional importance of the VTA–amygdala projection is suggested by the observation that typical and atypical neuroleptic agents have distinct effects on neuronal activity in the amygdala (Rebec et al., 1981), as in behavioural tests (Costall and Naylor, 1974; Bradbury et al., 1985). Also, increased DA levels in the left amygdala have been reported in the schizophrenic brain (Reynolds and Czudek, 1988). Current evidence suggests that DA acts in the amygdala to inhibit its output. Thus, both DA stimulation and lesions of the amygdala have been found to protect against gastric ulceration following stress (Henke, 1988), and both DA stimulation and tetrodotoxin (TTX) blockade of the amygdala decreased DA turnover in the nucleus accumbens (Louilot et al., 1985). In addition to supporting an inhibitory role for DA in the amygdala, the latter observation also suggests a reciprocal balance between DA activity in the amygdala and the accumbens. It is conceivable that a shift in this balance (from accumbens to amygdala) could mediate the transition from active to passive behaviour that occurs during and following consummatory behaviour. As the various projections of the VTA are to some extent under independent control, such a shift could involve changes in afferent input to the VTA: for example, an increase in the release of neurotensin (Cador et al., 1989a).

Interaction of DA with the Hippocampus-Accumbens Pathway

Lesions to the hippocampus cause a range of 'disinhibitory' effects, which include an inability to suppress an on-going behaviour in response to a change in environmental demands (Isaacson, 1984; Eichenbaum et al., 1986, 1988). These effects show several similarities to those of low doses of amphetamine or dysfunctions of the mesolimbic DA system, suggesting that the hyper-responsiveness seen after hippocampal lesions may stem from secondary changes at the level of the nucleus accumbens (Isaacson, 1984). (Indeed, the hippocampal-lesioned animal has been proposed as an animal model of schizophrenia (Schmajuk, 1987), and structural changes have been detected in the hippocampus of schizophrenic patients (Conrad and Scheibel, 1987).) Commonalities between hippocampal-lesioned and amphetamine-treated animals include: impairments of selective attention, latent inhibition, extinction and passive avoidance; high rates of responding in differential reinforcement of low rate (DRL) schedules; improvement of active avoidance performance; reduction of spontaneous alternation; and increased locomotor activity. DA antagonists have been shown to reverse several of these deficits in hippocampal-lesioned animals (Devenport et al., 1981; Isaacson, 1984; Schmajuk, 1987).

The role of the hippocampus–accumbens pathway has recently been investigated using tasks of spatial memory, such as the eight-arm radial maze (Kesner and Di Mattia, 1987) or the Morris water maze (Morris and Hagan, 1986), which are highly sensitive to lesions of the hippocampus. The glutamate antagonist kynurenic acid, locally injected into the nucleus accumbens, increased the latency to initiate exploratory movements in the eight-arm maze and increased reference memory errors, but surprisingly, was without effect on working memory (Schacter et al., 1989). This conflicting effect is difficult to interpret, but does indicate that the hippocampus–accumbens projection is not critically involved in the retention of spatial information. In the water maze (and in a T-maze), ibotenic acid lesions of the nucleus accumbens impaired, but did not abolish, spatial acquisition; the data were interpreted as an initial disruption of behaviour in response to external change (Annett et al., 1989).

In a recent study, performance during acquisition in the Morris water maze was impaired by blockade of glutamate transmission from the hippocampal formation to the nucleus accumbens, or from the prefrontal cortex to the anterior dorsal striatum. The NMDA antagonist AP7 (0.25 and 1 μg), locally injected into the nucleus accumbens or dorsal striatum, caused a dose-dependent inhibition of spatial performance without motor disturbances. The D2 antagonist l-sulpiride (10 and 25 ng), and the D1 antagonist SCH 23390 (100 ng), caused similar effects after injection into the nucleus accumbens; the dorsal striatum was far less sensitive to sulpiride. Interestingly, intra-accumbens injection of AP7 and the DA antagonists also antagonized the exploratory behaviours of rearing, and head and body turning, performed on the platform during the inter-trial intervals; no such impairments were found after injection of AP7 into the dorsal striatum. DA antagonists did not impair the performance of well trained rats, whereas the blockade of NMDA receptors in the nucleus accumbens still caused a dose-related impairment of performance. However, DA antagonists did impair performance in these animals if the platform was moved to a new position. Thus, the glutamate system from the hippocampus and the prefrontal cortex seems to carry specific information whereas DA receptor activation is mainly involved during the initial phase in the selection of appropriate new behaviours (Scheel-Kruger et al., in preparation). The maintenance of long-term changes may involve the induction of the D1 second messenger system (Beninger, Chapter 11, this volume) and/or activation of the nuclear c-fos oncogene (Robertson et al., 1989).

These results suggest that the nucleus accumbens is an important interface in the initiation and selection of behavioural strategies. Bos and Cools (1989a) also concluded (from experiments using a swim test in which escape was initially impossible, but was later made possible by the introduction of a rope) that DA within the nucleus accumbens is involved in switching behaviour under the control of external cues (see also Robbins et al., 1989). The dorsal–striatum–prefrontal cortex system, by contrast, is essential for the arbitrary internal selection of behaviour unassisted by currently available sensory information (Divac and Oberg, 1979; Cools, 1980; Hikosaka et al., 1989; Robbins et al., 1989).

The Mesocortical DA System

A substantial volume of information now suggests that the mesocortical DA neurons projecting to the prefrontal cortex are directly involved in the control of attention, emotional states, adaptive behaviour and cognitive abilities. Lesions of the prefrontal cortex, or depletion of mesocortical DA, produce severe deficits in behavioural tests of all of these functions, which are consistent with a regulatory role of the prefrontal cortex in the internal guidance and sequential planning of behaviour (Kolb, 1984; Goldman-Rakic, 1987a, b; Kesner and Di Mattia, 1987).

Schizophrenic patients also present several symptoms suggestive of prefrontal dysfunction, such as blunted affect, poor initiative, lack of motivation, difficulty in planning, and impairment of problem-solving ability (Robbins, Chapter 19, this volume). Some schizophrenic patients have been found to display hypometabolism of the prefrontal cortex, particularly under cognitively demanding conditions; these deficits were correlated with the concentration of the DA metabolite homovanillic acid (HVA) in the cerebrospinal fluid (Weinberger, 1988; Weinberger et al., 1988). In schizophrenic patients undergoing testing for sustained attention, an abnormality of the prefrontal cortex (detected by PET scanning methods) could be partially reversed by neuroleptic medication (Cohen et al., 1988).

The mesocortical DA projection is particularly sensitive to activation by a wide variety of stressors. In most circumstances, stressor-induced increases in DA turnover are considerably more marked in the prefrontal cortex than in the nucleus accumbens (Tassin et al., Chapter 7; Zacharko and Anisman, Chapter 16, this volume). This difference may arise from the lesser density of inhibitory autoreceptors on the cortical DA terminals (Altar et al., 1987; Abercrombie et al., 1989). From experiments examining stress-induced increases in DA turnover in two rat strains in relation to their emotional and coping behaviour, D'Angio et al. (1988) have suggested that the increase in cortical DA turnover should be seen as part of a preparatory coping process rather than as a manifestation of the emotional reaction to the aversive event. This conclusion is consistent with the observations of increased emotionality but decreased cortical DA metabolism after long-term isolation (Blanc et al., 1980).

An important role of mesocortical DA in cognitive function has also been seen in monkeys: for example, 6-OHDA lesions (Brozoski et al., 1979) or local injection of the D1 antagonist SCH 23390 into the prefrontal cortex (Goldman-Rakic, 1989) impaired performance in a delayed alternation task. Prefrontal cortical neurons that increased their activity prior to a voluntary movement have been identified: the signal to noise ratio of these neurons was increased by DA and decreased by DA antagonists (Aou et al., 1983; Sawaguchi et al., 1986). The anatomical basis of these effects is known: DA nerve terminals in the prefrontal cortex are in direct contact with dendritic spines of pyramidal cells projecting to other cortical and subcortical areas (Goldman-Rakic et al., 1989).

It is important to emphasize that the mesocortical, mesolimbic and mesostriatal systems must be viewed as both integrated and interdependent neural circuits (Simon and Le Moal, 1984; Bjorklund and Lindvall, 1986; Oades and Halliday, 1987; Louilot et al., 1989). The distinct DA cell groups innervating the various mesocortical or mesolimbic structures are subject to differential and complex feedback and feedforward loops. Thus, 6-OHDA lesions of the prefrontal cortex are known to increase DA activity in both the striatum and the nucleus accumbens (Pycock et al., 1980; Haroutunian et al., 1988; Tassin et al., Chapter 7, this volume). This inhibitory effect of prefrontal DA over the subcortical projection is consistent with a pre-eminent position of the prefrontal cortex in the hierarchy of neuronal systems controlling behaviour (Salamone, Chapter 23, this volume). However, the full functional significance of these interactions remains to be elucidated.

As a final comment, it should be emphasized that the prefrontal cortex does not work as a single unit but rather as a series of topographically organized parallel systems. The functionally separate sensory inputs from the parietal and temporal cortex may project through distinct input/output channels to dorsal and ventral striatum and other limbic targets, as well as to segregated autonomic and visceral systems (Alexander et al., 1986; Mogenson, 1987; Goldman-Rakic, 1987a, b; Krushel and Van der Kooy, 1988; Sesack et al., 1989; Groenewegen et al., Chapter 2, this volume).

OUTPUT SYSTEMS OF THE VENTRAL STRIATUM

At present, we remain ignorant of how a specific, motivationally significant stimulus is able to cause the selection of an appropriate action. We lack, in other words, these crucial details of how the limbic motor interface actually functions. However, at the level of gross anatomy, the major output pathways to the motor system are now relatively clear.

The major output stations of the nucleus accumbens are the ventral pallidum, the anterior lateral hypothalamus, the VTA and the A8 area of the substantia nigra zona compacta, which contains cell bodies of the nigrostriatal DA projection (Nauta et al., 1978). The ventral striatum may also project directly to the mesencephalic locomotor region of the pedunculopontine nucleus (Groenewegen and Russchen, 1984; Swanson et al., 1987). It is also quite well established that GABA, dynorphin, substance P and, to a minor degree, enkephalin, represent the neurotransmitters of the accumbens-ventral pallidal pathway, and also of the other output channels. These transmitters may also co-exist in various combinations within the accumbens output neurons (Groenewegen and Russchen, 1984; Haber and Watson, 1985; Sugimoto and Mizuno, 1987; Haber and Groenewegen, 1989; Zahm, 1989). The significance of this latter finding remains largely unknown (Reid et al., 1988; Tan and Tsou, 1988).

The major output of the ventral pallidum is a GABAergic projection directed towards the mediodorsal nucleus of the thalamus, the lateral habenula, the medial subthalamic nucleus, the substantia nigra zona compacta and the mesencephalic locomotor region of the pedunculopontine nucleus. The lateral preoptic area and the lateral hypothalamus also project to the lateral habenula, the VTA and the zona compacta (Mogenson et al., 1985; Mogenson, 1987; Swanson et al., 1987; Groenewegen, 1988; Groenewegen et al., Chapter 2, this volume).

The Ventral Pallidum

Recent behavioural and electrophysiological studies have established that the ventral pallidum represents an essential output structure for the behavioural expression of DA-dependent activation of the nucleus accumbens (Figure 3). Thus, electrolytic or ibotenic acid lesions of the ventral pallidum reduced or abolished the locomotor stimulant action of amphetamine or cocaine, or the locomotor response elicited by stimulation of supersensitive DA receptors in the nucleus accumbens (Swerdlow et al., 1986). The nucleus accumbens also represents a neuroanatomical substrate of both cocaine and heroin self-administration (Bozarth, Chapter 12; Cooper, Chapter 13; Pulvirenti et al., Chapter 5, this volume). The finding that an ibotenic acid lesion of the ventral pallidum also decreased the reinforcing effects of cocaine and heroin again suggests the essential nature of the accumbens–ventral pallidal circuit (Hubner and Koob, 1990; Pulvirenti et al., Chapter 5, this volume). Of particular interest in this context is the observation of Tsai et al. (1989) that identified ventral pallidal output neurons were inhibited by hippocampal stimulation and activated by amygdala stimulation. The combined activation of D1 and D2 receptors may be essential for these changes in ventral pallidal neurons (Yang and Mogenson, 1989; White, Chapter 3, this volume).

While it is well established that GABA represents a major efferent transmitter in the accumbens–ventral pallidal pathway, there has been some

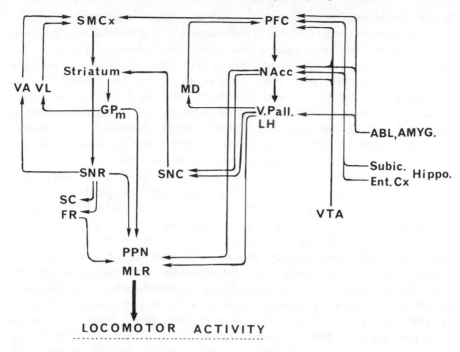

Figure 3. Simplified diagram showing the involvement of the mesolimbic VTA DA system in locomotor activity. The nucleus accumbens (NAcc) and the prefrontal cortex (PFC) are innervated by the VTA dopamine system, the entorhinal cortex (Ent. Cx) and the subiculum (Subic) from the hippocampus (Hippo.) and the basolateral nucleus (ABL) of amygdala (AMYG). The outputs from NAcc are directed towards the ventral pallidum (V. Pall.), lateral hypothalamus (LH), substantia nigra zona compacta (SNC) and the pedunculopontine nucleus (PPN) in the mesencephalic locomotor region (MLR). The mediodorsal thalamic nucleus (MD) provides the feed forward loop from V. Pall. to the PFC. The dorsal striatal loop includes the somatosensory motor cortex (SMCx), striatum, globus pallidus, medial segment (GPm), and subtantia nigra zona reticulata (SNR) and their efferents towards distinct regions of PPN, MLR and the ventroanterior (VA) and ventrolateral (VL) thalamic nuclei. The SNR efferents include the superior colliculus (SC) and formatio reticularis (FR)

disagreement over whether DA receptor stimulation within the nucleus accumbens excites or inhibits this pathway. Thus, local injection of GABA agonists into the ventral pallidum has been reported both to reduce (Mogenson et al., 1985; Swerdlow et al., 1986; Mogenson, 1987) and to stimulate (Scheel-Kruger, 1984, 1986; Baud et al., 1988) spontaneous or DA-stimulated locomotor activity. This controversy is resolved by the finding of Bos and Cools (1989b) that the GABAergic efferent outputs of the accumbens are heterogeneously organized. Thus, GABAergic stimulation in the rostral area of the ventral pallidum stimulated locomotor activity, whereas the more caudal (substantia innominata) ventral pallidal areas inhibited locomotion and produced tonic EMG activity and catalepsy. Catalepsy has also been reported following injection of GABA within the zona incerta region of the lateral hypothalamus (Ossowska et al., 1990). Functionally distinct interactions between GABA and encephalin have also been reported within the dorsal and ventral pallidal areas (Scheel-Kruger, 1984, 1986). These findings suggest that there are regionally distinct output channels in the nucleus accumbens–ventral pallidal system, which may perhaps be innervated by distinct combinations of limbic and/or prefrontal cortical afferents.

It also seems likely that, just as in the dorsal striatum (Gimenez-Amaya and Graybiel, 1990), distinct regional cell groups within the matrix-patch organization of the ventral striatum will be found to control the distinct output channels (the accumbens–pallido–thalamic–cortical 'cognitive loop', the pallidohabenula feedback loop, the pallidopedunculopontine locomotor loop, the accumbens–A8 zona compacta feedforward loop, and so on (Scheel-Krüger, 1986; Groenewegen, Chapter 2, this volume)). These distinct outputs of the nucleus accumbens, using different transmitters and/or combinations, may be subject to differential control by D1 and D2 receptors, again, as in the dorsal striatum (Voorn et al., 1987; Jiang et al., 1990). Further, distinct output channels may be triggered from the different cortical layers within a functional subunit of prefrontal cortex, as these relate differently to the striatal–accumbens matrix-patch compartments (Gerfen, 1989).

The Habenula

It has been suggested that the habenula may be a crucial nucleus through which outputs from the basal ganglia and the limbic forebrain may be relayed downstream to the midbrain monoamine-containing nuclei (locus coeruleus, raphe, VTA and substantia nigra zona compacta), as well as to premotor regions in the brainstem and pons (Figure 1; Araki et al., 1988; Bjorklund and Lindvall, 1986; Skagerberg et al., 1984). The lateral habenula receives a minor DA input and a major non-DA input from the VTA, in addition to inputs from the limbic output channels (via the ventral pallidum and the lateral hypothalamus) and the basal ganglia output channels (via the entopeduncular nucleus: in primates, the medial pallidal segment). The lateral habenula thus seems to be well placed to integrate information projecting back towards the VTA (see Figure 1 and Groenewegen, Chapter 2, this volume). Lisoprawski et al. (1980) originally reported that this inhibitory feedback system was specific for the mesocortical DA neurons, but more recent studies have suggested that the habenula also controls accumbens and striatal DA projections (Nishikawa et al., 1986; Christoph et al., 1986; Sasaki et al., 1990).

Behavioural studies by Thornton and colleagues strongly suggest that the habenula represents a critical relay for the integration of DA-related outputs of the dorsal and ventral striata (Thornton and Evans, 1982; Thornton et al., 1987). Carvey et al. (1987) also found that lesions of the habenula increased oral stereotypy but decreased locomotor activity in response to intermediate doses of apomorphine, and abolished the supersensitive locomotor response usually induced by chronic haloperidol treatment. These data suggest that it may be the habenula which is responsible for the expression of the 'supersensitive' locomotor response to DA receptor stimulation in the nucleus accumbens rather than the mediodorsal thalamic-prefrontal loop as suggested by Pulvirenti et al. (Chapter 5, this volume; Swerdlow and Koob, 1987): the lateral habenula is localized immediately posterior to the mediodorsal nucleus, and was probably damaged by their thalamic lesion. The lateral habenula projects to the essential premotor nuclei in the brainstem and pons, both directly and via its projection to non-DA neurons in the VTA (Figure 5, Araki et al., 1988; Figure 8, Skagerberg et al., 1984).

OVERVIEW

In this chapter, we have summarized and systematized our current understanding of the functional neuroanatomy of the mesolimbic DA system and its role in the interface between motivation and action. It is now reasonably clear that mesolimbic DA cells are activated by the same stimuli that activate the whole organism: broadly, incentive stimuli and stressors. Incentives are stimuli that have been associated with a primary reward, and now predict that reward will be delivered if the appropriate behaviour is performed (positive reinforcement). Stressors similarly require action to be taken, which, if successful, will cause stress reduction (negative reinforcement). In both cases, activation of the mesolimbic DA system appears to be the necessary and sufficient condition for behavioural activation by these stimuli.

In the case of incentive stimuli, the alerting signal that switches on the mesolimbic system originates in the amygdala, and, *en route* to the VTA, passes through a motivational gate in the hypothalamus (Alheid and Heimer, 1988; Wilson and Rolls, 1990). Stressful stimuli also reach the VTA via the amygdala, but in addition, have direct access via projections from a variety of brainstem and hypothalamic sites. Incentive stimuli and stressors not only activate, but also organize, behaviour. However, the DA system is not involved in the selection of appropriate responses: the organization of behaviour remains intact following treatment with DA antagonists or 6-OHDA lesions (Robbins et al., 1989; Salamone, Chapter 23, this volume). Rather, this information is transmitted directly from the amygdala to the ventral striatum, where DA modulates its intensity (Cador et al., Chapter 9, this volume). In addition to activating appropriate behaviours, motivationally significant stimuli also activate the visceral, autonomic and neuroendocrine systems. These effects may be mediated by the projections from the posterior part of the basolateral amygdala to the more medial parts of the ventral striatum (medial nucleus accumbens, bed nucleus of the stria terminalis and medial preoptic area), and from these structures to the VTA and brainstem (Mogenson, 1987; Swanson et al., 1987; Cools, 1988).

The concept of the ventral striatum as a limbic-motor interface (Stevens, 1973; Nauta et al., 1978; Mogenson et al., 1980; Heimer et al., 1982; Mogenson, 1987) is now generally accepted, and we have reviewed much of the relevant evidence. However, a major question that still remains open is whether specific information arriving in all the afferent systems is integrated in the ventral striatum or processed in parallel. The currently available anatomical information seems to favour the conclusion that the nucleus accumbens mainly operates by parallel processing with only a minor degree of integration (Zahm, 1989; Groenewegen et al., Chapter 2, this volume).

The afferents to the ventral striatum are subject to gating influences not only from the mesolimbic DA system, but also by NA, CCK, neurotensin and probably other neuromodulators. The transformed signals are then passed through the 'associative cognitive loop' (Goldman-Rakic and Porrino, 1985; Alexander et al., 1986; Groenewegen, 1988), which channels information via the ventral pallidum, and the midline and mediodorsal nuclei of the thalamus towards the prefrontal cortical areas. The midline and mediodorsal thalamic nuclei also receive specific sensory information from limbic, visceral, olfactory, visuomotor, premotor and brainstem nuclei (Groenewegen, 1988), which is integrated at the thalamic level with the corresponding afferents from the ventral pallidum before the final thalamic outputs are transmitted towards the frontal cortex. (The midline thalamic nuclei are also able to transmit specific information to the nucleus accumbens (Groenewegen, Chapter 2, this volume), and to enhance DA release within the accumbens (Jones et al., 1989).) A further input to the 'cognitive loop' arises from the DA-innervated 'extended amygdala', which controls the cholinergic neurons in the basal forebrain that project directly to the cortex (Alheid and Heimer, 1988; Wilson and Rolls, 1990). Subsequent processing involves integrative cortico-cortical associative loops (Goldman-Rakic, 1987a, b; Groenewegen et al., Chapter 2, this volume), and the prefrontal–parietal–temporal–entorhinal–subicular–basolateral amygdala loop, which carries the evaluated, integrated reponse back to the nucleus accumbens. It should also be emphasized that DA has an established neuromodulatory function in the cortical association areas: the multimodal sensory-related entorhinal cortex, the visceral motor-related prelimbic and infralimbic cortex, and the visceral sensory-related agranular insular cortex (Bjorklund and Lindvall, 1986).

Connections between the prefrontal–premotor and prefrontal–motor cortical loops and the dorsal striatum are probably involved in the establishment of complex, sequentially organized, internally guided motor programs (Cools, 1980, 1985). However, the basal ganglia system is also subject to limbic influences through two other routes: the direct (substance P and enkephalinergic) projection from the nucleus accumbens to the A8 DA cells (Nauta et al., 1978; Haber and Groenewegen, 1989), which may be considered as a feedforward system (Scheel-Kruger, 1986), and the ventral pallidum–zona compacta GABAergic feedback loop (Sugimoto and Mizuno, 1987; Figure 4, Groenewegen et al., Chapter 2, this volume). In addition to its outputs to the basal ganglia, the ventral striatum may also influence spontaneous or goal-directed locomotor activity by a direct projection to the mesencephalic locomotor region (Groenewegen and Russchen, 1984; Swanson et al., 1987), or via the 'classical' loops from the accumbens to the ventral pallidum, lateral hypothalamus and subthalamic zones, all of which project to the mesencephalic locomotor region (Mogenson et al., 1985; Mogenson, 1987; Swanson et al., 1987).

It seems of considerable significance, for this discussion of the role of DA in the motivational activation of behaviour, that this neuromodulator participates at nearly all levels of these hierarchically organized loops: at the cortical level, at the subcortical level (nucleus accumbens, septum and amygdala), in the feedback/feedforward loops (lateral habenula and lateral hypothalamus), and in the locus coeruleus (Bjorklund and Lindvall, 1986). The hypothalamic A11 DA cell group also provides an output directed towards the spinal cord (Bjorklund and Lindvall, 1986). This anatomy strongly suggests a role of DA in many aspects of motivation, emotion, cognition and behaviour. It must be emphasized that motivationally significant stimuli do not lead simply to the selection of appropriate responses, but rather create what Bindra (1969) has termed a 'central motive state', which biases perceptual processing, potentiates whole classes of response outputs, and alters the balance of visceral, autonomic and neuroendocrine activity. It is clear that the DA system may participate in many aspects of these central states.

The simple observation that DA acts to facilitate, or otherwise modulate, the processing of information in the structures receiving a dopaminergic innervation (Cools, 1985; Simon and Le Moal, 1984; Louilot et al., 1989; Cador et al., Chapter 9; Cools et al., Chapter 6, this volume) has a profoundly important implication: that the consequences of activating the mesolimbic DA system will vary according to the balance of on-going activity in other structures. Consider, for example, the well established observation that stressors activate the mesocortical projection more strongly than the mesoaccumbens projection (Altar et al., 1987; D'Angio et al., 1988; Tassin et al., Chapter 7; Zacharko and Anisman, Chapter 16, this volume). In conditions requiring the simple execution of a well learned response, we suppose that coping behaviour would be controlled largely by the amygdala–accumbens system, with relatively little input from the frontal cortex, and consequently, relatively little contribution of mesocortical DA. However, under novel conditions requiring the selection of an appropriate response strategy, or in tasks that call for the sequential execution of a series of actions, the frontal cortex exercises an essential supervisory function (Shallice, 1982; Kolb, 1984; Goldman-Rakic, 1987a), and we should expect the contributions of mesocortical DA and of cortico-subcortical interactions to be prominent. This type of analysis, which we believe will come increasingly to characterize the next generation of research, will require an adequate conceptualization of the hierarchical structure of behaviour and its neural control mechanisms (see Cools, 1985; Salamone, Chapter 23, this volume, for further discussion). The development along these lines of a more flexible and complex model of DA function is likely to have important implications for our understanding of the brain mechanisms of schizophrenia and the affective disorders (Fibiger, Chapter 24, this volume).

The construction, over the past two decades, of an understanding of the functions of the mesolimbic DA system has undoubtedly been one of the success stories of behavioural neuroscience: indeed, in almost every respect, our knowledge of this system far outweighs that of any other well defined pathway in the central nervous system. Nevertheless, this reflection serves only to underline the extent of our current ignorance. Our comprehension of the coordination between the mesolimbic DA system and the many other structures and systems with which it interacts to control and guide behaviour remains woefully inadequate. A broadening of the focus to encompass the integration of information processing within and between the structures that communicate with and through the 'limbic–motor interface' constitutes a major challenge for future research.

REFERENCES

Abercrombie, E., Keefe, K. and Zigmond, M. (1989) Evidence that nerve terminal density is an important contributor to apparent differences in the activation of central dopamine systems. *Behavioural Pharmacology* **1**, 26 (suppl 1).

Aggleton, J.P. and Mishkin, M. (1986) The amygdala: sensory gateway to the emotions. In: Plutchik, R. and Kellerman, H. (eds) *Emotion: Theory, Research and Experience, Vol. 3*. New York: Academic Press, pp. 281–299.

Alexander, G.E., DeLong, M.R. and Strick, P.L. (1986) Parallel organization of functionally segregated circuits linking basal ganglia and cortex. *Annual Review of Neuroscience* **9**, 357–381.

Alheid, G.F. and Heimer, L. (1988) New perspectives in basal forebrain organization of special relevance for neuropsychiatric disorders: the striatopallidal, amygdaloid, and corticopetal components of substantia innominata. *Neuroscience* **27**, 1–39.

Altar, C.A., Boyar, W.C., Oei, E. and Wood, P.L. (1987) Dopamine autoreceptors modulate the in vivo release of dopamine in the frontal, cingulate and entorhinal cortices. *Journal of Pharmacology and Experimental Therapeutics* **242**, 115–120.

Anand, B.K. and Brobeck, J.R. (1951) Hypothalamus control of food intake in rats and cats. *Yale Journal of Biology and Medicine* **24**, 123–140.

Annett, L.E., McGregor, A. and Robbins, T.W. (1989) The effects of ibotenic acid lesions of the nucleus accumbens on spatial learning and extinction in the rat. *Behavioral Brain Research* **31**, 231–242.

Antin, J., Gibbs, J., Holt, J., Young, R.C. and Smith, G.P. (1975) Cholecystokinin elicits the complete behavioural sequence of satiety in rats. *Journal of Comparative Physiology and Psychology* **89**, 784–790.

Aou, S., Oomura, Y., Nishino, H., Inokuchi, A. and Mizuno, Y. (1983) Influence of catecholamines on reward-related neuronal activity in monkey orbitofrontal cortex. *Brain Research* **267**, 165–170.

Araki, M., McGeer, P.L. and Kimura, H. (1988) The efferent projections of the rat lateral habenular nucleus revealed by the PHA-L anterograde tracing method. *Brain Research* **441**, 319–330.

Arbuthnott, G.W. (1980) The dopamine synapse and the notion of 'pleasure centres' in the brain. *Trends in Neuroscience* **3**, 199–200.

Arnt, J. and Scheel-Krüger, J. (1979) GABA in the ventral tegmental area: differential regional effects on locomotion, aggression and food intake after microinjection of GABA agonists and antagonists. *Life Sciences* **25**, 1351–1360.

Baud, P., Mayo, W., Le Moal, M. and Simon, H. (1988) Locomotor hyperactivity in the rat after infusion of muscimol and [D-A1a2]Met-enkephalin into the nucleus basalis magnocellularis. Possible interaction with cortical cholinergic projections. *Brain Research* **452**, 203–211.

Beckstead, R.M., Domesick, V.B. and Nauta, W.J.H. (1979) Efferent connections of the substantia nigra and ventral tegmental area in the rat. *Brain Research* **175**, 191–217.

Beninger, R.J. (1983) The role of dopamine in locomotor activity and learning. *Brain Research Reviews* **6**, 173–196.

Bindra, D. (1969) A unified interpretation of emotion and motivation. *Annals of the New York Academy of Sciences* **159**, 1071–1083.

Björklund, A. and Lindvall, O. (1986) Catecholaminergic brain stem regulatory systems. In: Bloom, F.B. and Geiger, S.R. (eds) *Handbook of Physiology: The Nervous System, Vol IV, Intrinsic Regulatory Systems of the Brain*. Bethesda: American Physiological Society, pp. 155–235.

Blanc, G., Hervé, D., Simon, H., Lisoprawski, A., Glowinski, J. and Tassin, J.-P. (1980) Response to stress of mesocortico-frontal dopaminergic neurones in rats after long-term isolation. *Nature* **284**, 265–267.

Blandina, P., Goldfarb, J., Craddock-Royal, B. and Green, J.P. (1989) Release of endogenous dopamine by stimulation of 5-hydroxytryptamine3 receptors in rat striatum. *Journal of Pharmacology and Experimental Therapeutics* **251**, 803–808.

Bos, R. van den and Cools, A.R. (1989a) The involvement of the nucleus accumbens in the ability of rats to switch to cue-directed behaviors. *Life Sciences* **44**, 1697–1704.

Bos, R. van den and Cools, A.R. (1989b) The ventral pallidum/substantia innominata complex: further evidence for heterogeneity as determined by the effects of GABA-ergic drugs. *Behavioural Pharmacology* **1**, 29 (suppl 1).

Bradbury, A.J., Costall, B., Domeney, A.M. and Naylor, R.J. (1985) Laterality of dopamine function and neuroleptic action in the amygdala in the rat. *Neuropharmacology* **24**, 1163–1170.

Brozoski, T.J., Brown, R.M., Rosvold, H.E. and Goldman, P.S. (1979) Cognitive deficit caused by regional depletion of dopamine in prefrontal cortex of rhesus monkey. *Science* **205**, 929–932.

Cador, M., Kelley, A.E., Le Moal, M. and Stinus L. (1986) Ventral tegmental area infusion of substance P, neurotensin and enkephalin: differential effects on feeding behavior. *Neuroscience* **18**, 659–669.

Cador, M., Kelley, A.E., Le Moal, M. and Stinus, L. (1988) d-Ala-met-enkephalin injection into the ventral tegmental area: effect on investigatory and spontaneous motor behaviour in the rat. *Psychopharmacology* **96**, 332–342.

Cador, M., Rivet, J.-M., Kelley, A.E., Le Moal, M. and Stinus L. (1989a) Substance P, neurotensin and enkephalin injections into the ventral tegmental area: comparative study on dopamine turnover in several forebrain structures. *Brain Research* **486**, 357–363.

Cador, M., Robbins, T.W. and Everitt, B.J. (1989b) Involvement of the amygdala in stimulus-reward associations: interaction with the ventral striatum. *Neuroscience* **30**, 77–86.

Carboni, E., Acquas, E., Frau, R. and Di Chiara, G. (1989) Differential inhibitory effects of a 5-HT3 antagonist on drug-induced stimulation of dopamine release. *European Journal of Pharmacology* **164**, 515–519.

Carvey, P.M., Kao, L.C. and Klawans, H.L. (1987) The effect of bilateral kainic acid-induced lateral habenula lesions on dopamine-mediated behaviors. *Brain Research* **409**, 193–196.

Christie, M.J., Bridge, S., James, L.B. and Beart, P.N. (1985) Excitotoxin lesions suggest an aspartatergic projection from rat medial prefrontal cortex to ventral tegmental area. *Brain Research* **333**, 169–172.

Christoph, G.R., Leonzio, R.J. and Wilcox, K.S. (1986) Stimulation of the lateral habenula inhibits dopamine-containing neurons in the substantia nigra and ventral tegmental area of the rat. *Journal of Neuroscience* **6**, 613–619.

Cohen, R.M., Semple, W.E., Gross, M., Nordahl, T.E., Holcomb, H.H., Dowling, M.S. and Pickar D. (1988) The effect of neuroleptics on dysfunction in a prefrontal substrate of sustained attention in schizophrenia. *Life Sciences* **43**, 1141–1150.

Conrad, A.J. and Scheibel, A.B. (1987) Schizophrenia and the hippocampus: the embryological hypothesis extended. *Schizophrenia Bulletin* **13**, 577–587.

Cools, A.R. (1980) Role of the neostriatal dopaminergic activity in sequencing and selecting behavioural strategies: facilitation of processes involved in selecting the best strategy in a stressful situation. *Behavioral Brain Research* **1**, 361–378.

Cools, A.R. (1985) Brain and behavior: hierarchy of feedback systems and control of input. In: Bateson, P.P.G. and Klopfer, P.H. (eds) *Perspectives in Ethology 6 (Mechanisms)*. New York: Plenum Press, pp. 109–168.

Cools, A.R. (1988) Transformation of emotion into motion: role of mesolimbic noradrenaline and neostriatal dopamine. In: Hellhammer, D., Florin, I. and Weiner, H. (eds) *Neurobiological Approaches to Human Disease*. Toronto: Hans Huber, pp. 15–28.

Cormier, S.M. (1981) A match-mismatch theory of limbic system function. *Physiological Psychology* **9**, 3–36.

Costall, B. and Naylor, R.J. (1974) The nucleus amygdaloideus centralis and neuroleptic activity in the rat. *European Journal of Pharmacology* **25**, 138–146.

Costall, B., Domeney, A.M., Naylor, R.J. and Tyers, M.B. (1987) Effects of the 5-HT3 receptor antagonist, GR38032F, on raised dopaminergic activity in the mesolimbic system of the rat and marmoset brain. *British Journal of Pharmacology* **92**, 881–894.

D'Angio, M., Serrano, A., Driscoll, P. and Scatton, B. (1988) Stressful environmental stimuli increase extracellular DOPAC levels in the prefrontal cortex of hypoemotional (Roman high-avoidance) but not hyperemotional (Roman low-avoidance) rats. An in vivo voltammetric study. *Brain Research* **451**, 237–247.

Daugé, V., Steimes, P., Derrien, M., Beau, M., Roques, B.P. and Féger, J. (1989) CCK8 effects on motivational and emotional states of rats involve CCKA receptors of the postero-median part of the nucleus accumbens. *Pharmacology Biochemistry and Behavior* **34**, 157–163.

Deutch, A.Y., Bean, A.J. and Roth, R.H. (1988) Regulation of A8 dopamine neurons by somatostatin. *European Journal of Pharmacology* **147**, 317–320.

Devenport, L.D., Devenport, J.A. and Holloway, F.A. (1981) Reward-induced stereotypy: modulation by the hippocampus. *Science* **212**, 1288–1289.

Divac, I. and Öberg, R.G.E. (1979) *The Neostriatum*. London: Pergamon Press.

Dunn, L.T. and Everitt, B.J. (1988) Double dissociations of the effects of amygdala and insular cortex lesions on conditioned taste aversion, passive avoidance, and neophobia in the rat using the excitotoxin ibotenic acid. *Behavioral Neuroscience* **102**, 3–23.

Durkin, T., Galey, D. Micheau, J., Beslon, H. and Jaffard, R. (1986) The effects of acute intraseptal injection of haloperidol in vivo on hippocampal cholinergic function in the mouse. *Brain Research* **376**, 420–424.

Eichenbaum, H., Fagan, A. and Cohen, N.J. (1986) Normal olfactory discrimination learning set and facilitation of reversal learning after medial-temporal damage in rats: implications for an account of preserved learning abilities in amnesia. *Journal of Neuroscience* **6**, 1876–1884.

Eichenbaum, H., Fagan, A., Mathews, P. and Cohen, N.J. (1988) Hippocampal system dysfunction and odor discrimination learning in rats: impairment or facilitation depending on representational demands. *Behavioral Neuroscience* **102**, 331–339.

Elliott, P.J., Alpert, J.E., Bannon, M.J. and Iversen, S.D. (1986) Selective activation of mesolimbic and mesocortical dopamine metabolism in rat brain by infusion of a stable substance P analogue into the ventral tegmental area. *Brain Research* **363**, 145–147.

Everitt, B.J., Cador, M. and Robbins, T.W. (1989) Interactions between the amygdala and ventral striatum in stimulus-reward associations: studies using a second-order schedule of sexual reinforcement. *Neuroscience* **30**, 63–75.

Ferssiwi, A., Cardo, B. and Velley, L. (1987) Gustatory preference-aversion thresholds are increased by ibotenic acid lesion of the lateral hypothalamus in the rat. *Brain Research* **437**, 142–150.

Fukuda, M., Ono, T. and Nakamura, K. (1987) Functional relations among inferotemporal cortex, amygdala, and lateral hypothalamus in monkey operant feeding behavior. *Journal of Neurophysiology* **57**, 1060–1077.

Gaffan, E.A., Gaffan, D. and Harrison, S. (1988) Disconnection of the amygdala from visual association cortex impairs visual reward-association learning in monkeys. *Journal of Neuroscience* **8**, 3144–3150.

Galey, D., Dukin, T., Sifakis, G., Kempf, E. and Jaffard, R. (1985) Facilitation of spontaneous and learned spatial behaviours following 6-hydroxydopamine lesions of the lateral septum: a cholinergic hypothesis. *Brain Research* **340**, 171–174.

Galey, D., Toumane, A., Durkin, T. and Jaffard, R. (1989) In vivo modulation of septo-hippocampal cholinergic activity in mice: relationships with spatial reference and working memory performance. *Behavioral Brain Research* **32**, 163–172.

Gariano, R.F. and Groves, P.M. (1988) Burst firing induced in midbrain dopamine neurons by stimulation of the medial prefrontal and anterior cingulate cortices. *Brain Research* **462**, 194–198.

Gerfen, C.R. (1989) The neostriatal mosaic: striatal patch-matrix organization is related to cortical lamination. *Science* **246**, 385–388.

Giménez-Amaya, J.M. and Graybiel, A.M. (1990) Compartmental origins of the striatopallidal projection in the primate. *Neuroscience* **34**, 111–126.

Goldman-Rakic, P.S. (1987a) Circuitry of primate prefrontal cortex and regulation of behavior by representational memory. In: Plum, F. and Mountcastle, V. (eds) *Handbook of Physiology. The Nervous System, Vol. 5.* Bethesda: American Physiol. Society, pp. 373–417.

Goldman-Rakic, P.S. (1987b) Circuit basis of a cognitive function in non-human primates. In: Stahl, S.M., Iversen, S.D. and Goodman, E.C. (eds) *Cognitive Neurochemistry.* Oxford: Oxford Science Publishers, pp. 90–109.

Goldman-Rakic, P.S. (1989) Dopamine innervation, receptors and functional correlates in primate prefrontal cortex. *Behavioural Pharmacology* 1, 23 (suppl 1).

Goldman-Rakic, P.S. and Porrino, L.J. (1985) The primate mediodorsal (MD) nucleus and its projection to the frontal lobe. *Journal of Comparative Neurology* 242, 535–560.

Goldman-Rakic, P.S., Leranth, C., Williams, S.M., Mons, N. and Geffard, M. (1989) Dopamine synaptic complex with pyramidal neurons in primate cerebral cortex. *Proceedings of the National Academy of Sciences of the USA* 86, 9015–9019.

Goomas, D.T., Hamm, C. and Skinner Jr, J. (1980) Runway performance of amygdalectomized rats: magnitude of reinforcement and delay of food reward. *Physiological Psychology* 8, 97–100.

Gould, E., Woolf, N.J. and Butcher, L.L. (1989) Cholinergic projections to the substantia nigra from the pedunculopontine and laterodorsal tegmental nuclei. *Neuroscience* 28, 611–623.

Grenhoff, J. and Svensson, T.H. (1989) Clonidine modulates dopamine cell firing in rat ventral tegmental area. *European Journal of Pharmacology* 165, 11–18.

Groenewegen, H.J. (1988) Organization of the afferent connections of the mediodorsal thalamic nucleus in the rat, related to the mediodorsal-prefrontal topography. *Neuroscience* 24, 379–431.

Groenewegen, H.J. and Van Dijk, C.A. (1984) Efferent connections of the dorsal tegmental region in the rat, studied by means of anterograde transport of the lectin phaseolus vulgaris-leucoagglutinin (PHA-L). *Brain Research* 304, 367–371.

Groenewegen, H.J. and Russchen, F.T. (1984) Organization of the efferent projections of the nucleus accumbens to pallidal, hypothalamic, and mesencephalic structures: a tracing and immunohistochemical study in the cat. *Journal of Comparative Neurology* 223, 347–367.

Groenewegen, H.J., Vermeulen-Van der Zee, E., Kortschot, A.T. and Witter, M.P. (1987) Organization of the projections from the subiculum to the ventral striatum in the rat. A study using anterograde transport of *Phaseolus vulgaris* leucoagglutinin. *Neuroscience* 23, 103–120.

Guan, X.-M. and McBride, J. (1989) Serotonin microinfusion into the ventral tegmental area increases accumbens dopamine release. *Brain Research Bulletin* 23, 541–547.

Haber, S.N. and Groenewegen, H.J. (1989) Interrelationship of the distribution of neuropeptides and tyrosine hydroxylase immunoreactivity in the human substantia nigra. *Journal of Comparative Neurology* 290, 53–68.

Haber, S.N. and Watson, S.J. (1985) The comparative distribution of enkephalin, dynorphin and substance P in the human globus pallidus and basal forebrain. *Neuroscience* 14, 1011–1024.

Hardy, S.G.P. (1986) Projections to the midbrain from the medial versus lateral prefrontal cortices of the rat. *Neuroscience Letters* 63, 159–164.

Haroutunian, V., Knott, P. and Davis, K.L. (1988) Effects of mesocortical dopaminergic lesions upon subcortical dopaminergic function. *Psychopharmacology Bulletin* **24**, 341–344.

Heimer, L., Switzer, R.D. and van Hoesen, G.W. (1982) Ventral striatum and ventral pallidum. Components of the motor system? *Trends in Neuroscience* **5**, 83–87.

Henke, P.G. (1977) Dissociation of the frustration effect and the partial reinforcement extinction effect after limbic lesions in rats. *Journal of Comparative and Physiological Psychology* **91**, 1032–1038.

Henke, P.G. (1988) Recent studies of the central nucleus of the amygdala and stress ulcers. *Neuroscience and Biobehavioral Reviews* **12**, 143–150.

Hernandez, L. and Hoebel, B.G. (1988) Feeding and hypothalamic stimulation increase dopamine turnover in the accumbens. *Physiology and Behavior* **44**, 599–606.

Hervé, D., Simon, H., Blanc, G., Le Moal, M., Glowinski, J. and Tassin, J.-P. (1981) Opposite changes in dopamine utilization in the nucleus accumbens and the frontal cortex after electrolytic lesion of the median raphe in the rat. *Brain Research* **216**, 422–428.

Herve, D., Blanc, G., Glowinski, J. and Tassin, J.-P. (1982) Reduction of dopamine utilization in the prefrontal cortex but not in the nucleus accumbens after selective destruction of noradrenergic fibers innervating the ventral tegmental area in the rat. *Brain Research* **237**, 510–516.

Hikosaka, O., Sakamoto, M. and Usui, S. (1989) Functional properties of monkey caudate neurons III. Activities related to expectation of target and reward. *Journal of Neurophysiology* **61**, 814–832.

Hirsh, R. (1974) The hippocampus and contextual retrieval of information from memory: A theory. *Behavioral Biology* **12**, 421–444.

Hubner, C.B. and Koob, G.F. (1990) The ventral pallidum plays a role in mediating cocaine and heroin self-administration in the rat. *Brain Research* **508**, 20–29.

Imperato, A. and Angelucci, L. (1989) 5HT3 receptors control dopamine release in the nucleus accumbens of freely moving rats. *Neuroscience Letters* **101**, 214–218.

Isaacson, R.L. (1984) Hippocampal damage: effects on dopaminergic systems of the basal ganglia. *International Review of Neurobiology* **25**, 339–359.

Jiang, H.-K., McGinty, J.F. and Hong, J.S. (1990) Differential modulation of striatonigral dynorphin and enkephalin by dopamine receptor subtypes. *Brain Research* **507**, 57–64.

Jiang, L.H. and Oomura, Y. (1988) Effect of catecholamine-receptor antagonists on feeding-related neuronal activity in the central amygdaloid nucleus of the monkey: a microiontophoretic study. *Journal of Neurophysiology* **60**, 536–548.

Jones, B. and Mishkin, M. (1972) Limbic lesions and the problem of stimulus-reinforcement associations. *Experimental Neurology* **36**, 362–377.

Jones, M.W., Kilpatrick, I.C. and Phillipson, O.T. (1989) Regulation of dopamine function in the nucleus accumbens of the rat by the thalamic paraventricular nucleus and adjacent midline nuclei. *Experimental Brain Research* **76**, 572–580.

Kalivas, P.W. and Abhold, R. (1987) Enkephalin release into the ventral tegmental area in response to stress: modulation of mesocorticolimbic dopamine. *Brain Research* **414**, 339–348.

Kalivas, P.W., Widerlöv, E., Stanley, D., Breese, G. and Prange Jr, A.J. (1983) Enkephalin action on the mesolimbic system: a dopamine-dependent and a dopamine-independent increase in locomotor activity. *Journal of Pharmacology and Experimental Therapeutics* **227**, 229–237.

Kelley, A.E., Lang, C.G. and Gauthier, A.M. (1988) Induction of oral stereotypy following amphetamine microinjection into a discrete subregion of the striatum. *Psychopharmacology* **95**, 556–559.

Kelley, A.E., Cador, M., Stinus, L. and Le Moal, M. (1989) Neurotensin, substance P, neurokinin-α, and enkephalin: injection into ventral tegmental area in the rat produces differential effects on operant responding. *Psychopharmacology* **97**, 243–252.

Kemble, E.D. and Beckman, G.J. (1970) Runway performance of rats following amygdaloid lesions. *Physiology and Behavior* **5**, 45–47.

Kesner, R.P. and Di Mattia, B.V. (1987) Neurobiology of an attribute model of memory. In: Epstein, A.N. and Morris, A. (eds) *Progress in Psychobiology and Physiological Psychology, Vol 12*. New York: Academic Press, pp. 207–275.

Kolb, B. (1984) Functions of the frontal cortex of the rat: a comparative review. *Brain Research Reviews* **8**, 65–98.

Krushel, L.A. and Van der Kooy, D. (1988) Visceral cortex: integration of the mucosal senses with limbic information in the rat agranular insular cortex. *Journal of Comparative Neurology* **270**, 39–54.

Lane, R.F., Blaha, C.D. and Rivet, J.M. (1988) Selective inhibition of mesolimbic dopamine release following chronic administration of clozapine: involvement of α-1-noradrenergic receptors demonstrated by in vivo voltammetry. *Brain Research* **460**, 398–401.

Lénárd, L., Oomura, Y., Nakano, Y. Aou, S. and Nishino, H. (1989) Influence of acetylcholine on neuronal activity of monkey amygdala during bar press feeding behavior. *Brain Research* **500**, 359–368.

Lisoprawski, A., Hervé, D., Blanc, G., Glowinski, J. and Tassin, J.-P. (1980) Selective activation of the mesocortico-frontal dopaminergic neurons induced by lesion of the habenula in the rat. *Brain Research* **183**, 229–234.

Louilot, A., Simon, H., Taghzouti, K. and Le Moal, M. (1985) Modulation of dopaminergic activity in the nucleus accumbens following facilitation or blockade of the dopaminergic transmission in the amygdala: a study by in vivo differential pulse voltammetry. *Brain Research* **346**, 141–145.

Louilot, A., Taghzouti, K., Simon, H. and Le Moal, M. (1989) Limbic system, basal ganglia, and dopaminergic neurons. *Brain Behavior and Evolution* **33**, 157–161.

Mantz, J., Milla, C., Glowinski, J. and Thierry, A.M. (1988) Differential effects of ascending neurons containing dopamine and noradrenaline in the control of spontaneous activity and of evoked responses in the rat prefrontal cortex. *Neuroscience* **27**, 517–526.

Margules, D.L. and Olds, J. (1962) Identical 'feeding' and 'reward' systems in the lateral hypothalamus of rats. *Science* **135**, 374–375.

Marighetto, A., Durkin, T., Toumane, A., Lebrun, C. and Jaffard, R. (1989) Septal α-noradrenergic antagonism in vivo blocks the testing-induced activation of septo-hippocampal cholinergic neurones and produces a concomitant deficit in working memory performance of mice. *Pharmacology Biochemistry and Behavior* **34**, 553–558.

McGaugh, J.L., Introini-Collison, I.B. and Nagahara, A.H. (1988) Memory-enhancing effects of posttraining naloxone: involvement of β-noradrenergic influences in the amygdaloid complex. *Brain Research* **446**, 37–49.

Meredith, G.E., Wouterlood, F.G. and Pattiselanno, A. (1990) Hippocampal fibers make synaptic contacts with glutamate decarboxylase-immunoreactive neurons in the rat nucleus accumbens. *Brain Research* **513**, 329–334.

Mogenson, G.J. (1987) Limbic-motor integration. In: Epstein, A.N. and Morris, A. (eds) *Progress in Psychobiology and Physiological Psychology, Vol. 12.* New York: Academic Press, pp. 117–170.

Mogenson, G.J., Jones, D.L. and Yim, C.Y. (1980) From motivation to action: functional interface between the limbic system and the motor system. *Progress in Neurobiology* **14**, 69–97.

Mogenson, G.J., Swanson, L.W. and Wu, M. (1985) Evidence that projections from substantia innominata to zona incerta and mesencephalic locomotor region contribute to locomotor activity. *Brain Research* **334**, 65–76.

Morris, R.G.M. and Hagan, J.J. (1986) Allocentric spatial learning by hippocampectomised rats: a further test of the 'spatial mapping' and 'working memory' theories of hippocampal function. *Quarterly Journal of Experimental Psychology* **38B**, 365–395.

Murray, E.A. and Mishkin, M. (1985) Amygdalectomy impairs cross-modal association in monkeys. *Science* **228**, 604–606.

Museo, E. and Wise, R.A. (1990) Locomotion induced by ventral tegmental microinjections of a nicotinic agonist. *Pharmacology Biochemistry and Behavior* **35**, 735–737.

Nakano, Y., Lénárd, L., Oomura, Y., Nishino, H., Aou, S. and Yamamoto, T. (1987) Functional involvement of catecholamines in reward-related neuronal activity of the monkey amygdala. *Journal of Neurophysiology* **57**, 72–91.

Nauta, W.J.H., Smith, G.P., Faull, R.L.M. and Domesick, V.B. (1978) Efferent connections and nigral afferents of the nucleus accumbens septi in the rat. *Neuroscience* **3**, 385–401.

Niijima, K. and Yoshida, M. (1988) Activation of mesencephalic dopamine neurons by chemical stimulation of the nucleus tegmenti pedunculopontinus pars compacta. *Brain Research* **451**, 163–171.

Nishikawa, T., Fage, D. and Scatton, B. (1986) Evidence for, and nature of, the tonic inhibitory influence of habenulointerpeduncular pathways upon cerebral dopaminergic transmission in the rat. *Brain Research* **373**, 324–336.

Nishino, H., Ono, T., Muramoto, K., Fukuda, M. and Sasaki, K. (1987) Neuronal activity in the ventral tegmental area (VTA) during motivated bar press feeding in the monkey. *Brain Research* **413**, 302–313.

Oades, R.D. (1985) The role of noradrenaline in tuning and dopamine in switching between signals in the CNS. *Neuroscience and Biobehavioral Reviews* **9**, 261–282.

Oades, R.D. and Halliday, G.M. (1987) Ventral tegmental (A10) system: neurobiology. 1. Anatomy and connectivity. *Brain Research Reviews* **12**, 117–165.

Olds, M.E. (1988) Amphetamine-induced increase in motor activity is correlated with higher firing rates of non-dopamine neurons in substantia nigra and ventral tegmental area. *Neuroscience* **24**, 477–490.

Ono, T., Luiten, P.G.M., Nishijo, H., Fukuda, M. and Nishino, H. (1985) Topographic organization of projections from the amygdala to the hypothalamus of the rat. *Neuroscience Research* **2**, 221–239.

Ono, T., Nakamura, K., Nishijo, H. and Fukuda, M. (1986) Hypothalamic neuron involvement in integration of reward, aversion, and cue signals. *Journal of Neurophysiology* **56**, 63–79.

Ono, T., Tamura, R., Nishijo, H., Nakamura, K. and Tabuchi, E. (1989) Contribution of amygdalar and lateral hypothalamic neurons to visual information processing of food and nonfood in monkey. *Physiology and Behavior* **45**, 411–421.

Ossowska, K., Wardas, J., Golembiowska, K. and Wolfarth, S. (1990) Lateral hypothalamus-zona incerta region as an output station for the catalepsy induced by the blockade of striatal D1 and D2 dopamine receptors. *Brain Research* **506**, 311–315.

Packard, M.G. and White, N.M. (1989) Memory facilitation produced by dopamine agonists: role of receptor subtype and mnemonic requirements. *Pharmacology Biochemistry and Behavior* **33**, 511–518.

Packard, M.G., Hirsh, R. and White, N.M. (1989) Differential effects of fornix and caudate nucleus lesions on two radial maze tasks: evidence for multiple memory systems. *Journal of Neuroscience* **9**, 1465–1472.

Papez, J.W. (1937) A proposed mechanism of emotion. *Archives of Neurology and Psychiatry* **38**, 725–745.

Phillips, A.G. and Fibiger, H.C. (1989) Neuroanatomical basis of intracranial self-stimulation. Untangling the Gordian Knot. In: Liebman, J.M. and Cooper, S.J. (eds) *The Neuropharmacological Basis of Reward*. Oxford: Oxford University Press, pp. 66–105.

Phillipson, O.T. (1979) Afferent projections to the ventral tegmental area of tsai and interfascicular nucleus: a horseradish peroxidase study in the rat. *Journal of Comparative Neurology* **187**, 117–144.

Piazza, P.V., Ferdico, M., Crescimanno, G., Benigno, A. and Amato, G. (1987) Inhibitory effect of the ventral tegmental A10 region on the hypothalamic defence reaction: evidence for a possible dopaminergic mediation. *Brain Research* **413**, 356–359.

Piazza, P.V., Ferdico, M., Russo, D., Crescimanno, G., Benigno, A. and Amato, G. (1988) Facilitatory effect of ventral tegmental area A10 region on the attack behaviour in the cat: possible dopaminergic role in selective attention. *Experimental Brain Research* **72**, 109–116.

Price, J.L., Russchen, F.T. and Amaral, D.G. (1987) The limbic region. II: The amygdaloid complex. In: Björklund, A., Hökfelt, T. and Swanson, L.W. (eds) *Handbook of Chemical Neuroanatomy Vol. 5: Integrated Systems of the CNS, Part I*. New York: Elsevier Science Publishers, pp. 272–388.

Pycock, C.J., Kerwin, R.W. and Carter, C.J. (1980) Effect of lesion of cortical dopamine terminals on subcortical dopamine receptors in rats. *Nature* **286**, 74–77.

Rebec, G.V., Alloway, K.D. and Bashore, T.R. (1981) Differential actions of classical and atypical antipsychotic drugs on spontaneous neuronal activity in the amygdaloid complex. *Pharmacology Biochemistry and Behavior* **14**, 49–56.

Reid, M., Herrera-Marschitz, M., Hökfelt, T., Terenius, L. and Ungerstedt, U. (1988) Differential modulation of striatal dopamine release by intranigral injection of δ-aminobutyric acid (GABA), dynorphin A and substance P. *European Journal of Pharmacology* **147**, 411–420.

Reynolds, G.P. and Czudek, C. (1988) Status of the dopaminergic system in post-mortem brain in schizophrenia. *Psychopharmacology Bulletin* **24**, 345–347.

Ridley, R.M., Aitken, D.M. and Baker, H.F. (1989) Learning about rules but not about reward is impaired following lesions of the cholinergic projection to the hippocampus. *Brain Research* **502**, 306–318.

Riolobos, A.S. (1986) Differential effect of chemical lesion and electrocoagulation of the central amygdaloid nucleus on active avoidance responses. *Physiology and Behavior* **36**, 441–444.

Robbins, T.W. (1988) Norepinephrine, dopamine, and selective attention: interactions in theory and practice. In: Belmaker, H., Sandler, M. and Dahlström, A. (eds) *Progress in Catecholamine Research, Part B: Central Aspects*. New York: Alan R. Liss, pp. 169–173.

Robbins, T.W., Cador, M., Taylor, J.R. and Everitt, B.J. (1989) Limbic-striatal interactions in reward-related processes. *Neuroscience and Behavioral Reviews* **13**, 155–162.

Robertson, A. (1989) Multiple reward systems and the prefrontal cortex. *Neuroscience and Biobehavioral Reviews* **13**, 163–170.

Robertson, H.A., Peterson, M.R., Murphy, K. and Robertson, G.S. (1989) D1-dopamine receptor agonists selectively activate striatal c-fos independent of rotational behaviour. *Brain Research* **503**, 346–349.

Rolls, E.T., Murzi, E., Yaxley, S., Thorpe, S.J. and Simpson, S.J. (1986) Sensory-specific satiety: food-specific reduction in responsiveness of ventral forebrain neurons after feeding in the monkey. *Brain Research* **368**, 79–86.

Rudy, J.W. and Sutherland, R.J. (1989) The hippocampal formation is necessary for rats to learn and remember configural discriminations. *Behavioural Brain Research* **34**, 97–109.

Salamone, J.D. (1986) Different effects of haloperidol and extinction on instrumental behaviours. *Psychopharmacology* **88**, 18–23.

Salamone, J.D. (1988) Dopaminergic involvement in activational aspects of motivation: effects of haloperidol on schedule-induced activity, feeding, and foraging in rats. *Psychobiology* **16**, 196–206.

Sasaki, K., Suda, H., Watanabe, H. and Tagi, H. (1990) Involvement of the entopeduncular nucleus and the habenula in the methamphetamine induced inhibition of dopamine neurons in the substantia nigra of rats. *Brain Research Bulletin* **25**, 121–127.

Sawaguchi, T., Matsumura, M. and Kubota, K. (1986) Dopamine modulates neuronal activities related to motor performance in the monkey prefrontal cortex. *Brain Research* **371**, 404–408.

Schacter, G.B., Yang, C.R., Innis, N.K. and Mogenson, G.J. (1989) The role of the hippocampal-nucleus accumbens pathway in radial-arm maze performance. *Brain Research* **494**, 339–349.

Scheel-Krüger, J. (1984) On the role of GABA for striatal functions. Interaction between GABA and enkephalin in the pallidal systems. *Neuropharmacology* **23**, 867–868.

Scheel-Krüger, J. (1986) Dopamine-GABA interactions: evidence that GABA transmits, modulates and mediates dopaminergic functions in the basal ganglia and the limbic system. *Acta Neurologica Scandinavica* **73**, 1–54 (suppl 107).

Schmajuk, N.A. (1987) Animal models for schizophrenia: the hippocampally lesioned animal. *Schizophrenia Bulletin* **13**, 317–327.

Selemon, L.D. and Goldman-Rakic, P.S. (1985) Longitudinal topography and interdigitation of corticostriatal projections in the rhesus monkey. *Journal of Neuroscience* **5**, 776–794.

Sesack, S.R., Deutch, A.Y., Roth, R.H. and Bunney, B.S. (1989) Topographical organization of the efferent projections of the medial prefrontal cortex in the rat: an anterograde tract-tracing study with phaseolus vulgaris leucoagglutinin. *Journal of Comparative Neurology* **290**, 213–242.

Shallice, T. (1982) Specific impairments of planning. *Philosophical Transactions of the Royal Society (London)* **B298**, 199–209.

Shizgal, P. and Murray, B. (1989) Neuronal basis of intracranial self-stimulation. In: Liebman, J.M. and Cooper, S.J. (eds) *The Neuropharmacological Basis of Rewards*. Oxford: Oxford University Press, pp. 106–163.

Siegel, A., Joyner, K. and Smith, G.P. (1988) Effect of bilateral ibotenic acid lesions in the basolateral amygdala on the sham feeding response to sucrose in the rat. *Physiology and Behavior* **42**, 231–235.

Simon, H. and Le Moal, M. (1984) Mesencephalic dopaminergic neurons: functional role. In: Usdin, E., Carlsson, A., Dahlström, A. and Engel, J. (eds) *Catecholamines: Neuropharmacology and Central Nervous System—Theoretical Aspects*. New York: Alan R. Liss, pp. 293–307.

Simon, H., Le Moal, M. and Calas, A. (1979) Efferents and afferents of the ventral tegmental-A10 region studied after local injection of [^{3}H]leucine and horseradish peroxidase. *Brain Research* 178, 17–40.

Skagerberg, G., Lindvall, O. and Bjöklund, A. (1984) Origin, course and termination of the mesohabenular dopamine pathway in the rat. *Brain Research* 307, 99–108.

Sorensen, S.M., Humphreys, T.M. and Palfreyman, M.G. (1989) Effect of acute and chronic MDL 73,147EF, a 5-HT3 receptor antagonist, on A9 and A10 dopamine neurons. *European Journal of Pharmacology* 163, 115–118.

Stevens, J.R. (1973) An anatomy of schizophrenia. *Archives of General Psychiatry* 29, 177–189.

Stinus, L., Herman, J.P. and Le Moal, M. (1982) GABAergic mechanisms within the ventral tegmental area: involvement of dopaminergic (A 10) and non-dopaminergic neurones. *Psychopharmacology* 77, 186–192.

Sugimoto, T. and Mizuno, N. (1987) Neurotensin in projection neurons of the striatum and nucleus accumbens, with reference to coexistence with enkephalin and GABA: an immunohistochemical study in the cat. *Journal of Comparative Neurology* 257, 383–395.

Swanson, L.W. (1982) The projections of the ventral tegmental area and adjacent regions: a combined fluorescent retrograde tracer and immunofluorescence study in the rat. *Brain Research Bulletin* 9, 321–353.

Swanson, L.W., Mogenson, G.J., Simerly, R.B. and Wu, M. (1987) Anatomical and electrophysiological evidence for a projection from the medial preoptic area to the 'mesencephalic and subthalamic locomotor regions' in the rat. *Brain Research* 405, 108–122.

Swerdlow, N.R. and Koob, G.F. (1987) Lesions of the dorsomedial nucleus of the thalamus, medial prefrontal cortex and pedunculopontine nucleus: effects on locomotor activity mediated by nucleus accumbens-ventral pallidal circuitry. *Brain Research* 412, 233–243.

Swerdlow, N.R., Vaccarino, F.J., Amalric, M. and Koob, G.F. (1986) The neural substrates for the motor-activating properties of psychostimulants: a review of recent findings. *Pharmacology Biochemistry and Behavior* 25, 233–248.

Taghzouti, K., Simon, H., Louilot, A., Herman, J.P. and Le Moal, M. (1985) Behavioral study after local injection of 6-hydroxydopamine into the nucleus accumbens in the rat. *Brain Research* 344, 9–20.

Tan, D.-P. and Tsou, K. (1988) Intranigral injection of dynorphin in combination with substance P on striatal dopamine metabolism in the rat. *Brain Research* 443, 310–414.

Tanner, T. (1979) GABA-induced locomotor activity in the rat, after bilateral injection into the ventral tegmental area. *Neuropharmacology* 18, 441–446.

Ter Horst, G.J., de Boer, P., Luiten, P.G.M. and van Willigen, J.D. (1989) Ascending projections from the solitary tract nucleus to the hypothalamus. A phaseolus vulgaris lectin tracing study in the rat. *Neuroscience* 31, 785–797.

Thornton, E.W. and Evans, J.C. (1982) The role of habenular nuclei in the selection of behavioral strategies. *Physiological Psychology* 10, 361–367.

Thornton, E.W., Evans, J.A.C. and Wickens, A. (1987) Changes in motor activities induced by microinjections of the selective dopamine agonists LY 171555, quinpirole hydrochloride, and SK&F 38393 into the habenula nucleus. *Pharmacology Biochemistry and Behavior* **26**, 643–646.

Totterdell, S. and Smith, A.D. (1989) Convergence of hippocampal and dopaminergic input onto identified neurons in the nucleus accumbens of the rat. *Journal of Chemical Neuroanatomy* **2**, 285–298.

Tsai, C.T., Mogenson, G.J., Wu, M. and Yang, C.R. (1989) A comparison of the effects of electrical stimulation of the amygdala and hippocampus on subpallidal output neurons to the pedunculopontine nucleus. *Brain Research* **494**, 22–29.

Turner, B.H., Mishkin, M. and Knapp, M. (1980) Organization of the amygdalopetal projections from modality-specific cortical association areas in the monkey. *Journal of Comparative Neurology* **191**, 515–543.

Ugedo, L., Grenhoff, J. and Svensson, T.H. (1989) Ritanserin, a 5-HT2 receptor antagonist, activates midbrain dopamine neurons by blocking serotonergic inhibition. *Psychopharmacology* **98**, 45–50.

Ungerstedt, U. (1971) Adipsia and aphagia after 6-hydroxydopamine induced degeneration of the nigro-striatal dopamine system. *Acta Physiologica Scandinavica* **367**, 95–122 (suppl).

Voorn, P., Roest, G. and Groenewegen, H.J. (1987) Increase of enkephalin and decrease of substance P immunoreactivity in the dorsal and ventral striatum of the rat after midbrain 6-hydroxydopamine lesions. *Brain Research* **412**, 391–396.

Wallace, D.M., Magnuson, D.J. and Gray, T.S. (1989) The amygdalobrainstem pathway: selective innervation of dopaminergic, noradrenergic and adrenergic cells in the rat. *Neuroscience Letters* **97**, 252–258.

Wang, R.Y. and Hu, X.-T. (1986) Does cholecystokinin potentiate dopamine action in the nucleus accumbens? *Brain Research* **380**, 363–367.

Weinberger, D.R. (1988) Schizophrenia and the frontal lobe. *Trends in Neuroscience* **11**, 367–370.

Weinberger, D.R., Berman, K.F. and Illowsky, B.P. (1988) Physiological dysfunction of dorsolateral prefrontal cortex in schizophrenia. *Archives of General Psychiatry* **45**, 609–615.

Willner, P., Chawla, K., Sampson, D., Sophokleous, S. and Muscat, R. (1988) Tests of functional equivalence between pimozide pretreatment, extinction and free feeding. *Psychopharmacology* **95**, 423–426.

Wilson, F.A.W. and Rolls, E.T. (1990) Neuronal responses related to reinforcement in the primate basal forebrain. *Brain Research* **509**, 213–231.

Wise, R. (1989) The brain and reward. In: Liebman, J.M. and Cooper S.J. (eds) *The Neuropharmacological Basis of Reward*. Oxford: Oxford University Press, pp. 377–424.

Witter, M.P., Groenewegen, H.J., Lopes da Silva, F.H. and Lohman, A.H.M. (1989) Functional organization of the extrinsic and intrinsic circuitry of the parahippocampal region. In: Kerkut, G.A. and Phillis, J.W. (eds) *Progress in Neurobiology*. Oxford: Pergamon Press, pp. 161–253.

Yamamoto, T., Matsuo, R., Kiyomitsu, Y. and Kitamura, R. (1989) Response properties of lateral hypothalamic neurons during ingestive behavior with special reference to licking of various taste solutions. *Brain Research* **481**, 286–297.

Yang, C.R. and Mogenson, G.J. (1989) Ventral pallidal neuronal responses to dopamine receptor stimulation in the nucleus accumbens. *Brain Research* **489**, 237–246.

Zahm, D.S. (1989) The ventral striatopallidal parts of the basal ganglia in the rat-II. Compartmentation of ventral pallidal efferents. *Neuroscience* **30**, 33–50.

23

Behavioral Pharmacology of Dopamine Systems: a New Synthesis

JOHN D. SALAMONE

Department of Psychology, University of Connecticut, Storrs
CT 06269-1020, USA

INTRODUCTION

Research into the behavioral functions of mesolimbic and striatal dopamine (DA) has been one of the most active areas of study in behavioral neuroscience. Particular emphasis has been placed on characterization of the behavioral effects of DA agonist and antagonist drugs. Numerous studies have described the response-suppressing effects of DA antagonists, and how these effects are particularly noticeable in appetitively motivated tasks. In addition, it is well documented that drugs acting directly or indirectly to facilitate DA transmission can act as motor stimulants, and will often be self-administered by animals or humans. Taken together, these results suggest that limbic and striatal DA is involved in motivational and motor processes, and indeed, these hypothesized functions have proven to be the focus of research into the behavioral pharmacology of DA systems.

However, it can be argued that reliance on such global terms as 'motivation', 'reward', or 'movement' can lead to an oversimplification and misrepresentation of the complex behavioral functions of DA systems and the structures they innervate. Motivation and motor control are complex and multifaceted processes. Three decades of research have demonstrated that systemic, intrastriatal or intra-accumbens administration of DA antagonists suppresses neither all aspects of motivation, nor all aspects of reward, nor all aspects of movement. For example, low doses of neuroleptic drugs can impair instrumental lever pressing even though food consumption remains

The Mesolimbic Dopamine System: From Motivation to Action.
Edited by P. Willner and J. Scheel-Krüger

© 1991 John Wiley & Sons Ltd

intact (Rolls et al., 1974; Fibiger et al., 1976). Moreover, interference with DA systems can suppress movement under some conditions (e.g. active avoidance), but the organism still retains considerable residual motor capacity, which can manifest under different stimulus conditions (e.g. escape responses; Posluns, 1962). Clearly, the terms motivation, reward and motor function are too broad to offer an adequate description of the behavioral functions of brain DA, and more specific hypotheses are required.

Several researchers have hypothesized functions of mesolimbic and striatal DA that are more specific than the global hypotheses described above. Mogenson and his colleagues (Mogenson et al., 1980) have emphasized that the nucleus accumbens represents a functional interface between the limbic system and the motor system, thereby providing a link between motivational and motor processes. Since it was originally offered, this view has gained considerable acceptance (Cools et al., Chapter 6; Mogenson and Yim, Chapter 4, this volume). Some investigators characterize the behavioral functions of striatal DA as being sensorimotor in nature, and have emphasized that the role of the striatum might be to allow various sensory and cognitive functions to influence motor control (Divac, 1972; Ungerstedt and Ljungberg, 1974; Lidsky et al., 1985; White, 1986). Cools (1980) suggested that striatal DA is involved in the temporal sequencing and selection of behavioral responses. DA in the striatum and accumbens has been implicated in the regulation of perseveration and switching in the temporal control of behavior (Evenden and Robbins, 1983b; Koob et al., 1978).

It has been hypothesized by Beninger (1983) that DA is involved in the process of reward-related or incentive learning. According to this view, release of DA in the striatum and accumbens is able to modify the efficacy of synapses that were recently active, which would promote the acquisition of reward-related learning. DA is hypothesized to act via stimulation of D1 receptors, and the neuronal changes produced by formation of cyclic-AMP would modulate the cellular processes involved in these synaptic changes (Beninger, Chapter 11, this volume). As well as being involved in the acquisition of incentive learning, DA may also be involved in responding to established incentive stimuli. Horvitz and Ettenberg (1989), demonstrated that haloperidol blocked the response-reinstating effects of food presentation during extinction: haloperidol administered at the time of food presentation was able to suppress the increase in run speeds observed 24 hours later in untreated animals, suggesting that it may have blocked an incentive process.

To specify more precisely the effects of DA antagonists on motivated behavior, some investigators have made distinctions between various aspects of motivated behavior that are differentially affected by DA-related manipulations. Phillips and his co-workers (Blackburn et al., 1987, 1989; Phillips et al., Chapter 8, this volume) have emphasized the distinction between preparatory behaviors which are more easily disrupted by administration of DA antagonists, and consummatory behaviors, which are less easily disrupted. Salamone (1988) noted that motivational theorists have often emphasized the distinction between activational (e.g. response rate, vigor or persistence) and directional (goal-directed) aspects of motivation. Several studies have demonstrated that indices of response activation can be impaired at doses of DA antagonists that leave intact directional aspects of responding. For example, paradigms that offer separate measures of response-rate or speed and response choice have shown that DA antagonists can impair response rate or speed at doses that do not impair choice (Evenden and Robbins, 1983a; Tombaugh et al., 1983; Bowers et al., 1985). Also, haloperidol impaired food-induced locomotor activity at doses that did not disrupt simple instrumental approach responses (Salamone, 1986, 1988).

The research generated by these and other specific hypotheses of DA function has stimulated a significant re-evaluation of the role of DA in aspects of motor control and motivation. In turn, the continuing assessment of the behavioral functions of DA can lead investigators to re-examine our basic ideas about motor control and motivation, and to consider how these processes are related.

MOTOR CONTROL PROCESSES

Central nervous system control of movement is organized in a complex hierarchical manner. Therefore, there is no precise uniformity to the term 'motor deficit'. It is often mistakenly assumed that an impairment of motor function implies paralysis or a complete loss of motor capacity. Of course, the exact nature of a motor deficit depends upon where in the nervous system the dysfunction is situated, and which functions are subserved by the impaired structure. Impairments at various levels of this hierarchically organized motor system can lead to flaccid paralysis, spastic paralysis, tremor, apraxia or motor aphasia, all very different types of deficits that describe aspects of motor dysfunction.

The striatum and nucleus accumbens are involved in aspects of motor function, and these structures influence brain stem and ultimately spinal mechanisms that more directly control motor output (Garcia-Rill, 1986). However, interference with mesolimbic and nigrostriatal DA does not produce a true paralysis. Reports of 'paradoxical kinesia' in Parkinson's disease, in which akinetic or bradykinetic patients show movement in response to intense stimuli, underscores the capability for movement present in these patients. It is well documented that rats made akinetic with lesions of the nigrostriatal bundle are capable of being activated by cold baths or tail-pinch (Antleman et al., 1976; Marshall et al., 1976). Keefe et al. (1989) demonstrated that rats that had received DA-depleting lesions with

6-hydroxydopamine (6-OHDA) plus 1.0 mg/kg haloperidol were still capable of swimming in a forced-swim test, and of escaping from an ice bath. These data all demonstrate that the response-suppressing effects of interference with DA systems, even in extreme cases, can be overridden by increasing sensory input to the organism.

The observation that increased sensory input can reverse motor suppression in extreme instances of DA dysfunction is also of relevance to the involvement of DA systems in motivational processes. In some experiments, it has been demonstrated that neuroleptic-treated animals which have 'extinguished' responding in operant tasks will show increased responding if they are exposed to a stimulus paired with reinforcement (Franklin and McKoy, 1979; Wise, 1982). Another paradigm that has been used to assess the behavioral effects of DA antagonists is response-reinforcement matching, in which it can be demonstrated that the relation between responding and reinforcement density on variable interval schedules is described by a rectangular hyperbola (Herrnstein, 1974). Low doses of neuroleptics have been shown in some studies to change the response-reinforcement relation (Heyman, 1983; Heyman et al., 1986; Willner et al., Chapter 10, this volume) by causing an increase in the density of reinforcement necessary to maintain a half-maximal rate of responding. Usually these effects are presumed to reflect a blunting of 'reward' produced by the neuroleptic. One possible interpretation of these data, as well as experiments showing similar shifts in the consumption of sucrose solutions (Willner et al., Chapter 10, this volume), is that they represent a complete reversibility of the effects of low doses of neuroleptics by increasing the sensory stimulation proved by the reinforcing stimulus.

The implications of the reversibility of the effects of DA antagonists or DA depletion on behavior are very important. Does this mean that the akinesia of Parkinson's disease is really a motivational deficit? Do the matching and sucrose-consumption experiments reflect a mild and reversible suppression of responsiveness to stimuli which leaves residual motor capacity intact? Perhaps the best way to summarize these data is to emphasize that the absolute distinction between motor and motivational processes may be a false dichotomy, and that the behavioral deficits produced by DA antagonists reflect impairments of brain processes that represent areas of overlap between motor control and motivation.

MOTIVATIONAL PROCESSES

P.T. Young defined motivation as the process of 'arousing activity, maintaining the activity in progress, and regulating the pattern of activity'. Motivational theorists such as Duffy (1963) and Cofer (1972) have emphasized that an important aspect of motivation is the activation of responding produced by motivationally relevant stimuli. Salamone (1988) suggested that low doses of DA antagonists impair activational aspects of motivation, but basically leave intact the directed, goal-oriented features of motivated behavior. Low doses of haloperidol suppressed schedule-induced motor activity, but did not impair simple approach responses for food (Salamone, 1986, 1988). In paradigms that yielded separate measures of response rate and response choice, DA antagonists impaired indices of response rate but not response choice (Evenden and Robbins, 1983a; Tombaugh et al., 1983; Bowers et al., 1985). The notion that DA in the nucleus accumbens is involved in the activating effects of motivationally significant stimuli is consistent with elements of both the motor and the motivational interpretations of the behavioral functions of DA systems.

Of course, there are other significant features of motivation that must also be considered. One aspect of motivated behavior is that some of the responses in which organisms engage represent direct interactions with motivationally relevant stimuli. These responses, such as feeding and drinking, are usually the terminal or consummatory behaviors in a sequence of responses. To engage in these consummatory responses, organisms must first engage in some instrumental responses that enable them to have access to the relevant stimulus. This distinction between instrumental and consummatory responses is another important dimension of behavior for understanding the role of DA systems in motivation. It has been hypothesized that complex chains of instrumental behaviors are more sensitive to disruption by DA antagonists than are consummatory behaviors, and moreover, indices of DA release in the nucleus accumbens show greater increases during the instrumental phase of behavior than the consummatory phase (Blackburn et al., 1987, 1989; Phillips et al., Chapter 8, this volume).

It is possible to relate these various aspects of motivated behavior to each other by considering that both instrumental and consummatory responses have activational and directional characteristics. For example, one can observe indices of vigorous, persistent responding both in lever pressing for food and in food consumption. One way of integrating the views of Salamone (1988) and Phillips et al. (Chapter 8, this volume) is to propose that the activational aspects of instrumental behavior are very sensitive to disruption by DA antagonists, and that consummatory responses directed at particular stimuli are much less sensitive to disruption. This position is consistent with previous studies showing that vigorous instrumental responses such as lever pressing, hoarding large numbers of food pellets, and highly active schedule-induced and preparatory behaviors, are easily disrupted by low doses of DA antagonists (Rolls et al., 1974; Fibiger et al., 1976; Keehn and Riusech, 1977; Ettenberg et al., 1981; Salamone, 1986, 1988; Sanger, 1986; Blackburn et al., 1987) or mesolimbic DA depletion (Robbins and Koob, 1980; Wallace et al., 1983; Kelley and Stinus, 1985). In contrast to these more vigorous instrumental or preparatory responses, very simple approach or consummatory responses directed towards food are much less sensitive to disruption by interference with DA systems (Rolls et al., 1974; Fibiger et al., 1976; Salamone, 1986, 1988; Blackburn et al., 1987).

In addition to the aspects of motivation described above, other important features of motivated behavior also bear some relevance to the behavioral functions of mesolimbic and nigrostriatal DA. The data outlined above, describing the reversibility of the motor effects of DA antagonists or DA-depleting lesions, emphasize the importance of the intensity of the stimuli that elicit the responses observed. White (1986) suggested that depletion of forebrain DA increased the threshold for responding to stimuli that elicit orientation, approach and consumption. Thus, higher levels of stimulation are necessary to induce activity in DA-depleted animals. Clody and Carlton (1980) hypothesized that increases in the efficacy (proximity or intensity) of reinforcing stimuli attenuated the behavioral effects of chlorpromazine.

It has been suggested that DA is more involved in the execution of learned, as opposed to unlearned, motor acts (Marsden, 1982). There is also evidence that DA antagonists may more easily disrupt behavior that is elicited by conditioned, as opposed to unconditioned, stimuli. For example, avoidance behavior, which represents locomotion to a particular locus in reponse to a conditioned stimulus, is very sensitive to disruption by DA antagonists (Posluns, 1962; Janssen et al., 1965). However, escape behavior, which is a similar motor response to avoidance but which is elicited by the unconditioned aversive stimulus, is relatively insensitive to disruption by DA antagonists (Posluns, 1962). Gramling and Fowler (1985) demonstrated that a conditioned licking response was more easily disrupted by haloperidol, chlorpromazine and clozapine than was a reflexive licking response.

Even when one considers just the effects of conditioned stimuli on motivated behavior, it should be emphasized that various characteristics of conditioned stimuli can be dissociated. For example, the work of Cador et al. (Chapter 9, this volume) has clearly demonstrated that the secondary reinforcing effects of conditioned stimuli are dissociable from the ability of conditioned stimuli to control responding in a discrimination paradigm. There is considerable evidence that DA is involved in secondary reinforcement. Systemic administration of pimozide was shown to disrupt the establishment of conditioned reinforcement (Beninger and Phillips, 1980). Injection of amphetamine into the nucleus accumbens increased the effects of secondary reinforcement (Taylor and Robbins, 1984), and depletion of DA from the nucleus accumbens attenuated the effect of amphetamine on responding to secondary reinforcement (Taylor and Robbins, 1986). Administration of amphetamine into the nucleus accumbens reversed the deficit in responding for secondary reinforcement that resulted from amygdala lesions (Cador et al., 1989; Everitt et al., 1989; see Cador et al., Chapter 9, this volume). However, systemic administration of DA antagonists does not generally impair discrimination or stimulus–stimulus associative mechanisms (Beninger et al., 1980; Beninger, 1982; Tombaugh et al., 1983; Bowers et al., 1985).

Combination of all the aspects of motivation described above into a multidimensional model may prove to be a useful way of summarizing the behavioral pharmacology of mesolimbic and nigrostriatal DA systems. The behaviors that are most easily disrupted by DA antagonists are highly activated, and complex learned instrumental responses that are elicited or supported by mild conditioned stimuli (e.g. lever pressing on a VI schedule that produces submaximal response rates, or lever pressing for secondary reinforcement). The behaviors that are most resistant to disruption by DA antagonists are relatively simple and often unlearned responses to intense unconditioned stimuli (e.g. locomotion in response to shock or forced swimming). This summary statement is in general agreement with most of the available literature.

A MULTIPROCESS MODEL OF MOTIVATION

Motivation is defined in different ways by different researchers, but for the present discussion it is defined as follows: motivation is the set of processes that enable the organism to control the availability, probability or proximity of stimuli. Defined in this way, motivation is not defined in terms of hypothetical states, drives, desires or euphoria. Rather, motivation is meant to describe the set of sensory, motor and other processes that characterize the regulation of behavior. Of course, this is a very broad definition, which includes most behaviors demonstrated by whole organisms (as opposed to isolated preparations). It is precisely because of this breadth that one cannot simply state that a drug impairs motivation, but instead one must identify the specific aspects of motivation that are influenced by a particular manipulation.

As shown in Figure 1, the motor system of the organism, which is organized in a complex hierarchical manner, is the means through which organisms control their environment. Sensory systems, also organized hierarchically, monitor the condition of the external and internal environments. The behavior of organisms is characterized by sensory-motor loops at various levels of function. At the most complex level (response allocation/stimulus selection), organisms are capable of allocating time and responses in relation to a vast array of stimuli. The idea that organisms allocate behavior with relation to the characteristics of a variety of stimuli is at the heart of several important behavioral theories, including optimal foraging theory (Krebs, 1978), the matching equation (Herrnstein, 1974), and economic models of operant conditioning (Staddon, 1979).

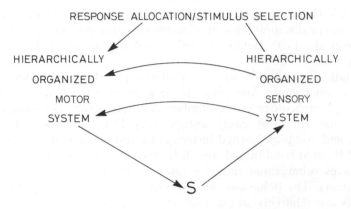

Figure 1. Schematic representation of the proposed model of behavioral control in motivational processes. Motor and sensory processes are hierarchically organized, and behavior is regulated by sensory-motor loops at various levels. At the highest level of motivational control is the process that regulates allocation of responses with relation to the value of various stimuli in the environment

Figure 2 shows the suggested role of mesolimbic and nigrostriatal DA in the model described above. DA in the ventral and dorsal striatum is seen as modulating the ability of some sensory, associative and affective processes to influence complex aspects of motor function. Increases in indices of DA release are associated with the presentation of motivationally relevant stimuli (Church et al., 1987; Hernandez et al., 1988; Blackburn et al., 1986, 1989; Salamone et al., 1989). DA release modulates aspects of motor function, including the local rate of responding and the duration of periods of responding. In addition, DA systems modulate the extent to which organisms will overcome obstacles, or 'response costs', in order to obtain access to significant stimuli (Neill and Justice, 1981; Salamone, 1987, 1988).

According to the model described in Figure 2, nigrostriatal and mesolimbic DA have little direct involvement in sensory, affective and stimulus–stimulus associative processes. The residual motor capacity present after severe DA dysfunction occurs because, although DA modulates motor function, striatal DA synapses are still several steps removed from the motor neurons themselves. Also, intense stimuli can activate movement through processes that do not require DA. Emotional reactivity to positive and aversive tastes was preserved after DA antagonists or DA-depleting lesions (Berridge et al., 1989), perhaps because relatively simple responses related to affective processes do not require intact DA systems. Because these sensory, affective and associative processes are basically intact, and have some access to motor areas of the brain, interference with accumbens or striatal DA is less likely

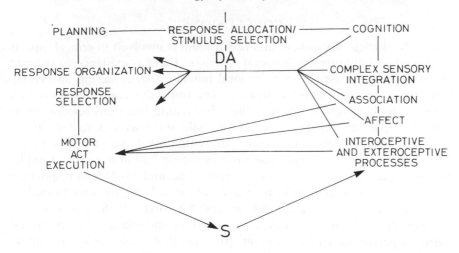

Figure 2. The proposed role of neostriatal and accumbens DA in the proposed model of motivation. DA in these structures modulates the ability of some sensory, affective, associative and cognitive processes to influence complex aspects of motor function. The connections drawn are highly oversimplified, and this figure is not meant to imply that neostriatal and accumbens DA serve exactly the same function. Note that some sensory processes have access to motor mechanisms through routes that do not require DA. S, Stimuli

to impair relatively simple responses to unconditoned stimuli (i.e. terminal or consummatory responses, forced swimming).

In behavioral terms, it can be said that the responses that are most sensitive to disruption after interference with mesolimbic or striatal DA are highly active or complex learned instrumental responses elicited or supported by conditioned stimuli. Some of the processes involved in these responses, such as coordination of learned motor acts in a temporal sequence, conditioning, evaluation of density or rate of various reinforcers, or decision-making processes based on cost/benefit analyses, probably depend heavily on neocortical and limbic processes. These processes must eventually gain access to the brain areas directly involved in the execution of motor acts. It is proposed that DA in the accumbens and striatum is importantly involved in the process that allows neocortical and limbic areas to influence complex aspects of motor function. Thus, interference with DA systems produces a 'subcortical apraxia' which dissociates complex stimulus processes from complex motor processes, but leaves aspects of those sensory and motor processes essentially intact.

CONCLUSIONS

DA in the nucleus accumbens and neostriatum is involved in critical aspects of normal and abnormal behavioral function. There is evidence to indicate an involvement in aspects of behavioral function that represent an overlap between motor control and motivation. The respective contributions of DA in the accumbens and striatum to these behavioral functions remains to be explained. The model described above could serve as a basis for further experiments that could demonstrate differential involvement of one or the other DA system in the particular functions described above. For example, evidence indicates a selective involvement of accumbens DA in responding to secondary reinforcement (Taylor and Robbins, 1986). As emphasized by Le Moal and his colleagues (Simon and Le Moal, 1988; Cador et al., Chapter 9, this volume), DA is involved in modulating the particular functions performed by the different structures that receive DA innervation. In addition to the motor and motivational functions performed by the striatum and accumbens, there is evidence that prefrontal cortex DA could be involved in learning or memory functions (Brozoski et al., 1979; Simon et al., 1980; Sahakian et al., 1985).

Mesolimbic and striatal DA is involved in Parkinson's disease, and may be involved in depression (Willner et al., Chapter 15, this volume) and drug abuse (Bozarth, Chapter 12; Cooper, Chapter 13; Di Chiara et al., Chapter 14, this volume). One possible way to interpret the role of accumbens DA in drug self-administration is to suggest that DA directly mediates the subjective euphoria produced by positive reinforcers. This interpretation is consistent with the hypothesis (Wise, 1982) that DA mediates the rewarding effects of natural rewards and drugs, and that administration of DA antagonists produces an extinction-like effect. However, it has been demonstrated that the effects of neuroleptics differ substantially from those of extinction (Evenden and Robbins, 1983a; Salamone, 1986, 1987, 1988; Willner et al., 1988). It is also important to consider that interference with DA systems can impair performance on aversive as well as appetitive motivational tasks (Posluns, 1962; Janssen et al., 1965; Sanger, 1986). Moreover, aversive stimuli can increase DA turnover in the accumbens and frontal cortex (Thierry et al., 1976; Fada et al., 1978; D'Angio et al., 1987; Abercrombie et al., 1989a, b; Zacharko and Anisman, Chapter 16, this volume), and, under some conditions, the striatum as well (Abercrombie et al., 1989a, b).

As stated above, reinforcement and motivation are very complex processes. Thus, it is probably too simplistic to equate the concepts of 'reward' and 'euphoria'. Several different types of conditions can reinforce behavior. Rats will run in alleyways to gain access to complex mazes that they can explore

(Montgomery, 1954). Various types of arousing stimulus changes are reinforcing (Berlyne, 1967). It is possible that some drugs are abused because of the changes in internal and external stimuli they produce. In addition, it is possible that behavioral activation is itself rewarding (Wise, 1988; Beninger, Chapter 11, this volume).

Because emotions such as euphoria are very complex, it is difficult to determine the particular aspect of the emotional response in which DA may be involved. The work of Schacter (Schacter and Singer, 1962; Schacter, 1964) demonstrated that emotions in humans have complex cognitive and autonomic physiological determinants. The cognitive processes involved in emotions are necessary for evaluating the situations in which the emotion takes place, and the labeling of events as positive or negative. Physiological arousal represents the activation of physiological (e.g. autonomic) responses that can occur in both positive or negative situations. Schacter's experiments indicated that people could experience arousal after injections of adrenaline, and that the emotion they experienced could be anger or euphoria depending on the environmental conditions they were exposed to in the experiment. Because mesolimbic DA is involved in both appetitive and aversive motivation, it is possible that this system is an important component of the brain mechanisms involved in the arousal of positive and negative emotional responses.

Taking all these data into consideration, it is plausible to suggest that accumbens DA is involved in aspects of motivation that are common to appetitive and aversive emotional states. Organisms actively engage in instrumental activities to obtain positive reinforcers and to avoid aversive stimuli. Viewed in this manner, a major function of DA in the accumbens would be to promote interaction with, and adaptation to, the environment. Although this mechanism can be viewed as common to appetitive and aversive conditions, manipulation of DA systems could have powerful indirect effects on the affective state of the organism. Reduced functional activity in accumbens and striatal DA would leave the organism less able to avoid aversive stimuli and less able to obtain positive stimuli; both of these consequences would generate a less positive affective state (Willner, 1985). In addition, a mild activation of DA, as produced by low doses of stimulant drugs, would render the organism more able to avoid aversive stimuli and more able to obtain positive stimuli, which would generate a more positive affective state. Indeed, these effects could contribute to the positive reinforcing effects of some drugs. Mild psychomotor stimulation may be positively reinforcing, partly because it promotes interaction with the environment and generates internal and external stimuli that are consistent with the ability to adapt to and control the environment.

REFERENCES

Abercrombie, E.A., Keefe, K.A., DiFrischia, D.A. and Zigmond, M.J. (1989a) Differential effect of stress on in vivo dopamine release in striatum, nucleus accumbens and medial frontal cortex. *Journal of Neurochemistry* **52**, 1655–1658.

Abercrombie, E., Keefe, K. and Zigmond, M. (1989b) Evidence that nerve terminal density is an important contributor to apparent differences in the activation of central dopamine systems. *Behavioural Pharmacology* **1**, 26 (suppl 1).

Antleman, S.M., Rowland, R.E. and Fisher, A.E. (1976) Stress related recovery from lateral hypothalamic aphagia. *Brain Research* **102**, 346–350.

Beninger, R.J. (1982) A comparison of the effects of pimozide and nonreinforcement on discriminated operant responding in rats. *Pharmacology Biochemistry and Behavior* **16**, 667–669.

Beninger, R.J. (1983) The role of dopamine activity in locomotor activity and learning. *Brain Research Reviews* **6**, 173–196.

Beninger, R.J. and Phillips, A.G. (1980) The effect of pimozide on the establishment of conditioned reinforcement. *Psychopharmacology* **68**, 147–153.

Beninger, R.J., Maclennan, A.J. and Pinel, J.P.J. (1980) The use of conditioned defensive burying to test the effects of pimozide on associative learning. *Pharmacology Biochemistry and Behavior* **12**, 445–448.

Berlyne, D.E. (1967) Arousal and reinforcement. In: Levine, D. (ed.) *Nebraska Symposium on Motivation*. Lincoln, Nebraska: University of Nebraska Press, pp. 1–110.

Berridge, K.C., Venier, I.L. and Robinson, T.E. (1989) Taste reactivity analysis of 6-hydroxydopamine-induced aphagia: implications for arousal and anhedonia hypotheses of dopamine function. *Behavioral Neuroscience* **103**, 36–45.

Blackburn, J.R., Phillips, A.G., Jakubovic, A. and Fibiger, H.C. (1986) Increased dopamine metabolism in nucleus accumbens and striatum following consumption of a nutritive meal but not a palatable non-nutritive saccharin solution. *Pharmacology Biochemistry and Behavior* **25**, 1095–1100.

Blackburn, J.R., Phillips, A.G. and Fibiger, H.C. (1987) Dopamine and preparatory behavior: I. Effects of pimozide. *Behavioral Neuroscience* **101**, 352–360.

Blackburn, J.R., Phillips, A.G., Jakubovic, A. and Fibiger, H.C. (1989) Dopamine and preparatory behavior: II. A neurochemical analysis. *Behavioral Neuroscience* **103**, 15–23.

Bowers, W., Hamilton, M., Zacharcho, R.M. and Anisman, H. (1985) Differential effects of pimozide on response-rate and choice accuracy in a self-stimulation paradigm in mice. *Pharmacology Biochemistry and Behavior* **22**, 521–526.

Brozoski, T.J., Brown, R.M., Rosvold, H.E. and Goldman, P.S. (1979) Cognitive deficit caused by regional depletion of dopamine in prefrontal cortex of rhesus monkey. *Science* **205**, 929–932.

Cador, M., Robbins, T.W. and Everitt, B.J. (1989) Involvement of the amygdala in stimulus-reward associations: interactions with the ventral striatum. *Neuroscience* **30**, 77–86.

Church, W.H., Justice, J.B. and Neill, D.B. (1987) Detecting behaviorally relevant changes in extracellular dopamine with microdialysis. *Brain Research* **412**, 397–399.

Clody, D.E. and Carlton, P.L. (1980) Stimulus efficacy, chlorpromazine, and schizophrenia. *Psychopharmacology* **69**, 127–131.

Cofer, C.N. (1972) *Motivation and Emotion*. Glenview, Illinois: Scott, Foresman.

Cools, A.R. (1980) Role of neostriatal dopaminergic activity in sequencing and selecting behavioural strategies: facilitation of processes involved in selecting the best strategy in a stressful situation. *Behavioral Brain Research* **1**, 361–378.

D'Angio, M.D., Serrano, A., Rivy, J.P. and Scatton, B. (1987) Tail-pinch stress increases extracellular DOPAC levels (as measured by in vivo voltammetry) in rat nucleus accumbens but not frontal cortex: antagonism by diazepam and zolpidem. *Brain Research* **409**, 169–174.

Divac, I. (1972) Neostriatum and functions of prefrontal cortex. *Acta Neurobiologica Experimentalis* **32**, 461–477.

Duffy, E. (1963) *Activation and Behavior*. New York: Wiley.

Ettenberg, A., Koob, G.F. and Bloom, F. (1981) Response artifact in the measurement of neuroleptic-induced anhedonia. *Science* **209**, 357–359.

Evenden, J.L. and Robbins, T.W. (1983a) Dissociable effects of d-amphetamine, chlordiazepoxide and alpha-flupenthixol on choice and rate measures of reinforcement in the rat. *Psychopharmacology* **79**, 180–186.

Evenden, J.L. and Robbins, T.W. (1983b) Increased response switching, perseveration and perseverative switching following d-amphetamine in the rat. *Psychopharmacology* **80**, 67–73.

Everitt, B.J., Cador, M. and Robbins, T.W. (1989) Interactions between the amygdala and ventral striatum in stimulus-reward associations: studies using a second-order schedule of sexual reinforcement. *Neuroscience* **30**, 63–75.

Fada, F., Argiolas, A., Melis, M.R., Tissari, A.H., Onali, P.C. and Gessa, G.L. (1978) Stress-induced increase in 3,4-dihydroxyphenylacetic acid (DOPAC) levels in the cerebral cortex and in nucleus accumbens: reversal by diazepam. *Life Science* **23**, 2219–2224.

Fibiger, H.C., Carter, D.A. and Phillips, A.G. (1976) Decreased intracranial self-stimulation after neuroleptics or 6-hydroxydopamine: evidence for mediation by motor deficits rather than by reduced reward. *Psychopharmacology* **47**, 21–27.

Franklin, K.B.T. and McCoy, S.H. (1979) Pimozide-induced extinction in rats: stimulus control of responding rules out motor deficit. *Pharmacology Biochemistry and Behavior* **11**, 71–75.

Garcia-Rill, E. (1986) The basal ganglia and the locomotor regions. *Brain Research Reviews* **11**, 47–63.

Gramling, S.E. and Fowler, S.C. (1985) Effects of neuroleptics on rate and duration of operant versus reflexive licking in rats. *Pharmacology Biochemistry and Behavior* **22**, 541–545.

Hernandez, L., Auerbach, S. and Hoebel, B.G. (1988) Food reward and cocaine increase extracellular dopamine in the nucleus accumbens as measured by microdialysis. *Life Science* **42**, 1705–1712.

Herrnstein, R.J. (1974) Formal properties of the matching law. *Journal of the Experimental Analysis of Behavior* **21**, 159–164.

Heyman, G.M. (1983) A parametric evaluation of hedonic and motoric effects of drugs: pimozide and amphetamine. *Journal of the Experimental Analysis of Behavior* **40**, 113–122.

Heyman, G.M., Kinzie, D.L. and Seiden, L.S. (1986) Chlorpromazine and pimozide alter reinforcement efficacy and motor performance. *Psychopharmacology* **88**, 346–353.

Horvitz, J.C. and Ettenberg, A. (1989) Haloperidol blocks the response-reinstating effects of food reward: a methodology for separating neuroleptic effects on reinforcement and motor processes. *Pharmacology Biochemistry and Behavior* **31**, 861–865.

Janssen, P.A., Niemegeers, C.J.F. and Schellekens, K.H.L. (1965) Is it possible to predict the clinical effects of neuroleptic drugs (major tranquilizers) from animal data? *Arzneimittel-Forschung* **15**, 104–117.

Keefe, K.A., Salamone, J.D., Zigmond, M.J. and Stricker, E.M. (1989) Paradoxical kinesia in Parkinsonism is not caused by dopamine release: studies in an animal model. *Archives of Neurology* **46**, 1070–1075.

Keehn, J.D. and Riusech, R. (1977) Schedule-induced water and saccharin polydipsia under haloperidol. *Bulletin of the Psychonomic Society* **9**, 413–415.

Kelley, A.E. and Stinus, L. (1985) Disappearance of hoarding behavior after 6-hydroxydopamine lesions of the mesolimbic dopamine neurons and its reinstatement with L-DOPA. *Behavioral Neuroscience* **99**, 531–535.

Koob, G.F., Riley, S.J., Smith, S.C. and Robbins, T.W. (1978) Effects of 6-hydroxydopamine lesions of the nucleus accumbens septi and olfactory tubercle on feeding, locomotor activity, and amphetamine anorexia in the rat. *Journal of Comparative and Physiological Psychology* **92**, 917–927.

Krebs, J.R. (1978) Optimal foraging: decision rules for predators. In: Krebs, J.R. and Davies, W.B. (eds) *Behavioral Ecology*. Sunderland, Massachusetts: Sinauer Associates, pp. 23–63.

Lidsky, T.I., Buchwald, N.A., Manetto, C. and Schneider, J.S. (1985) A consideration of sensory factors involved in the motor functions of the basal ganglia. *Brain Research Reviews* **9**, 133–146.

Marsden, C.D. (1982) The mysterious motor function of the basal ganglia *Neurology* **32**, 514–539.

Marshall, J.F., Levitan, D. and Stricker, E.M. (1976) Activation-induced restoration of sensorimotor functions in rats with dopamine-depleting brain lesions. *Journal of Comparative and Physiological Psychology* **90**, 536–546.

Mogenson, G., Jones, D. and Yim, C.Y. (1980) From motivation to action: functional interface between the limbic system and the motor system. *Progress in Neurobiology* **14**, 69–97.

Montgomery, K.C. (1954) The role of the exploratory drive in learning. *Journal of Comparative and Physiological Psychology* **44**, 582–589.

Neill, D.B. and Justice, J.B. (1981) An hypothesis for a behavioral function of dopaminergic transmission in nucleus accumbens. In: Chronister, R.B. and DeFrance, J.F. (eds) *The Neurobiology of the Nucleus Accumbens*. Brunswick, ME: Haer Institute.

Posluns, D. (1962) An analysis of chlorpromazine-induced suppression of the avoidance response. *Psychopharmacology* **3**, 361–373.

Robbins, T.W. and Koob, G.F. (1980) Selective disruption of displacement behaviour by lesions of the mesolimbic dopamine system. *Nature* **285**, 409–412.

Rolls, E.T., Rolls, B.J., Kelly, P.H., Shaw, S.G., Wood, R.J. and Dale, R. (1974) The relative attenuation of self-stimulation, eating and drinking produced by dopamine-receptor blockade. *Psychopharmacology* **38**, 219–230.

Sahakian, B.J., Sarna, G.S., Kantameneni, B.D., Jackson, A., Hutson, P.H. and Curzon, G. (1985) Association between learning and cortical catecholamines in non-drug-treated rats. *Psychopharmacology* **86**, 339–343.

Salamone, J.D. (1986) Different effects of haloperidol and extinction on instrumental behaviors. *Psychopharmacology* **88**, 18–23.

Salamone, J.D. (1987) The actions of neuroleptic drugs on appetitive instrumental behaviors. In: Iversen, L.L., Iversen, S.D. and Snyder, S.H. (eds) *Handbook of Psychopharmacology*. New York: Plenum Press, pp. 575–608.

Salamone, J.D. (1988) Dopaminergic involvement in activational aspects of motivation: effects of haloperidol on schedule-induced activity, feeding and foraging in rats. *Psychobiology* **16**, 196–206.

Salamone, J.D., Keller, R.W., Zigmond, M.J. and Stricker, E.M. (1989) Behavioral activation in rats increases striatal dopamine metabolism measured by dialysis perfusion. *Brain Research* **487**, 215–224.

Sanger, D.J. (1986) Response decrement patterns after neuroleptic and non-neuroleptic drugs. *Psychopharmacology* **89**, 98–104.

Schacter, S. (1964) The interaction of cognitive and physiological determinants of emotional state. In: Berkowitz, L. (ed.) *Advances in Experimental Social Psychology*. New York: Academic Press, pp. 49–80.

Schacter, S. and Singer, J.E. (1962) Cognitive, social and physiological determinants of the emotional state. *Psychological Reviews* **69**, 379–399.

Simon, H. and Le Moal, M. (1988) Mesencephalic dopaminergic neurons: role in the general economy of the brain. *Annals of the New York Academy of Science* **537**, 235–253.

Simon, H., Scatton, B. and Le Moal, M. (1980) Dopaminergic A10 neurons are involved in cognitive function. *Nature* **286**, 150–151.

Staddon, J.D. (1979) Operant behavior as adaptation to constraint. *Journal of Experimental Psychology: General* **108**: 48–67.

Taylor, J.R. and Robbins, T.W. (1984) Enhanced behavioral control by conditioned reinforcers following microinjections of D-amphetamine into the nucleus accumbens. *Psychopharmacology* **84**, 405–412.

Taylor, J.R. and Robbins, T.W. (1986) 6-Hydroxydopamine lesions of the nucleus accumbens but not the caudate nucleus attenuate responding with reward-related stimuli produced by intra-accumbens D-amphetamine. *Psychopharmacology* **90**, 390–397.

Thierry, A.M., Tassin, J.-P., Blanc, G. and Glowinski, J. (1976) Selective activation of mesocortical dopaminergic system by stress. *Nature* **263**, 242–244.

Tombaugh, T.N., Szostak, C. and Mills, P. (1983) Failure of pimozide to disrupt acquisition of light–dark and spatial discrimination problems. *Psychopharmacology* **79**, 161–168.

Ungerstedt, U. and Ljungberg, T. (1974) Central dopamine neurons and sensory processing. *Journal of Psychiatry Research* **55**, 149–150.

Wallace, M., Singer, J., Finlay, J. and Gibson, S. (1983) The effect of 6-OHDA lesions of the nucleus accumbens septi on schedule-induced drinking, wheel running and corticosterone levels in the rat. *Pharmacology Biochemistry and Behavior* **18**, 129–136.

White, N.M. (1986) Control of sensorimotor functions by dopaminergic nigrostriatal neurons: influence on eating and drinking. *Neuroscience and Biobehavioral Reviews* **10**, 15–36.

Willner, P. (1985) *Depression: A Psychobiological Synthesis*. New York: Wiley.

Willner, P., Chawla, K., Sampson, D., Sophokleous, S. and Muscat, R. (1988) Tests of functional equivalence between pimozide pretreatment, extinction and free feeding. *Psychopharmacology* **95**, 423–426.

Wise, R.A. (1982) Neuroleptics and operant behavior: the anhedonia hypothesis. *Behavioral and Brain Sciences* **5**, 39–87.

Wise, R.A. (1988) Psychomotor stimulant properties of addictive drugs. *Annals of the New York Academy of Science* **537**, 228–234.

24

The Dopamine Hypotheses of Schizophrenia and Mood Disorders: Contradictions and Speculations

H.C. FIBIGER

Division of Neurological Sciences, Department of Psychiatry, The University of British Columbia, 2255 Wesbrook Mall, Vancouver BC, Canada V6T 1W5

The broad forms of the dopamine (DA) hypotheses of schizophrenia and of mood disorders seem mutually contradictory. The former postulates that schizophrenia is associated with heightened dopaminergic activity in mesolimbic and/or mesocortical systems, and the latter proposes that mood disorders are due in part to either sustained decreases (depression) or increases (mania) in mesolimbic dopaminergic tone. When these hypotheses are considered together, a number of questions immediately become apparent. For example, why are schizophrenic patients, whose mesocortico-limbic systems are hypothetically hyperactive, not also manic as the DA hypothesis of affective illness might predict? On the contrary, dysphoric mood is common in schizophrenia (Barnes et al., 1989). How is it that depression, which is hypothesized to be associated with reduced mesolimbic dopaminergic activity, can co-exist in the same patient diagnosed as schizophrenic? Why does depression not preclude an individual from having schizophrenia as the two hypotheses might predict? Although these contradictions are undoubtedly due primarily to the inadequacies of both hypotheses, they raise a number of interesting and potentially important issues that may help to guide future thinking and research on these syndromes. Before addressing specific sources of these contradictions, it will be useful to review briefly the strengths and weaknesses of each hypothesis.

The Mesolimbic Dopamine System: From Motivation to Action.
Edited by P. Willner and J. Scheel-Krüger

© 1991 John Wiley & Sons Ltd

THE DA HYPOTHESIS OF MOOD DISORDERS

The DA hypothesis of mood disorders is considered in detail elsewhere in this volume (Willner et al., Chapter 15, Post et al., Chapter 17). Unlike the DA hypothesis of schizophrenia, which derives largely from the clinical observation that DA receptor antagonists have anti-psychotic properties, the DA hypothesis of mood disorders is based on both clinical and preclinical findings. The core support for the hypothesis is found in the following observations: (*1*) the meso-accumbens DA projection is a component of the neural circuitry of reward and/or incentive motivation, and both of these processes are dysfunctional in mania and major depression; (*2*) some anti-depressant treatments enhance the functional status of the mesolimbic DA system; (*3*) acute administration of drugs such as amphetamine produces, via a dopaminergic mechanism, effects in humans that are remarkably similar to the early phase of an idiopathic manic episode; (*4*) idiopathic mania can be treated with neuroleptic drugs; and (*5*) acute administration of DA receptor antagonists produces effects in normal volunteers that share important features with endogenous depression; these include restlessness, paralysis of volition, lack of physical and psychic energy, and anxiety (Belmaker and Wald, 1977).

Other observations seem incompatible with the DA hypothesis of mood disorders. First, despite extensive investigation there is no firm biochemical or physiological evidence that DA systems are dysfunctional during major depressive episodes. Thus, although there are numerous (but not invariant) reports of decreased DA metabolite concentrations in the CSF of depressed patients, it is uncertain whether this is simply a reflection of reduced motoric output in these patients or whether it is related to the affective disturbances *per se* (see Willner et al., Chapter 15, this volume). Despite the considerable effort that has been invested in this approach, it is at best a very crude test of the hypothesis because only a small, perhaps insignificant, fraction of homovanillic acid (HVA) and dihydroxyphenylacetic acid (DOPAC) in the CSF originates from the nucleus accumbens. Even if substantial abnormalities in DA release or metabolism in the nucleus accumbens of depressed or manic patients existed, it is quite conceivable that this would not be detected in CSF. It is worth mentioning here that there is strong evidence that the various components of the mesotelencephalic DA system can be regulated differentially (Thierry et al., 1976; Fadda et al., 1978; Miller et al., 1984). Abnormalities in meso-accumbens DA neurons need not, therefore, be accompanied by similar changes in nigrostriatal DA neurons. Another potential problem for the hypothesis is that attempts to detect functional abnormalities in central DA systems on the basis of neuroendocrine measures of hypothalmic DA activity during mood disorders have produced inconsistent or negative results (Jimerson, 1987). However, because hypothalamic DA neurons have physiological, pharmacological and neurochemical characteristics that are distinct from mesotelencephalic DA neurons (Moore, 1987), it is inappropriate and unwarranted to make inferences about the latter on the basis of data obtained on the former. The absence of consistent abnormalities in hypothalamic–pituitary DA function in psychiatric disease is irrelevant, therefore, to hypotheses concerning the role(s) of mesotelencephalic DA systems in such conditions. The third, and perhaps most serious potential problem with the DA hypothesis of mood disorders is that major depressive episodes with psychotic features (delusions or hallucinations) are often treated successfully with neuroleptic drugs. If a major depressive episode is associated with reduced dopaminergic tone in the nucleus accumbens, how then could DA receptor antagonists possibly be of therapeutic value to such patients? This important paradox will be addressed in detail after the DA hypothesis of schizophrenia is briefly reviewed.

THE DA HYPOTHESIS OF SCHIZOPHRENIA

The DA hypothesis of schizophrenia is based primarily on the fact that drugs that block central DA receptors are effective in treating some of the symptoms of this syndrome. It is also supported by evidence indicating that compounds such as d-amphetamine and cocaine, which increase synaptic concentrations of DA and noradrenaline, can, when administered repeatedly over a few days, produce a syndrome which has been claimed to have much in common with idiopathic paranoid schizophrenia (Snyder, 1973; but see below). Given that this drug-induced syndrome can be treated with DA receptor antagonists (Angrist et al., 1974; Gawin, 1986), and given the absence of evidence implicating noradrenergic mechanisms in schizophrenia (Crow and Johnstone, 1986), a dopaminergic substrate for these effects of d-amphetamine and cocaine seems likely. However, a combined action of these stimulants on dopaminergic and noradrenergic systems cannot be excluded as the neurochemical substrate for this syndrome.

The DA hypothesis of schizophrenia has received considerable support from the post-mortem findings of several laboratories, indicating that the caudate nucleus, putamen and nucleus accumbens of schizophrenic patients, some of whom were never treated with neuroleptics or were not so treated for many months, have elevated numbers (B_{max}) of D2DA receptors compared to controls (Cross et al., 1983; Seeman et al., 1987, Joyce et al., 1988). Positron emission tomography (PET) studies have also been used to test the hypothesis and to date have generated mixed results, with one group reporting elevated [^{11}C] n-methylspiperone binding in schizophrenia (Wong et al., 1986), while other workers, using raclopride as the radioligand, failed to confirm such differences between schizophrenic patients and controls (Farde et al., 1987). At present, therefore, there is accumulating post-mortem evidence for an increased number of D2DA receptors in the striatum and nucleus accumbens of schizophrenic patients, and some of this increase is apparently not neuroleptic-induced. Additional PET studies are required to determine whether such increases can reliably be demonstrated *in vivo*. This is of considerable importance because the biological significance of results based on *in vitro* binding techniques, where the incubation conditions often bear little or no semblance to the *in vivo* receptor environment, is open to question (Bennett and Wooten, 1986; Perlmutter and Raichle, 1986).

A number of objections can be raised to the DA hypothesis of schizophrenia. First, substantial numbers of schizophrenic patients do not benefit from neuroleptic drugs, suggesting that abnormalities in dopaminergic transmission do not contribute significantly to the expression of symptoms in these patients. Second, there is controversy as to whether only some or all types of symptoms in schizophrenia respond to DA receptor blockade. For example, Crow and his colleagues (Johnstone et al., 1978; Crow, 1980a, b) have indicated that neuroleptics are selectively effective against positive symptoms (delusions, hallucinations and florid thought disorder), but have little beneficial effect on what have been termed the negative symptoms of the syndrome (flattening of affect, poverty of speech, loss of drive and motor retardation). This elegantly simple hypothesis is supported by reports that there is a correlation between the presence of positive symptoms and increased numbers of DA receptors in the striatum and nucleus accumbens (Crow et al., 1981), and that negative symptoms are more often associated with structural changes in the brain (Crow and Johnstone, 1986). Unfortunately, however, others have failed to confirm an association between positive symptoms and increased D2 receptor binding in the brains of schizophrenic patients (Kornhuber et al., 1989). In addition, at present there is little agreement as to whether neuroleptics do indeed specifically target positive symptoms (Kane and Mayerhoff, 1989). This problem is no doubt due in large part to the absence of consensus concerning the definition and measurement of negative symptoms. As Sommers (1985) has pointed out: 'Negative symptoms . . . represent arguably the most difficult class of clinical phenomena to measure with acceptable validity and reliability', and as a result, '. . . there is no clear consensus about exactly which symptoms should be included in a "negative symptom score" for research purposes . . .'. Until there is substantial progress regarding the definition, measurement and validation of negative symptoms, the specificity of neuroleptics with respect to actions on positive and negative symptoms cannot be addressed in a meaningful manner. In the context of the DA hypotheses of schizophrenia and major depression, it is also important to appreciate that the vegetative signs of depression can be difficult to distinguish from the negative symptoms in schizophrenia (Andreasen, 1979).

A third limitation of the DA hypothesis of schizophrenia is that many of the symptoms seen in this condition can also occur in other psychiatric syndromes such as mania and major depression, and that here too the symptoms are responsive to neuroleptic treatment. Thus, there is no particular specificity of DA receptor antagonists for the symptoms of schizophrenia. The drugs are not specifically 'anti-schizophrenic'. Instead, neuroleptics are efficacious in the treatment of symptoms associated with a variety of psychotic disorders, not only when these symptoms form the basis of a diagnosis of schizophrenia.

SOME LIMITATIONS OF SCHIZOPHRENIA AND THE MOOD DISORDERS AS PSYCHIATRIC SYNDROMES

With this brief review of the DA hypotheses of mood disorders and schizophrenia, it is appropriate to consider the possible bases of their contradictory predictions. First, it must be recognized that schizophrenia and mood disorders are hypothetical constructs. Both are syndromes, a syndrome being a group of signs and symptoms that usually occur together and characterize a particular abnormality. I will argue that a large part of the confusion concerning the DA hypotheses stems from the primitive state of understanding of psychiatric syndromes. The problem is essentially twofold: (*1*) there is considerable variability with respect to the signs and symptoms displayed by patients diagnosed as having the same psychiatric syndrome; and (*2*) there is substantial overlap between the signs and symptoms that form the basis of psychiatric syndromes such as schizophrenia and mood disorders. As Pope and Lipinski (1978) have so cogently pointed out, because they also commonly occur in other psychiatric syndromes such as bipolar disorder, the classic 'schizophrenic' symptoms such as delusions, ideas of reference, hallucinations and catatonia are by themselves of no diagnostic or prognostic significance. It is only when these symptoms are considered in the context of age of onset, premorbid adjustment, duration of illness, marital status, family history and the presence or absence of affective symptoms that they may be of diagnostic and prognostic value. In a similar vein, Kendell (1987) has pointed out that: 'None of the functional psychoses has yet been shown to be a "disease entity" . . . . None of them is yet demarcated from its neighbours by clear boundaries. All are still defined by their clinical syndromes, and these syndromes merge imperceptibly into one another'. It must also be recognized that much psychiatric research is limited by the fact that it is often difficult to quantify and to generate operational definitions of the signs and symptoms that are used to formulate a psychiatric syndrome. These issues are discussed below; each suggests that it is premature to attempt to address the neurobiological substrates of psychiatric syndromes as they are currently conceived. Instead, I will argue that, because psychiatric syndromes presently lack the confirmatory biochemical, morphological or histological evidence that is of critical diagnostic value in other branches of medicine, a more fruitful approach would be to reorientate psychiatric research in a manner that begins to address the possible neurochemical and structural correlates of specific signs and symptoms, and to limit these investigations to those signs and symptoms that can be operationally defined and quantified.

Variability of Signs and Symptoms

According to the DSM-IIIR classification there is no single sign or symptom that is both necessary and sufficient for a diagnosis of major depression. Instead, for patients to be diagnosed as suffering from a major depressive episode, they must show evidence of at least five of the following: (*1*) depressed mood; (*2*) markedly diminished interest or pleasure in most, if not all, activities; (*3*) weight loss; (*4*) insomnia or hypersomnia; (*5*) psychomotor agitation or retardation; (*6*) fatigue, loss of energy; (*7*) guilt, feelings of worthlessness; (*8*) diminished ability to think or concentrate; and (*9*) recurrent thoughts of death or suicide. Depressed mood or diminished interest or pleasure must be among the five positive categories. In addition, the above may occur either with or without psychotic features (delusions or hallucinations). One important consequence of this and other current approaches to psychiatric syndromes is that individuals showing substantially different symptom patterns could be admitted to the same diagnostic research group. The group, for example, could conceivably contain Mrs Smith who showed the following symptoms: (*1*) diminished interest and pleasure in most activities; (*2*) fatigue; (*3*) psychomotor retardation; (*4*) diminished ability to think; (*5*) recurrent thoughts of suicide. The same group could also include Mr Jones whose symptoms included: (*1*) markedly depressed mood; (*2*) weight loss; (*3*) insomnia; (*4*) psychomotor agitation; (*5*) feelings of worthlessness; and (*6*) mood-incongruent delusions and auditory hallucinations. While these are admittedly somewhat extreme examples, they serve to illustrate the problem. It is not surprising that PET scans, CSF HVA measures, MRI scans, or any other biological measure for that matter, might fail to show consistent abnormalities in patients with the diagnosis of major depression but whose specific symptoms differed so considerably.

Although the situation is somewhat better in the case of schizophrenia, according to the DSM-IIIR classification there can be considerable heterogeneity in the symptoms required for a diagnosis of schizophrenia. For example, negative symptoms have been claimed to occur in less than half of chronically institutionalized schizophrenic patients (Johnstone et al., 1978; Owens and Johnstone, 1980). Here again, therefore, patients with significant qualitative differences in symptomatology can, according to this classification, be included in the same diagnostic research group and can be expected to generate substantial variation in biological measures. A case in point is the controversy about the prevalence of lateral ventricular enlargement in patients suffering from schizophrenia. Thus, while some researchers have noted that a high proportion of schizophrenic patients have such abnormalities (Weinberger et al., 1979; Golden et al., 1980), others have failed to confirm this (Jernigan et al., 1982; Benes et al., 1982). As has been noted by Luchins (1982), these inconsistencies are likely to be due to clinical differences (i.e. type, severity and duration of symptoms) in the populations under study. In this context, Crow's (1980a, b) proposal to view positive symptoms in terms of biochemical (dopaminergic) abnormalities and negative symptoms in terms of structural changes represents a significant advance that is very much in line with what is being advocated here. What the positive/negative symptom classification does is to narrow down the specific symptoms in schizophrenia that are investigated with respect to particular neurobiological correlates. What it fails to do, however, is to consider these symptoms as phenomena to be studied in their own right, regardless of whether they occur in the context of schizophrenia, bipolar disorder or major depression.

An alternative to the major syndrome-orientated approach that is so predominant in modern psychiatric research is to study the neurobiological correlates of specific symptoms, or clusters of symptoms that have by factor analytic techniques been shown to have a very high probability of occurring together, and can therefore be assumed to have common etiological origins. An important example of this approach has recently been contributed by Liddle (1987a) who studied the correlations between symptoms in a group of 40 patients with chronic schizophrenia. The symptoms were found to segregate into three clusters which were identified as: (*1*) psychomotor poverty (poverty of speech, flatness of affect and decreased spontaneous movement); (*2*) disorganization (disorders of form of thought and inappropriate affect); and (*3*) reality distortion (hallucinations and delusions). To quote Liddle et al. (1989): 'The correlations between symptoms in each factor were high but the correlations between symptoms from different syndromes were low. The syndromes were not mutually exclusive. Some patients suffered from more than one syndrome . . . the findings suggest that there are several distinguishable but overlapping pathological processes in chronic schizophrenia'. Liddle (1987b) subsequently reported that neuropsychological tests indicated that psychomotor poverty and disorganization, but not reality distortion, are associated with impaired neurological function, perhaps specifically in the frontal lobes (Liddle et al., 1989; see also Robbins, Chapter 19, this volume). As will be discussed later, a strong case can be made for an association between central dopaminergic mechanisms and Liddle's psychomotor poverty and reality distortion syndromes.

Shared Symptomatology of Schizophrenia and Mood Disorders

Although it is now almost 100 years since Kraepelin proposed his classic distinction between dementia praecox (schizophrenia) and manic-depressive psychosis, the differential diagnosis of these syndromes in individual cases is often still uncertain and the subject of debate (Ollerenshaw, 1973; Pope and Lipinski, 1978). It is common clinical experience, for example, to observe periods in a manic episode during which a patient's symptoms are indistinguishable from those occurring in the active phase of schizophrenia (Carlson and Goodwin, 1973). In addition, symptoms such as delusions and hallucinations which have classically been associated with schizophrenia also commonly occur in both manic and major depressive episodes (Winokur et al., 1969; Carlson and Goodwin, 1973). Pope and Lipinski (1978) estimate, for example, that: 'Classical "schizophrenic" symptoms, including many types of hallucinations, delusions, catatonic symptoms, and Schneiderian first rank symptoms, are reported in 20% to 50% of well-validated cases of manic-depressive illness'. Negative symptoms are also not unique to schizophrenia, occurring in bipolar mood disorder and in major depression (Andreasen, 1979; Pearlson et al., 1984; Pogue-Geile and Harrow, 1984). Schizophrenic patients often complain of anhedonia, a defect in pleasure capacity which is shared by patients who are depressed. The failure of many of the core symptoms of schizophrenia and major depression to respect each other's boundaries has recently been extended to biological measures of cerebral function. Thus, according to PET studies, patients with major affective disorders show the same decreases in mid-prefrontal cortex glucose utilization and the same increases in superior posterior parietal metabolism (i.e. a reduced anteroposterior gradient) that have been identified in some schizophrenic patients (Buchsbaum et al., 1984; Cohen et al., 1989). Similarly, CT studies indicate that lateral ventricular enlargement is not unique to schizophrenia but also occurs in patients with bipolar affective disorder (Pearlson et al., 1984). At present, therefore, it is quite clear that neither the symptoms of schizophrenia and mood disorders, nor the neurobiological correlates of these syndromes, are unique to, or pathognomonic of, these conditions. It is interesting in this regard that eminent contributors to this field have previously questioned whether there may be: 'A general biology of psychosis that would cut across traditional diagnostic lines' (Freedman, 1975), and have raised the possibility that: 'there is a core biological dysfunction common to schizophrenia, the affective psychoses and the paranoid state' (Meltzer, 1982). The literature reviewed in this chapter is entirely consistent with such speculations.

The above discussion serves to illustrate some of the shortcomings of current conceptualizations of schizophrenia, bipolar disorder and major depression. In so far as these syndromes have not been adequately defined, and because the symptoms associated with each are neither necessary for nor unique to any of these conditions, it should not be surprising that neurobiological formulations of these syndromes might be inconsistent and even contradictory. Given the historical and continuing lack of agreement concerning appropriate definitions of these syndromes, the failure to find consistent biochemical, hormonal or neuropathological abnormalities associated with them is highly predictable. Furthermore, under these circumstances, significant progress towards identification of specific neurobiological correlates of these conditions cannot be anticipated. Their definitions are too diffuse, too unspecific and too inconsistent to allow such investigations to be usefully pursued. Homogeneous populations of patients are required in research on the etiology and treatment of the psychoses. Current formulations of these major psychiatric syndromes fall so far short of meeting this essential requirement that their continued use in research is likely to continue mainly to confuse and obscure the issues.

As mentioned earlier, an alternative is to abandon the major syndrome-orientated approach and to attempt to specify the biological substrates of some specific symptoms or clusters of symptoms in schizophrenia and mood disorders, regardless of the syndromal context in which they occur. When this is done, the contradictions of the DA hypotheses of schizophrenia and major depression become somewhat less apparent and can be partially reconciled. The first step in this approach is to specify the particular symptoms occurring in schizophrenia and mood disorders that can be reasonably demonstrated to have dopaminergic substrates. This can be approached: (*1*) by identifying psychiatric symptoms that can be reproduced in normal individuals by stimulants such as d-amphetamine, methylphenidate and cocaine, drugs that are known to increase central catecholaminergic transmission; and (*2*) by specifying the symptoms occurring in schizophrenia, bipolar disorder and major depression that are sensitive to DA receptor antagonists. With regard to the former, it is of course necessary to demonstrate that the stimulant-induced symptoms have a dopaminergic rather than a noradrenergic basis.

STIMULANT-INDUCED PSYCHOSES

There is much literature on the response of non-psychiatric patients to acute and chronic administration of psychomotor stimulants such as d-amphetamine, methamphetamine and cocaine. With one notable exception, there is substantial agreement in this literature concerning the nature and sequence of the symptoms that can be elicited during continued exposure to these compounds. The exception, which is discussed further below, concerns the controversy regarding the extent to which these drugs can produce formal thought disorder. The initial sequence of events that commonly occurs during chronic administration of d-amphetamine and cocaine closely resembles what Carlson and Goodwin (1973) have identified as the 'initial phase' of an idiopathic manic episode. The characteristic features of this and the two subsequent phases of the manic episode are summarized in Table 1. Importantly, Carlson and Goodwin (1973) concluded that, although there is variability in the rate at which individual patients progress from the initial to the final phase of a manic episode, the sequence of symptoms is 'remarkably consistent'. On reviewing the progression of the signs and symptoms that occur during the course of a manic episode, the extent to which both the symptoms and their order of appearance are mimicked by chronically administered stimulants such as d-amphetamine, methamphetamine and cocaine is striking. Post (1975) has presented evidence for a continuum model of cocaine-induced psychosis in which chronic administration of this compound produces an orderly progression of effects that begins with euphoria, evolves to dysphoria, and ends in psychosis (i.e. delusions and hallucinations) (see also Post et al., Chapter 17, this volume). The rate at which this sequence progresses depends upon a variety of factors, including the dose and duration of drug administration. This continuum appears to be identical for other chronically administered stimulants such as d-amphetamine and methylphenidate (Table 1), and can therefore be considered a general property of these compounds. It is surprising in this regard that the stimulant-induced psychoses have historically been viewed as a model of paranoid schizophrenia (Connell, 1958; Angrist and Gershon, 1970; Griffith et al., 1972; Snyder, 1973); in fact, the sequence of symptoms produced by chronically administered stimulants much more closely models the prototypical psychotic manic episode described by Carlson and Goodwin (1973). The only major difference between the two is that the evolution of the idiopathic manic episode is generally slower, typically running its course from the 'initial' to the 'final' phase over a period of weeks, while in the stimulant-induced syndrome, the onset and sequential progression of the symptoms are considerably compressed, occurring in some individuals over a period of 1 or 2 days.

That there exists this apparent confusion as to whether chronic stimulant exposure models paranoid schizophrenia or a manic episode serves once again to underscore the shortcomings of past and current formulations of these psychiatric syndromes. More importantly, however, the remarkable similarities between the natural history of an idiopathic manic episode and stimulant-induced psychoses are of considerable theoretical significance. DA receptor antagonists are effective in the treatment of symptoms associated with both an idiopathic manic episode and those produced by chronically administered stimulants. A dopaminergic substrate for these symptoms, regardless of whether they occur in the context of a manic episode or during extended exposure to stimulants, can therefore be strongly inferred.

Table 1. Comparison of the sequence of symptoms occurring in a psychotic manic episode and during chronic stimulant administration

	Manic episode	Chronic stimulants
Phase I *(initial)*	↑ Psychomotor activity ↑ Speech Euphoria, irritability Expansiveness Grandiosity Overconfidence ↑ Sexuality Paranoid trends	↑ Psychomotor activity ↑ Speech Euphoria, emotional lability ↑ Mental agility Grandiosity Overconfidence ↑ Sexuality
Phase II *(intermediate)*	↑↑ Psychomotor activity and ↑ Pressure of speech pressure of speech Predominant dysphoria and depression, occasional euphoria Hostility, anger Disorganization of cognitive state, flight of ideas Delusions	Dysphoria, apathy, loss of interest Hostility, irritability Flight of ideas Suspiciousness
Phase III *(final)*	Desperate, panic-stricken, hopeless state Clearly dysphoric Frenzied, bizarre psychomotor activity Incoherent thought processes Loosening of associations Disorientation to time and place Bizarre, idiosyncratic delusions Hallucinations	Agitation, restlessness, fear Affectual flattening, cold, distant affect Motor stereotypy Thought disorder Tangentiality, irrelevance Paranoid delusions Auditory, visual, olfactory hallucinations

The left-hand column lists the progression of symptoms recorded by Carlson and Goodwin (1973) in their study of the stages of a manic episode. The right-hand column lists the symptoms produced by chronically administered stimulants (mainly amphetamines) in human subjects (Bell, 1965; Ellinwood, 1967; Angrist and Gershon, 1970; Griffith et al., 1972; Post, 1975). Although none of the latter studies systematically recorded the course of stimulant-induced symptoms in as detailed a manner as Carlson and Goodwin (1973) reported for idiopathic mania, on the basis of the information provided in these reports, it is possible to deduce the temporal sequence of stimulant-induced symptoms as listed above. It should be emphasized that the symptoms listed in both columns are unmodified and taken verbatim from the reports in question

For example, Jonsson (1972) has reported that, whereas α-adrenergic (phenoxybenzamine) and β-adrenergic (propranolol) blockade are without effect, chlorpromazine and pimozide attenuate the intense euphoria produced by large, intravenous doses of d, l-amphetamine. Angrist et al. (1974) have observed that haloperidol produces a 'striking antagonism' of the psychopathology produced by chronically administered amphetamine. Similarly, the delusions and hallucinations occurring in patients diagnosed as schizophrenic can also be inferred to have a dopaminergic basis because these symptoms are rapidly and acutely exacerbated by d-amphetamine and methylphenidate (Janowsky et al., 1973; Janowsky and Davis, 1976), and are among the symptoms in schizophrenia that respond well to DA receptor antagonists (Johnstone et al., 1978; Crow, 1980a). Leaving aside, therefore, whether they occur in the context of schizophrenia, bipolar disorder or major depression, both the early (e.g. euphoria) and later occurring symptoms (e.g. dysphoria and psychosis) produced by chronically administered stimulants can be considered to have dopaminergic substrates, because in each condition they respond to neuroleptic drugs. Thus, euphoria, dysphoria, delusions and hallucinations, at least as they occur in these syndromes, appear to be reflections of disturbed dopaminergic transmission. The role of DA in 'flatness of affect' is less clear and will be discussed further below.

RAPPROCHEMENT, SYNTHESIS AND SPECULATIONS

The literature reviewed above indicates that, when the ambiguities concerning definitions of schizophrenia and mood disorders are taken into consideration, and when it is understood that many symptoms are shared by these syndromes, the contradictions generated by the DA hypotheses of schizophrenia and mood disorder become more apparent than real. Why, then, are schizophrenic patients, whose mesocorticolimbic systems are hypothetically hyperactive, not also manic as the DA hypothesis of affective illness would predict? A substantial part of the answer appears to be that many patients diagnosed as being in the 'active phase' of schizophrenia are misdiagnosed and are indeed suffering a manic episode just as the DA hypothesis predicts. Ollerenshaw (1973) and Pope and Lipinski (1978) have argued compellingly that many patients diagnosed as 'schizophrenic' are in fact suffering from manic-depressive psychosis. On the basis of the similarity of the response to treatment (neuroleptics, lithium, electroconvulsive therapy), and on the basis of prognostic, family history and genetic studies, these authors have proposed that: 'What is currently classed as "acute schizophrenia" is really what might be termed a "manic equivalent" in a manic-depressive psychosis' (Ollerenshaw, 1973). It is of considerable interest in this regard that it is common for patients who suffer an acute 'schizophrenic' illness to develop subsequently a depressive episode indistinguishable from depression in bipolar disorder (Roth, 1970). Viewed in this light, patients diagnosed with 'good prognosis', 'remitting', 'schizo-affective', 'reactive' or 'acute' schizophrenia may in fact be suffering from bipolar disorder, especially mania. This classification: (*1*) broadens somewhat the symptomatic features of a psychotic manic episode as currently formulated in DSM-IIIR to include the possible presence of incoherence or marked loosening of associations and flat or grossly inappropriate affect; and (*2*) drops the requirement that a manic episode must feature a distinct period of abnormally and persistently elevated, expansive or irritable mood. In any event, if it is the case that a substantial percentage of patients diagnosed as schizophrenic are misdiagnosed and suffer instead from bipolar disorder, then one of the apparent contradictions between DA hypotheses of schizophrenia and mood disorders immediately evaporates because the symptoms observed in 'acute schizophrenia' (Ollerenshaw, 1973), currently termed the 'active phase' of schizophrenia (DSM-IIIR), are most appropriately viewed as variants of a manic episode. These symptoms (changes in psychomotor activity, delusions, hallucinations, ideas of reference, dysphoria and perhaps some forms of thought disorder) have, at least in part, dopaminergic substrates because all can be reproduced by indirectly acting DA receptor agonists, and all are blocked DA receptor antagonists.

Although the misdiagnosis of bipolar disorder as schizophrenia partly reconciles one important contradiction between the DA hypotheses of these two syndromes, this does not, of course, deny the possibility that some types of 'schizophrenia' will ultimately prove to be diseases that are different from bipolar disorder, and that all of these conditions share, to a greater or lesser extent, abnormalities in the function of mesotelencephalic DA systems. Indeed, while classical 'schizophrenic' symptoms do not reliably differ between these conditions (Pope and Lipinski, 1978), other factors, including age of onset, premorbid adjustment, duration of illness, family history, employment history and marital status, suggest that schizophrenia and bipolar disorder can be differentiated on these grounds.

The paradox that major depressive episodes with psychotic features are often treated successfully with DA receptor antagonists will now be considered. At a superficial level, this clinical fact would appear to devastate the DA hypothesis of mood disorders. If anything, the hypothesis predicts that neuroleptics should exacerbate major depression because addition of DA receptor blockade when mesolimbic DA activity is already compromised should only further impair the function of this system (see also Willner et al., Chapter 15, this volume). In addressing this contradiction, it should first be pointed out that many investigations of the effects of neuroleptics in depression have studied patients who were not endogenously depressed (i.e. 'anxious', 'neurotic', 'reactive' depression) and often employed doses of neuroleptics substantially below anti-psychotic ranges (Nelson, 1987). In this regard, recent reports that low, presumably 'DA autoreceptor specific' doses of neuroleptics are useful in the treatment of depression are of interest because the net effect of such treatments would be to enhance the activity of mesotelencephalic DA neurons and would, on this basis, be predicted to have anti-depressant effects (Del Zompo et al., 1990). Neuroleptic dose appears, therefore, to be an important variable in considering the effects of these compounds, and limits the extent to which it is possible to make general statements about the role of these compounds in the treatment of depression.

Another equally important part of the answer to this paradox appears to be the inappropriate use of syndromal concepts as opposed to a more symptom-orientated approach. For example, when one asks what symptoms of a major psychotic depressive episode respond to neuroleptics, the answer is reasonably clear. Neuroleptics are useful in treating psychotic symptoms (delusions and hallucinations), and perhaps the symptoms associated with 'agitation' (Nelson, 1987), but are of no value in alleviating the mood-related symptoms of this syndrome. In reviewing the literature on the efficacy of neuroleptics in the treatment of depression, Nelson (1987) concluded that: 'Antipsychotic drugs were useful in the treatment of agitation and delusional thinking and resulted in considerable improvement; however, depressive symptoms such as anhedonia, lack of energy, and motor retardation frequently persisted until a tricyclic was added'. Since they are not effective in treating anhedonia, Nelson (1987) further concluded that neuroleptics are not true anti-depressants. It is probably for this reason that the current pharmacological treatment of a major depressive episode with psychotic features typically involves a combination of neuroleptic and anti-depressant drugs. In the context of the DA hypothesis it is noteworthy that tricyclic anti-depressants can precipitate or exacerbate psychotic (delusional) symptoms in patients suffering from a major depressive episode (Nelson et al., 1979).

It must be acknowledged that even the symptom-orientated analysis is only partly satisfactory in dealing with the above issue; the DA hypothesis of depression would reasonably still predict that neuroleptics should prevent the mood-enhancing effects of the anti-depressant drugs. It would also predict that, when given alone, neuroleptics should exacerbate the mood-related symptoms (anhedonia, loss of interest, and so on) of a psychotic depressive episode. At present, there appears to be no obvious solution to these issues, but many possibilities exist. It is quite possible, for example, that neuroleptics do indeed worsen some symptoms of major depression with psychotic features and attenuate the mood-enhancing effects of anti-depressant drugs. In fact, a recent study has reported striking improvements in depressed patients on withdrawal of the haloperidol component of a chlorimipramine–haloperidol cocktail (Del Zompo et al., 1990). Unfortunately, the author has not been able to identify other clinical studies in which these questions have been specifically addressed.

If, as is proposed above, central DA mechanisms are neural substrates for the euphoria, dysphoria, depression, delusions and hallucinations that can occur both in idiopathic functional psychoses and in the evolution of stimulant-induced psychosis, it is reasonable to ask how such disparate phenomena could possibly be mediated by a single neurochemical substrate. Although it is only possible to speculate on this point, recent discoveries about the regulation and functions of different components of the mesotelencephalic DA system provide a theoretical framework which may help to explain the divergent effects of acutely and chronically enhanced DA activity. Specifically, it can be suggested that these symptoms reflect alterations in the activity of different terminal regions of these ascending DA neurons. There is, for example, substantial information indicating that meso-accumbens DA neurons are an important neural substrate of reward and incentive motivation. Animals will work to stimulate electrically DA neurons in the ventral tegmental area (Fibiger et al., 1987). DA release is enhanced in the nucleus accumbens during the anticipatory and consummatory phases of motivated behavior in the rat (Damsma et al., 1990). The rewarding effects of cocaine and d-amphetamine are mediated by dopaminergic mechanisms in the nucleus accumbens (Lyness et al., 1979; Roberts et al., 1980). Given these findings, the euphoria produced by stimulants and observed during the early stages of mania may be the result of enhanced DA release in the nucleus accumbens. The biological mechanisms responsible for this increased dopaminergic tone in idiopathic mania are not presently known and their identification would be of fundamental importance. In addition, while stimulant-induced euphoria has a presynaptic basis, the idiopathic condition may be due to changes either in presynaptic regulation leading to increased DA release or to abnormalities in postsynaptic DA receptor-mediated mechanisms.

Because dysphoria reliably follows euphoria in both idiopathic and stimulant-induced mania episodes (Table 1), dysphoria may be the inevitable consequence of prolonged, excessive activity of the meso-accumbens DA projection. Whether the transition from the euphoric to the dysphoric condition is due to a presynaptic effect such as a gradual depletion of DA stores, or to postsynaptic effects such as DA receptor subsensitivity or alterations in second messenger systems, is not known. Whatever molecular mechanisms are involved, it appears that enhanced dopaminergic tone leading to euphoria can only be maintained in the nucleus accumbens for a limited time, and that compensatory mechanisms are eventually engaged so that this enhanced activity evolves into a net decrease in the effects of DA on postsynaptic neurons in the nucleus accumbens. The depression that follows a manic episode in bipolar disorder, or that occurs after withdrawal from stimulant drugs, would similarly be viewed as reflecting a net reduction in dopaminergic tone in the nucleus accumbens. The mechanisms underlying the decreased dopaminergic activity during dysphoria associated with either a manic episode or during chronic exposure to stimulant drugs need not be the same as those leading to depression after a manic episode or to that occurring after stimulant drug withdrawal. What the two conditions have in common is that the net dopaminergic tone in the nucleus accumbens is reduced and this would lead to the depressed mood that is present in the dysphoric and depressive states.

Dopaminergic mechanisms in the amygdala may mediate the paranoid delusions that are common to stimulant-induced and idiopathic functional psychoses. There is considerable evidence that the amygdaloid complex, especially the central nucleus, plays an important role in fear-motivated behavior (Hitchcock and Davis, 1986; Davis et al., 1987). The central nucleus is also heavily innervated by mesencephalic dopaminergic neurons (Kilts et al., 1988). Paranoid delusions can be viewed as inappropriate fear responses to neutral, normally non-threatening stimuli in the environment. For example, the delusional patient who is convinced that other patients on the ward are plotting to poison him considers these individuals to be sources of harm and responds fearfully. The demonstrated dopaminergic involvement in stimulant-induced and idiopathic paranoid delusions (see above), and the role of the amygdala in fear-motivated behaviour, make this structure, particularly its central nucleus, a plausible candidate for mediating such delusional processes. It is clear, however, that it cannot be simply an increase in DA release in the amygdala that leads directly to paranoid delusions, for although suspiciousness can increase rapidly (Sherer et al., 1988), delusions are not typically observed acutely after stimulant administration. Similarly, delusions are not normally observed during the early, euphoric phase of an idiopathic manic episode (Table 1). It is only later that delusions become prominent features of both conditions. For this reason, it can be proposed that delusions must be the result of chronically enhanced DA activity in the amygdala, perhaps reflecting a gradual change in dopaminergic tone in this structure after a sustained period of increased activity. What are the possible behavioural correlates of the initial increase in dopaminergic activity? To a certain extent, expansiveness, overconfidence and grandiosity are the antithesis of a paranoid delusional state, and it is interesting that these are the terms that have been used to describe the early phases of manic episodes and the initial response to chronically administered stimulants (Table 1). Could delusions simply be the result of a net decrease in dopaminergic activity in the amygdala that occurs after prolonged exposure to stimulants or during the natural progression of a psychotic episode? This seems most unlikely because such a hypothesis would predict that DA receptor antagonists should also cause delusions in humans. Since this does not happen, other consequences of chronically administered stimulants on DA neurotransmission must underlie paranoid delusions. These could include gradually developing changes in: (*1*) the ratio of DA release to cholecystokinin (CCK) and/or neurotensin (NT) release; and (*2*) in the ratio of D1 and D2 receptor-mediated events in the amygdala. With regard to the former, CCK and NT are co-localized with DA in subpopulations of mesencephalic dopaminergic neurons (Hokfelt et al., 1980, 1984). With regard to the latter, it is possible that D1 and D2 receptors, as well as their second messenger systems, adapt differentially to prolonged, excessive exposure to DA.

Attributing euphoria and depression to DA-mediated events in the nucleus accumbens, and delusions to related processes in the amygdala is, of course, highly speculative. Identification of the anatomical locus of the dopaminergic mechanisms responsible for the auditory and visual hallucinations that can occur in functional and stimulant-induced psychoses is even more uncertain. Dopaminergic neurons in the mesencephalon have been known for some time to project to restricted parts of the rodent neocortex (Thierry et al., 1973; Lindvall et al., 1974). In contrast, recent evidence suggests that the dopaminergic innervation of the primate neocortex is substantially more extensive, being distributed to virtually every cortical region (Lewis et al., 1987). In cynomolgus monkey neocortex, the density of the dopaminergic innervation is greater in sensory association than in primary sensory regions of both the visual and auditory cortical systems (Lewis et al., 1987). Given the complexity of visual and auditory hallucinations, abnormalities in DA function in these cortical association areas are potential candidates for the neural substrates of these phenomena. If this conjecture has any validity, it is interesting that, given the more restricted distribution of DA afferents in the rodent neocortex, rodent models of dopaminergically mediated visual and auditory hallucinations may not exist. As is the case for dysphoria and delusions, stimulant-induced hallucinations are not an early consequence of drug administration; they take time to emerge. This indicates that hallucinations must be a result of prolonged increases in extracellular concentrations of DA. It is not possible to specify whether these hallucinations might be a consequence of slowly emerging changes in presynaptic or postsynaptic mechanisms produced by the sustained increases in extracellular DA. Furthermore, if hallucinations are due to chronic increases in cortical DA release, the behavioral consequences of acute increases in DA release are not currently apparent. Unfortunately, very little is known about the functions of DA in the primate neocortex (Brozoski et al., 1979). This issue is an important priority for future research, partly because it may be germane to understanding the neurobiology of hallucinations in functional and stimulant-induced psychoses.

The scheme proposed above can be summarized as follows: mesotelencephalic DA neurons innervate large and disparate regions of the primate forebrain. Certain symptoms that are common to schizophrenia and major affective illness may be due to persistent abnormalities in dopaminergic tone in different terminal regions of the mesotelencephalic DA system. These abnormalities may be presynaptic, postsynaptic or both. It is hypothesized that mood disturbance is associated with the meso-accumbens DA projection, delusions with the meso-amygdala DA system, and hallucinations with the mesocortical DA projection. Because components of the mesotelencephalic DA system are under separate regulation, abnormalities in the function of one need not be accompanied by similar changes in others. It is perhaps for this reason that mood disturbance, delusions and hallucinations do not invariably occur together in either idiopathic or stimulant-induced psychotic episodes. Instead, both the expression and the severity of these dopaminergically mediated symptoms can vary considerably within and between patients. Similarly, stimulant-induced psychotic symptoms have been reported to occur in the presence of either euphoric or dysphoric mood (Bell, 1973; Griffith et al., 1972). The author is the first to acknowledge the tentative, potentially neuromythological nature of these speculations (Fibiger, 1987). They should be viewed as an attempt to provide a framework within which to consider the broad spectrum and evolving nature of the symptoms that occur in the course of idiopathic and stimulant-induced psychoses. Although a symptom-orientated approach is advocated here as an alternative to what, by any standard, must be considered to be a disappointing if not failed syndromal approach in biological psychiatry, the author is well aware that attempts to determine the biological correlates of specific psychiatric symptoms is not without its limitations and potential pitfalls. It is obviously theoretically possible that similar symptoms might occur in patients suffering from completely different neurobiological disorders. For example, Slater and Roth (1969) have pointed out that temporal lobe epilepsy is sometimes: 'Completely indistinguishable from schizophrenic psychoses'. In a similar vein, it is possible that hallucinations occurring in schizophrenia are mediated by brain mechanisms that are quite different from those underlying the same symptoms in bipolar disorder. However, until such time that it can be demonstrated that this is indeed the case, neurobiological investigations of specific symptoms or symptom clusters (Liddle, 1987a, b) can be offered as a viable alternative to the long-suffering use of major syndromes in biological psychiatric research.

ACKNOWLEDGEMENTS

This manuscript is dedicated to Daniel Kai Fibiger. Work in the author's laboratory was supported by the Medical Research Council of Canada. The excellent secretarial assistance of C. Pires and S. Sturgeon is gratefully acknowledged.

REFERENCES

Andreasen, N.C. (1979) Affective flattening and the criteria for schizophrenia. *American Journal of Psychiatry* **136**, 944–947.

Angrist, B.M. and Gershon, S. (1970) The phenomenology of experimentally induced amphetamine psychosis—preliminary observations. *Biological Psychiatry* **2**, 95–107.

Angrist, B., Lee, H.K. and Gershon, S. (1974) The antagonism of amphetamine-induced symptomatology by a neuroleptic. *American Journal of Psychiatry* **131**, 817–819.

Barnes, T.R.E., Liddle, P.F., Curson, D.A. and Patel, M. (1989) Negative symptoms, tardive dyskinesia and depression in chronic schizophrenia. *British Journal of Psychiatry* **155**, 99–103 (Suppl 7).

Bell, D.S. (1965) Comparison of amphetamine psychosis and schizophrenia. *British Journal of Psychiatry* **3**, 701–707.

Bell, D.S. (1973) The experimental reproduction of amphetamine psychosis. *Archives of General Psychiatry* **29**, 35–40.

Belmaker, R.H. and Wald, D. (1977) Haloperidol in normals. *British Journal of Psychiatry* **131**, 222–223.

Benes, F., Sunderland, P. and Jones, B.D. (1982) Normal ventricles in young schizophrenics. *British Journal of Psychiatry* **141**, 90.

Bennett Jr, J.P. and Wooten, G.F. (1986) Dopamine denervation does not alter in vivo ^{3}H-spiperone binding in rat striatum: implications for external imaging of dopamine receptors in Parkinson's disease. *Annals of Neurology* **19**, 378–383.

Brozoski, T.J., Brown, R.M., Rosvold, H.E. and Goldman, P.S. (1979) Cognitive deficit caused by regional depletion of dopamine in prefrontal cortex of rhesus monkey. *Science* **205**, 929–932.

Buchsbaum, M.S., DeLisi, L.E., Holcomb, H.H., Cappelletti, J., King, A.C., Johnson, J., Hazlett, E., Dowling-Zimmerman, S., Post, R.M., Morihisa, J., Carpenter, W., Cohen, R., Pickar, D., Weinberger, D.R., Margolin, R. and Kessler, R.M. (1984) Anteroposterior gradients in cerebral glucose use in schizophrenia and affective disorders. *Archives of General Psychiatry* **41**, 1159–1166.

Carlson, G.A. and Goodwin, F.K. (1973) The stages of mania. A longitudinal analysis of the manic episode. *Archives of General Psychiatry* **28**, 221–228.

Cohen, R.M., Semple, W.E., Gross, M., Nordahl, T.E., King, A.C., Pickar, D. and Post, R.M. (1989) Evidence for common alterations in cerebral glucose metabolism in major affective disorders and schizophrenia. *Neuropsychopharmacology* **2**, 241–254.

Connell, P.H. (1958) *Amphetamine Psychosis*. London: Oxford University Press.

Cross, A.J., Crow, T.J., Ferrier, I.N., Johnstone, E.C., McCreadie, R.M., Owen, F., Owens, D.G.C. and Poulter, M. (1983) Dopamine receptor changes in schizophrenia in relation to the disease process and movement disorder. *Journal of Neural Transmission* **18**, 265–272 (suppl).

Crow, T.J. (1980a) Molecular pathology of schizophrenia: more than one disease? *British Medical Journal* **280**, 66–68.

Crow, T.J. (1980b) Positive and negative schizophrenic symptoms and the role of dopamine. *British Journal of Psychiatry* **137**, 383–386.

Crow, T.J. and Johnstone, E.C. (1986) Schizophrenia: nature of the disease process and its biological correlates. In: Mountcastle, V.B. and Plum, F. (eds) *Handbook of Physiology—The Nervous System V*. Baltimore: American Physiological Society, pp. 843–869.

Crow, T.J., Owen, F., Cross, A.J., Ferrier, I.N., Johnstone, E.C., McCreadie, R.M., Owens, D.G.C. and Poulter, M. (1981) Neurotransmitters, enzymes and receptors in post-mortem brain in schizophrenia: evidence that an increase in D2 dopamine receptors is associated with the type I syndrome. In: Riederer, P. and Usdin, E. (eds) *Transmitter Biochemistry of Human Brain Tissue*. London: Macmillan, pp. 85–96.

Damsma, G., Pfaus, J.G., Nomikos, G.G., Wenkstern, D.G., Blaha, C.D., Phillips, A.G. and Fibiger, H.C. (1990) Sexual behavior enhances dopamine transmission in the nucleus accumbens and striatum of the male rat. *Brain Research* (in press).

Davis, M., Hitchcock, J.M. and Rosen, J.B. (1987) Anxiety and the amygdala: pharmacological and anatomical analysis of the fear-potentiated startle paradigm. In: Bower, G.H. (ed.) *The Psychology of Learning and Motivation: Advances in Research and Theory*. New York: Academic Press, pp. 263–305.

Del Zompo, M., Bocchetta, A., Bernardi, F., Burrai, C. and Corsini, G.U. (1990) Clinical evidence for a role of dopaminergic system in depressive syndromes. In: Gessa, G.L. and Serra, G. (eds) *Dopamine and Mental Depression*. Oxford: Pergamon, pp. 177–184.

Ellinwood, Jr, E.H. (1967) Amphetamine psychosis: I. description of the individuals and process. *Journal of Nervous and Mental Disorders* **144**, 273–283.

Fadda, F., Argiolas, A., Melis, M.R., Tissaari, A.H., Onali, P.L. and Gessa, G.L. (1978) Stress-induced increase in 3,4-dihydroxyphenylacetic acid (DOPAC) levels in cerebral cortex and in N. accumbens: reversal by diazepam. *Life Science* **23**, 2219–2224.

Farde, L., Wiesel, F.-A., Hall, H., Halldin, C., Stone-Elander, S. and Sedvall, G. (1987) No D2 receptor increase in PET study of schizophrenia. *Archives of General Psychiatry* **44**, 671–672.

Fibiger, H.C. (1987) Neural circuit models of psychopathology: dancing on the precipice of neuromythology? *Behavioral and Brain Sciences* **10**, 212–213.

Fibiger, H.C., LePiane, F.G., Jakubovic, A. and Phillips, A.G. (1987) The role of dopamine in intracranial self-stimulation of the ventral tegmental area. *Journal of Neuroscience* **7**, 3888–3896.

Freedman, D.X. (ed.) (1975) Biology of the major psychoses: a comparative analysis. *Research Publications of the Association for Research in Nervous and Mental Disorders* **54**, vii–viii.

Gawin, F.H. (1986) Neuroleptic reduction of cocaine-induced paranoia but not euphoria? *Psychopharmacology* **90**, 142–143.

Golden, C.J., Moses, J.A., Zelazowski, R., Graber, B., Zatz, L.M., Horvath, T.B. and Berger, P.A. (1980) Cerebral ventricular size and neuropsychological impairments in young schizophrenics. *Archives of General Psychiatry* **37**, 619–623.

Griffith, J.D., Cavanaugh, J., Held, J. and Oates, J.A. (1972) Dextroamphetamine evaluation of psychomimetic properties in man. *Archives of General Psychiatry* **26**, 97–100.

Hitchcock, J.M. and Davis, M. (1986) Lesions of the amygdala, but not of the cerebellum or red nucleus, block conditioned fear as measured with the potentiated startle paradigm. *Behavioral Neuroscience* **100**, 11–22.

Hokfelt, T., Skirboll, L., Rehfeld, J.F., Goldstein, M., Marey, K. and Dann, O. (1980) A subpopulation of mesencephalic dopamine neurons projecting to limbic areas contains a cholecystokinin-like peptide: evidence from immunohistochemis* combined with retrograde tracing. *Neuroscience* **5**, 2093–2124.

Hokfelt, T., Everitt, B.J., Theodorsson-Norheim, E. and Goldstein, M. (1984) Occurrence of neurotensin like immunoreactivity in subpopulation of hypothalamic, mesencephalic and medullary catecholamine neurons. *Journal of Comparative Neurology* **222**, 543–559.

Janowsky, D.S. and Davis, J.M. (1976) Methylphenidate, dextroamphetamine, and levanfetamine. *Archives of General Psychiatry* **33**, 304–308.

Janowsky, D.S., El-Yousef, M.K., Davis, J.M. and Sekerke, J.H. (1973) Provocation of schizophrenic symptoms by intravenous administration of methylphenidate. *Archives of General Psychiatry* **28**, 185–191.

Jernigan, T.L., Zatz, L.M., Moses, J.A. and Berger, P.A. (1982) Computer tomography in schizophrenics and normal volunteers: 1. Fluid volume. *Archives of General Psychiatry* **39**, 765–770.

Jimerson, D.C. (1987) Role of dopamine mechanisms in the affective disorders. In: Meltzer, H.Y. (ed.) *Psychopharmacology The Third Generation of Progress*. New York: Raven Press, pp. 505–511.

Johnstone, E.C., Crow, T.J., Frith, C.D., Carney, M.W.P. and Price, J.C. (1978) Mechanism of the antipsychotic effect in the treatment of acute schizophrenia. *Lancet* **i**, 848–851.

Jonsson, L.-E. (1972) Pharmacological blockade of amphetamine effects in amphetamine dependent subjects. *European Journal of Clinical Psychopharmacology* **4**, 206–211.

Joyce, J.N., Lexow, N., Bird, E. and Winokur, A. (1988) Organization of dopamine D1 and D2 receptors in human striatum: receptor autoradiographic studies in Huntington's disease and schizophrenia. *Synapse* **2**, 546–557.

Kane, J.M. and Mayerhoff, D. (1989) Do negative symptoms respond to pharmacological treatment? *British Journal of Psychiatry* **155**, 115–118 (suppl 7).

Kendell, R.E. (1987) Diagnosis and classification of functional psychoses. *British Medical Bulletin* **43**, 499–513.

Kilts, C.D., Anderson, C.M., Ely, T.D. and Mailman, R.B. (1988) The biochemistry and pharmacology of mesoamygdaloid dopamine neurons. *Annals of the New York Academy of Sciences* **537**, 173–187.

Kornhuber, J., Riederer, P., Reynolds, G.P., Beckmann, H., Jellinger, K. and Gabriel, E. (1989) 3H-spiperone binding sites in post-mortem brains from schizophrenic patients: relationship to neuroleptic drug treatment, abnormal movements, and positive symptoms. *Journal of Neural Transmission* **75**, 1–10.

Lewis, D.A., Campbell, M.J., Fotte, S.L., Goldstein, M. and Morrison, J.H. (1987) The distribution of tyrosine hydroxylase-immunoreactive fibers in primate neocortex is widespread but regionally specific. *Journal of Neuroscience* **7**, 279–290.

Liddle, P.F. (1987a) The symptoms of chronic schizophrenia. A re-examination of the positive-negative dichotomy. *British Journal of Psychiatry* **151**, 145–151.

Liddle, P.F. (1987b) Schizophrenic syndromes, cognitive performance and neurological dysfunction. *Psychological Medicine* **17**, 49–57.

Liddle, P.F., Barnes, T.R.E., Morris, D. and Haque, S. (1989) Three syndromes in chronic schizophrenia. *Psychological Medicine* **155**, 119–122 (suppl 7).

Lindvall, O., Bjorklund, A., Moore, R.Y. and Stenevi, V. (1974) Mesencephalic dopamine neurons projection to neocortex. *Brain Research* **81**, 325–331.

Luchins, D.J. (1982) Computed tomography in schizophrenia: disparities in the prevalence of abnormalities. *Archives of General Psychiatry* **39**, 859–860.

ness, W.H., Friedle, N.M. and Moore, K.E. (1979) Destruction of dopaminergic nerve terminals in nucleus accumbens: effect on d-amphetamine self-administration. *Pharmacology Biochemistry and Behavior* **11**, 553–556.

Meltzer, H.Y. (1982) What is schizophrenia. *Schizophrenia Bulletin* **8**, 433–434.

Miller, J.D., Speciale, S.G., McMillen, B.A. and German, D.C. (1984) Naloxone antagonism of stress-induced augmentation of frontal cortex dopamine metabolism. *European Journal of Pharmacology* **98**, 437–439.

Moore, K.E. (1987) Hypothalamic dopaminergic neuronal systems. In: Meltzer, H.Y. (ed.) *Psychopharmacology The Third General of Progress*. New York: Raven Press, pp. 127–139.

Nelson, J.C. (1987) The use of antipsychotic drugs in the treatment of depression. In: Zohar, J. and Belmaker, R.H. (eds) *Treating Resistant Depression*. New York: PMA Publishing Corporation, pp. 131–146.

Nelson, J.C., Bowers, M.B. and Sweeney, D.R. (1979) Exacerbation of psychosis by tricyclic antidepressants in delusional depression. *American Journal of Psychiatry* **136**, 574–576.

Ollerenshaw, D.P. (1973) The classification of the functional psychoses. *British Journal of Psychiatry* **122**, 517–530.

Owens, D.G.G. and Johnstone, E.C. (1980) The disabilities of chronic schizophrenia: their nature and the factors contributing to their development. *British Journal of Psychiatry* **136**, 384–395.

Pearlson, G.D., Garbacz, D.J., Breakey, W.R., Ahn, H.S. and DePaulo, J.R. (1984) Lateral ventricular enlargement associated with persistent unemployment and negative symptoms in both schizophrenia and bipolar disorder. *Psychiatry Research* **12**, 1–9.

Perlmutter, J.S. and Raichle, M.E. (1986) In vitro or in vivo receptor binding: where does the truth lie? *Annals of Neurology* **19**, 384–385.

Pogue-Geile, M.F. and Harrow, M. (1984) Negative and positive symptoms in schizophrenia and depression: a follow up. *Schizophrenia Bulletin* **10**, 371–387.

Pope Jr, H.G. and Lipinski Jr, J.F. (1978) Diagnosis in schizophrenia and manic-depressive illness. *Archives of General Psychiatry* **35**, 811–828.

Post, R.M. (1975) Cocaine psychoses: a continuum model. *American Journal of Psychiatry* **132**, 225–231.

Roberts, D.C.S., Koob, G.F., Klonoff, P. and Fibiger, H.C. (1980) Extinction and recovery of cocaine self-administration following 6-hydroxydopamine lesions of the nucleus accumbens. *Pharmacology Biochemistry and Behavior* **12**, 781–787.

Roth, S. (1970) The seemingly ubiquitous depression following acute schizophrenic episodes, a neglected area of clinical discussion. *American Journal of Psychiatry* **127**, 91–98.

Seeman, P., Bzowej, N.H., Guan, H.C., Bergeron, C., Reynolds, G.P., Bird, E.D., Riederer, P., Jellinger, K. and Tourtellotte, W.W. (1987) Human brain D1 and D2 dopamine receptors in schizophrenia, Alzheimer's, Parkinson's and Huntington's diseases. *Neuropsychopharmacology* **1**, 5–15.

Sherer, M.A., Kumor, K.M., Cone, E.J. and Jaffe, J.H. (1988) Suspiciousness induced by four-hour intravenous infusions of cocaine. *Archives of General Psychiatry* **45**, 673–677.

Slater, E. and Roth, M. (1969) *Clinical Psychiatry* 3rd ed. London: Cassell.

Snyder, S.H. (1973) Amphetamine psychosis: a 'model' schizophrenia mediated by catecholamines. *American Journal of Psychiatry* **130**, 61–67.

Sommers, A.A. (1985) 'Negative symptoms': conceptual and methodological problems. *Schizophrenia Bulletin* **11**, 364–379.

Thierry, A.M., Blanc, G., Sobel, A., Stinus, L. and Glowinski, J. (1973) Dopaminergic terminals in the rat cortex. *Science* **182**, 499–501.

Thierry, A.M., Tassin, J.-P., Blanc, G. and Glowinski, J. (1976) Selective activation of the mesocortical DA system by stress. *Nature* **263**, 242–244.

Weinberger, D.R., Torrey, E.F., Neophytides, A.N. and Wyatt, R.J. (1979) Lateral cerebral ventricular enlargement in chronic schizophrenia. *Archives of General Psychiatry* **36**, 735–739.

Winokur, G., Clayton, P.J. and Reich, T. (1969) *Manic Depressive Illness*. St Louis: Mosby Co.

Wong, D.F., Wagner, H.N., Tune, L.E., Dannals, R.F., Pearlson, G.D., Links, J.M., Tamminga, C.A., Broussole, E.P., Ravert, H.T., Wilson, A.A., Toung, J.K.T., Malat, J., Williams, J.A., O'Tuama, L.A., Snyder, S.H., Kuhar, M.J. and Gjedde, A. (1986) Positron emission tomography reveals elevated D2 dopamine receptors in drug-naive schizophrenics. *Science* **234**, 1558–1563.

Index

Index compiled by Liza Weinkove